Equine Anesthesia and Co-Existing Disease

Equine Anesthesia and Co-Existing Disease

First Edition

Stuart Clark-Price, DVM, MS

Diplomate, American College of Veterinary Internal Medicine, Large Animal
Diplomate, American College of Veterinary Anesthesia and Analgesia
Associate Professor
College of Veterinary Medicine
Auburn University
Auburn, Alabama, USA

Khursheed Mama, DVM

Diplomate, American College of Veterinary Anesthesia and Analgesia
Professor, Veterinary Anesthesiology
College of Veterinary Medicine and Biomedical Sciences
Colorado State University
Fort Collins, Colorado, USA

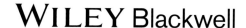

This first edition first published 2022
© 2022 John Wiley & Sons, Inc.

The right of Stuart Clark-Price and Khursheed Mama to be identified as the authors of the editorial material in this work has been asserted in accordance with law.

Registered Office
John Wiley & Sons, Inc., 111 River Street, Hoboken, NJ 07030, USA

Editorial Office
111 River Street, Hoboken, NJ 07030, USA

For details of our global editorial offices, customer services, and more information about Wiley products visit us at www.wiley.com.

Wiley also publishes its books in a variety of electronic formats and by print-on-demand. Some content that appears in standard print versions of this book may not be available in other formats.

Limit of Liability/Disclaimer of Warranty
The contents of this work are intended to further general scientific research, understanding, and discussion only and are not intended and should not be relied upon as recommending or promoting scientific method, diagnosis, or treatment by physicians for any particular patient. In view of ongoing research, equipment modifications, changes in governmental regulations, and the constant flow of information relating to the use of medicines, equipment, and devices, the reader is urged to review and evaluate the information provided in the package insert or instructions for each medicine, equipment, or device for, among other things, any changes in the instructions or indication of usage and for added warnings and precautions. While the publisher and authors have used their best efforts in preparing this work, they make no representations or warranties with respect to the accuracy or completeness of the contents of this work and specifically disclaim all warranties, including without limitation any implied warranties of merchantability or fitness for a particular purpose. No warranty may be created or extended by sales representatives, written sales materials or promotional statements for this work. The fact that an organization, website, or product is referred to in this work as a citation and/or potential source of further information does not mean that the publisher and authors endorse the information or services the organization, website, or product may provide or recommendations it may make. This work is sold with the understanding that the publisher is not engaged in rendering professional services. The advice and strategies contained herein may not be suitable for your situation. You should consult with a specialist where appropriate. Further, readers should be aware that websites listed in this work may have changed or disappeared between when this work was written and when it is read. Neither the publisher nor authors shall be liable for any loss of profit or any other commercial damages, including but not limited to special, incidental, consequential, or other damages.

Library of Congress Cataloging-in-Publication Data

Names: Clark-Price, Stuart, 1972- editor. | Mama, Khursheed, 1964- editor.
Title: Equine anesthesia and co-existing disease / [edited by] Stuart
    Clark-Price, Khursheed Mama.
Description: First edition. | Hoboken, NJ : Wiley-Blackwell, 2022. |
    Includes bibliographical references and index.
Identifiers: LCCN 2021048465 (print) | LCCN 2021048466 (ebook) | ISBN
    9781119307150 (paperback) | ISBN 9781119307396 (adobe pdf) | ISBN
    9781119307419 (epub)
Subjects: MESH: Horse Diseases–surgery | Anesthesia–veterinary |
    Anesthesia–adverse effects | Anesthetics–adverse effects |
    Intraoperative Complications–veterinary
Classification: LCC SF951 (print) | LCC SF951 (ebook) | NLM SF 951 | DDC
    636.1/0896796–dc23/eng/20211005
LC record available at https://lccn.loc.gov/2021048465
LC ebook record available at https://lccn.loc.gov/2021048466

Cover Design: Wiley
Cover Image: Courtesy of Stuart Clark-Price and Khursheed Mama

Set in 9.5/12.5pt STIXTwoText by Straive, Pondicherry, India

Printed in Singapore
M069535_070122

The path to veterinary medicine for me is unique and personal, as I suspect it is for most veterinarians. There are a great many people that mentored me along the way, and, to all of them, I say thank you! *The following individuals were particularly influential in helping me reach my goals. I would like to sincerely thank Dr. Joseph Coli and Dr. Stephen Damonte for edifying integrity and dedication; Dr. Alan Reich, Dr. Kathy Yvorchuk, and Dr. Roger Warren for inspiring me; and Dr. Christine Schweizer, Dr. Bonne Rush, and Dr. Robin Gleed for taking a chance on me. Finally, I would like to dedicate this textbook to my father, Charles Price. It was his suggestion that I pursue veterinary medicine. While he was far from a prefect human, he was my dad.*

Stuart Clark-Price

This is dedicated to family, mentors, colleagues, trainees, and friends who have enhanced my career. You encouraged me to pursue my passion, challenged me to continually strive to provide outstanding care, supported me in accomplishing my goals, and encouraged me when I wavered in my commitment. I remain grateful to you all. Gene, you are a constant source of support and, through your actions, remind me that excellence is a worthy goal. I consider it a privilege to be entrusted with the anesthesia care of these amazing and sometimes fragile animals and acknowledge all who are dedicated to advancing their management.

Khursheed Mama

Content

Contributing Authors

Jennifer Carter, DVM, MClinEd
Diplomate, American College of Veterinary
Anesthesia and Analgesia
Senior Lecturer
University of Melbourne
Melbourne, Australia

Sathya Chinnadurai, DVM, MS
Diplomate, American College of Zoological
Medicine
Diplomate, American College of Veterinary
Anesthesia and Analgesia
Diplomate, American College of
Animal Welfare
Director of Animal Health
Saint Louis Zoo
Saint Louis, Missouri

Stuart Clark-Price, DVM, MS
Diplomate, American College of Veterinary
Internal Medicine, Large Animal
Diplomate, American College of Veterinary
Anesthesia and Analgesia
Associate Professor
College of Veterinary Medicine
Auburn University
Auburn, Alabama

Jeremiah Easley, DVM
Diplomate, American College of Veterinary
Surgeons
Associate Professor
College of Veterinary Medicine and
Biomedical Sciences
Colorado State University
Fort Collins, Colorado

Ryan Fries, DVM
Diplomate, American College of Veterinary
Internal Medicine, Cardiology
Assistant Professor
College of Veterinary Medicine
University of Illinois
Urbana, Illinois

Kirsty Gallacher, BVMS
Diplomate, American College of
Theriogenologists.
Lecturer
School of Animal and Veterinary Sciences
The University of Adelaide
Roseworthy campus, Australia

Santiago Gutierrez-Nibeyro, DVM, MS
Diplomate, American College of Veterinary
Surgeons
Diplomate, American College of Veterinary
Sports Medicine and Rehabilitation
Clinical Associate Professor
College of Veterinary Medicine
University of Illinois
Urbana, Illinois

Eileen Hackett, DVM, PhD
Diplomate, American College of Veterinary
Surgeons,
Diplomate, American College of Veterinary
Emergency and Critical Care,
American College of Veterinary Surgeons
Founding Fellow Minimally Invasive Surgery
(Large Animal Soft Tissue)
Professor

College of Veterinary Medicine and
Biomedical Sciences
Colorado State University
Fort Collins, Colorado

Diana Hassel, DVM, PhD
Diplomate, American College of Veterinary
Surgeons
Diplomate, American College of Veterinary
Emergency & Critical Care
Professor
College of Veterinary Medicine and
Biomedical Sciences
Colorado State University
Fort Collins, Colorado

Bonnie Hay Kraus, DVM
Diplomate, American College of Veterinary
Surgeons
Diplomate, American College of Veterinary
Anesthesia and Analgesia
Associate Professor
College of Veterinary Medicine
Iowa State University
Ames, Iowa

Rachel Hector, DVM, MS
Diplomate, American College of Veterinary
Anesthesia and Analgesia
Assistant Professor
College of Veterinary Medicine and
Biomedical Sciences
Colorado State University
Fort Collins, Colorado

Dean Hendrickson, DVM, MS
Diplomate, American College of Veterinary
Surgeons
ACVS Founding Fellow, Minimally Invasive
Surgery (Large Animal Soft Tissue)
Professor
College of Veterinary Medicine and
Biomedical Sciences
Colorado State University
Fort Collins, Colorado

Klaus Hopster, DVM
Diplomate, European College of Veterinary
Anaesthesia and Analgesia

Assistant Professor
School of Veterinary Medicine
University of Pennsylvania
Kennett Square, Pennsylvania

Philip Johnson, BVSc (Hons), MS, MRCVS
Diplomate, American College of Veterinary
Internal Medicine, Large Animal
Diplomate, European College of Equine
Internal Medicine
Professor
College of Veterinary Medicine
University of Missouri
Columbia, Missouri

Stephanie Keating, DVM, DVSc
Diplomate, American College of Veterinary
Anesthesia and Analgesia
Clinical Assistant Professor
College of Veterinary Medicine
University of Illinois
Urbana, Illinois

Kara Lascola, DVM, MS
Diplomate, American College of Veterinary
Internal Medicine, Large Animal
Associate Professor
College of Veterinary Medicine
Auburn University
Auburn, Alabama

Khursheed Mama, BVSc, DVM
Diplomate, American College of Veterinary
Anesthesia and Analgesia.
Professor
College of Veterinary Medicine and
Biomedical Sciences
Colorado State University
Fort Collins, Colorado

Bianca Martins, DVM, MS, PhD
Diplomate, American College of Veterinary
Ophthalmology
Associate Professor
University of California, Davis
School of Veterinary Medicine
Davis, California

Manuel Martin-Flores, MV
Diplomate, American College of Veterinary
Anesthesia and Analgesia
Associate Professor
College of Veterinary Medicine
Cornell University
Ithaca, New York

Nora Matthews, DVM
Diplomate, American College of Veterinary
Anesthesia and Analgesia
Professor Emeritus
College of Veterinary Medicine & Biomedical
Sciences
Texas A & M University
College Station, Texas
Adjunct Professor
College of Veterinary Medicine
Cornell University
Ithaca, New York

Erica McKenzie, BSc, BVMS, PhD
Diplomate, American College of Veterinary
Internal Medicine, Large Animal
Diplomate, American College of Veterinary
Sports Medicine and Rehabilitation
Professor
College of Veterinary Medicine
Oregon State University
Corvallis, Oregon

Valerie Moorman, DVM, PhD
Diplomate, American College of Veterinary
Surgeons (Large Animal)
Clinical Associate Professor
College of Veterinary Medicine
University of Georgia
Athens, Georgia

Daniel Pang, BVSc, MSc, PhD, MRCVS
Diplomate, American College of Veterinary
Anesthesia and Analgesia
Diplomate, European College of Veterinary
Anaesthesia and Analgesia
EBVS European Specialist in Veterinary
Anaesthesia & Analgesia
Associate Professor

Faculty of Veterinary Medicine
University of Calgary
Calgary, Alberta, Canada
Adjunct Professor
Faculty of Veterinary Medicine
Université de Montréal
St-Hyacinthe, Quebec, Canada

Marlis Rezende, DVM, MS, PhD
Diplomate, American College of Veterinary
Anesthesia and Analgesia
Associate Professor
College of Veterinary Medicine and
Biomedical Sciences
Colorado State University
Fort Collins, Colorado

**Eugene Steffey, VMD, PhD, MRCVS (hon) and
Dr.h.c.(U Bern).**
Diplomate, American College of Veterinary
Anesthesia and Analgesia
Diplomate, European College of Veterinary
Anaesthesia and Analgesia
Professor Emeritus
School of Veterinary Medicine
University of California, Davis
Davis, California
Affiliate Faculty
College of Veterinary Medicine and
Biomedical Sciences
Colorado State University
Fort Collins, Colorado

Alexander Valverde, DVM, DVSc
Diplomate, American College of Veterinary
Anesthesia and Analgesia
Professor
Ontario Veterinary College
University of Guelph
Ontario, Canada

Tom Yarbrough DVM
Diplomate, American College of Veterinary
Surgeons
Senior Veterinarian
Dubai Equine Hospital
Dubai, UAE

Preface

Textbooks solely dedicated to veterinary anesthesia became widely available in the early 1960s, and many have been published since. More recent textbooks contain detailed information on clinical disease and management of small animal patients with specific conditions. A few excellent books related to anesthetic management of equine patients have also been published. However, there are no comprehensive textbooks addressing anesthetic management of horses for specific surgical procedures and diseases. The editors are excited to present this book, which aims to fill that void by providing both a review of the pathogenesis of specific diseases, and procedural considerations relevant to equine anesthesia management.

Recognizing that teamwork is important when providing medical care, most chapters are co-authored by anesthesiologists and known experts in their field including internal medicine, surgery, dentistry, ophthalmology, cardiology, reproduction and zoological medicine. Each chapter combines traditional and cutting-edge knowledge with practical information related to peri-anesthetic management to provide the reader with unparalleled information in a single source. Our hope is that specialists, general practitioners, residents, trainees, and students will find this textbook helpful when managing their equine patients. In addition to chapters focusing on gastrointestinal and orthopedic diseases, considerations for horses undergoing laparoscopy, thoracoscopy, and interventional cardiac procedures, as well as those with co-morbidities unrelated to the need of anesthesia such as inherited muscular diseases, endocrinopathies, and inflammatory respiratory diseases, are included. Considerations for neonatal foals, domestic and non-domestic equids, and a discussion of accidents and error management round out the compilation. The goal is for this to be a broad-based and comprehensive resource relevant to the advances in anesthesia in both healthy and compromised horses.

No such work is possible without the involvement of many. The editors wish to thank the contributing authors for their time, experience, and dedication to this project. The completion of this work is particularly notable given that much of it was accomplished during a global pandemic that had an immeasurable impact on personal and working lives. The editors also thank Merryl Le Roux and the team at Wiley for their assistance, support, and patience.

Stuart Clark-Price
Khursheed Mama

1

Anesthetic Management for Dental and Sinus Surgery

Santiago Gutierrez-Nibeyro[1] and Jennifer Carter[2]

[1] *Department of Veterinary Clinical Medicine, College of Veterinary Medicine, University of Illinois, 1008 W. Hazelwood Dr., Urbana, IL, 61802, USA*
[2] *Faculty of Veterinary and Agricultural Sciences, Melbourne Veterinary School, University of Melbourne, 250 Princes Highway, Werribee, VIC, 3030, Australia*

Introduction

Most adult horses have 36–44 teeth by the time they reach 5 years of age. In general, the dental arcades are composed of 12 incisors, 12 premolars, and 12 molars (some horses will also have additional teeth including canine and wolf teeth). Due to the grinding nature of eating, horse teeth must continue to grow at approximately 1/8″ per year until the individual horse reaches old age where teeth can then be completely shed. Throughout the maxillary and frontal areas of the skull, air-filled sinus cavities developed to allow for a large number of premolar and molar teeth without adding significant weight. The linings of the sinuses are rich in vasculature and may play a role in thermoregulation. Significant disease requiring surgical intervention can occur in the teeth or sinus.

Relevant Anatomy

The nasal cavity is a voluminous cavity divided by the nasal septum and vomer bone (Hillmann 1975). The nasal cavity contains the reserve crowns of the maxillary cheek teeth and a portion of the paranasal sinuses of which the major clinically significant sinuses are the frontal and maxillary sinuses (Hillmann 1975). Two major nasal conchae in each nasal cavity divide the nasal passage into the dorsal, middle, ventral, and common meatus.

The frontal sinus has a large communication with the dorsal conchal sinus, and thereby both are known as the conchofrontal sinus (Hillmann 1975). The ventral conchal sinus communicates with the rostral maxillary sinus over the infraorbital canal and is separated from the caudal maxillary sinus by a thin osseous sheet, the caudal bulla of the ventral conchal sinus. The conchae (or turbinates) are delicate scrolls of bone that are attached laterally in the nasal passage and contain the conchal sinuses (Hillmann 1975).

The maxillary sinus is divided by a thin septum into rostral and caudal compartments or rostral and caudal maxillary sinuses, respectively (Hillmann 1975). The rostral maxillary sinus contains the root of the maxillary first molar and the caudal maxillary sinus contains the roots of the second and third molars (Dixon 2005). The caudal maxillary sinus is partially divided by the infraorbital canal, which may be distorted by a disease process within the sinus. The caudal and rostral maxillary sinuses have separate openings into the middle nasal meatus and the caudal maxillary

Equine Anesthesia and Co-Existing Disease, First Edition. Stuart Clark-Price and Khursheed Mama.
© 2022 John Wiley & Sons, Inc. Published 2022 by John Wiley & Sons, Inc.

sinus communicates with the frontal sinus through the large frontomaxillary opening (Hillmann 1975).

Diagnostic Techniques

Complete history and physical examination of the horse, including assessment of mental status, cardiopulmonary functions, hydration status, and body temperature are mandatory prior to sedation, anesthesia, and/or local anesthetic techniques for dental and sinus surgery. Frontonasal and maxillary bone flaps are indicated to remove of a wide variety of lesions that may develop in the paranasal sinuses or turbinates, such as paranasal sinus cysts, neoplasia, progressive ethmoid hematomas, and apical infections of maxillary cheek teeth (Nickels 2012). The lesions typically cause unilateral epistaxis or mucopurulent nasal drainage, in contrast with diseases of the pharynx or lungs in which the drainage is typically bilateral. However, appropriate diagnostic techniques are indicated to rule out concurrent diseases of the pharynx and lungs that may affect patient management either under general anesthesia or under standing sedation.

On endoscopy, narrowed nasal meati, purulent material, masses, or blood can be seen in the nasal passage and/or draining from the sinus openings (Nickels 2012). Radiography of the skull may reveal free fluid lines, radiodense masses, paranasal sinus cysts, and lucency and/or proliferation associated with dental disease (Figure 1.1). Sinocentesis can be used to obtain fluid sample for culture and cytological examination. Sinuscopy with the horse standing and sedated is useful for the examination, diagnosis, and treatment of some disorders of the paranasal sinuses (Nickels 2012).

Local Anesthetic Techniques for the Equine Teeth and Sinuses

Locoregional anesthesia can be performed prior to many dental and surgical procedures for horses under both standing sedation and general anesthesia. It is routinely accomplished using either lidocaine 2% or mepivacaine 2% solutions with mepivacaine providing a longer duration of action compared to lidocaine (two to four hours versus one to two hours). It is generally advisable to infuse a small amount (1–2 ml) of local anesthetic into the skin at the site of the nerve block to desensitize the skin prior to attempting the locoregional block. This is especially important under standing sedation conditions. Approximately 5–10 minutes should

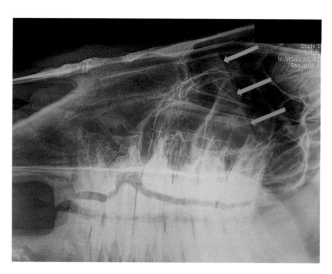

Figure 1.1 Lateral radiograph of a horse skull showing a fluid line (blue arrows) running through the caudal maxillary sinuses. The horse's nose was angled downward resulting in the gravity-dependent fluid line being parallel to the ground. The sinusitis likely resulted from a periapical infection of a cheek tooth (red arrow). Maxillary nerve blockade can be used to desensitize the area for surgical removal of the tooth and drainage and lavage of the sinus.

be allowed to elapse after administration of the local anesthetic to achieve desensitization of the region.

Infraorbital Block

The infraorbital block desensitizes the maxillary teeth to the level of the first molar, the maxillary sinus, the skin from the lip nearly to the medial canthus, and the rostral nose as well as the roof of the nose (Skarda et al. 2010) (Figure 1.2). The infraorbital canal is palpated as the midpoint on a line between the nasoincisive notch and the rostral most aspect of the facial crest (Rice 2017). The levator labii superioris muscle must be manually elevated to facilitate placement of the needle into the canal (Rice 2017). For local anesthesia of the upper lip and nose, a 20 gauge, 2.5 cm needle can be advanced perpendicularly to the skin at the opening of the infraorbital canal using 5 ml of local anesthetic (Skarda et al. 2010). For

blockade of the maxillary teeth and sinus, a 25–20 gauge, 3.8–5 cm needle should be advanced into the canal and 3–5 ml of local anesthetic should be injected (Rice 2017; Skarda et al. 2010).

Maxillary Nerve Block

Blocking the maxillary nerve within the pterygopalatine fossa results in blockade of the maxillary teeth, the paranasal sinus, and the nasal cavity (Woodie 2013) (Figure 1.3). Multiple techniques have been described for performing this block, owing in part to relatively vague surface landmarks for injection. The first involves the injection of local anesthetic into the extraperiorbital fat body (Staszyk et al. 2008). This technique uses a 18 gauge, 3.5″ spinal needle to inject approximately 10 ml of local anesthetic into the fat body surrounding the maxillary nerve (Staszyk et al. 2008). The injection site is made

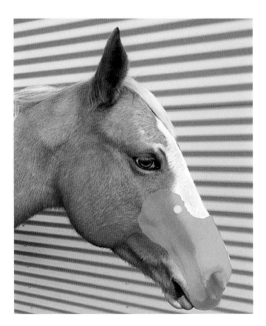

Figure 1.2 The infraorbital block in the horse. The yellow circle indicates the location of the infraorbital canal, and stippling indicates the area of desensitization following administration of local anesthetic.

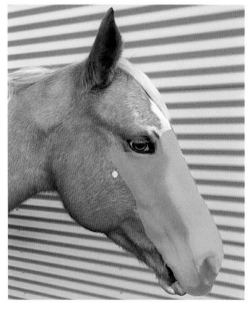

Figure 1.3 The maxillary nerve block in the horse. The yellow circle indicates the location of the infraorbital canal, and stippling indicates the area of desensitization following administration of local anesthetic.

perpendicular to the skin at a point located 10 mm ventral to the zygomatic arch transverse to the plane between the middle and caudal 1/3 of the eye and the needle is advanced until it pops through the masseter muscle for a total depth of approximately 4.5–5 cm (Staszyk et al. 2008). The technique was used in horses under standing sedation using a 20 gauge, 3.5″ spinal needle and reported generally successful blockade with no reaction of mechanical or thermal stimulus with mild chewing, bleeding, swelling, and turgor at the injection site as the only complications (Rieder et al. 2016a). Another study evaluating the volume of lidocaine necessary to produce anesthesia with the extraperiorbital fat body technique and found that 2 ml/100 kg of body weight should result in sufficient local anesthesia while minimizing side effects (Rieder et al. 2016b).

Another technique involves the use of a 19 gauge, 2.5″ spinal needle with an injection site along the ventral border of the zygomatic arch at the narrowest point of the arch (Newton et al. 2000). The needle is inserted into the skin on a rostromedial and ventral angle and is directed along this angle toward the 6th cheek tooth on the contralateral side to a depth of approximately 2″ at which 5 ml of local anesthetic is injected (Newton et al. 2000). At a landmark slightly rostral to that described by Newton, an injection can be made perpendicular to the skin, ventral to the zygomatic process at a point on the skin found on the line running perpendicular to the dorsal head contour and through the temporal canthus of the eye (Bemis 1917). These two techniques were compared using cadaver heads and new methylene blue dye and failed to elucidate a significant difference between the two, with both techniques resulting in at least partial success in "blockade" of the maxillary nerve approximately 80% of the time (Bardell et al. 2010). It is worth noting that the authors reported inadvertent deposition of dye into the deep facial vein on two instances (Bardell et al. 2010). This reinforces the need to aspirate the needle at the injection site prior to injection for any local anesthesia technique.

Another approach to locoregional anesthesia of the maxillary nerve is accomplished by directing a long (8–9 cm, 21–19 gauge) Touhy spinal needle through the infraorbital canal, using the landmarks described previously and injecting 10 ml of local anesthetic (Nannarone et al. 2016). This technique was evaluated using CT of cadaver heads and contrast medium and noted that the needle placement and injection were reasonably easy and that the contrast medium reached the maxillary nerve sufficiently such that it would be expected to result in blockade of the nerve (Nannarone et al. 2016).

In an attempt to minimize complications, including inadvertent puncture of vascular structures in the pterygopalatine fossa, a technique for ultrasound-guided perineural injections of the maxillary nerve has been described (O'Neill et al. 2014). Using a 6 mHz ultrasound probe facilitated visual identification of all relevant anatomical structures, allowing the operator to position the 18 gauge, 3.5″ spinal needle tip in close proximity to the maxillary nerve (O'Neill et al. 2014). In cadavers injected with new methylene blue, ultrasound guidance resulted in successful staining of the maxillary nerve with all injections while cutaneous desensitization of the ipsilateral nose was achieved in all live horses injected with mepivacaine (O'Neill et al. 2014).

Lastly, a recent study evaluated veterinary students performing contrast injection maxillary nerve blocks using the Bemis (1917) or Newton et al. (2000) techniques for surface landmark locations with O'Neill's et al. (2014) ultrasound-guided technique and a technique using a new needle guidance tool (SonixGPS) (Stauffer et al. 2017). Compared to a success rate of 50% with surface landmark techniques, ultrasound guidance resulted in 65.4% success and the GPS tool increased the success rate to 83.3%; however, there was no difference in complication rates between the three (53.9%) (Stauffer et al. 2017).

It is important to note that both the infraorbital and maxillary nerves arise from the trigeminal nerve and are responsible for sensation. However, the facial nerve supplies motor function to the muscle of the face, and branches can run in proximity to the infraorbital and maxillary nerves. Inadvertent blockade of the facial nerve can result in paralysis of the levator labii superioris, levator nasolabialis, and levator anguli oris muscles. As a result, a horse may lose the ability to "flair" its nostrils during inspiration and can even result in nasal collapse during inspiration leading to upper airway obstruction, particularly if blockade is bilateral. Short endotracheal tubes or cut syringe cases can be inserted into the nostrils to provide stenting of the nasal passage until the nerve blockade wears off and normal nerve function resumes.

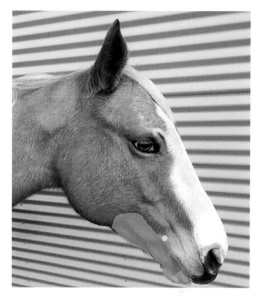

Figure 1.4 The mental nerve block in the horse. The yellow circle indicates the location of the infraorbital canal, and stippling indicates the area of desensitization following administration of local anesthetic.

Mental Nerve Blocks

Blockade of the mental nerve at the mental foramen results in desensitization of the lower lip while advancement of a needle into the mandibular canal results in blockade of the mandibular alveolar nerve leading to desensitization of the ipsilateral incisors and premolars (Skarda et al. 2010; Rice 2017) (Figures 1.4 and 1.5). The block is achieved by elevating the depressor labii inferioris muscle and depositing approximately 5 ml of local anesthetic with a 22 gauge, 1″ needle at the palpable ridge along the mandible at approximately the middle of the interdental space (Skarda et al. 2010). A 25–20 gauge, 1–2.5″ needle and 3–10 ml of local anesthetic is described blockade of the mandibular alveolar nerve within the mandibular canal (Skarda et al. 2010; Rice 2017).

Figure 1.5 Lateral radiograph of a horse skull with severe dental disease. The mental foramen (red arrow) can be seen where the mental nerve exits to innervate the rostral aspect of the mandible. Mental nerve blockade can be used to desensitize the mandible rostral to the mental foramen to the level of the mandibular symphysis.

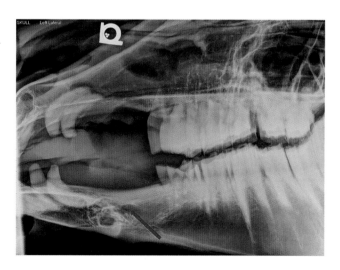

Inferior Alveolar (Mandibular) Nerve Blocks

Desensitization of the inferior alveolar nerve prior proximal to its entrance into the mandibular canal results in blockade of the entire hemi-mandible including teeth, mandibular bone, skin, and gingiva (Figures 1.6 and 1.7). Due to the close anatomical proximity of the lingual branch of the trigeminal nerve, it is also possible to inadvertently desensitize the tongue, potentially resulting in self-trauma on recovery (Caldwell and Easley 2012; Harding et al. 2012). Smaller volumes of local anesthetic may minimize this risk (Harding et al. 2012). Much like the maxillary nerve, multiple techniques have been proposed to achieve desensitization of this nerve in the horse. The earliest was by Bemis who suggested that a vertical line be drawn from the lateral canthus of the eye ventrally to the mandible and a horizontal line be drawn from the occlusal surface of the mandibular molars caudally to the ramus of the mandible with the mandibular foramen located on the medial aspect of the mandible at the junction of the two lines (1917). The technique suggested inserting a spinal needle 3 cm ventral to the temporomandibular junction and advancing it medially to the mandibular foramen (Bemis 1917). Modifications of this technique include approaching the foramen

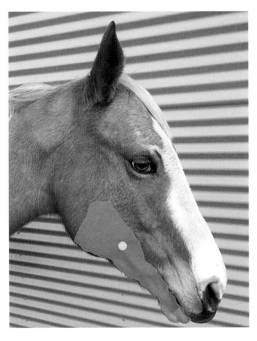

Figure 1.6 The inferior alveolar/mandibular nerve block in the horse. The yellow circle indicates the location of the infraorbital canal, and stippling indicates the area of desensitization following administration of local anesthetic.

from the ventral border of the ramus and inserting a long spinal needle along the imaginary horizontal line from the caudal aspect of the vertical ramus, medially along the mandible to a depth of 9 cm and injecting

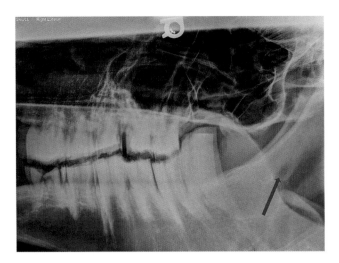

Figure 1.7 Lateral radiograph of a horse skull with severe dental disease. The mandibular foramen (red arrow) can be seen where the mandibular nerve enters on the medial aspect to innervate the entire hemi-mandible. Mandibular nerve blockade can be used to desensitize the entire hemi-mandible.

10 ml of local anesthetic (Fletcher 2004; Harding et al. 2012).

A recent cadaver study compared inferior alveolar nerve blocks performed using the landmarks suggested by Bemis and advancing an 18 gauge, 20 cm spinal needle either from the ventral border of the vertical ramus at Bemis' imaginary vertical line to the mandibular foramen or rostrodorsal from the angle where the horizontal and vertical rami meet the foramen (Harding et al. 2012). The study reported successful dye staining of the nerve in 59% of the vertical injections and 73% of the angled injections; however, there was no significant difference between the two techniques (Harding et al. 2012).

Lastly, another recent study has described the use of an intraoral approach to the inferior alveolar nerve block in the horse. The intraoral approach is used quite frequently in other species; however, the anatomy and relatively narrow gape of the horse make manual palpation of the mandibular foramen impossible. The study described the use of a custom-made tool that was essentially a 20-gauge needle attached to a length of extension tubing and secured to a bent metal rod to allow the needle to be directed through the mouth and to the medial mandibular location of the foramen (Henry et al. 2014). In the study, a total of 51 blocks using 5 ml of 2% mepivacaine were administered and procedures including endodontics, mucosal elevation, and dental extractions were performed successfully following all blocks (Henry et al. 2014). One horse was reported to develop an abscess in the pterygoid fossa two weeks after the procedure (Henry et al. 2014).

Dental Extractions and Repulsions

Extractions and repulsions of teeth can be done either with standing sedation and local anesthesia techniques or under a general anesthetic. The choice is a matter of the horse's personality and health status, the perceived invasiveness of the procedure, as well as the surgeon's preference; however, the obvious benefit of performing the procedure in a standing horse is the avoidance of the inherent risk and complications associated with general anesthesia. In addition, standing sedation avoids having an orotracheal tube in the mouth where it may obstruct the surgeon's view and/or make access to the tooth with extraction equipment difficult. Multiple studies have described the successful use of a combination of standing sedation and local anesthesia blocks in order to accomplish oral extraction or sinus repulsion of both retained fragments and intact teeth (MacDonald et al. 2006; Coomer et al. 2011; Dixon et al. 2005). There are no procedure-specific considerations when choosing a general anesthesia protocol for dental procedures in the horse. To facilitate adequate access to the oral cavity, a total intravenous (TIVA) protocol such as "triple-drip" (guaifenesin, ketamine, xylazine) can be used while supplementing oxygen via a nasotracheal tube. TIVA techniques should be reserved for procedures in healthy horses lasting less than 45 minutes to 1 hour. During the general anesthetic, care should be taken when positioning the horse for the extraction or repulsion to avoid pressure on the contralateral facial nerve. Lastly, recovery should be facilitated with either a nasotracheal or orotracheal tube left in place to maintain the airway and partially guard the airway against any remaining bleeding from the procedure.

Standing sedation protocols have been reviewed elsewhere in this book; however, it is worth highlighted a recent study describing the use of romifidine-based standing sedation for cheek tooth extraction (Müller et al. 2017). The authors evaluated the use of a romifidine continuous rate infusion alone (0.05 mg/kg/h) and in combination with butorphanol (0.04 mg/kg/h), midazolam (0.06 mg/kg/h), or ketamine (1.2 mg/kg/h). All drugs received appropriate loading doses (romifidine 0.03 mg/kg; butorphanol 0.02 mg/kg; midazolam 0.02 mg/kg; ketamine 0.5 mg/kg) prior to commencement of the CRI and lidocaine-based maxillary or mandibular nerve blocks. The protocol achieved sufficient sedation for completion of the extractions in all groups other than group receiving romifidine alone. The combination of romifidine with midazolam produced substantial ataxia compared to combination with ketamine although both produced good surgical conditions. Combination with butorphanol resulted in a reduced cortisol stress response (Müller et al. 2017). The study concludes that romifidine should not be used alone for standing sedation for dental extractions (Müller et al. 2017).

Surgical Diseases of Paranasal Sinuses

Primary Sinusitis

Primary sinusitis is caused by an upper respiratory tract infection (most commonly, Streptococcus species) that has involved the paranasal sinuses, and secondary sinusitis is caused by an apical infection of maxillary cheek teeth (Tremaine and Dixon 2001a). Systemic antibiotic therapy is very effective but sinus lavage once or twice daily with an indwelling catheter introduced into the infected sinus through a trephine opening may be clinically necessary to fully resolve the infection or remove inspissated pus. The skin over the trephination site is locally infiltrated with 2–3 ml of 2% mepivacaine prior to surgery (Tremaine 2007).

Paranasal Sinus Cysts

Paranasal sinus cysts are single or loculated fluid-filled lesions that typically develop in the maxillary sinuses and ventral concha and can extend into the conchofrontal sinus (Woodford and Lane 2006). The etiology and pathogenesis are unknown (Tremaine et al. 1999); however, extirpation of the cyst and the involved conchal lining through a frontonasal or maxillary bone flap is curative (Woodford and Lane 2006).

Ethmoid Hematoma

Ethmoid hematoma is a progressive and locally destructive idiopathic mass that may arise from the ethmoid labyrinth or the floor of the paranasal sinuses. These lesions are characterized by endoturbinate or a sinus submucosal hemorrhage and concurrent stretching and thickening of the mucosa that becomes the capsule of the hematoma (Tremaine et al. 1999). Ethmoid hematomas can extend into the frontal sinus, the maxillary sinus, the nasal cavity, or the sphenopalatine sinus by disrupting the tectorial plate (Nickels 2012). If the ethmoid hematoma extends into one of the paranasal sinuses, a frontonasal bone flap is indicated to remove the lesion, but it can be associated with profuse intraoperative hemorrhage (Nickels 2012). Typically, ethmoid hematoma causes mild and spontaneous intermittent epistaxis; however, anemia is very rare.

Neoplasia

Neoplasia in the nasal cavity or paranasal sinuses are uncommon (Tremaine and Dixon 2001a). Squamous cell carcinoma is the most common neoplasia of the paranasal sinuses; however, other types of sarcoma tumors (osteogenic sarcoma, lymphosarcoma, poorly differentiated carcinoma, fibrosarcoma, hemangiosarcoma, and adenocarcinoma) have been reported.

Surgery of the Paranasal Sinuses

Sinoscopy

Sinoscopy of the paranasal sinuses is usually performed with the horse standing and adequately sedated. The examination is performed with a flexible endoscope using portals created with a 15-mm Galt trephine following local infiltration of 3–4 ml of 2% mepivacaine at the surgery sites. The endoscopic portal for the **conchofrontal sinus** is located 60% of the distance from midline toward the medial canthus and 0.5 cm caudal to the medial canthus of the eye, whereas the endoscopic portal for the maxillary sinuses is located 2 cm rostral and 2 cm ventral to the medial canthus of the eye (**caudal maxillary sinus**) or 50% of the distance from the rostral end of the facial crest to the level of the medial canthus and 1 cm ventral to a line joining the infraorbital foramen and the medial canthus (**rostral maxillary sinus**).

Frontonasal and Maxillary Bone Flap Technique

A frontonasal bone flap approach is used to gain access to the **conchofrontal** and **caudal maxillary sinuses** and, by additional steps, the rostral maxillary and ventral conchal sinuses. If there is bilateral disease, a tracheotomy should be performed prior to induction and the horse should be intubated through the tracheostomy incision; the animal is otherwise intubated routinely. In addition, sufficient analgesia of the cheek teeth and sinus is a prerequisite for procedures performed on standing horses under chemical sedation. To provide anesthesia of the paranasal sinuses and maxillary cheek teeth, the maxillary branch of the trigeminal nerve in the pterygopalatine fossa should be desensitized using one of the locoregional maxillary nerve block techniques described in the previous section. This block should be performed regardless of whether the surgical procedure is done under standing sedation or general anesthesia.

The frontonasal or maxillary bone flap procedure consists of incising the skin, periosteum, and bone on three sides. For a frontonasal bone flap, the caudal margin is a line drawn at right angle to the dorsal midline and midway between the supraorbital foramen and the medial canthus of the eye, the lateral margin is a line 2.5 cm medial to the medial canthus of the eye that runs slightly dorsal to another line from the medial canthus to the nasoincisive notch, and the rostral margin is caudal to the point at which the nasal bones become parallel. For a maxillary bone flap, the rostral margin of the maxillary bone flap is a line drawn from the rostral end of the facial crest to the infraorbital foramen, the dorsal margin is a line from the infraorbital foramen to the medial canthus of the eye, the caudal margin is a line (parallel to the rostral margin) from the medial canthus of the eye to the caudal aspect of the facial crest, and the ventral margin is the facial crest (Nickels 2012). The bone flap is then elevated, the affected cheek teeth are repelled by placing a dental punch onto the roots or the lesion (paranasal cyst, ethmoid hematoma, neoplasia, etc.) and removed while controlling intraoperative bleeding.

Following a frontonasal or maxillary bone flap, a surgical opening into the nasal cavity is created and then saline-soaked rolled gauze is inserted immediately into the sinus and nasal passages to control hemorrhage and the end of the gauze is pulled through the sinuses and out the nostril. The packing is removed at 48–72 hours after surgery. Historically, frontonasal and maxillary bone flaps have been associated with profuse hemorrhage so that having a potential blood donor identified by cross-match is recommended. However, in recent publications of the surgical procedure this complication was infrequent (Tremaine and Dixon 2001a, b; Woodford and Lane 2006; Hart and Sullins 2011).

Surgical Diseases of the Nasal Cavity

Nasal Septum Deformity

Although it is clinically infrequent, nasal septum resection is indicated for treatment of malformations, cystic degeneration, fungal infections, traumatic thickening secondary to septal fracture, and neoplasia among others (Valdez et al. 1978; Watt 1970; Doyle and Freeman 2005; Schumacher et al. 2008). The cartilage of the nasal septum responds in an exaggerated fashion to trauma and heals with deformity, thickening, and deviation which produces decreased airflow or complete unilateral obstruction and nasal stertor. Diagnosis can generally be made with endoscopic and radiographic examination. The abnormality may be rostral enough to palpate digitally; however, advanced diagnostic imaging may be useful in same cases to plan the surgical treatment (Auer 2012).

Campylorrhinus Lateralis (Wry Nose)

Campylorrhinus lateralis is a congenital abnormality consisting of dysplasia of one side of the maxilla and premaxilla that results in deviation of the maxillae, premaxillae, nasal bones, vomer, and the nasal septum to the dysplastic side (Schumacher et al. 2008). The deviation usually results in malocclusion of the incisors of the mandible and maxilla. Depending on the degree of deviation foals may have difficulty breathing and stridor due to progressive airway obstruction secondary to deviation of the nasal septum to the convex side of the deformity (Schumacher et al. 2008). Radiography supports the clinical diagnosis; however, computed tomography may be useful to assess if there is rotational component in the deviation (Auer 2012). Slight nasal deviation may straighten with growth, but horses with moderate or severe deviation require surgical treatment to resolve respiratory obstruction and to improve incisor occlusion and cosmetic appearance (Auer 2012).

Choanal Atresia

This is a rare maxillofacial malformation in which one or both nasal cavities fail to communicate with the nasopharynx due to persistence of the buccopharyngeal septum, which separates the nasal cavities from the nasopharynx during the embryonic development (James et al. 2006; Hogan et al. 1995). Although there are multiple theories proposed for its embryological origin, it appears that buccopharyngeal membrane persistence is due to misdirection of mesodermal flow caused by errors in neural crest migration in the nasal cavities during embryogenesis.

Affected animals may have partial (unilateral atresia) or complete (bilateral atresia) airflow obstruction through the nasal cavity (James et al. 2006; Hogan et al. 1995; Richardson et al. 1994). Given that horses are obligate nasal breathers, bilateral choanal atresia in foals can cause immediate asphyxia upon birth unless an airway is immediately established by a temporary tracheostomy (James et al. 2006). When the atresia occurs unilaterally, foals exhibit loud respiratory noise, exercise intolerance, and asymmetry of airflow from the nostrils can be detected (James et al. 2006; Hogan et al. 1995, Richardson et al. 1994). The diagnosis is typically made by endoscopic examination but other modalities such as skull radiography, contrast radiography, and computed tomography can be helpful to plan the surgical approach (Gerros and Stone 1994; Nykamp et al. 2003). The treatment is resection of the buccopharyngeal membrane.

Surgery of the Nasal Cavity

Nasal Septum Resection

The nasal septum is covered with a highly vascular mucosa, consequently excision of the septum may cause severe intraoperative hemorrhage, hypotension, and hypoxia. Administration of large volumes of intravenous fluids during surgery is recommended to help alleviate the hypotension. However, it is advisable to identify a suitable blood donor and collect 4–8 l of blood before surgery in case a blood transfusion is necessary. A tracheotomy should be performed before surgery for maintenance of ventilation and inhalational agent delivery thereby allowing adequate surgical access to the oral cavity during surgery.

This procedure should be performed under general anesthesia; however, no specific protocol is indicated and, instead, should be chosen based on the needs of the horse. As the horse will be placed in lateral recumbency for the procedure, administration of a bilateral maxillary block can be challenging. The anesthetist should consider positioning the horse in dorsal recumbency on the surgical table initially to facilitate blockade of the "down" nerve prior to repositioning to lateral recumbency. Alternatively, consideration could be made for performing the bilateral maxillary blocks in the standing horse under sedation/premedication and possibly at the same time as the temporary tracheostomy is performed.

The horse is positioned in lateral recumbency, and the obstetrical wire is passed up one nasal passage. The most commonly used technique involves transecting the nasal septum dorsally, ventrally, and caudally with obstetrical wire and the most rostral incision is made with a scalpel leaving 5 cm of septum to support the nostrils and alar folds (Doyle and Freeman 2005). The mouth is held open with a speculum, a hand passed back into the oral cavity, and the wire is retrieved around the edge of the soft palate. Another wire is introduced in similar manner up the other nasal passage and is also brought out through the mouth. The ends of the wires are connected outside the mouth, and one is drawn back through a nasal passage until the splice is brought out of the nostril. The wires are then disconnected and the one is left in place so that it passes around the ventral edge of the vomer bone and out both nostrils; this wire is used to transect the nasal septum ventrally.

Next, a trephine hole is placed in the nasal bones immediately rostral to the point at which these bones diverge on the face toward the eyes. A Chamber's mare catheter is introduced into the nasal passage to exit through the trephine hole. A length of obstetrical wire is then threaded down this catheter and the catheter is removed so that the wire runs from the trephine hole to exit at the nostril. The catheter is introduced into the other nostril and the same wire is threaded down it so that it loops around the septum at the level of the trephine hole and both ends exit the nostril; this wire is used to transect the septum dorsally.

Another length of obstetrical wire is now passed through the trephine hole and into one nasal passage, in a direction toward the caudal edge of the soft palate. The mouth is held open with a speculum, a hand passed back into the oral cavity, and the wire is retrieved around the edge of the soft palate. Another wire is introduced in similar manner through the trephine hole into the other nasal passage and is also brought out the mouth. The ends of the wires are then taped together outside the mouth, and one is drawn back through a nasal passage until the splice is brought out of the trephine hole. The remaining wire is left in place so that it passes around the ventral edge of the vomer bone and out the trephine hole; this wire is used to transect the septum caudally. The ventral and dorsal cuts are made simultaneously taking care and completed rapidly once started so that hemorrhage is minimal before packing is inserted. The septum is extracted by grasping it with long forceps at the rostral end and pulling it through one of the nostrils. The nasal cavity is packed similarly as for sinuses following surgery and the horse should be allowed to recover with a temporary tracheostomy tube secured in place. The nasal packing and temporary tracheostomy tube may be removed after 48 or 72 hours.

Wry Nose (Campylorrhinus Lateralis)

Successful surgical treatment can improve cosmetic appearance and alleviate airway obstruction (Schumacher et al. 2008). This reconstructive surgery is recommended when the foal is two to three months of age to allow the facial bones to gain enough strength to support implant. The foal is anesthetized using a routine protocol and positioned in dorsal or lateral recumbency on the surgery table (Schumacher et al. 2008). The endotracheal tube is inserted ideally through a tracheostomy approach, the cuff is inflated, and the mouth is thoroughly washed. A bilateral maxillary block can be performed at this time; however, there are currently no studies reporting on this technique in foals.

The first step consists of resecting the nasal septum leaving sufficient septum to support the nostrils and alar folds; the section of septum to be removed is centered on the middle of the bend in the nasal septum. The nasal passages are packed with rolled gauze to control the hemorrhage and the nostrils are sutured closed to retain the packing. The second step consists of transecting the rami of the maxilla at the level of the interalveolar space to allow re-alignment of the maxillae and premaxillae followed by stabilization with bone plates or Steinmann pins. During surgery, symmetry of the upper and lower jaws is maintained by temporarily wiring the incisors of the maxilla and mandible. The third step consists of correcting the nasal bone deviation and stabilize with reconstruction bone plates. Some surgeons use an autogenous cortical bone graft in the form of a rib to fit the gap in the concave side of the premaxilla; therefore, a section of rib can be harvested before straightening the maxillae/premaxillae, with the horse positioned in left or right lateral recumbency, or in dorsal recumbency (Schumacher et al. 2008).

Choanal Atresia

Treatment options for choanal atresia include transendoscopic laser excision of the buccopharyngeal membrane, or via bilateral frontonasal bone flap (if the buccopharyngeal membrane is osseous, or the condition is bilateral), or via laryngotomy with endoscopic assistance to gain access to the obstructed choanae (Aylor et al. 1984; James et al. 2006; Ducharme 2012).

In horses with unilateral choanal atresia, transendoscopic laser excision can be done with the patient standing and seated with detomidine and butorphanol, and topical anesthesia with phenylephrine (2% lidocaine or mepivacaine hydrochloride and 10 ml of 0.15% phenylephrine) applied to the buccopharyngeal membrane and nasal cavity. Choanal stenosis is a frequent complication, so the use of stents is mandatory post-operatively to prevent stricture (James et al. 2006). This can be done with a silicone endotracheal tube threaded over the wire, pushed through the puncture site in the choanal membrane, and left in place to serve as a stent. If resection of the buccopharyngeal membrane via frontonasal bone flap with the animal anesthetized is elected, a temporary tracheostomy should be performed to allow tracheal intubation during surgical manipulations of the head and should be left in place with the cuff inflated during recovery to assure an adequate airway and protect it from surgical site bleeding.

Equine Blood Typing and Transfusion Considerations

As stated earlier in this chapter, significant acute hemorrhage is a potential risk associated with surgical procedures of the nose. Acute blood loss of >20% of the blood volume and/or clinical signs of hypovolemia should be used to assess the need for emergency transfusions as changes in packed cell volume (PCV) or total protein may lag behind by several hours due to splenic contraction (Hardy 2009). Transfusions of whole blood should be reserved for lifesaving situations however as transfused red blood cells only last in recipient circulation for two to six days (Hardy 2009; Kallfelz et al. 1978). Transfusion medicine in horses is more complicated than in humans or small companion animals owing to the lack of a universal blood type in horses. Horses have eight different blood groups, A, C, D, K, P, Q, U, and T as well as more than 30 different surface marker factors on the red blood cells. As a result, the likelihood of a perfect match between donor and recipient is estimated to be upward of 1 in 400 000. Fortunately, the vast majority of transfusion reactions are attributable to two specific blood types, Aa and Qa, and horses that possess Ca antigens also pose a theoretical risk (Schmotzer 1985). As stored equine blood samples are only stable for a few weeks, blood banking is not common, and donors must typically be either kept on site or available at short notice (Mudge et al. 2004). Ideal donors must be healthy adult horses, up to date on vaccines and free from any diseases. Unrelated geldings of the same breed or mares who have never foaled can be chosen for blood donors as long as their PCV is greater than 35% and they test negative for Aa, Qa, and Ca antigens. Related horses or mares who have foaled previously are more likely to possess antibodies that could lead to transfusion reactions. In larger practice settings where donor horses are maintained, blood typing should be performed prior to donation to avoid Aa, Qa, and Ca antigens; however, Quarter horses and standardbreds are reported as breeds less likely to possess Aa or Qa antigens if prior blood typing is not possible (Nolen-Walston, n.d.).

Cross-matching should be performed, if possible, prior to blood transfusion administration. A major cross-match involves combining washed donor red blood cells with recipient serum while a minor cross-match combines donor serum with washed recipient red blood cells. Signs of incompatibility include auto-agglutination and hemolysis.

Donor horses should have a large gauge, short catheter placed aseptically in the jugular vein and connected to a bag containing anticoagulant. Adult horses greater than 450 kg can donate between 15 and 20 ml/kg of whole blood which should be replaced with at least an equivalent volume of crystalloid fluids after donation (Malikides et al. 2001; Nolen-Walston, n.d.).

When estimating the amount of donor blood needed for transfusion, one can calculate with the following general estimate:

Donor blood needed =
  Estimated Recipient blood volume
  $\times \left(\text{Desired PCV\%} - \text{Actual PCV\%/Donor PCV\%} \right)$

A more general estimate assumes that 2–3 ml/kg of whole blood from a donor with a PCV of 40% will raise the recipient's PCV by 1% (Hardy 2009). In general, adult horse's blood volumes can be estimated as 80 ml/kg. The technique for administration of the actual transfusion is not dissimilar to that of small animals or humans where the transfusion is started at a slow rate for the first 15 minutes to closely observe for transfusion reactions after while time the remainder of the volume can be administered at 5–20 ml/kg/h with the goal of completing the transfusion in less than four hours to maintain sterility (Hardy 2009; Nolen-Walston, n.d.). Signs of transfusion reactions include hypotension, skin wheals, sweating, tachycardia, fever, diarrhea, colic, and piloerection (Hardy 2009; Nolen-Walson, n.d.). Transfusions should be stopped if signs of reaction occur and treatment, including fluids and epinephrine if needed, should be instituted. If the transfusion reaction is mild and the signs resolve with discontinuation of the infusion, restarting the infusion at a slower rate can be considered, especially if no other suitable donor is available.

References

Auer, J.A. (2012). Craniomaxillofacial disorders. In: *Equine Surgery*, 4e (eds. J.A. Auer and J.A. Stick), 1456–1482. St. Louis, MO: Elsevier Saunders.

Aylor, M.K., Campbell, M.L., Goring, R.L., and Hillidge, C.J. (1984). Congenital bilateral choanal atresia in a standardbred foal. *Equine Veterinary Journal* 16 (4): 396–398.

Bardell, D., Iff, I., and Mosing, M. (2010). A cadaver study comparing two approaches to perform a maxillary nerve block in the horse. *Equine Veterinary Journal* 42 (8): 721–725.

Bemis, H.E. (1917). Local anaesthesia in animal dentistry. *American Veterinary Journal* 51: 188.

Caldwell, F.J. and Easley, K.J. (2012). Self-inflicted lingual trauma secondary to inferior alveolar nerve block in 3 horses. *Equine Veterinary Education* 24: 119–123.

Coomer, R.P., Fowke, G.S., and McKane, S. (2011). Repulsion of the maxillary and mandibular cheek teeth in standing horses. *Veterinary Surgery* 40: 590–595.

Dixon, P.M. (2005). Dental anatomy. In: *Equine dentistry*, 2e (eds. G.J. Baker and J. Easley), 25–66. St. Louis MO: Elsevier.

Dixon, P.M., Dacre, I., Dacre, K. et al. (2005). Standing oral extraction of cheek teeth in 100 horses (1998–2003). *Equine Veterinary Journal* 37: 105–112.

Doyle, A.J. and Freeman, D.E. (2005). Extensive nasal septum resection in horses using a 3-wire method. *Veterinary Surgery* 34 (2): 167–173.

Ducharme, N.G. (2012). Pharynx. In: *Equine Surgery*, 4e (eds. J.A. Auer and J.A. Stick), 569–591. St. Louis, MO: Elsevier Saunders.

Fletcher, B.W. (2004). How to perform effective equine dental nerve blocks. In: *Proceedings of the Convention of the American Association of Equine Practitioners*, Denver, CO.

Gerros, T.C. and Stone, W.C. (1994). What is your diagnosis? Complete bilateral choanal atresia. *Journal of the American Veterinary Medical Association* 205 (2): 179–180.

Harding, P.G., Smith, R.L., and Barakzai, S.Z. (2012). Comparison of two approaches to performing an inferior alveolar nerve block in the horse. *Australian Veterinary Journal* 90: 146–150.

Hardy, J. (2009). Venous and arterial catheterization and fluid therapy. In: *Equine Anesthesia: Monitoring and Emergency Therapy*, 2e (eds. W.W. Muir and J.A.E. Hubbell), 131–148. St. Louis, MO: Saunders.

Hart, S.K. and Sullins, K.E. (2011). Evaluation of a novel postoperative treatment for sinonasal disease in the horse (1996–2007). *Equine Veterinary Journal* 43 (1): 24–29.

Henry, T., Pusterla, N., Guedes, A.G.P., and Vertraete, F.J.M. (2014). Evaluation and clinical use of an intraoral inferior alveolar nerve block in the horse. *Equine Veterinary Journal* 46: 706–710.

Hillmann, D.J. (1975). Skull. In: *Sisson and Grossman's the Anatomy of the Domestic Animals*, 5e (ed. R. Getty), 255–348. Philadelphia, PA: W. B. Saunders Company.

Hogan, P.M., Embertson, R.M., and Hunt, R.J. (1995). Unilateral choanal atresia in a foal. *Journal of the American Veterinary Medical Association* 207 (4): 471–473.

James, F.M., Parente, E.J., and Palmer, J.E. (2006). Management of bilateral choanal atresia in a foal. *Journal of the American Veterinary Medical Association* 229 (11): 1784–1789.

Kallfelz, F.A., Whitlock, R.H., and Schultz, R.D. (1978). Survival of 59 Fe-labeled erythrocytes in cross-transfused equine blood. *American Journal of Veterinary Research* 39: 617–620.

MacDonald, M.H., Basile, T., Wilson, W.D. et al. (2006). Removal of maxillary tooth fragments and root remnants in standing horses. In: *American Association of Equine Practitioners Dental Focus Meeting Proceedings*, 148–155. Indianapolis, IN.

Malikides, N., Hodgson, J.L., Rose, R.J., and Hodgson, D.R. (2001). Cardiovascular, haematological and biochemical responses after large volume blood collection in horses. *Veterinary Journal* 162 (1): 44–55.

Mudge, M.C., MacDonald, M.H., Owens, S.D., and Tablin, F. (2004). Comparison of 4 blood storage methods in a protocol for equine pre-operative autologous donation. *Veterinary Surgery* 33 (5): 475–486.

Müller, T.M., Hopster, K., Bienert-Zeit, A. et al. (2017). Effect of butorphanol, midazolam or ketamine on romifidine based sedation in horses during standing cheek tooth removal. *BMC Veterinary Research* 13: 381.

Nannarone, S., Bini, G., Vuerich, M. et al. (2016). Retrograde maxillary nerve perineural injection: a tomographic and anatomical evaluation of the infraorbital canal and evaluation of needle size in equine cadavers. *The Veterinary Journal* 217: 33–39.

Newton, S.A., Knottenbelt, D.C., and Eldridge, P.R. (2000). Headshaking in horses: possible aetiopathogenesis suggested by the results of diagnostic tests and several treatment regimes used in 20 cases. *Equine Veterinary Journal* 32 (2): 208–216.

Nickels, F.A. (2012). Nasal passages and paranasal sinuses. In: *Equine Surgery*, 4e (eds. J.A. Auer and J.A. Stick), 557–568. St. Louis, MO: Elsevier Saunders.

Nolen-Walston, R.D. (n.d.) Equine blood transfusion- what you need to know to get the job done. https://vvma.org/resources/ Conferences/2016%20VVC%20Notes/ Nolen-Walston-%20Blood%20Transfusions.pdf

Nykamp, S.G., Dykes, N.L., Cook, V.L. et al. (2003). Computed tomographic appearance of choanal atresia in an alpaca cria. *Veterinary Radiology & Ultrasound* 44 (5): 534–536.

O'Neill, H.D., Garcia-Pereira, F.L., and Mohankumar, P.S. (2014). Ultrasound-guided injection of the maxillary nerve in the horse. *Equine Veterinary Journal* 46 (2): 180–184.

Rice, M.K. (2017). Regional nerve blocks for equine dentistry. *Journal of Veterinary Dentistry* 34: 106–109.

Richardson, J.L., Lane, J.G., and Day, M.J. (1994). Congenital choanal restriction in 3 horses. *Equine Veterinary Journal* 26: 162–165.

Rieder, C.M., Zwick, T., Hopster, K. et al. (2016a). Maxillary nerve block within the pterygopalatine fossa for oral extraction of cheek teeth in 80 horses. *Pferdeheilkunde* 32: 587–594.

Rieder, C.M., Staszyk, C., Hopster, K., and Bienert-Zeit, A. (2016b). Maxillary nerve block within the equine pterygopalatine fossa with different volumes: practicability, efficacy and side-effects. *Pferdeheilkunde* 32 (2): 132–140.

Schmotzer, W.B. (1985). Time-saving techniques for the collection, storage, and administration of equine blood and plasma. *Veterinary Medicine* 80: 89–94.

Schumacher, J., Brink, P., Easley, J., and Pollock, P. (2008). Surgical correction of wry nose in four horses. *Veterinary Surgery* 37 (2): 142–148.

Skarda, R.T., Muir, W.W., and Hubbell, J.A.E. (2010). Local anesthetic drugs and techniques. In: *Equine Anesthesia: Monitoring and Emergency Therapy*, 2e (eds. W.W. Muir

and J.A.E. Hubbell), 210–242. St. Louis, MO: Saunders.

Staszyk, C., Bienert, A., Bäumer, W. et al. (2008). Simulation of local anaesthetic nerve block of the infraorbital nerve within the pterygopalatine fossa: anatomical landmarks defined by computed tomography. *Research in Veterinary Science* 85: 399–406.

Stauffer, S., Cordner, B., Dixon, J., and Witte, T. (2017). Maxillary nerve blocks in horses: an experimental comparison of surface landmark and ultrasound-guided techniques. *Veterinary Anaesthesia and Analgesia* 44: 951–958.

Tremaine, W.H. (2007). Local analgesic techniques for the equine head. *Equine Veterinary Education* 19 (9): 495–503.

Tremaine, W.H. and Dixon, P.M. (2001a). A long-term study of 277 cases of equine sinonasal disease. Part 1: details of horses, historical, clinical and ancillary diagnostic findings. *Equine Veterinary Journal* 33 (3): 274–282.

Tremaine, W.H. and Dixon, P.M. (2001b). A long-term study of 277 cases of equine sinonasal disease. Part 2: treatments and results of treatments. *Equine Veterinary Journal* 33 (3): 283–289.

Tremaine, W.H., Clarke, C.J., and Dixon, P.M. (1999). Histopathological findings in equine sinonasal disorders. *Equine Veterinary Journal* 31 (4): 296–303.

Valdez, H., McMullan, W.C., Hobson, H.P., and Hanselka, D.V. (1978). Surgical correction of deviated nasal septum and premaxilla in a colt. *Journal of the American Veterinary Medical Association* 173 (8): 1001–1004.

Watt, D.A. (1970). A case of cryptococcal granuloma in the horse. *Australian Veterinary Journal* 46: 493.

Woodford, N.S. and Lane, J.G. (2006). Long-term retrospective study of 52 horses with sinunasal cysts. *Equine Veterinary Journal* 38 (3): 198–202.

Woodie, J.B. (2013). How to use local and regional anesthesia for procedures of the head and perineum in the horse. *Proceedings of the American Association of Equine Practitioners Annual Conference*, 59, 464–466.

2

Anesthetic Management for Ocular Interventions

Bianca Martins[1] and Manuel Martin-Flores[2]

[1] *Department of Surgical and Radiological Sciences, School of Veterinary Medicine, University of California, One Garrod Drive, Davis, CA, 95616, USA*
[2] *Department of Clinical Sciences, College of Veterinary Medicine, Cornell University, 930 Campus Road, Ithaca, NY, 14853, USA*

Introduction

Resolution of ocular procedures in horses can present several particular challenges to the anesthesia provider: many surgeries that are performed under general anesthesia require a central and immobile eye, which is best achieved by the use of neuromuscular blockers. The introduction of these agents to the anesthetic protocol adds a new level of complexity, as it will be reviewed in following paragraphs. In some instances, the procedure might be completed with the horse awake and standing, facilitated by the use of sedatives and locoregional anesthesia. In that case, the anesthetist must be experienced in the use of sedatives to provide a state of "conscious sedation" that allows sufficient cooperation from the animal (or tolerance to the surgery) while retaining the ability to stand with as minimal ataxia as possible. For this approach, knowledge of the relevant anatomy and locoregional techniques is necessary. Aside from these technical challenges, complications might arise from manipulation of the eye during surgery (i.e. cardiac dysrhythmias), or secondary to topical ophthalmic medication. Therefore, a basic understanding of ocular physiology and therapeutics is also necessary.

Several ocular pathologies are resolved through surgical interventions in horses. These involve extraocular procedures, such as those involving the eyelids, removal of the globe, and ocular/intraocular surgeries.

Anatomy and Physiology of the Eye

The globe is located within the orbit and surrounded by periorbital tissues (extraocular muscles [EOMs], retrobulbar fat, among others) and periocular structures (such as the conjunctiva and eyelids). The eyelids are modified upper and lower folds of skin, which form the palpebral fissure (opening), provide mechanical protection for the globe, and spread the tear film. Several muscles are responsible for the closure and opening of the eyelids (Table 2.1). However, in a simplistic way, closure of the eyelids is achieved by contraction of the *orbicularis oculi* muscle, while the opening of the eyelids is done by a combination of relaxation of the *orbicularis oculi* muscle, and contraction of the *levator palpebrae superioris* muscle. All other muscles aid in those movements. In general, motor innervation to the eyelids is provided by the oculomotor nerve (CN III) and

Table 2.1 Muscles of the eyelids, associated function and cranial nerve (CN) innervation.

Eyelid muscle	Function	Innervation
Orbicularis oculi	Closure of eyelids	Facial (CN VII)
Levator palpebrae superioris	Elevation of upper eyelid	Oculomotor (CN III)
Retractor anguli oculi	Lengthening palpebral fissure	Facial (CN VII)
Corrugator supercilli	Assist in elevation of upper eyelid	Facial (CN VII)
Malaris	Depression of lower eyelid	Facial (CN VII)
Levator anguli oculi medialis	Lengthening palpebral fissure	Facial (CN VII)
Müller	Elevate upper eyelid	Sympathetic fibers

facial nerve (CN VII), while the sensory innervation to all aspects of the eyelids is provided by the ophthalmic branch of the trigeminal nerve (CN V).

The orbit is a bony fossa that separates the globe from the cranial cavity. In addition to mechanical protection, the orbit provides several foramina and fissures, which are pathways for blood vessels and nerves involved with ocular maintenance. Within the orbit, a total of seven EOMs are responsible for providing ocular motility – four recti (dorsal, ventral, lateral, and medial rectus), two obliques (dorsal oblique and ventral oblique), and one retractor bulbi muscle (Table 2.2). The four rectus muscles (dorsal, ventral, lateral, and medial rectus) move the globe in the direction of their respective names; the dorsal oblique muscle pulls the dorsal aspect of the globe medially and ventrally; the ventral oblique muscle moves the globe medially and dorsally; and the retractor bulbi, which forms a "cone shape" behind the eye, is responsible for retracting the globe into the orbit. The dorsal, ventral, and medial rectus muscles, as well as the ventral oblique muscle, are innervated by cranial nerve III (oculomotor). The dorsal oblique muscle is innervated by cranial nerve IV (trochlear), while the lateral rectus and the retractor bulbi muscles are innervated by cranial nerve VI (abducens).

The globe itself is separated into three layers or tunics. The external or outmost wall of the globe consists of the *fibrous tunic*, composed by the cornea and sclera, which provides the shape and mechanical support for the intraocular structures. The second, middle layer is the highly vascular *uveal tunic or tract*, composed by the iris, ciliary body, and the choroid. The third and innermost layer is the *neural tunic* of the eye, composed by the retina. The lens is

Table 2.2 Extraocular muscle responsible for movement of the globe, associated movement and cranial nerve (CN) innervation.

Extraocular muscle	Function	Innervation
Dorsal rectus	Pull globe upward	Oculomotor (CN III)
Ventral rectus	Pull globe downward	Oculomotor (CN III)
Medial rectus	Pull globe medially	Oculomotor (CN III)
Lateral rectus	Pull globe laterally	Abducens (CN VI)
Dorsal oblique	Move globe medially and ventrally	Trochlear (CN IV)
Ventral oblique	Move glove medially and dorsally	Oculomotor (CN III)
Retractor bulbi	Retract globe	Abducens (CN VI)

located just posterior to the iris and is attached to the ciliary body by the lenticular zonules. The anterior segment comprises all structures from the cornea to the lens (including the cornea itself, the iris, ciliary body, and the lens), and is bathed by the aqueous humor. The anterior segment is divided into two spaces: the anterior chamber (from the cornea to the iris), and the posterior chamber (from the iris to the lens). The posterior segment comprises all structures from the lens to the retina, including the vitreous humor, the choroid, and the retina itself.

The cornea, the anterior outermost structure of the globe, is one of the most densely innervated tissues in the body, richly supplied in sensory nerves (mainly pain receptors) to provide corneal protection, with a neuronal density that is 300–600 times greater than the skin epithelium (Rozsa and Beuerman 1982; Brooks et al. 2000). Sensory innervation of the cornea originates from the long ciliary nerves, which are derived from the ophthalmic branch of the trigeminal nerve (CN V). Most of the nerve endings are located on the subepithelial and anterior stromal layers of the cornea and, in the horse, the cornea appears to be most sensitive in the center and less so toward the periphery.

The innervation of the uveal tract is made by both sympathetic and parasympathetic fibers. The iris sphincter muscle is partly responsible for controlling the pupil size, while the ciliary body muscle is partly responsible for the lens accommodation and focus. The ciliary body muscle and iris sphincter muscle are supplied by parasympathetic fibers from the oculomotor nerve (CN III) via the short ciliary nerves, and by sympathetic nerve fibers via the long ciliary nerves. Medications that may stimulate or paralyze those neuronal pathways may alter the pupil size, either facilitating or precluding some intraocular procedures, such as cataract removal.

Tear Production

The preocular tear film (POTF) is responsible for maintaining an optically uniform ocular surface, lubricating the cornea and conjunctiva, and providing nutrients to the cornea. The tears are mainly composed of three layers: (i) the outer lipid layer, produced by the meibomian glands, and responsible for preventing the evaporation of the tear film; (ii) the intermediate aqueous layer, produced by the orbital (or principal) gland and by the third eyelid gland, composed mainly by water, plus electrolytes, glucose, urea, globulins, lysozymes, and other solids, and responsible for providing the lubrication and nutrients to the cornea; (iii) the inner mucin layer, produced by the conjunctival goblet cells, responsible for anchoring the aqueous film to the corneal epithelium. Also, the POTF contains antibacterial cytokines and exerts some control over the ocular surface flora; therefore, the incidence of ocular surface infections is elevated in tear-deficient patients.

Even though the innervation to the lacrimal gland is not yet completely understood, it is known that the lacrimal gland receives sensory input from the lacrimal nerve, which is a branch of the trigeminal nerve (CN V). Also, the lacrimal branch of the facial nerve (CN VII), sympathetic and parasympathetic fibers are involved in the process. In general, some cholinergic drugs stimulate lacrimation, while anticholinergic drugs decrease the tear production. Even though keratoconjunctivitis sicca ("dry eye") is rare in horses (and usually related to trauma), it is important to remember that general anesthesia may decrease or completely temporarily stop tear production in horses, increasing the risk of corneal erosions and ulcers. Tear replenishment with lacrimomimetics during anesthetic procedures is, therefore, recommended. Artificial tears in ointment or gel formulations are preferable over drops or solutions since those forms stay longer on the eye.

Aqueous Humor and Intraocular Pressure

The aqueous humor is a transparent fluid that resembles an ultrafiltration of plasma and fills and nourishes the anterior segment structures. This fluid is produced by the ciliary body, flows from the posterior chamber through the pupil, into the anterior chamber, and drains out of the eye via the iridocorneal angle into the intrascleral venous plexus (conventional outflow) or via the supraciliary-suprachoroidal space into the scleral vessels (unconventional outflow). In healthy conditions, aqueous humor is constantly produced and drained, establishing a normal intraocular pressure (IOP). Decreased IOPs are usually associated with intraocular inflammation (uveitis), while elevated IOP is one of the main and most devastating components of the glaucoma syndrome, a progressive condition that leads to blindness.

The aqueous humor is formed by three mechanisms: (i) *diffusion* of solutes following a down concentration gradient; (ii) *ultrafiltration* from plasma by hydrostatic force; (iii) *active secretion* by the ciliary body epithelium, utilizing energy to secrete solutes against a concentration gradient. This active process is catalyzed by the carbonic anhydrase enzyme, leading to entry of sodium (Na^+) and bicarbonate (HCO_3^-) into the aqueous, establishing an osmotic gradient leading to the entry of water into the posterior chamber. Topical and systemic carbonic anhydrase inhibitors will thus decrease the rate of aqueous humor formation, resulting in lower IOP values. Even though no significant diurnal IOP variation has been detected in horses, the effect of head position on IOP is well documented, with increased IOPs detected when the head is below heart level (Komaromy et al. 2006). This phenomenon is particularly relevant during hoisting after induction of anesthesia, with IOP values up to 80 mmHg obtained while the horse is hoisted. This should be taken into consideration when anesthetizing and hoisting patients where an increase in IOP could be detrimental, such as those suffering from glaucoma, deep corneal ulcers, descemetocele, or corneal rupture (Monk et al. 2017).

Oculocardiac Reflex

Any sensory stimulation to the eye and its periocular structures may result in stimulation of

the vagal nucleus, leading to a slowing of the heart. This oculocardiac reflex has been documented secondary to traction of the globe during enucleations, and during intraocular surgeries in the dog, cat, horses, humans, and other species. Sensory fibers of the ophthalmic branch of the trigeminal nerve (CN V) to its nucleus make up the afferent pathway of this reflex, while the efferent pathway is via the vagus nerve (CN X) to the heart. The most common clinical sign associated with this phenomenon is bradycardia; however, cardiac arrest and ventricular fibrillation have also been documented (Raffe et al. 1986; Oel et al. 2014).

Sedation for Ocular Procedures

Several ophthalmic procedures, such as surgical correction of defects in the eyelids (often of traumatic origin), placement of episcleral cyclosporine implants for immune-mediated keratitis, intra-stromal injections for corneal abscesses, and even removal of the globe, can be performed under sedation and regional anesthesia. Sedation is tailored to produce a cooperative horse that can tolerate surgical manipulation while standing as stable as possible. Regional anesthesia is also provided to achieve sensory blockade, motor blockade, or both.

Sedation in horses is most commonly achieved with the use of α2-agonist agents. These agents provide reliable sedation, analgesia, and result in an animal that typically stands with minimal ataxia. While some minor clinical differences are reported between the use of different agents [e.g. less ataxia reported with romifidine (England et al. 1992)], all α2-agonists in clinical use are suitable sedatives for these purposes, and all can be administered either as repeated boluses or infused over time to prolong the duration of sedation. If sedation is insufficient during stimulating periods of the procedure, boluses of the agent can be administered without altering the infusion rate. Alternatively, the infusion can be titrated according to a horse's response to surgical

Table 2.3 Alpha 2-agonist drugs loading dosages and infusion rates for standing sedation for ophthalmic procedures.

Drug	Loading dosage	Infusion rate	References
Xylazine	0.5–1.0 mg/kg	0.7 mg/kg/h	Ringer et al. (2012)
Detomidine	0.008–0.01 mg/kg	0.006–0.02 mg/kg/h	Gozalo-Marcilla et al. (2019)[a]
Romifidine	0.08 mg/kg	0.03 mg/kg/h	Marly et al. (2014)

[a] The range has been expanded based on the dosages and experiences at the author's institution.

stimuli. Doses for constant rate infusions of these agents are summarized in Table 2.3. The author commonly uses opioids such as morphine (0.05–0.1 mg/kg) or butorphanol (0.01–0.02 mg/kg), or the phenothyazine agent acepromazine (0.005–0.01 mg/kg), to enhance sedation from α2-agonists in horses that respond to surgical stimulation.

When choosing which a2-agonist to use, it is important to discuss with the ophthalmologist or surgeon the expected duration of the procedure. In general, detomidine and romifidine are most commonly used for longer procedures (>60 minutes), while xylazine is usually chosen for shorter procedures.

While ketamine can be utilized at lower dosages to provide standing sedation, it has been shown to increase the IOP in horses (Ferreira et al. 2013). On the other hand, sedation with xylazine and detomidine decreases the IOP (Holve 2012) and are likely safer options for patients with increased IOP, such as those with glaucoma or deep corneal ulcers.

Locoregional Anesthesia of the Eye and Surrounding Structures

Locoregional Anesthesia of the Eyelid

Anesthesia of the eye and/or surrounding structures is also necessary, in addition to sedation, for performing ocular procedures in the standing horse. Moreover, a combination of sedation and local anesthesia might be used to facilitate ocular exams by decreasing muscular tone of the eyelid and allowing better exposure of the globe.

Akinesia of the eyelids is achieved by the desensitization of the auriculopalpebral nerve, a branch of the facial nerve, which innervates the *orbicularis oculi* muscle. Desensitization of this nerve facilitates examination of the eye and improves the surgical field, but does not provide anesthesia (sensory block) to the lids. The auriculopalpebral nerve runs superficial over the temporalis muscle and dorsal orbit and can be palpated dorsal to the zygomatic process of the temporal bone (Figure 2.1). It can be desensitized at this location, or alternatively, at the depression found caudally to the mandible and ventral to the temporal portion of the zygomatic arch. Surgical procedures involving the lids that are expected to produce pain also require sensory blockade, which may be achieved by desensitizing four nerves that surround the eye (Figure 2.2). The supraorbital (or frontal) nerve can be desensitized as it emerges from the supraorbital foramen, on the dorsolateral aspect of the orbit (Figure 2.1). Desensitization of this nerve provides sensory block to the central portion of the upper eyelid. Anesthesia of the lacrimal nerve, located dorsolateral to the lateral canthus, provides sensory block to the lateral canthus and lateral portion of the eyelid. The medial canthus and medial aspect of the lids are desensitized by anesthetizing the infratrochlear nerve, located dorsomedial to the medial canthus of the eye. The zygomatic nerve, located on the ventrolateral aspect of the orbit, provides sensory block to the central portion of the lower lid. Each nerve may be blocked individually to provide complete sensory block of these structures. Alternatively, a ring block may be performed

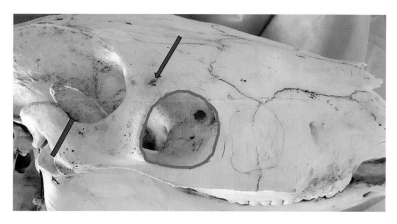

Figure 2.1   Lateral view of an equine skull. The blue line indicates where the auriculopalpebral nerve can be palpated and blocked as it courses over the zygomatic arch. The red arrow indicated the supraorbital foramen where the supraorbital (frontal) nerve emerges and can be blocked. The green circle indicated the bony orbit.

so that all four nerves are involved. Excessive use of local anesthetics during infiltration, however, can disrupt the anatomy and result in edema, which may complicate the conditions of the surgical field.

Locoregional Anesthesia of the Globe

Procedures involving not only the surrounding structures but also the globe itself can be performed in many horses under sedation. Foreign bodies might be removed under a combination of sedative and locoregional techniques as mentioned above. In addition, topical desensitization of the cornea should be performed and can be achieved with topical ophthalmic anesthetics, such as tetracaine 0.5% and propa-racaine 0.5% ophthalmic solutions, applied directly to the ocular surface. In general, the maximum anesthetic effect is achieved within 5–10 minutes when either tetracaine or propa-racaine are used, and last approximately 20–25 minutes. If one drop is used, full desensitization of the cornea is not achieved with aqueous solutions of proparacaine and tetracaine, and some sensation (though minimal) might still be present. However, the instillation of two drops of aqueous 0.5% tetracaine, one minute apart, results in full desensitization of the cornea, with the same duration of action (Monclin et al. 2011). A viscous preparation of 0.5% tetracaine is currently available. It

Figure 2.2   Lateral view of an equine head. Colored dots indicate the location where blockade can be performed to provide local anesthesia of the skin and structures surrounding the eye. Green is the supraorbital (frontal) nerve, blue is the lacrimal nerve, orange is the infratrochlear nerve, and red is the zygomatic nerve.

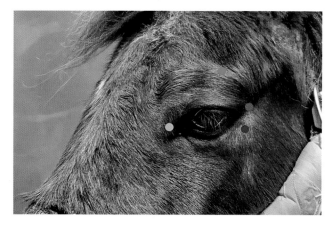

provides complete desensitization of the cornea within 10 minutes, with a duration of approximately 30 minutes after initial administration (Kalf et al. 2008; Sharrow-Reabe and Townsend 2012). A Subconjunctival injection of anesthetic agents is also a viable option for ocular surface anesthesia, and usually increases the duration of the anesthetic effect. The administration of 2% mepivacaine into the subconjunctival space leads to almost complete corneal anesthesia in around 10 minutes, for a total duration of 120 minutes. Bupivacaine and lidocaine can also be used, with maximum effect reached between 15 and 25 minutes after administration, and total duration of around 70–80 minutes (Jinks et al. 2018). Topical 1% morphine sulfate, and topical 1% nalbuphine solution do not result in analgesia of the cornea in horses (Gordon et al. 2018; Wotman and Utter 2010).

In addition to procedures involving the surface of the globe, removal of the eye can also be performed in the standing horse. There are different techniques for desensitizing the relevant structures required for enucleation. Several nerves must be desensitized if complete akinesia and anesthesia of the eyeball is to be achieved, including the optic, oculomotor, abducens, and trochlear nerves, and the maxillary an ophthalmic branches of the trigeminal nerve. In addition, the surrounding structures may also be desensitized, as described above.

Retrobulbar Block

A retrobulbar block is likely the most commonly used locoregional technique for achieving anesthesia of the globe. Retrobulbar anesthesia requires injection of the anesthetic agent into the extraocular muscle cone (EOMC), that is, the EOMC needs to be punctured (Figure 2.3). Retrobulbar injection of local anesthetics occurs at close proximity of the target nerves, and hence, it is expected to produce reliable conduction blockade of those nerves. The injection is also performed in close proximity of other structures, such as blood vessels and the

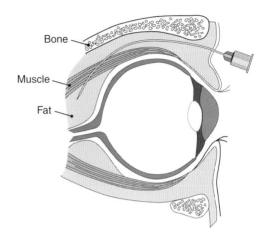

Figure 2.3 Diagram of needle placement for a retrobulbar block. *Source:* Taken from Shilo-Benjamini 2019 with permission from ELSEVIER.

dural cuff that surrounds the optic nerve. Hence, the retrobulbar block carries the risks of direct injury to the nerves enclosed by the EOMC, retrobulbar hemorrhage and hematoma, intrameningeal injection of local anesthetic, and perforation of the globe. In people, the use of long sharp needles, injection of large volumes, or an uncooperative patient, increase the risks for these complications. Application of the local anesthetic outside the EOMC is referred to as peribulbar anesthesia, which likely carries a lower risk of injury to the structures mentioned above (Figure 2.4).

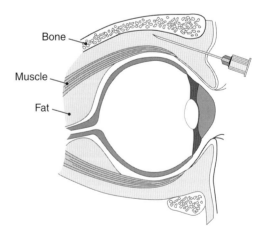

Figure 2.4 Diagram of needle placement for a peribulbar block. *Source:* Taken from Shilo-Benjamini 2019 with permission from ELSEVIER.

Different approaches have been described to perform anesthesia of the globe. The simplest approach is likely the insertion of a needle in four points around the rim of the orbit; midline at the dorsal and ventral aspects of the orbital rim, and at the medial and lateral canthi. The needle is advanced distally, in close proximity to the globe, along the curve of the orbit. For this technique, some authors prefer the use of a pre-bent needle (Hewes et al. 2007; Pollock et al. 2008). There are no clear landmarks to assess depth of insertion, nor is there a method to ensure that important structures are not penetrated or injured by the needle. Because of the "blind" nature of this puncture, the risk for the complications mentioned above is substantial. Injection of local anesthetics typically results in exophthalmos. Reports of successful cases anesthetized with 8–15 ml per point of local anesthetics have been recently described (Hewes et al. 2007; Pollock et al. 2008).

Anesthesia of the globe can also be performed by a modified Peterson technique, whereby a needle is inserted at the supraorbital fossa, caudal and medial to the posterior portion of the zygomatic process. The needle is advanced in a craniomedial direction. This technique allows for guidance with ultrasound (Morath et al. 2013). A curved array transducer can be placed over the closed upper eyelid, and identification of the structures within the EOMC space, including the optic nerve, was possible in a cadaveric study (Figures 2.5 and 2.6) (Morath et al. 2013). Tomographic evaluation of those specimens suggested that sufficient spread of the solution was achieved. It is important to note that the authors of that study reported that even with US guidance, puncture of the nerve sheath could not be excluded in one case. This observation highlights the risks of nerve blocks, especially when performed in sedated animals that may move during the procedure.

Sub-Tenon's Block

Sub-Tenon anesthesia is a technique first introduced to clinical (human) practice in the 1990s as a safer alternative to retrobulbar or peribulbar block (Hansen et al. 1990; Mein and Woodcock 1990; Kumar et al. 2011). Tenon's capsule is a fibrous layer that envelopes the outside of the sclera and fasciae of the EOMs, originating at the limbus and extends caudally around the optic nerve, where it connects to the peridural fascia. Injection of anesthetics into the sub-Tenon's space results in akinesia

Figure 2.5 Diagram of needle placement for a modified Peterson technique using ultrasound guidance. The zygomatic process of the frontal bone and the lateral rectus muscle are removed. A, ultrasound transducer; B, needle with tip positioned within the cone of the retractor bulbi muscle; C, retractor bulbi muscle; D, optic nerve; E, orbital fissure. *Source:* Taken from Morath et al. 2013 with permission from ELSEVIER.

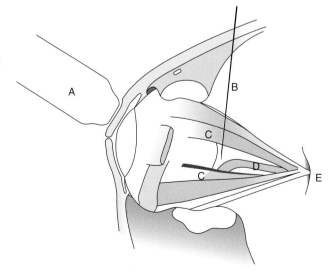

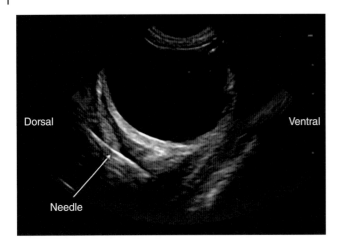

Dorsal

Ventral

Needle

Figure 2.6 Ultrasound image of a needle being directed caudal to the globe during a modified Peterson technique for local blockade of the eye and surrounding structures. *Source:* Used with permission, Dr. Ute Morath.

and anesthesia of the globe that is no different from that obtained with atracurium or a retrobulbar block in dogs (Figure 2.7) (Ahn et al. 2013). The agent injected acts on the anterior motor nerves, the optic nerve, ciliary nerves, and the oculomotor, abducens, and trochlear nerves, resulting in akinesia, mydriasis, and sensory block. Vision may also be interrupted.

The technique for injection of anesthetic in the sub-Tenon's space has been described in dogs and horses (Ahn et al. 2013; Stadler et al. 2017). Because anesthetics are injected using a blunt cannula, a small incision is performed in the conjunctiva, approximately

5 mm posterior to the limbus. The blunt cannula is then inserted, after blunt dissection, along the globe. An alternative technique has been described in humans, where the blunt cannula was replaced by an over-the-needle catheter (Amin et al. 2002). In a cadaveric study on horses, 7–10 ml of solution was sufficient to distribute over the anterior and posterior sub-Tenon's space; however, the injectate did not distribute to the optic nerve in most specimens (Figure 2.8). The authors of that study also reported that globe puncture

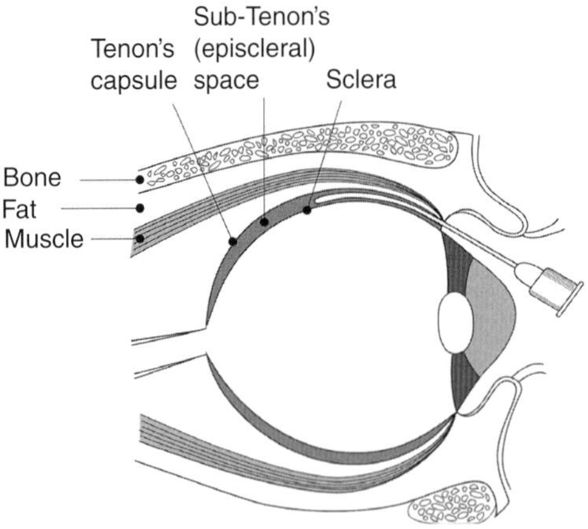

Sub-Tenon's
Tenon's (episcleral)
capsule space   Sclera

Bone
Fat
Muscle

Figure 2.7 Diagram of needle placement for a sub-Tenon's block. *Source:* Taken from Shilo-Benjamini 2019 with permission from ELSEVIER.

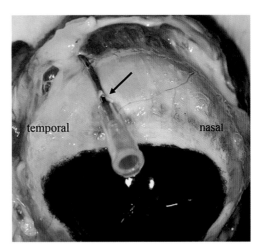

temporal   nasal

Figure 2.8 Equine cadaver eye after enucleation showing the temporo-dorsal position of a sub-Tenon's cannula. The site of Tenon's capsule perforation is indicated by the arrow. *Source:* Taken from Stadler et al. 2017.

occurred in one eye (Stadler et al. 2017). At the time this chapter was written, clinical experience performing the sub-Tenon's block in awake, sedated animals have not been yet evaluated, and the risk of globe perforation resulting from inexperience or sudden movements needs to be considered. However, due to its benefits over retrobulbar blocks in humans, sub-Tenon's anesthesia might be indicated for providing akinesia and analgesia in anesthetized horses, as an alternative to the use of neuromuscular blocking agents (NMBA).

General Anesthesia for Ocular Procedures

Several ophthalmic procedures may require the use of general anesthesia. Procedures such as conjunctival and corneal grafts for the correction of corneal ulcers, perforations, iris prolapse, and for stromal abscesses removal, suprachoroidal cyclosporine implants for management of equine recurrent uveitis (ERU), and phacoemulsification for cataract removal are some of the most common ophthalmic procedures performed that requires general anesthesia.

Corneal ulcers are one of the most common ophthalmic conditions affecting horses. Superficial, non-complicated ulcers should heal fast with the aid of topical therapy. However, deep and infected ulcers may rapidly progress to corneal melting and perforation of the cornea, with or without iris prolapse, and may lead to permanent blindness if not promptly corrected. Keratectomy, conjunctival graft placement, corneal grafts or transplants, and grafts utilizing biological or synthetic materials are surgical options for the correction of corneal wounds. Due to the fragile nature of deep ulcers and imminent risk of perforation, drugs and procedures that result in elevated IOP should be avoided.

Corneal abscesses are also commonly observed in horses, especially in the Southeast of the United States. The current hypothesis for the development of corneal abscesses is the inoculation of microorganisms (bacteria or fungi) into the stroma of the cornea, as a result of a microtrauma. This is a painful condition, and the abscess may dive deeper, perforate through the cornea, and lead to a severe intraocular uveitis, which may result in blindness. If not treatable, enucleation is often recommended, due to the intense pain provoked by the condition. Since these abscesses are solid, drainage is not possible, and topical medications including antibacterial and antifungal drugs are recommended as a therapeutical plan. In some cases, intra-stromal injection of antifungals is also recommended and can be performed under sedation and topical anesthetic in a standing horse (see the preceding text). However, cases refractory to medical management are candidates for surgical removal of the abscess via keratectomy/keratoplasty, or corneal grafts/transplants.

Cataracts are opacities in the lens that blocks the light from reaching the retina. In advance stages, cataract leads to blindness, but in several cases, vision can be restored after surgery for cataract removal. The removal of cataracts in foals have a better prognosis compared to the same procedure in adult horses. The reason behind that observation is that, in general, cataracts in foals are congenital and not associated with other co-morbidities, while cataracts in adult horses are generally acquired and secondary to ERU or trauma, which leads to several other alterations of the globe, resulting in a less favorable prognosis. To date, no medication has been able to remove cataracts or delay their progression, and surgical removal is the only therapeutic option. Currently, phacoemulsification is the accepted standard of care for cataract removal in veterinary medicine.

Corneal surgical procedures (keratectomy, conjunctival graft, corneal graft or transplants, etc.) and phacoemulsification for cataract removal should be performed with the patient under general anesthesia, and utilize a surgical microscope for magnification, due to the precise and millimetric nature of those procedures.

The position of the eye is also of crucial importance, as the globe should be centrally positioned to allow visualization and access to the area to be manipulated. Optimal eye position is usually achieved with NMBA, which act by paralyzing the EOMs. This results in a centrally positioned globe and minimizes the anterior displacement of intraocular structures since the EOM tone is reduced. In patients undergoing cataract surgery, mydriasis (pupil dilation) is also imperative to allow access to the entire lens, and medications that lead to pupil constriction should be avoided.

ERU, commonly known as moon blindness or periodic ophthalmia, is one of the most devastating ocular condition in horses. This immune-mediated disease is characterized by recurrent episodes of severe inflammation of the uveal tract, resulting in cataract, blindness, and, in some cases, globe atrophy. Each flare-up should be treated with medical therapy, including topical steroids, atropine, and systemic non-steroidal anti-inflammatory drugs. However, there is no cure for the condition, and the more frequent and severe the flare-ups, the more likely for the patient to become blind. Cyclosporine, an immune-modulator agent, surgically placed into the suprachoroidal space is a newer therapeutic approach for the condition, aiming to decrease the frequency and severity of the flare-ups. The implant is placed underneath the sclera, above the choroid, on the dorsal aspect of the globe. This procedure should be done with the patient under general anesthesia, due to its precise and millimetric nature. However, since the dorsal sclera is the area to be approached during surgery, paralysis is not required, as the horse's globe usually rotates ventromedially during general anesthesia, exposing the desired surgical site.

General Anesthesia

General anesthesia for ocular procedures represents a number of unique challenges. A recent single-center study reported that ocular procedures were associated with longer anesthesia and recovery times. Moreover, the rate of post-operative morbidity was higher for ocular procedures than for horses undergoing other types of procedures (Curto et al. 2018). In particular, the use of preoperative fluconazole in horses undergoing certain ocular procedures was associated with worse outcomes, including poor quality of recovery. In addition to the observations of that retrospective, there are other challenges directly related to anesthesia for these type of interventions: as mentioned above, topical ophthalmic medication can have cardiovascular effects, even if that medication was administered preoperatively. In dogs, preoperative administration of topical medication containing scopolamine and phenylephrine resulted in significantly higher systemic arterial pressures than in those not receiving those agents (Martin-Florcs et al. 2010).

General anesthesia in adult horses also imposes other complications that should not be overlooked. Hoisting horses, which is necessary during initial positioning following induction, or prior to recovery, substantially elevates the IOP; values up to 80 mmHg have been recorded (Monk et al. 2017). Moreover, ketamine, likely the most commonly used induction agent, has also been linked with increased IOP in horses when administered preceded by guaifenesin (Ferreira et al. 2013). While these complications may be impossible to avoid in many circumstances, the potential deleterious effects of increased IOP needs to be considered as part of the risks associated with general anesthesia in these animals.

In addition to an immobile patient, intraocular surgery may require an immobile and relaxed eye. Relaxation of the EOMs facilitates manipulation of the globe by the use of sutures and improves the surgical conditions. Relaxation of the globe might be achieved by the use of local anesthesia as described above. However, it is important to consider the potential risks of such techniques, as it may promote inflammation of structures around the globe, or the formation of hematomas should accidental vascular puncture occur.

Relaxation of the eye may also be achieved with the administration of muscle relaxants, more precisely named NMBA. Neuromuscular block, while providing a central and relaxed globe and preventing sudden movement of an anesthetized patient, adds a new level of complexity to anesthesia care. Neuromuscular block suppresses reflexes and eliminates muscle tone, signs that are often used to assess depth of anesthesia. Furthermore, residual effects of NMBA may extend into the early post-operative period, where in humans, NMBA have been shown to contribute to upper airway collapse and hypoxia (Murphy et al. 2008). Hence, the use of NMBA implies that close attention must be paid to ensure a proper level of hypnosis, and a complete return of neuromuscular function prior to recovery. The latter, as will be discussed, requires the use of objective monitoring of neuromuscular transmission and/or the use of reversal agents.

Neuromuscular Blocking Agents

A small number of competitive, nondepolarizing neuromuscular blocking agents are used routinely in clinical anesthesia of horses. The benzylisoquinoline agent atracurium is likely the most commonly used drug, owing to its short duration and reliable metabolism. At the time this chapter was prepared, atracurium was also the most cost-effective agent at the author's institution. Atracurium's metabolism, which is in part independent of organ function, typically results in a predictable duration of action. However, longer than expected duration can be observed in individual horses putting them at risk of residual block (Martin-Flores et al. 2008).

Cisatracurium is one of the 10 isomers from atracurium. The potential for histamine release with cisatracurium is less than with its parent compound atracurium. This agent is also more potent, and it is characterized by a slower onset time. Little data on the use of cisatracurium in

horses is available. Pilot data suggests that doses of 0.04–0.05 mg/kg will often produce complete block in horses.

From the aminosteroid compounds, rocuronium is likely the most frequently used; moreover, thanks to availability of a specific reversal agent (see the following text), its use is likely to increase. The onset of rocuronium is possibly faster than for atracurium. Doses of 0.2–0.6 mg/kg have been evaluated in horses, with the lowest dose producing close to complete block (Auer et al. 2007b). In a study investigating the use of rocuronium in horses undergoing ocular procedures, 0.3 mg/kg of this agent resulted in complete block in all horses, and a clinical duration of 32 ± 18 minutes (Auer and Moens 2011). It should be noted that the range of clinical duration was wide: 7.7–56 minutes, and the time until complete recovery of neuromuscular function ranged between 20 and 84 minutes. Such variation results in unpredictable recovery times and may contribute to increased risk of residual block if monitoring is not performed.

Vecuronium, also an aminosteroid agent, has long been used in humans and small animals, and is characterized by cardiovascular stability and a predictable duration of action. Its use in horses, however, is scarcely documented. A dose-finding study in horses showed that the doses required to reliably produce complete neuromuscular block in horses also resulted in long duration of block, and required large doses of anticholinesterase agents during reversal (Martin-Flores et al. 2012). These characteristics make it an unlikely agent for routine clinical use.

Monitoring of Neuromuscular Function

There are different techniques used to monitor neuromuscular function, all of which represent minor alterations of the same fundamental principle: the stimulation of a motor nerve and the assessment of the evoked muscular contraction. In horses, and in particular for ocular surgery, the peroneal and radial nerves can be used interchangeably to monitor neuromuscular block (Mosing et al. 2010). Figure 2.9

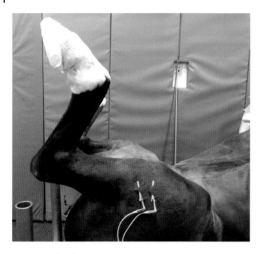

Figure 2.9 Placement of a nerve stimulator electrodes for stimulation of the peroneal nerve in an anesthetized horse in dorsal recumbency.

shows positioning of the stimulating electrodes for the peroneal nerve.

Motor nerves can be stimulated in different patterns. The train-of-four (TOF) is the pattern most commonly used in the clinical setting: four stimuli are delivered at a frequency of 2 Hz (2 per second), with a pulse duration of 0.1–0.3 milliseconds. Each TOF can be repeated no more frequently than every 10 seconds. The TOF, which was originally described almost half a century ago (Ali et al. 1970), offers a great advantage for clinical use: observation of a progressive decrease in the magnitude of twitches within the TOF – that is, the presence of fade – is indicative of incomplete neuromuscular function. By opposition, if no fade is observed in the TOF, neuromuscular function is normal. In other words, each TOF acts as its own control, and a baseline measurement is not required. When NMBA are used, a fade in the TOF develops during onset of block. If the dose is sufficient, complete block occurs and no responses are elicited with TOF stimulation (TOF count of zero). During offset of block, the first twitch of the train (T1) is initially restored, followed in order by the remaining responses. Once all four twitches have reappeared during offset of block, neuromuscular function recovers progressively until all four twitches reach

their maximum value and no more fade can be observed.

The most rudimentary form for assessing the magnitude of the evoked responses is by observing or palpating those contractions. This method, while commonly used, is unreliable, as only the most evident degrees of fade can be reliably observed (Martin-Flores et al. 2008). There are several methods to quantify the muscular response, mechanomyography – the measurement of isometric force – being the gold standard. The most commonly used method in the clinical setting is acceleromyography (AMG), whereby the acceleration of a free-moving extremity is measured in response to nerve stimulation. AMG has been used extensively in anesthetized horses, and has been applied to pelvic and thoracic limbs, and to the *orbicularis oris* muscle (Figure 2.10) (Mosing et al. 2010). AMG is affordable, easy to apply, and can detect fade when observation fails to recognize it. Given the potential risks of neuromuscular function impairment during recovery from anesthesia in horses, AMG is an essential monitor when NMBA are used during general anesthesia.

Quantification of the magnitude of the evoked contractions during TOF allows the measurement of the TOF ratio (T4 : T1). Historically, it was considered that once the TOF ratio reached 0.7 during recovery,

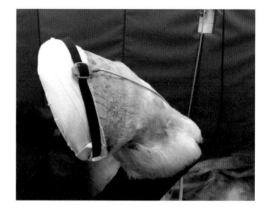

Figure 2.10 Placement of a nerve stimulator accelerometer on the hind leg hoof for acceleromyography in an anesthetized horse in dorsal recumbency.

neuromuscular function was sufficiently restored to safely allow extubation, as only minor discomfort was reported with those values. In humans, a TOF ratio of at least 0.9 is currently accepted as a better threshold, given that even low degrees of residual block can contribute to a blunted response to hypoxia and aspiration of materials into the airway (Eriksson et al. 1993; Eriksson 1996; Eriksson et al. 1997; Sundman et al. 2000). Moreover, some authors suggest that a TOF ratio of 1.0 should be achieved before neuromuscular transmission is considered adequate (Capron et al. 2004). In dogs, laryngeal dysfunction was still observed when the TOF ratio measured at the limb was 0.9 (Sakai et al. 2017). While these findings have not been corroborated in horses, all efforts to avoid residual block should be made if complications secondary to inadequate neuromuscular function are to be minimized.

Other patterns of stimulation have been described but have not replaced the TOF in clinical anesthesia. Measurement of the magnitude of T1, or of a single twitch, is often used in research to calculate the potency of a given agent, or to describe the characteristics of recovery from neuromuscular blockade by calculating the recovery index: the time between T1 reaching 25% and 75% of its control value. Therefore, monitoring the single twitch require that the magnitude of the twitch be measured objectively, and that a baseline value be obtained. Double burst stimulation (DBS) is a stimulating pattern consisting of two short tetanic stimuli (or bursts) at 50 Hz separated by a short interval (750 milliseconds) (Engbaek et al. 1989). The result is two contractions of larger magnitude than those evoked with TOF. Despite this, and similarly to using TOF, fade cannot always be detected by the subjective observation of DBS (Samet et al. 2005; Capron et al. 2006).

Reversal of Neuromuscular Block

Pharmacological reversal of neuromuscular blockade is most commonly achieved with the use of acetylcholinesterase inhibitors, such as edrophonium or neostigmine. These agents reduce the activity of the acetylcholinesterase enzyme, which is responsible for the hydrolysis of acetylcholine in the neuromuscular cleft. As a result, the concentration of acetylcholine increases. It is this concentration of acetylcholine that will ultimately competitively antagonize the effects of the NMBA at the nicotinic cholinergic receptor in the neuromuscular cleft. The effects of these reversal agents are, therefore, indirect. This particular mechanism of action has two important implications for the anesthesia provider: First, once sufficient anticholinesterase inhibitor has been administered and the enzymatic activity has been completely abolished, no more effect will be achieved by any further administration of these agents. In other words, once the enzymatic activity has been fully inhibited, the ceiling effect has been reached. Second, the rate of rise of acetylcholine in the cleft secondary to inhibition of the cholinesterase enzyme is determined by the rate of synthesis and release of acetylcholine by the presynaptic cell. This rate is not accelerated by the administration of these reversal agents. The consequence of these characteristics is that the depth of neuromuscular block that can be reversed, and the speed of reversal are limited by the aforementioned mechanisms. From a practical point of view, during deep neuromuscular block, a large number of molecules of the relaxant is present at the neuromuscular cleft. The concentration of ACh that can be achieved during reversal is not enough to competitively antagonize block. This explains why profound block cannot be effectively reversed with these agents.

Aside from these limitations, reversal of block with cholinesterase inhibitor drugs has other drawbacks. The increase in ACh concentration that results from enzymatic inhibition can result in systemic effects, most commonly characterized by bradyarrhythmias. Co-administration of atropine is common practice when these agents are used in people or small animals. The use of atropine in horses remains controversial. The resulting situation is difficult to reconcile, as avoidance of reversal administration carries the risk of residual block, and the use of reversal agents carries the risk of observing side effects from those agents or from atropine. Different approaches have been used to avoid these situations. Both neostigmine and edrophonium have been successfully used in horses in the absence of atropine (Hildebrand and Howitt 1984). However, gastrointestinal signs and increased airway secretions were observed, and of larger magnitude with neostigmine than edrophonium. Neostigmine and edrophonium have been used in horses at doses of 0.007–0.04 mg/kg, and 0.5–1.0 m/kg, respectively. While both agents can produce side effects secondary to increases in acetylcholine, both have been used successfully in horses without pretreatment with atropine or glycopyrrolate (Hildebrand and Howitt 1984; Auer and Moens 2011). Slow, incremental dosing may help prevent or minimize the impact of acetylcholine.

An alternate approach is to avoid unnecessarily profound block, by closely monitoring neuromuscular function. With the use of AMG, the minimal effective dose of the NMBA that produces the desired effect can be administered by the injection of small boluses. For most ocular procedures, sufficient relaxation of the eye can be achieved with submaximal relaxant doses. In dogs, centralization of the eye was achieved with subclinical doses of rocuronium that did not produce profound paralysis and did not result in apnea (Auer et al. 2007a). In horses, the eye remained central throughout the recovery period from rocuronium, even when the TOF ratio had reached 0.9 (Auer and Moens 2011). Sufficient relaxation of the eye can therefore be achieved with small doses, and even when responses to TOF are decreased but not completely suppressed. A shallow level of block can then be maintained by either infusing the NMBA or by administering small boluses in order to prevent both complete block and complete reversal. This approach relies almost completely on the use of monitoring. By maintaining a shallow level of block, spontaneous recovery can occur more rapidly and more predictably than when deeper levels of block are achieved.

The (Present and) Future of Reversal

Sugammadex: A new concept for reversing neuromuscular blockers was developed and introduced to clinical practice in the past decade (de Boer et al. 2006a; de Boer et al. 2006b). Sugammadex is a selective relaxant-binding agent (SRBA) now available worldwide. This modified cyclodextrin binds to aminosteroid agents (1 : 1 ratio) to form a complex devoid of neuromuscular blocking properties with a very low dissociation rate. Formation of this complex promptly decreases the plasma concentration of free NMBA creating a gradient that promotes diffusion away from the neuromuscular junction. The end result is a rapid termination of the neuromuscular blocking effects of the aminosteroid agent. Because this mechanism circumvents any of the limitations of the acetylcholinesterase inhibitors, the effect is not only quick, but this agent is also able to reverse profound block, providing sufficient sugammadex is administered to bind to the NMBA. Moreover, there is no concern with increased levels of circulating ACh and a need for atropine or glycopyrrolate. Sugammadex has been successfully used in ponies paralyzed with rocuronium and in dogs paralyzed with rocuronium and vecuronium (Mosing et al. 2010; Mosing et al. 2012). Sugammadex has no effect on benzylisoquinolinium agents such as atracurium.

Calabadion: Calabadion 1 is a member of the cucurbit[n]uril family or molecular containers that, similarly to sugammadex, can form complexes with NMBA. Unlike sugammadex, however, calabadion 1 can bind to both steroidal and benzyisoquinoline agents. (Ma et al. 2012; Hoffmann et al. 2013). In laboratory studies, calabadion 1 has shown to be substantially faster than neostigmine for reversing both cistacurium and rocuronium (Hoffmann et al. 2013). At the time this chapter was prepared, calabadion 1 was not yet commercially available.

Fumarates and cysteine: Fumarates (olefinic isoquinolinium diester) compounds are a new group of NMBA with a unique mechanism of deactivation (Lien ct al. 2009; Lien 2011). Two agents are being researched for clinical applications; gantacurium and CW002 (Heerdt et al. 2015). These agents produced nondepolarizing block, but distinguish themselves in the mechanisms for deactivation. Gantacurium undergoes rapid hydrolysis but also interacts with endogenous L-cysteine to yield an adduction product practically devoid of neuromuscular blocking effects. This reaction is fast. In addition, pH-sensitive ester hydrolysis also occurs. Gantacurium is thus an ultrashortacting blocker, with a profile that resembles that of succinylcholine. CW002 differs from gantacurium in that interaction with L-cysteine is slower, resulting in an intermediate-acting NMBA. While gantacurium, at clinical useful doses, produces block of approximately 10 minutes in people, CW002 results in block of approximately 1 hour (Heerdt et al. 2016). However, this duration can be abbreviated by the administration of exogenous L-cysteine. In a study in Rhesus monkeys receiving supraclinical doses of CW002, L-cysteine restored neuromuscular function in two to four minutes (Sunaga et al. 2016). In cats, L-cysteine accelerated the recovery index of CW002 from 27 minutes to 6 minutes.

With sugammadex being already commercially available, and calabadion 1 and fumarates being under different phases of investigation, the future armamentarium for relaxing and reversing horses is likely to be expanded. It is likely that these agents will allow more freedom to increase the use of relaxants by simplifying reversal of block and decreasing the risks associated with it.

References

Ahn, J., Jeong, M., Park, Y. et al. (2013). Comparison of systemic atracurium, retrobulbar lidocaine, and sub-Tenon's lidocaine injections in akinesia and mydriasis in dogs. *Veterinary Ophthalmology* 16 (6): 440–445.

Ali, H.H., Utting, J.E., and Gray, C. (1970). Stimulus frequency in the detection of neuromuscular block in humans. *British Journal of Anaesthesia* 42 (11): 967–978.

Amin, S., Minihan, M., Lesnik-Oberstein, S. et al. (2002). A new technique for delivering sub-Tenon's anaesthesia in ophthalmic surgery. *British Journal of Ophthalmology* 86 (1): 119–120.

Auer, U. and Moens, Y. (2011). Neuromuscular blockade with rocuronium bromide for ophthalmic surgery in horses. *Veterinary Ophthalmology* 14 (4): 244–247.

Auer, U., Mosing, M., and Moens, Y.P. (2007a). The effect of low dose rocuronium on globe position, muscle relaxation and ventilation in dogs: a clinical study. *Veterinary Ophthalmology* 10 (5): 295–298.

Auer, U., Uray, C., and Mosing, M. (2007b). Observations on the muscle relaxant rocuronium bromide in the horse -- a dose-response study. *Veterinary Anaesthesia and Analgesia* 34 (2): 75–81.

de Boer, H.D., van Egmond, J., van de Pol, F. et al. (2006a). Reversal of profound rocuronium neuromuscular blockade by sugammadex in anesthetized rhesus monkeys. *Anesthesiology* 104 (4): 718–723.

de Boer, H.D., van Egmond, J., van de Pol, F. et al. (2006b). Sugammadex, a new reversal agent for neuromuscular block induced by rocuronium in the anaesthetized rhesus monkey. *British Journal of Anaesthesia* 96 (4): 473–479.

Brooks, D.E., Clark, C.K., and Lester, G.D. (2000). Cochet-bonnet aesthesiometer determined corneal sensitivity in neonatal foals and adult horses. *Veterinary Ophthalmology* 3 (2-3): 133–137.

Capron, F., Alla, F., Hottier, C. et al. (2004). Can acceleromyography detect low levels of residual paralysis? A probability approach to detect a mechanomyographic train-of-four ratio of 0.9. *Anesthesiology* 100 (5): 1119–1124.

Capron, F., Fortier, L.P., Racine, S. et al. (2006). Tactile fade detection with hand or wrist stimulation using train-of-four, double-burst stimulation, 50-hertz tetanus, 100-hertz tetanus, and acceleromyography. *Anesthesia and Analgesia* 102 (5): 1578–1584.

Curto, E.M., Griffith, E.H., Posner, L.P. et al. (2018). Factors associated with postoperative complications in healthy horses after general anesthesia for ophthalmic versus non-ophthalmic procedures: 556 cases (2012-2014). *Journal of the American Veterinary Medical Association* 252 (9): 1113–1119.

Engbaek, J., Ostergaard, D., and Viby-Mogensen, J. (1989). Double burst stimulation (DBS): a new pattern of nerve stimulation to identify residual neuromuscular block. *British journal of Anaesthesia* 62 (3): 274–278.

England, G.C., Clarke, K.W., and Goossens, L. (1992). A comparison of the sedative effects of three alpha 2-adrenoceptor agonists (romifidine, detomidine and xylazine) in the horse. *Journal of Veterinary Pharmacology and Therapeutics* 15 (2): 194–201.

Eriksson, L.I. (1996). Reduced hypoxic chemosensitivity in partially paralysed man. A new property of muscle relaxants? *Acta Anaesthesiologica Scandinavica* 40 (5): 520–523.

Eriksson, L.I., Sato, M., and Severinghaus, J.W. (1993). Effect of a vecuronium-induced partial neuromuscular block on hypoxic ventilatory response. *Anesthesiology* 78 (4): 693–699.

Eriksson, L.I., Sundman, E., Olsson, R. et al. (1997). Functional assessment of the pharynx at rest and during swallowing in partially paralyzed humans: simultaneous videomanometry and mechanomyography of awake human volunteers. *Anesthesiology* 87 (5): 1035–1043.

Ferreira, T.H., Brisnan, R.J., Shilo-Benjamini, Y. et al. (2013). Effects of ketamine, propofol, or thiopental administration on intraocular pressure and qualities of induction of and

recovery from anesthesia in horses. *American Journal of Veterinary Research* 74 (8): 1070–1077.

Gordon, E., Sandquist, C., Cebra, C.K. et al. (2018). Esthesiometry evaluation of corneal analgesia after topical application of 1% morphine sulfate in normal horses. *Veterinary Ophthalmology* 21 (3): 218–223.

Gozalo-Marcilla, M., de Oliveira, A.R., Fonseca, M.W. et al. (2019). Sedative and antinociceptive effects of different detomidine constant rate infusions, with or without methadone in standing horses. *Equine Veterinary Journal* 51 (4): 530–536.

Hansen, E.A., Mein, C.E., and Mazzoli, R. (1990). Ocular anesthesia for cataract surgery: a direct sub-Tenon's approach. *Ophthalmic Surgery* 21 (10): 696–699.

Heerdt, P.M., Sunaga, H., and Savarese, J.J. (2015). Novel neuromuscular blocking drugs and antagonists. *Current Opinion in Anaesthesiology* 28 (4): 403–410.

Heerdt, P.M., Sunaga, H., Owen, J.S. et al. (2016). Dose-response and cardiopulmonary side effects of the novel neuromuscular-blocking drug CW002 in man. *Anesthesiology* 125 (6): 1136–1143.

Hewes, C.A., Keoughan, G.C., and Gutierrez-Nibeyro, S. (2007). Standing enucleation in the horse: a report of 5 cases. *Canadian Veterinary Journal* 48 (5): 512–514.

Hildebrand, S.V. and Howitt, G.A. (1984). Antagonism of pancuronium neuromuscular blockade in halothane-anesthetized ponies using neostigmine and edrophonium. *American Journal of Veterinary Research* 45 (11): 2276–2280.

Hoffmann, U., Grosse-Sundrup, M., Eikermann-Haerter, K. et al. (2013). Calabadion: a new agent to reverse the effects of benzylisoquinoline and steroidal neuromuscular-blocking agents. *Anesthesiology* 119 (2): 317–325.

Holve, D.L. (2012). Effect of sedation with detomidine on intraocular pressure with and without topical anesthesia in clinically normal horses. *Journal of the American Veterinary Medical Association* 240 (3): 308–311.

Jinks, M.R., Fontenot, R.L., Wills, R.W. et al. (2018). The effects of subconjunctival bupivacaine, lidocaine, and mepivacaine on corneal sensitivity in healthy horses. *Veterinary Ophthalmology* 21 (5): 498–506.

Kalf, K.L., Utter, M.E., and Wotman, K.L. (2008). Evaluation of duration of corneal anesthesia induced with ophthalmic 0.5% proparacaine hydrochloride by use of a Cochet-bonnet aesthesiometer in clinically normal horses. *American Journal of Veterinary Research* 69 (12): 1655–1658.

Komaromy, A.M., Garg, C.D., Ying, G. et al. (2006). Effect of head position on intraocular pressure in horses. *American Journal of Veterinary Research* 67 (7): 1232–1235.

Kumar, C.M., Eid, H., and Dodds, C. (2011). Sub-Tenon's anaesthesia: complications and their prevention. *Eye (Lond)* 25 (6): 694–703.

Lien, C.A. (2011). Development and potential clinical impairment of ultra-short-acting neuromuscular blocking agents. *British Journal of Anaesthesia* 107 (suppl 1): i60–i71.

Lien, C.A., Savard, P., Belmont, M. et al. (2009). Fumarates: unique nondepolarizing neuromuscular blocking agents that are antagonized by cysteine. *Journal of Critical Care* 24 (1): 50–57.

Ma, D., Zhang, B., Hoffmann, U. et al. (2012). Acyclic cucurbit[n]uril-type molecular containers bind neuromuscular blocking agents in vitro and reverse neuromuscular block in vivo. *Angewandte Chemie* 51 (45): 11358–11362.

Marly, C., Bettschart-Wolfensberger, R., Nussbaumer, P. et al. (2014). Evaluation of a romifidine constant rate infusion protocol with or without butorphanol for dentistry and ophthalmologic procedures in standing horses. *Veterinary Anaesthesia and Analgesia* 41 (5): 491–497.

Martin-Flores, M., Campoy, L., Ludders, J.W. et al. (2008). Comparison between acceleromyography and visual assessment of train-of-four for monitoring neuromuscular blockade in horses undergoing surgery. *Veterinary Anaesthesia and Analgesia* 35 (3): 220–227.

Martin-Flores, M., Mercure-McKenzie, T.M., Campoy, L. et al. (2010). Controlled retrospective study of the effects of eyedrops containing phenylephrine hydrochloride and scopolamine hydrobromide on mean arterial blood pressure in anesthetized dogs. *American Journal of Veterinary Research* 71 (12): 1407–1412.

Martin-Flores, M., Pare, M.D., Adams, W. et al. (2012). Observations of the potency and duration of vecuronium in isoflurane-anesthetized horses. *Veterinary Anaesthesia and Analgesia* 39 (4): 385–389.

Mein, C.E. and Woodcock, M.G. (1990). Local anesthesia for vitreoretinal surgery. *Retina* 10 (1): 47–49.

Monclin, S.J., Farnir, F., and Grauwels, M. (2011). Duration of corneal anaesthesia following multiple doses and two concentrations of tetracaine hydrochloride eyedrops on the normal equine cornea. *Equine Veterinary Journal* 43 (1): 69–73.

Monk, C.S., Brooks, D.E., Granone, T. et al. (2017). Measurement of intraocular pressure in healthy anesthetized horses during hoisting. *Veterinary Anaesthesia and Analgesia* 44 (3): 502–508.

Morath, U., Luyet, C., Spadavecchia, C. et al. (2013). Ultrasound-guided retrobulbar nerve block in horses: a cadaveric study. *Veterinary Anaesthesia and Analgesia* 40 (2): 205–211.

Mosing, M., Auer, U., Bardell, D. et al. (2010). Reversal of profound rocuronium block monitored in three muscle groups with sugammadex in ponies. *British Journal of Anaesthesia* 105 (4): 480–486.

Mosing, M., Auer, U., West, E. et al. (2012). Reversal of profound rocuronium or vecuronium-induced neuromuscular block with sugammadex in isoflurane-anaesthetised dogs. *Veterinary Journal* 192 (3): 467–471.

Murphy, G.S., Szokol, J.W., Marymont, J.H. et al. (2008). Residual neuromuscular blockade and critical respiratory events in the postanesthesia care unit. *Anesthesia and Analgesia* 107 (1): 130–137.

Oel, C., Gerhards, H., and Gehlen, H. (2014). Effect of retrobulbar nerve block on heart rate variability during enucleation in horses under general anesthesia. *Veterinary Ophthalmology* 17 (3): 170–174.

Pollock, P.J., Russell, T., Hughes, T.K. et al. (2008). Transpalpebral eye enucleation in 40 standing horses. *Veterinary Surgery* 37 (3): 306–309.

Raffe, M.C., Bistner, S.I., Crimi, A.J., and Ruff, J. (1986). Retrobulbar block in combination with general anesthesia for equine ophthalmic surgery. *Veterinary Surgery* 15 (1): 139–141.

Ringer, S.K., Portier, K.G., Fourel, I. et al. (2012). Development of a xylazine constant rate infusion with or without butorphanol for standing sedation of horses. *Veterinary Anaesthesia and Analgesia* 39 (1): 1–11.

Rozsa, A.J. and Beuerman, R.W. (1982). Density and organization of free nerve endings in the corneal epithelium of the rabbit. *Pain* 14 (2): 105–120.

Sakai, D.M., Martin-Flores, M., Romano, M. et al. (2017). Recovery from rocuronium-induced neuromuscular block was longer in the larynx than in the pelvic limb of anesthetized dogs. *Veterinary Anaesthesia and Analgesia* 44 (2): 246–253.

Samet, A., Capron, F., Alla, F. et al. (2005). Single acceleromyographic train-of-four, 100-hertz tetanus or double-burst stimulation: which test performs better to detect residual paralysis? *Anesthesiology* 102 (1): 51–56.

Sharrow-Reabe, K. and Townsend, W.M. (2012). Effects of action of proparacaine and tetracaine topical ophthalmic formulations on corneal sensitivity in horses. *Journal of the American Veterinary Medical Association* 241 (12): 1645–1649.

Shilo-Benjamini, Y. (2019). A review of ophthalmic local and region anesthesia in dogs and cats. *Veterinary Anaesthesia and Analgesia* 46 (1): 14–27.

Stadler, S., Dennler, M., Hetzel, U. et al. (2017). Sub-Tenon's injection in equine cadaver eyes: MRI visualization of anesthetic fluid distribution and comparison of two different volumes. *Veterinary Ophthalmology* 20 (6): 488–495.

Sunaga, H., Savarese, J.J., McGilvra, J.D. et al. (2016). Preclinical pharmacology of CW002: a nondepolarizing neuromuscular blocking drug of intermediate duration, degraded and antagonized by l-cysteine-additional studies of safety and efficacy in the anesthetized rhesus monkey and cat. *Anesthesiology* 125 (4): 732–743.

Sundman, E., Witt, H., Olsson, R. et al. (2000). The incidence and mechanisms of pharyngeal and upper esophageal dysfunction in partially paralyzed humans: pharyngeal videoradiography and simultaneous manometry after atracurium. *Anesthesiology* 92 (4): 977–984.

Wotman, K.L. and Utter, M.E. (2010). Effect of treatment with a topical ophthalmic preparation of 1% nalbuphine solution on corneal sensitivity in clinically normal horses. *American Journal of Veterinary Research* 71 (2): 223–228.

3

Anesthetic Management for Inflammatory or Infectious Respiratory Diseases

Kara Lascola and Stuart Clark-Price

Department of Clinical Sciences, College of Veterinary Medicine, Auburn University, 1220 Wire Road, Auburn, AL, 36849, USA

Introduction

Respiratory disease is common in horses. Infectious respiratory viruses or bacteria are easily transmitted from horse to horse, particularly with those that are regularly transported or housed in densely populated barns or pastures. As such, practitioners will be required to anesthetize horses with clinical and subclinical respiratory conditions that may impact or be impacted by general anesthesia. Additionally, as horses live longer lives because of progressive veterinary care, horses with chronic respiratory diseases such as asthma may present for anesthesia. Knowledge of the potential interaction between disease and anesthesia will improve the anesthetic care of these horses.

Respiratory Physiology

The primary function of the respiratory system is gas exchange, specifically the diffusion of CO_2 and O_2 across the alveolar-capillary membrane. Ventilatory mechanics and the anatomy of the respiratory system, including airways, pulmonary vasculature, and respiratory muscles, are specifically designed to support this function and to optimize delivery of air to the gas exchange regions of the lung. This is particularly important in the adult horse. As an athletic species, horses have relatively higher mass-specific O_2 consumption (Katz et al. 2000). At rest, minute ventilation is approximately 60–70 l/min corresponding to a minimum of 2 l/min of O_2 consumed and 1.7 l/min of CO_2 production. With strenuous exercise minute ventilation can increase 10-fold (Hornicke et al. 1987; Art et al. 1990; Connally and Derksen 1994).

The generation of respiratory drive and the control of breathing are primarily under central control with modulation from the cortex, central and peripheral chemoreceptors, and peripheral mechanoreceptors in response to changes in pH, $PaCO_2$, and PaO_2, respiratory disease, or other stimuli (Cunningham et al. 1986; Hazari and Farraj 2015). Neuronal networks within the brainstem provide central control of breathing and include the ventral and dorsal respiratory centers, central pattern generator, and pre-Bötzinger complex within the medulla and the pneumotactic and apneustic centers within the pons (Garcia et al. 2011; Feldman et al. 2013; Hazari and Farraj 2015; Guyenet and Bayliss 2015; Del Negro et al. 2018; Hines 2018; Beyeler et al. 2020). These centers, particularly those in the medulla, control inspiratory drive and establish the basic rhythm of breathing as well as the volume and rate of respiration (Feldman et al. 2003; Feldman et al. 2013;

Hazari and Farraj 2015). Rate and depth of respiration during automatic breathing are controlled via efferent output from the medullary respiratory center to the muscles of respiration including the diaphragm, as well as intercostal and abdominal muscles (Feldman et al. 2013; Hazari and Farraj 2015). In awake adult horses, inspiration and expiration are biphasic with each having active and passive phases (Koterba et al. 1988; Koterba et al. 1995).

Modification of depth and rate of respiration in response to hypercapnia and hypoxemia are mediated by sensory afferent signals from central and peripheral sites delivered to the respiratory center (Feldman et al. 2013; Guyenet and Bayliss 2015; Prabhakar and Peng 2017; Beyeler et al. 2020). Increases in $PaCO_2$ represent a primary stimulus for breathing. The central chemoreceptors within the ventral medulla are the most responsive to changes in $PaCO_2$ (Hazari and Farraj 2015; Guyenet and Bayliss 2015; Beyeler et al. 2020). These receptors detect decreases in CSF and interstitial fluid pH that are consistent with increased $PaCO_2$ and signal to the respiratory center to increase alveolar ventilation via increased inspiratory and expiratory muscle activity (Hazari and Farraj 2015; Guyenet and Bayliss 2015). Peripheral chemoreceptors include the carotid and aortic bodies which detect changes in both $PaCO_2$ and PaO_2. These receptors are most sensitive to changes in PaO_2, mediating the hypoxic ventilatory drive, but will also trigger centrally mediated increases in alveolar ventilation in response to changes in pH associated with metabolic acidosis (Hazari and Farraj 2015; Prabhakar and Peng 2017).

Additional sensory input to the respiratory centers comes from peripheral receptors located throughout the upper and lower respiratory tract and pulmonary tissue. Pulmonary slow adapting stretch receptors located in the walls of the bronchi and bronchioles help regulate the onset and termination of inspiration and the *Hering-Breuer Reflex* in response to increases in lung volume (Coleridge and Coleridge 1986; Widdicombe 2006; Dempsey and Smith 2014; Hazari and Farraj 2015; Hines 2018). Rapidly adapting stretch (irritant) receptors are also found throughout the airways. These receptors play a minor role in modifying respiration in healthy animals but respond to mechanical and irritant stimuli from endogenous and exogenous sources (Hazari and Farraj 2015). In the upper airway, these receptors help modulate ventilation in response to pressure changes associated with airway obstruction. Stimulation of receptors in the lower airway may modify ventilation, induce bronchoconstriction, and other inflammatory responses in association with respiratory disease (Canning et al. 2006; West 2011; Hines 2018). C-fiber receptors, when stimulated, also trigger alterations in ventilatory pattern, bronchoconstriction, and other inflammatory responses. These receptors are found within the pulmonary tissue and are stimulated in conditions of lung hyperinflation, edema, or inflammation (Hazari and Farraj 2015). Finally, carotid sinus or aortic arch baroreceptor stimulation results in hyperventilation in response to hypotension as part of the baroreceptor reflex (Hazari and Farraj 2015).

The lungs of the horse are divided into the left cranial and caudal lobe and right cranial, intermediate, and caudal lobe. Horse's lungs are poorly lobated and have incompletely developed interlobular connective tissue septa. Despite this, collateral (interlobular) ventilation is almost completely absent and, as a result, horses are less tolerant of obstructive lung disease (Robinson and Sorenson 1978). Anatomically, airway division within the lung of the horses follows the same general pattern as other species with some distinctions. The relatively straight division of right bronchus off the trachea may predispose horses to right-sided pulmonary disease (Ainsworth and Hackett 2004) and respiratory bronchioles are poorly developed, delegating the majority of gas exchange to the alveolar-capillary unit (McLaughlin et al. 1961; Tyler et al. 1971;

Ainsworth and Hackett 2004). Similar to other athletic species, alveolar surface density is quite large in the equine lung with over 10 million alveoli and an even greater number of associated capillaries within the alveolar-capillary network (Gehr et al. 1981).

Pulmonary circulation is the predominate source of blood flow to the lung, receiving approximately 99% of cardiac output. Its primary role is delivering blood to the alveolar-capillary network for gas exchange. In the standing horse a vertical perfusion gradient exists with blood flow favoring the ventral lung relative to the dorsal lung. Bronchial circulation accounts for only 1–2% of cardiac output and is responsible for providing O_2 and nutrients to the airways and other lung structures and contributing to thermoregulation. Pulmonary lymphatic drainage is via deep and superficial lymphatics found in close approximation to the airways and in the visceral pleura, respectively (Breeze and Turk 1984).

Bronchial smooth muscle activity is integral to bronchoconstriction and bronchodilation and is under control of the autonomic nervous system. Changes in airway diameter influence airway resistance and subsequently airflow to the lung. Parasympathetic input mediates smooth muscle contraction primarily via acetylcholine stimulation of M2 and M3 muscarinic receptors and resultant increases in intracellular Ca^{2+} concentration. In contrast, sympathetic input mediates bronchial smooth muscle relaxation primarily via stimulation of β_2-agonist receptors found in airway smooth muscle and subsequent cAMP mediated decreases in intracellular Ca^{2+}. Other important functions under influence of the autonomic nervous system include secretion of tracheobronchial mucus, fluid transport and blood flow, immunologic regulation, and interaction with the central respiratory control networks.

The mucosal lining of the trachea and bronchi consists primarily of tall columnar pseudostratified ciliated epithelium with lesser numbers of serous and goblet cells (Lopez 2001). Goblet cells and submucosal mucous glands are responsible for the production of the mucus layer. This mucus hydrates the tracheobronchial epithelial layer and is an essential component of the mucociliary apparatus involved in defense against respiratory pathogens. Immunoglobulins (IgA and IgG) as well as other immunomodulatory proteins are found in tracheal secretions.

Within the bronchioles and terminal bronchioles, goblet cells and ciliated cells are gradually replaced by Clara cells which predominate within the epithelium (Lopez 2001). Clara cells produce the pulmonary epithelial lining fluid throughout this region of the lung. Cartilage within airway walls is also gradually lost (Lopez 2001) and can increase the risk of collapse of peripheral airways especially under conditions of forced expiration, such as in equine asthma.

Within the alveoli, alveolar type I and type II pneumocytes predominate. Type I pneumocytes are the larger and more common cell type and are responsible for gas exchange. Although large, these cells form a very thin barrier (0.2–0.5 μm) with the capillary endothelium (Breeze and Turk 1984; West 2011). Type II pneumocytes are responsible for the production of surfactant and the replacement of damaged Type I pneumocytes. Pulmonary surfactant is comprised of 80–85% phospholipids and is essential for decreasing alveolar surface tension, providing alveolar stability, and maintaining gas exchange. The phospholipids within surfactant also have important immunologic functions (Christmann et al. 2006; Christmann et al. 2009). Thus, surfactant deficiency or loss of components can result in atelectasis, edema, and impaired pulmonary immunity.

In addition to the mucociliary apparatus, other essential immunologic defenses within the lung include bronchus associated lymphatic tissue (BALT) and alveolar macrophages. BALT represents a network of lymphoid tissue tract that protects the respiratory tract from invading pathogens and supports alveolar macrophage function. Alveolar macrophages represent the most important component of pulmonary immunologic defense and are the predominant cell found within the alveolar lining fluid. Alveolar macrophages are the first line of defense against pathogens reaching the lower airways, possessing phagocytic, antigen presenting, and microbicidal properties. Important threats to their function include hypoxia, glucocorticoids (endogenous and exogenous), and viral infections (equine influenza virus [EIV], equine herpes virus).

General Considerations for Anesthesia of Horses with Inflammatory/Infection Respiratory Disease

Pre-anesthetic Evaluation

Pre-anesthetic evaluation of horses with respiratory disease should begin with a standard physical examination and progress to more advanced diagnostics as warranted. Gathered information will provide a baseline for future comparison as well as guide anesthetic and therapeutic decision-making. If the horse is suspected to have respiratory disease, viewing the horse at rest may give indication of severity. Changes in rate and character of ventilatory efforts may be seen as well as phenotypic changes, such as a "heaves line" that may indicate chronicity. Additional focus on the respiratory tract should include auscultation of all lung field as well as the cervical portion of the trachea noting the location and character of unusual findings. Use of a rebreathing technique (bag) may further amplify lung sounds and facilitate finding abnormalities, particularly in horses with a thick chest wall. Simply, a large plastic trash bag is fitted securely around the horse's muzzle and as the horse continues to breath, increased CO_2 rebreathing will result in subsequent breaths with a larger tidal volume and effort. The phase of ventilation (inspiratory versus expiratory) and the

presence of stertor, stridor, crackles, wheezes, or rhonchi, or the absence of normal sounds, can help differentiate upper versus lower airway disease and help with further focused examination. Complete blood count with fibrinogen may be useful for identification of inflammatory conditions and arterial blood gas analysis can be particularly useful for characterizing conditions in which alveolar gas diffusion or ventilation are affected. Diagnostic imaging including thoracic, cervical, and head radiographs and thoracic ultrasonography are particularly useful for localizing disease to anatomical locations and for sample collection (i.e. thoracocentesis). Findings from upper airway endoscopy, including the guttural pouches, and bronchoalveolar lavage for cytology and tracheal aspirates for microbe culture, may further clarify upper versus lower airway conditions as well as help differentiate inflammatory and infectious diseases.

Anesthetic, Analgesic, and Adjunctive Drugs

Many of the anesthetic and analgesic medications commonly used in the anesthetic care of horses have some effect on the respiratory system. These effects can occur either locally in the respiratory tree or in lungs, systemically in the pulmonary or cardiovascular systems, or centrally in the higher centers of the central nervous system (CNS). Knowledge of the interplay between utilized drugs and the respiratory system can help identify potential adverse events that may arise in horses with specific respiratory system conditions. Drugs that may be utilized in the peri-anesthetic period in horses that may affect the respiratory system include anticholinergics, α_2-adrenergic receptor agonists, phenothiazines, opioids, benzodiazepines, guaifenesin, dissociatives, barbiturates, propofol, alfaxalone, and volatile anesthetics.

Anticholinergics
Anticholinergic drugs used in veterinary anesthesia consist mainly of atropine and glycopyrrolate and exert their action through

antagonism of postganglionic muscarinic cholinergic receptors of the parasympathetic nervous system. Although not routinely used in the anesthesia of horses, the effects of this class of drugs on the respiratory system has been documented. Atropine has been used in the treatment of disorders of bronchoconstriction in the equine lung and has been shown to completely inhibit neurogenic contraction of previously contracted bronchi (Menozzi et al. 2014). Thus, atropine may be a beneficial treatment for horses where bronchoconstriction is impacting airway gas flow. However, due to the potential for adverse events (ileus, CNS toxicity, tachycardia, increased viscosity of mucous secretion, and impaired mucociliary clearance), atropine is recommended to be limited to a single rescue therapy dose for bronchodilation (Rush and Mair 2004). In anesthetized horses, bronchodilation of poorly perfused lung from anticholinergic administration may increase dead space ventilation and reduce arterial oxygen tension offsetting the benefit of bronchodilation (Lerche 2015).

α_2-Adrenergic Receptor Agonists

Xylazine is one of the most common sedative agents used in equine anesthesia; however, other α_2-adrenergic receptor agonists (detomidine, romifidine, and dexmedetomidine) are used for sedation, analgesia, and balanced anesthesia in horses. The popularity of this class of drugs is owed to the relatively rapid and reliable sedation associated with their use. However, this class of agents can have profound effects on the respiratory system. Of primary concern is the impairment of pulmonary gas exchange that can result in significant decreases of arterial oxygen and increases of arterial carbon dioxide tensions (Freeman et al. 2000; Nyman et al. 2009). This occurs from an increase in pulmonary vascular resistance and a resulting ventilation/perfusion mismatching. Xylazine, and likely other α_2-adrenergic receptor agonists, decrease respiratory rate, minute ventilation, and peak airflows after administration in horses (Raidal

et al. 2017). Administration of α_2-adrenergic receptor agonists increases upper airway resistance and increases work of breathing in horses (Tomasic et al. 1997). This may be related to decreased muscle tone and collapse of the nasopharynx and oropharynx as nasotracheal or endotracheal intubation returns work of breathing to baseline effort.

Phenothiazines

Acepromazine is a widely used sedative and essentially the only agent in the class of drugs that is regularly used in equine patients. Acepromazine has minimal effects on the respiratory system when used at clinically relevant doses (Steffey et al. 1985; Raidal et al. 2017). In fact, in horses experiencing pulmonary ventilation/perfusion mismatch after sedation with an α_2-adrenergic receptor agonists, administration of acepromazine may reduce the fall in arterial oxygen tension (Marntell et al. 2005). This is thought to occur due to the ability of acepromazine to counteract the vasoconstrictive effects of the α_2-adrenergic receptor agonists through blockade of vascular α_1-adrenergic receptors. Acepromazine appears to have no effect on bronchial diameter but can cause pronounced muscle relaxation which may be problematic in horses with respiratory muscle fatigue.

Opioids

The use of opioids in horses, particularly full μ-agonists, continues to be debated due to questions on analgesic efficacy. However, the respiratory depressant effects of opioids are well recognized in veterinary species. In awake horses, the respiratory depression associated with opioids is generally not problematic and usually does not require intervention (Muir et al. 1978; Robertson et al. 1981). However, in anesthetized animals, respiratory depression manifests as decreased minute ventilation with a concomitant rise in arterial carbon dioxide tension. Subsequently, arterial pH drops below optimal and acidemia ensues. At lower doses of opioids, the respiratory rhythm is disturbed, characterized as a slower rate and increased inspiratory periods. As opioid doses increase, tidal volume becomes reduced due to decreased inputs from opioid sensitive chemoreceptors. Interestingly, this respiratory pattern has been described as "quantal" due to the nature in which action potentials are not transmitter further in the respiratory centers similar to Mobitz type-II second-degree heart block (Pattinson 2008). The effects of opioids on the respiratory system are not limited to central control of ventilation. Opioids can exert effects locally on the lungs including generation of pulmonary edema through endothelial dysfunction, dose-related bronchoconstriction, and immunosuppression of host cellular and innate defenses (Yamanaka and Sadikot 2013).

Benzodiazepines

Benzodiazepines are frequently used in the anesthesia of horse for combination with other medications for muscle relaxing effects. On their own, benzodiazepines, at clinically relevant doses, have negligible effects on the respiratory system.

Guaifenesin

Similar to benzodiazepines, guaifenesin is used in combination with other anesthetic drugs to provide muscle relaxation. Useful for total intravenous anesthesia with ketamine and xylazine, respiratory depression from this combination can occur resulting in hypoventilation and hypoxemia (Greene et al. 1986).

Dissociatives

Ketamine is one of the most commonly used anesthetic induction agents and intravenous maintenance agents in horses. It is also used as an anesthetic adjunctive agent during inhalant anesthesia either as bolus injections or a continuous infusion. Thus, the effects of this class of drugs on the equine respiratory system have been studied. In general ketamine does not cause respiratory depression, in fact, appropriate responses to hypoxemia and increased carbon dioxide are maintained during ketamine anesthesia (Soliman et al. 1975). However, respiratory patterns do change after ketamine administration and are frequently described as an "apneustic" pattern. This is characterized as a breath-holding pattern during inspiration and a relatively quick expiration immediately followed by a prolonged inspiration again (Jaspar et al. 1983). Ketamine has also been shown to be a potent bronchodilator. The use of ketamine in patients with status asthmaticus showed improved outcomes in patients with asthma unresponsive to conventional treatments (Goyal and Agrawal 2013). Ketamine may be a preferred agent in horses with bronchial obstructive diseases such as equine asthma.

Barbiturates

Barbiturates have been utilized as anesthesia induction and maintenance agents for veterinary patients since at least the 1940s and thiopental is probably the more favored barbiturate agent for equine induction. In general, barbiturates can have profound dose-dependent depressant effects on the respiratory system. Direct depression of the ventilatory centers occur after administration and animals have decreased responsiveness to both hypoxemia and hypercapnia (Tyagi et al. 1964; Hirshman et al. 1975; Quandt et al. 1998).

Propofol

Propofol as a sole induction agent in adult and/or large horses is problematic due to the large volumes necessary; however, it can be useful in smaller horses and foals and when combined with other agents such as ketamine (Mama et al. 1995). The effects of propofol on the respiratory system are very similar to the barbiturates in that direct respiratory depression occurs as well as sensitivity to changes in arterial oxygen and carbon dioxide tensions. These effects appear to be both dose and rate of administration dependent. Decreases in tidal volume and respiratory rate can be expected and supplemental oxygen and ventilatory support should be made available when propofol is used (Mama et al. 1995; Quandt et al. 1998).

Alfaxalone

Alfaxalone is one of the newest induction agents available in veterinary medicine, and limited comparative data is available with regard to its use in horses. The depressant effects of alfaxalone on the respiratory system are expected to be similar to or slightly less than propofol. When using alfaxalone in horses, there should be an expectation of clinically relevant respiratory depression, and options for ventilatory support should be available (Ohmura et al. 2016).

Volatile Anesthetics

Clinically useful volatile anesthetics in veterinary medicine include isoflurane and sevoflurane with halothane continuing to be utilized in some countries. Volatile anesthetics have various effects on the respiratory system that are widely considered dose dependent and to some degree, species dependent. Horses in particular can have profound changes in respiratory physiology and function related to volatile anesthetic exposure due to the complex nature and anatomy of the equine lung and recumbency during anesthesia (Auckburally and Nyman 2017). As dose of volatile anesthetics are increased (i.e. increased minimum alveolar concentration or MAC), respiratory rate and tidal volume decrease to the point where ventilation ceases and death ensues without intervention. Additionally, central and peripheral chemoreceptors become less sensitive to carbon dioxide tension further decreasing the drive to ventilate. Hypoxic pulmonary vasoconstriction is an important component to maintaining ventilation/perfusion matching in the equine lung. All modern volatile anesthetics inhibit hypoxic pulmonary vasoconstriction in a dose-dependent manner (Lumb and Slinger 2015). This can lead to a significant amount of blood perfusion to underventilated lung. Blood flow returning to the pulmonary circulation from this area has not had the opportunity to become oxygenated and, when combining with oxygenated blood, can result in a hypoxic mixture. Horses tend to suffer from hypoxemia during anesthesia at a higher rate than most veterinary species, and techniques that reduce the amount of inhalant anesthetic utilized may improve oxygenation (Auckburally and Nyman 2017). Interestingly, injectable anesthetics do not appear to affect hypoxic pulmonary vasoconstriction (Lumb and Slinger 2015).

Monitoring and Support During Anesthesia

General considerations for vital signs monitoring and support of anesthetized horses can be found elsewhere but should be in place as a starting point when anesthetizing horses with respiratory diseases. Horses with specific respiratory tract conditions (discussed blow) may require more intensive monitoring and support of gas exchange and diffusion or ventilation of alveoli. In general, upper airway diseases and conditions are more commonly associated with obstruction of airflow while lower airway diseases and conditions are more commonly associated with impaired gas exchange and diffusion. Airway management for upper airway conditions is focused on minimizing resistance to airflow and may include alternatives to orotracheal intubation including nasotracheal intubation or intubation though a tracheotomy (Figure 3.1). Management for lower airway conditions may include application of specific ventilator strategies or use of aerosolized medications to improve oxygenation.

Use of pulse oximetry, capnography, and arterial blood gas analysis can be useful to determine when intervention is necessary and how effective intervention strategies are. Pulse oximetry can be helpful for determining oxygen content in the arterial blood of a horse before, during, and after anesthesia (recovery) and can be used to indicate need for supplemental oxygen. Caution must be used when interpreting a pulse oximeter reading as skin thickness and pigmentation in horse skin may interfere with the reading. An arterial blood gas may be necessary for verification. Placement of an arterial

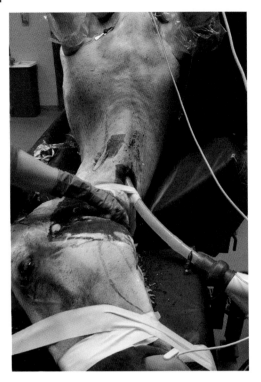

Figure 3.1 Intubation of an anesthetized horse through a tracheotomy due to inability to pass an orotracheal tube. The horse is being prepared for surgical drainage of the guttural pouch.

catheter for direct blood pressure measurements facilitates collection of arterial blood for gas analysis. However, it is frequently not practical to place the catheter in an awake horse; therefore, direct puncture of an artery may be necessary for sample collection. Sites for sample collection in the awake horse include the various branched of the facial artery with the branch palpated just caudal and ventral to the ventral aspect of the rim of the orbit being most convenient. Arterial blood gas analysis for PaO_2 and $PaCO_2$ are the most important variable for assessing respiratory function. Venous blood gas analysis may be useful for P_vO_2 and lactate concentrations and can be acquired from the jugular vein or transverse facial venous sinus (Lascola et al. 2017). Respiratory function can also be monitored with capnometry. Sampling of airway gases during anesthesia can provide graphical representation of CO_2 during inspiration and expiration. This graph (capnography) can be analyzed for airway status and spontaneous or mechanical ventilatory function. Real-time information on airway obstruction, hypoventilation, hyperventilation, rebreathing, and anesthesia breathing circuit integrity are some examples of available information. Other methods of respiratory and ventilatory monitoring of horses include spirometry and electrical impedance tomography, although this technology may not be practical for routine clinical use (Moens 2013; Auer et al. 2019). Detailed review information on respiratory monitoring in anesthetized horses can be found in previous publications (Hubbell and Muir 2009; Moens 2013). Additionally, information on the use and interpretation of capnography can be found at www.capnograph.com.

During the induction process, an amount of time will elapse between a horse becoming recumbent and intubation and initiation of oxygen and inhalant administration from an anesthesia machine. During this period, secondary to recumbency and the effect of anesthetic drugs, a decrease in PaO_2 may occur (van Oostrom et al. 2015). In horses with respiratory diseases that are associated with hypoxemia, a decrease in PaO_2 during induction may result in a critical hypoxemia that could affect health status. Placement of an intranasal cannula to the level of the medial canthus of the eye and provision of oxygen at 15 l/min for 3 minutes prior to induction may maintain PaO_2 above concentrations considered to indicate hypoxemia (van Oostrom et al. 2015). This may allow for a safer transition of horses from induction to maintenance with inhalant delivered in oxygen.

Mechanical ventilation (intermittent positive pressure ventilation) is frequently required for anesthetized adult horses. Moreover, horses with respiratory diseases, particularly diseases of the lower respiratory tract, may benefit from mechanical ventilation initiated shortly after induction. In fact, horses that are placed on mechanical ventilation immediately after induction of anesthesia maintain more normal

Figure 3.2 A wye piece with a fitting for administration of albuterol into the anesthetic breathing circuit.

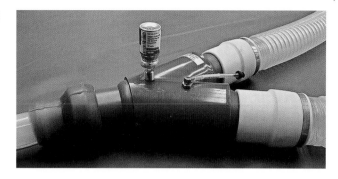

$PaCO_2$, pH, and PaO_2 compared to spontaneously breathing horses or those that are allowed to initially spontaneously breathe and then be subsequently mechanically ventilated (Day et al. 1995; Kerr and McDonell 2009). Ventilation techniques for improvement in ventilatory variables, particularly PaO_2, are widely reported and include the use of continuous positive airway pressure (CPAP), recruitment maneuvers, and use of various amounts of positive end-expiratory pressure (PEEP) (Hopster et al. 2011; Mosing et al. 2013; Andrade et al. 2019). Description and direction on the use of each ventilatory technique is beyond the scope of this chapter, and the reader is directed to the references for further reading.

Beyond mechanical ventilation, inhaled medications may be useful for improving PaO_2 in anesthetized horses. In hypoxemic horses, albuterol ($2\,\mu g/kg$) administered via inhalation can increase PaO_2 (Robertson and Bailey 2002). Administration of each actuation or "puff" must coincide with the beginning of the inhalation cycle of mechanical ventilation or a spontaneous breath and adaptation of a wye piece with a port facilitates administration (Figure 3.2). The improvement of PaO_2 may be the result of bronchodilation and improved aeration of alveoli or increased cardiac output to ventilated lung. Pulsed administration of inhaled nitric oxide can similarly improve PaO_2 in anesthetized horses. Although specialized equipment is necessary to administer nitric oxide into a breathing circuit, PaO_2 increases via reduction in the amount of blood shunted away from ventilated alveoli thus increasing the amount of blood available for gas exchange (Wiklund et al. 2020).

Recovery

The recovery period has the potential to be one of the most complicated areas of anesthesia of horses with respiratory diseases. Once placed in a recovery box, respiratory support and monitoring become challenging. The goal for recovery is a move to a standing position that is free from excitement and delirium which may exacerbate respiratory compromise. While continuation of mechanical ventilation is not feasible, assisted ventilation with a demand valve prior to extubation can provide continued oxygen support (Figure 3.3). Once extubated, nasal insufflation with

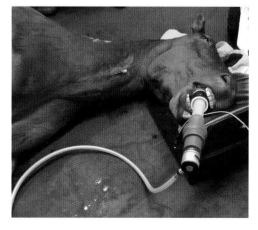

Figure 3.3 Use of a demand valve to support ventilation of a horse in a recovery stall.

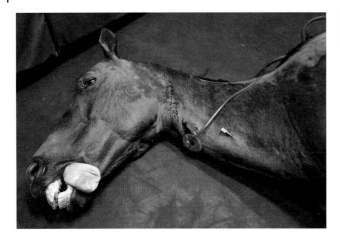

Figure 3.4 Insufflation of oxygen though a self-retaining tracheostomy in a horse recovering from anesthesia.

oxygen (15 l/min) can be utilized for oxygen support. For horses with a tracheostomy, a self-retaining tracheotomy can be placed and an oxygen line can be inserted through it directly into the trachea (Figure 3.4). Acepromazine can be used to reduce anxiety during recovery and improve arterial oxygenation (Marntell et al. 2005). If alpha-2 agonist drugs are used for sedation during recovery, the addition of acepromazine may counteract the vascular effect that can exacerbate ventilation to perfusion mismatching associated with alpha-2 agonists (Marntell and Nyman 1996; Nyman et al. 2009).

Anesthetic Consideration of Horses with Specific Infectious or Inflammatory Diseases of the Upper Respiratory System

While information on the pathophysiology and treatment of inflammatory and infectious diseases are well known, there is minimal published research data on anesthetic techniques for horses with respiratory diseases. Much of the information in this chapter regarding anesthetic techniques is derived from data in other species including humans, and clinical experience and anecdotal information from the veterinary anesthesia community.

Streptococcus equi subsp. *equi* (Equine Strangles)

Streptococcus equi subsp. *equi* (Equine Strangles) is one of the most common infectious upper respiratory tract diseases in horses and is reportable within the United States. *S. equi* is a gram-positive β-hemolytic coccoid bacterium and, unlike *S. equi* subsp. *zooepidemicus*, is a primary pathogen in horses, donkeys, and mules. Clinical disease is most common in horses one to six years of age, but can also develop in older horses and foals (Duffee et al. 2015). *S. equi* is highly infectious with morbidity reaching 100% in naïve horses. Following infection, protective immunity develops in approximately 75% of horses and persists for approximately five years (Hamlen et al. 1994; Boyle et al. 2018).

Transmission of *S. equi* is via direct contact with infected horses or contaminated fomites. Horses with obvious signs of clinical disease, asymptomatic carriers, and horses recovering from infection but no longer demonstrating clinical signs all contribute to disease outbreaks and persistence of the organism within a population. Chronic carriers continue to shed *S. equi* for more than six weeks and sometimes for months-to-years after infection (Mallicote 2015). Carrier prevalence has been reported to be between 10% and 40% in naturally infected horses (Newton et al. 2000;

Duffee et al. 2015; Boyle et al. 2018). In a recent report (Duffee et al. 2015), approximately 30% of horses diagnosed with strangles via upper airway endoscopy did not present with typical clinical signs of disease suggesting that acutely infected horses may also serve as silent shedders.

The pathogenesis of strangles has been well described (Timoney and Kumar 2008; Waller 2014; Mallicote 2015; Boyle et al. 2018). Bacteria gain entry to the upper respiratory tract primarily via inhalation, adhere to the mucosal surface of pharyngeal tonsillar tissue, rapidly translocate to deeper tonsillar tissues, and subsequently colonize regional lymph nodes within a few hours of infection. Bacterial replication and neutrophil influx with subsequent lymphadenopathy and abscessation characterize clinical strangles. Spread of *S. equi* beyond the upper respiratory via lymphatic or hematogenous routes is responsible for metastatic strangles and abscess formation elsewhere in the body (Mallicote 2015; Boyle et al. 2018). Bacterial virulence factors contribute to *S. equi* pathogenicity and evasion of host defenses. These factors include surface proteins such as the *Strep equi* M-like (SeM) protein, antiphagocytic proteins, and several bacterial toxins (Timoney et al. 2014; Boyle et al. 2018). The SeM protein not only plays a central role in virulence but the identification of SeM protein DNA or antibodies is also used to diagnose strangles.

Potential complications associated with *S. equi* infection are numerous. The most frequently reported include airway obstruction, guttural pouch empyema and chondroid formation, metastatic abscesses, and the immunologic sequelae of purpura hemorrhagica and *S. equi*–associated myositis (Mallicote 2015; Boyle et al. 2018). Airway obstruction most often occurs with pharyngeal compression secondary to lymphadenopathy and abscessation of the retropharyngeal lymph nodes. Tracheal compression from abscesses located in the cranial mediastinum or at the thoracic inlet has been reported more rarely. Metastatic *S. equi* can involve lymph nodes and organ systems throughout the body including the CNS, abdomen, lungs, and other thoracic cavity structures (Duffee et al. 2015; Boyle et al. 2018).

Empyema of the guttural pouch is caused by accumulation within the pouch of purulent material, debris, and exudate associated with bacterial infection (Judy et al. 1999; Freeman 2015). Strangles represents the most significant cause of empyema and involves rupture and drainage of a retropharyngeal lymph node abscess into the floor of the pouch. Less common causes of empyema include other bacterial infections of the upper respiratory tract (especially *S. equi* subsp. *zooepidemicus*), and, more rarely, trauma, stenosis of the pharyngeal orifice, or infusion of irritating substances into the pouch (Freeman 2015). In horses with strangles, empyema is typically bilateral, with unilateral disease more common with other causes (Sweeney et al. 1987; Pascoe 2019). Purulent material can become inspissated resulting in chondroid formation and the development of a *S. equi* carrier state in horses with chronic empyema.

Characteristic signs of strangles become evident 2–14 days after infection and include pyrexia ($\geq$103 °F), lethargy, serous progressing to mucopurulent nasal discharge, and lymphadenopathy with lymph node abscessation of the submandibular and/or retropharyngeal lymph nodes (Boyle et al. 2018). Pyrexia, usually the first clinical sign noted, may not always be identified in horses with clinical strangles (Duffee et al. 2015). In most horses, bacterial shedding begins within 2–3 days of fever and continues for a minimum of 2 weeks. Maturation and rupture of abscesses occurs in 7–14 days after the onset of clinical signs. Specific signs associated with metastatic strangles typically correspond to the organ system involved. Clinical presentation suggesting empyema include mucopurulent nasal discharge that is most prominent with the head lowered, swelling over the parotid region, cough, upper respiratory noise, and occasionally dyspnea (Judy et al. 1999). Inflammation or irritation of the cranial nerves within the guttural pouches may also cause dysphagia or other neuropathies.

Because of the highly infectious nature of *S equi*, timely and accurate diagnosis of strangles is critical. Horses with confirmed or suspected *S. equi* infection should be isolated and placed under strict biosecurity protocols until cleared of infection. In many states, diagnostic protocols and quarantine regulations are under the direction of the state veterinarian. In animals with overt clinical signs, direct sampling and culture of abscess or purulent exudate is ideal but not always possible. Culture or polymerase chain reaction (PCR) to detect SeM protein DNA can also be performed on guttural pouch (preferred) or nasopharyngeal washes. Serologic testing of SeM antibodies can be useful in horses suspected of complications associated with *S. equi* infection (Boyle et al. 2009). Hematologic findings are typically nonspecific and indicative of an inflammatory process. Endoscopic evaluation of the upper airways and guttural pouches is useful for evaluating horses with strangles, and can provide a definitive diagnosis when guttural pouch empyema is suspected. Both pouches should be evaluated, especially in horses with confirmed or suspected equine strangles infection. Exudate should be collected and submitted for microbial culture and

PCR testing. Radiography can be useful to identify fluid lines within the pouches when endoscopy is not available (Figure 3.5). Additional diagnostics such as ultrasound, or other advanced imaging, may be warranted in horses with metastatic strangles, depending on body systems involved.

Treatment of horses with strangles depends on the stage and manifestation of disease. In horses with uncomplicated strangles, treatment is primarily supportive and the prognosis for full recovery is generally very good. Administration of antimicrobials remains controversial as it may prolong the course of disease or interfere with the development of lasting immunity. For this reason, antimicrobial use is generally restricted to treating horses with complications associated with *S. equi* infection such as dyspnea or significant systemic inflammation, and when metastatic strangles, purpura hemorrhagica, or *S. equi* associated myositis are identified. Horses with dyspnea associated with pharyngeal compression may require tracheostomy and in rare cases, intensive supportive care (intravenous fluids, placement of indwelling feeding tube, antimicrobial drugs) is warranted. Surgical removal or drainage of abscesses may be performed in horses with metastatic strangles.

In horses with guttural pouch empyema, specific medical management involves removal

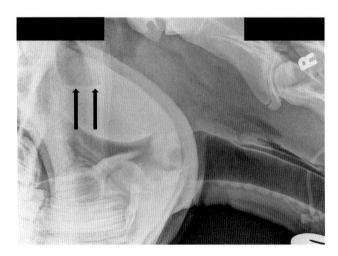

Figure 3.5 A lateral radiograph of a horse with guttural pouch empyema. The black arrows indicate a fluid line in the guttural pouch.

of exudate through repeated guttural pouch lavage using polyionic or other non-irritating solution. Endoscopic guided removal of chondroids can be attempted (Freeman and Hardy 2012). Surgical drainage of affected pouches is reserved for severe or chronic cases nonresponsive to lavage, cases with numerous chondroids, or cases where stenosis of the pharyngeal orifice is identified (Freeman 2015). Local or systemic antimicrobial therapy is controversial, especially in horses with strangles (Boyle et al. 2018), but may be useful in select cases with accompanying microbial culture. Additional therapy may be needed in horses with dysphagia, or other neurologic deficits.

Anesthetic Considerations

The vast majority of horses with strangles will not require surgical intervention, thus anesthesia is usually not necessary. However, horses with certain complications previously described may require anesthesia or sedation for tracheostomy or surgical approach and drainage of internal abscesses. When formulating an anesthetic plan, minimization of contamination of equipment and surrounding spaces is paramount to prevent infection of subsequently anesthetized horses. Use of personal protective equipment including face-masks and gloves should be routine as *Streptococcus equi* subsp. e*qui* has the potential for zoonotic infection (Baracco 2019). Biosecurity includes isolation of infected or suspected infected horses, use of footbaths and protective clothing and deep cleaning any area that may have had exposure. *Streptococcus equi* subsp. *equi* is susceptible to most standard disinfectants (diluted bleach or quaternary ammonium compounds); however all organic debris must be diligently removed as bacteria can survive for as long as three days (Mallicote 2015).

For surgical removal of chondroids or drainage of guttural pouch empyema, surgery can be performed in the standing horse facilitated by sedation and local anesthesia (Perkins et al. 2006). Sedation can be performed with xylazine or detomidine with butorphanol added for additional analgesia/sedation. After preparing the area for surgery, 20–30 ml of local anesthetic can be infused directly into the tissue, and an approach can be made via the modified Whitehouse approach to the guttural pouch. For deeper abscess in other areas of the body or large numbers of chondroids within the guttural pouches, general anesthesia may be necessary (Furniss et al. 2007).

During recovery of horses that have had diseases of the guttural pouch, neurologic complication such as dysphagia, abnormal soft palate positioning, laryngeal paralysis, and Horner syndrome can occur (Borges and Watanabe 2011). Airway obstruction may occur, and horses should be monitored closely as re-intubation or tracheostomy may be required to re-establish patency.

Disorders of the Guttural Pouch

Guttural Pouch Anatomy

The guttural pouches are anatomical structures that are unique to equids and a few other species and whose exact function is unknown (Baptiste et al. 2000). They represent paired diverticula of the auditory tubes that are located anatomically in the retropharyngeal space and that communicate with the pharynx through slit-like openings (Freeman and Hardy 2012; Pascoe 2019). Each pouch has a capacity of approximately 300 ml in the adult horse, but can distend to accommodate larger volumes of air or fluid. Each guttural pouch is divided into a larger medial and smaller lateral compartment by the stylohyoid bone. The mucosal lining consists of ciliated pseudostratified epithelium, goblet cells, and subepithelial aggregates of lymphocytic tissue. Several important structures within or in close proximation to the guttural pouch can become damaged in infectious or inflammatory conditions such as guttural pouch empyema or mycosis. Within the medial compartment, neural and vascular structures include cranial nerves IX, X, XI, XII, the cranial cervical ganglion, the cervical sympathetic trunk, and internal carotid artery. The pharyngeal branch of the vagus (CN X), the cranial laryngeal nerve, and the retropharyngeal lymph nodes are found ventral to the floor of the medial compartment. Within the lateral compartment neural and vascular structures include the facial (CN VII) and chorda tympani nerves, branches of the mandibular nerve, the external carotid and maxillary arteries, and the maxillary vein. The most significant medical disorders of the guttural pouches include guttural pouch empyema (see Section on Equine Strangles) and guttural pouch mycosis.

Guttural Pouch Mycosis

Pathophysiology Guttural pouch mycosis is defined as fungal invasion of the mucosal lining within one or both guttural pouches (Freeman 2015; Pascoe 2019). While epistaxis represents the most common clinical sign associated with this condition (Freeman 2015), the clinical manifestation of this condition varies among affected horses depending on the severity and location of fungal invasion and the specific involvement of underlying neuro-vascular structures. The etiopathogenesis of guttural pouch mycosis remains incompletely defined (Pascoe 2019). Age, breed, and sex predilections are not recognized among affected horses (Freeman 2015). The condition does appear to be more common in stabled horses residing in the northern hemisphere and during warmer seasons (Freeman 2015). While Aspergillus species (*A. fumigatus, A. nidulans*) are most frequently isolated (Freeman 2015; Pascoe 2019), other fungal species can be identified.

Fungal plaques can develop anywhere within the guttural pouch. One of the more common locations for plaque formation is dorsally in the medial compartment in association with the internal carotid artery (Cook 1968; Freeman 2015; Pascoe 2019). Plaques can involve additional neuro-vascular or other structures anywhere within the guttural pouch such as the maxillary artery, cranial nerves,

muscle, or bone. Fungal plaques attach to the underlying tissue through a diphtheritic membrane within which necrotic tissue and numerous bacterial and fungal organisms can be found (Freeman 2015; Pascoe 2019). These plaques cause significant inflammation, erosion, and necrosis of underlying tissue which can ultimately result in hemorrhage, neuropathy, or other tissue damage (Cook 1968).

Specific clinical signs of guttural pouch mycosis correspond to the location of fungal invasion. Epistaxis is most common (Freeman 2015) and may start as mild and intermittent and progressing over time, or can present acutely with severe-to-fatal hemorrhage. After epistaxis, dysphagia represents the second most common clinical abnormality and develops when there is involvement of cranial nerves IX, X, and XII (Cook 1968; Freeman 2015; Pascoe 2019). Dysphagic horses typically present with nasal discharge that contains feed or saliva and may become mucopurulent. Cough while eating and tongue paralysis may be noted. Other less common clinical presentations associated with cranial nerve neuropathy may include Horner's syndrome, respiratory noise secondary to recurrent laryngeal neuropathy, and signs of facial nerve paralysis (ear droop, muzzle deviation) (Cook 1968; Cook et al. 1968; Freeman and Hardy 2012). Horses may appear painful when palpated over the parotid region and may present with abnormal head posture or demonstrate head or neck extension.

Clinical signs of epistaxis or dysphagia should warrant inclusion of guttural pouch mycosis as a differential. Endoscopy of both guttural pouches is performed to confirm the diagnosis (Lepage and Piccot-Crézollet 2005). Fungal plaques vary in color and may appear as discrete lesions or as diffusely distributed patches (Cook 1968; Cook et al. 1968; Pascoe 2019). Significant hemorrhage or the presence of a large blood clot within the guttural pouch can limit visualization and localization of fungal plaques but can support a presumptive diagnosis. In horses with neuropathy, additional findings may include feed material in nasopharynx or trachea, dorsal displacement of the soft palate, decreased pharyngeal tone, and laryngeal hemiplegia. In horses with a surgical option for treatment, effort should be made to identify the source of hemorrhage as this will impact surgical technique and approach (Freeman and Hardy 2012, Freeman 2015; Pascoe 2019).

The preferred treatment for guttural pouch mycosis is surgical occlusion of the affected artery, and several surgical approaches have been described (Lepage and Piccot-Crézollet 2005; Freeman and Hardy 2012, Freeman 2015; Watkins and Parente 2018). Medical therapy requires systemic and repeated topical antifungal therapy in awake or anesthetized animals (Greet 1987; Dobesova et al. 2012; Pascoe 2019). This approach is time consuming and of variable efficacy and may increase the risk of severe or fatal hemorrhage in some horses. Prognosis for recovery is good with surgical therapy in uncomplicated cases. The presence of dysphagia or other significant neurologic deficits carries guarded prognosis for recovery irrespective of treatment.

Anesthetic Considerations Arterial occlusion has been described in both anesthetized and standing horses. Depending on the extent of the lesion, the common carotid, external carotid, internal carotid, or the maxillary artery, or a combination may require occlusion. Multiple techniques have been described but most require placement of an intra-arterial occlusion plug or device. Risk for general anesthesia is mainly centered on hemorrhage associated with rupture of the affected artery or arteries or reverse flow of blood from the cerebral arterial circle (Colles and Cook 1983; Freeman 2015). In severe cases, whole blood transfusion may be necessary. Aminocaproic acid (30 mg/kg, IV over 15 minutes), an antifibrinolytic drug may be useful to slow breakdown and stabilize formed clots and reduce the chance for further bleeding (Heidmann et al. 2005). The author has administered aminocaproic acid after arterial occlusion and prior to recovery in anesthetized horses. For standing procedures, sedation with a continuous infusion of detomidine or repeated doses of detomidine have been used (Genton et al. 2021). Blood loss in standing procedures appears to be minimal and position of the head may be partially responsible. In anesthetized horses, the head is closer to the level of the heart and results in a greater mean blood pressure in the arteries that are the focus of occlusion than in a standing horse where the vessels are elevated above the heart and have a lower mean blood pressure (Genton et al. 2021). If the surgical procedure is to be performed in a horse under general anesthesia, elevating the head or placing the horse in reverse Trendelenburg position may be advantageous. Deficits in cranial nerves leading to dysphagia and laryngeal paralysis have been reported and horses having either a procedure standing or under general anesthesia should be observed for upper airway respiratory compromise.

Tracheal Disorders and Tracheitis (Viral Diseases)

Pathophysiology

The trachea extends from the larynx to its termination at the carina where it branches into the right and left primary bronchi. Tracheal length varies from 45 to 55 cm in ponies to 70–80 cm in average sized horses (Dixon et al. 2007; Barakzai and Dixon 2019). Tracheal stability and rigidity is achieved through concentric hyaline cartilage rings along the length of the trachea (Pirie et al. 1990). The predominant cell types of the luminal mucous membrane include ciliated pseudostratified columnar epithelial cells, which are most numerous, and goblet cells (Pirie et al. 1990; Dixon 1992; Lopez 2001). Together, these cells play a critical role in mucus production and in forming the mucociliary apparatus that is important in the defense of the lower airways from exposure to inhaled foreign particulates or pathogens.

Disorders of the trachea are rare in horses (Barakzai and Dixon 2019). Trauma (intra- and extra-luminal), neoplasia, and inhaled foreign bodies are occasionally reported, and associated with focal lesions or obstructions. Tracheal collapse or stenosis occurs and can be associated with congenital malformation, degenerative conditions, previous trauma, or secondary to chronic inflammatory disease of the lower respiratory tract (Dixon et al. 2007; Barakzai and Dixon 2019). Primary tracheitis is rare; however, intraluminal inflammation has been reported in association with granulomatous disease and following endotracheal intubation. Damage to the tracheal and bronchial epithelial cells and cilia can also accompany infection with certain respiratory viruses.

Congenital malformation of the trachea, although relatively rare, is most often reported in miniature horses, ponies, and donkeys and frequently involves deformities associated with the cartilaginous tracheal rings (Mair and Lane 1990; Couëtil et al. 2004; Dixon et al. 2007; Aleman et al. 2008; Rickards and Thiemann 2019). In donkeys, the prevalence of tracheal deformities is relatively high compared to other equid species (Powell et al. 2010; Rickards and Thiemann 2019) but clinical signs are not more common. In general, unless lesions are severe or there is accompanying lower respiratory disease, animals with congenital malformations often remain asymptomatic until they reach middle age (Barakzai and Dixon 2019). This may reflect their less intense physical activity but may also correspond to a degenerative component to the condition.

Tracheitis has been reported in horses in association with the use of endotracheal tubes during general anesthesia. Inflammation and necrosis of the tracheal mucosa occurs at the site of cuff contact with the mucosa (Holland et al. 1986; Saulez et al. 2009; Trim 2015). Although histological evidence of inflammation and tissue damage can be identified experimentally in horses with endotracheal cuffs maintained by clinically appropriate pressures (<120 cm H_2O), significant damage is typically associated with use of excessive cuff pressures (Touzot-Jourde et al. 2005; Trim 2015). More rarely, residual sterilization or cleaning agents can cause tissue damage. Mild cases typically resolve without complications. More severe cases may result in tracheal perforation, excessive formation of granulation tissue, and potentially circumferential fibrosis and stenosis of the tracheal lumen (Holland et al. 1986; Dixon et al. 2007). Focal granulomatous lesions within the tracheal lumen are reported and are generally of little clinical concern. Isolated cases of diffuse granulomatous tracheitis have been reported in association with *Conidiobolus cornonatus* infection, after a tracheobronchial aspirate and secondary to intratracheal antibiotic instillation (Charlton and Tulleners 1991; Steiger and Williams 2000). Replication of respiratory viruses (EIV, EHV) within tracheobronchial epithelial cells can cause tracheitis and damage to the mucociliary apparatus. These will be discussed elsewhere in the chapter.

Clinical signs will depend on the cause. Dyspnea and stridor are common with obstructive lesions or with collapse. In horses with congenital malformations associated with dynamic collapse, clinical signs may be intermittent, more common during hot or humid weather, or during stressful events and exercise (Barakzai and Dixon 2019). More rarely, pulmonary hemorrhage has been reported in severe cases of collapse in response to increased negative intrathoracic pressure (Dixon et al. 2007; Barakzai and Dixon 2019). Cough is a common presenting sign with tracheal inflammation, and head or neck extension may be present if horses are painful. Endoscopy is ideal for the evaluation of the tracheal lumen. Palpation of tracheal irregularities may be possible and lateral radiographs of the trachea can also be diagnostic. Fluoroscopy is possible for diagnosis of tracheal collapse, but is infrequently performed in horses.

Anesthetic Considerations

Correct inflation of an endotracheal tube cuff is recommended to prevent aspiration of materials and to ensure effective mechanical ventilation can be delivered without loss of pressure or contamination or the environment with waste anesthetic gas. As mentioned, overinflation may compromise mucosal perfusion and result in tracheal irritation and inflammation. There is no consensuses on the proper technique for cuff inflation that minimizes adverse events. Factors associated with adverse outcomes include tube size, cuff position, type of tube, cuff contours, multiple attempts at intubation, duration of intubation, type of surgery, use of nasogastric tubes, type of lubrication used, and down folding of the epiglottis (Hockey et al. 2016). In humans, subjective assessment or standardizing cuff inflation pressure is associated with more adverse events than when periodic adjustments are made to cuff inflation using objective assessments such as length of anesthesia, change in cuff pressure, and transport of patients (Hockey et al. 2016). In horses, cuff pressures as high as $120\,cm\ H_2O$ have been studied (Touzot-Jourde et al. 2005). Cuff pressures between 80 and $120\,cm\ H_2O$ appear to prevent leakage and higher pressures caused more tracheal wall damage. Cuff pressures tend to change over time, and it is recommended that pressures be checked and adjusted at frequent intervals during anesthesia.

Viral Respiratory Disease of the Horse

Viral respiratory disease is a significant cause of respiratory disease in horses worldwide. Outbreaks are associated with significant morbidity, loss of athletic performance and economic impact (Gilkerson et al. 2015; Landolt 2019). Infection with respiratory viruses can predispose horses to the development of bacterial pneumonia and may increase the risk for development of equine asthma in athletic horses (Willoughby et al. 1992; Wood et al. 2005; Houtsma et al. 2015; Rossi

et al. 2019a,b). Viral respiratory disease can affect horses of all ages but is most common in weanling to five-year-old horses, particularly those with increased comingling and experiencing stressful conditions, such as in racing or training barns. Equine respiratory viruses include EIV, the alphaherpesviruses EHV1 and EHV4, equine arteritis virus (EVA), equine rhinitis A virus (ERAV), and equine adenovirus (EAdV). Of these, EIV and EHV-1 and EHV-4 are of greatest clinical significance because of their highly contagious nature, associated outbreaks, severity of disease, and for EHV-1, the potential for other disease manifestations. EHV-1 is reportable in many states within the USA.

EVA is of greatest significance for reproductive manifestations of disease including abortion. Infected geldings and non-pregnant mares usually have subclinical disease but may occasionally develop mild signs of rhinitis or tracheitis. Fatal pneumonia can develop in infected foals (Landolt 2019). Both ERAV and EAdV are considered of questionable significance as a cause of respiratory disease. These viruses are often isolated from healthy horses, and earlier reports of respiratory disease were primarily in immunocompromised individuals (Landolt 2019). More recently, ERAV has been isolated in association with upper and lower respiratory tract disease with similar clinical presentation as EIV or the alphaherpesviruses (Li et al. 1997; Diaz-Méndez et al. 2010; Lynch et al. 2013; Diaz-Méndez et al. 2014; Rossi et al. 2019a,b).

Equine influenza (A/equine type-2 H3N8) is an RNA orthomyxovirus endemic in many countries including the USA. The alphaherpesviruses EHV-1 and EHV-4 are DNA viruses and along with EIV represent the most common causes of viral associated acute rhinopharyngitis and tracheobronchitis (Gilkerson et al. 2015).

Transmission of respiratory viral particles is primarily via inhalation of respiratory secretions particularly among horses in close contact. Fomites may also serve as important contributors to transmission and thus appropriate biosecurity protocols should be utilized when working with infected animals. In horses infected with ERAV, urine and feces may serve as a potential route of transmission (Lynch et al. 2013; Rossi et al. 2019a,b). Viral latency and recrudescence characterize EHV 1 and 4 and maintain these viruses within the general equine population. Previously infected horses may develop clinical or subclinical disease during stressful events (illness, transport, and anesthesia) and infect naïve horses (Gilkerson et al. 2015). The incubation period is relatively short, as little as 1 day for EIV. Most horses shed for <7 days with longer periods noted occasionally with EHV infection (Landolt 2019).

Viral replication occurs within the respiratory epithelial cells and for EIV, EHV-4, and ERAV, viral infection is limited to the respiratory tract. Lymphocyte-mediated viremia and viral dissemination to the CNS and uterus can occur with EHV-1 infection with associated vasculitis, hemorrhage, thrombosis, ischemic necrosis and resultant abortion, and the neurologic disease equine herpes myeloencephalopathy (EHM) (Kydd et al. 1996; Allen et al. 2004; Landolt 2019). Viral replication within the respiratory tract causes epithelial degeneration and necrosis and loss of ciliated epithelia and goblet cells within the tracheobronchial tree (Wilson 1993) and produces an environment favoring bacterial attachment and colonization. Decreased alveolar type II pneumocytes (surfactant producing cells) and alveolar macrophage dysfunction are also identified. Together, these changes result in rhinitis and tracheitis; the most common clinical manifestations of viral respiratory infection. The impaired mucociliary clearance and pulmonary defenses also increase the risk for development of bacterial bronchopneumonia. After infection, the respiratory epithelium begins to regenerate within three to five days of illness onset but may require several weeks for complete recovery (Willoughby et al. 1992).

With uncomplicated disease, clinical presentation is very similar among respiratory viruses. During an outbreak, the severity of disease often varies among horses (Landolt 2019). Common clinical signs include fever, dry cough, serous nasal discharge, and nonspecific signs of malaise, mild anorexia, and lethargy. In uncomplicated cases, signs of disease usually resolve within five to seven days (Landolt 2019). Nasal discharge that becomes mucopurulent can be seen with EHV 1 and 4 infection and should also warrant investigation for secondary bacterial respiratory disease. Lymphadenopathy can be noted, especially with EHV 1 and 4 infection (Gilkerson et al. 2015; Landolt 2019). Rarely, foals infected with EIV can develop fatal pneumonia, and adult horses may present with myositis, myocarditis, and edema. In donkeys, EIV infection typically results in more severe respiratory disease and a greater risk for the development of bacterial bronchopneumonia (Rickards and Thiemann 2019). With EHV-1 infection, close monitoring for signs of neurologic disease or abortion is important.

Diagnosis of respiratory viruses is most often performed using real-time PCR testing of nasopharyngeal or nasal swabs. Current multiplex techniques allow for the testing of multiple pathogens as once. In horses with suspected EHV-1 infection, paired whole blood samples are often submitted for PCR to identify viremia. Treatment for uncomplicated cases is primarily supportive. Antiviral drugs have been evaluated for treatment during outbreaks and in horses with EHV-1 associated EHM (Maxwell et al. 2017). Vaccination remains the cornerstone of prevention for these diseases.

Anesthetic Consideration

The major concerns associated with anesthetizing horses with respiratory viral disease include transmission of infection to other horses in the hospital environment, contamination of anesthetic equipment, and delayed clearance of the viral infection and development of post-anesthetic complications from viral respiratory disease (i.e. bacterial colonization and bronchopneumonia).

Prior to anesthesia, general physical examination should identify symptoms of clinical infection, and signalment (i.e. young horses from training environments) may provide further support of viral respiratory infection. Particularly for elective procedures, horses with fever, cough, and/or nasal discharge should be suspected of having a viral infection and anesthesia should be postponed and the horse isolated for testing. Horses from barns or stables with known outbreaks of EIV, EHV-1, or EVA should not be permitted to enter the hospital unless being admitted directly to an isolation environment for treatment of clinical signs associated with viral infection. Once diagnostic testing is complete, negative horses can proceed with anesthesia for elective procedures. For positive horses, anesthesia should be postponed until at least two weeks after clinical signs have resolved. Horses with disrupted respiratory epithelium may have reduced ability to clear contaminants and may be at higher risk of post-anesthesia bacterial bronchopneumonia. In humans with uncomplicated influenza virus infection, pulmonary mechanics measured by forces expiratory spirometry and total pulmonary resistance continue to be altered up to five weeks after illness (Hall et al. 1976). Children with upper respiratory tract infections are 11 times more likely to have a respiratory-related event in the peri-operative period including laryngospasm, bronchoconstriction, altered respiratory patterns, and hypoxemia (Cohen and Cameron 1991). Airways can become hyperresponsive secondary to viral infections and can exacerbate chronic lung diseases and in humans it is recommended to avoid anesthesia when possible for at least several weeks after recovery (Jacoby and Hirshman 1991). If anesthesia cannot be delayed, clinicians should be prepared for complications associated with decreased airway microbial defenses and airway hyper-reactivity leading to hypoxemia.

Prophylactic use of broad-spectrum antibiotics, anti-inflammatory drugs, albuterol, and oxygen supplementation in the peri-anesthetic period may be beneficial.

Anesthetic Consideration of Horses with Specific Infectious or Inflammatory Diseases of the Lower Respiratory System

Equine Asthma (RAO, IAD)

Pathophysiology

Equine asthma is a chronic, inflammatory disease of the lower airways. This condition is recognized as the three related conditions of Inflammatory Airway Disease (IAD), Recurrent Airway Obstruction (RAO, heaves), and Summer Pasture Recurrent Airway Obstruction (SPRAO), each of which is distinguished by unique characteristics in disease manifestation. Equine Asthma represents a collective term recently adopted to define these conditions (Couëtil et al. 2016; Pirie et al. 2016; Bullone and Lavoie 2017; Bond et al. 2018; Couëtil et al. 2020). Severe equine asthma is a chronic respiratory disease of older horses and includes RAO and SPRAO. Mild-to-moderate equine asthma is diagnosed in younger athletic horses and includes IAD. The estimated prevalence of severe asthma is approximately 14–17% in mature horses in northern, temperate geographical regions (Hotchkiss et al. 2007; Wasko et al. 2011; Pirie 2014). In athletic horses (pleasure and racehorses), mild-to-moderate asthma represents one of the most common causes of reduced performance with an estimated prevalence of 60–80% (Gerber et al. 2003; Couëtil et al. 2016). Unlike severe asthma, clinical signs are often absent or very subtle at rest.

The etiology of equine asthma is multifactorial. Affected horses demonstrate hypersensitivity to aerosolized substances in the environment. In stabled horses, particularly those with severe equine asthma, respirable components of organic dust in hay or bedding such as thermophilic molds (*Aspergillus fumigatus*, *Faenia rectivirgula*) or bacterial endotoxins are most often implicated in triggering disease (Pirie et al. 2003; Séguin et al. 2012; Pirie 2014). Clinical exacerbations are episodic and most common when horses are indoors for extended periods of time. The average age of onset of severe asthma is >7 years and a heritable component has been described in some breeds (Gerber et al. 2015). In horses with SPRAO, seasonal (primarily summer) hypersensitivity to grass pollen or fungal spores is suspected (Costa et al. 2006; Ferrari et al. 2018). This condition is recognized in pastured horses and is most common in the Southeastern United States. Mild-to-moderate asthma is the most heterogenous form of equine asthma and is recognized in younger, athletic horses. Although hypersensitivity to aerosolized particles plays an important role in development of disease, other triggers have been proposed including strenuous training, viral or bacterial respiratory pathogens, and various immunologic or genetic factors (Couëtil et al. 2016; Bullone and Lavoie 2017; Couëtil et al. 2020). Horses with mild-to-moderate asthma may experience transient disease of several weeks-to-months or may progress to severe equine asthma later in life (Couëtil et al. 2016; Bullone and Lavoie 2017). In contrast, severe equine asthma is a progressive and lifelong condition.

Although disease manifestation is heterogenous, the shared clinical features of equine asthma include allergen mediated airway inflammation, airway hyper-responsiveness, and airway remodeling (Couëtil et al. 2016). In the horse with asthma, these features manifest as expiratory airflow limitations, increased work of breathing, and hypoxemia secondary to altered gas exchange. Chronic neutrophilic airway inflammation characterizes severe equine asthma while neutrophilic, eosinophilic, and/or mastocytic inflammation develop in mild-to-moderate asthma. Influx of inflammatory cells to the lungs is rapid and can be detected in the airways within hours of allergen exposure (Couëtil et al. 2016). Increased goblet cells and mucus hypersecretion accompany airway inflammation, contributing to lower airway obstruction.

Airway hyper-responsiveness is triggered by inflammatory mediators, bronchospasm, and dysfunction of the airway smooth muscle. Increased sensitivity of the peripheral airways to irritants or antigens promotes excessive bronchospasm which is exacerbated by dysfunction in airway smooth muscle relaxation (Yu et al. 1994; Derksen et al. 1999). Horses with severe asthma generally have some degree of bronchoconstriction at rest. Airway remodeling occurs to a variable degree throughout the lower airways and is more prominent in horses with severe asthma. Remodeling develops in response to chronic inflammation and recurrent injury to the airway walls and ultimately results in narrowing of the airway lumen. Changes become irreversible in long-standing cases of severe asthma and may include smooth muscle hypertrophy of the airways and pulmonary arteries, hyperinflation of the alveoli, alterations in collagen content, and potentially fibrosis (Leclere et al. 2011; Bullone et al. 2015; Couëtil et al. 2016; Bullone et al. 2018; Bullone and Lavoie 2020; Ceriotti et al. 2020). Occasionally, focal areas of emphysema can be identified in cases of severe asthma.

The clinical presentation differs between severe and mild-to-moderate asthma. In horses with severe asthma, clinical signs are present at rest and include episodic periods of expiratory dyspnea, expiratory wheezes detected on auscultation, cough (occasionally paroxysmal) and nasal discharge. In horses in remission, these signs may be subtle. In horses with poorly controlled disease, hypertrophy of the abdominal muscles of expiration appears as the characteristic "heave line" and body condition is often poor. Recognition of mild-to-moderate asthma is more challenging as clinical signs at rest are uncommon and presenting complaints of exercise intolerance are nonspecific. Occasionally, cough, mild tachypnea at rest, or mucoid nasal discharge is reported in horses with moderate asthma (Gy et al. 2019). Signs of respiratory compromise are recognized during work or with pulmonary function testing combined with histamine bronchoprovocation.

History and clinical signs can be used to make a presumptive diagnosis of equine asthma. Clinical scoring systems exist for horses with severe asthma in exacerbation (Tilley et al. 2012; Lavoie et al. 2019). Cytological evidence of non-septic lower airway inflammation in bronchoalveolar lavage (BAL) fluid is the preferred method for the diagnosis of asthma in horses (Table 3.1) (Couëtil et al. 2016; Couëtil et al. 2020) with controversy existing over the utility of tracheal wash cytology (Couëtil et al. 2020). Endoscopic retrieval of BAL fluid can yield additional information such as presence and degree of mucus accumulation, edema, and mucosal inflammation. Tracheal and bronchial mucus scoring systems, although subjective, are sometimes used in the diagnosis of equine asthma (Couëtil et al. 2016; Rossi et al. 2018). Additional diagnostic tools that are limited to referral or research settings include pulmonary function testing with histamine bronchoprovocation to quantify lung dysfunction and airway hyper-reactivity and endobronchial biopsy to characterize airway inflammation and remodeling (Bullone et al. 2015; Couëtil et al. 2016; Bullone et al. 2018; Couëtil et al. 2020). Standard hematologic evaluation and thoracic imaging (ultrasound, radiography) are ancillary diagnostics used to rule out infectious or other causes of lower respiratory disease.

Treatment and control of equine asthma, especially in severe cases, includes environmental management to reduce exposure to aerosolized allergens and medical management to target airway inflammation and hyper-reactivity. Environmental management is an essential component of treatment and in some horses can lead to resolution of clinical signs. Current recommendations for medical management include administration of corticosteroids to reduce pulmonary inflammation and bronchodilators to reduce bronchoconstriction. Systemic and aerosolized formulations are available for both types of medications with specific devices developed for the delivery of aerosolized formulations in horses. Systemic corticosteroids include dexamethasone and prednisolone. Aerosolized formulations include fluticasone, beclomethasone, and ciclesonide. Bronchodilators are used to provide relief of airway obstruction until asthma is controlled by corticosteroids and environmental management. Beta-2 adrenergic agonists (clenbuterol, albuterol) are used most often in horses. Tachyphylaxis has been observed with some formulations (Read et al. 2012). Muscarinic receptor antagonists (atropine, glycopyrrolate, Buscopan[*], ipratropium) are also described for use in horses but an increased risk of side effects may occur with certain formulations. Glycopyrrolate, a selective

Table 3.1 Cytologic findings on bronchoalveolar lavage (BAL) fluid analysis for horses with equine asthma

	Normal	Severe Asthma	Mild-moderate asthma
Neutrophils	< 5%	25–90%	> 5 – < 25%
Mast cells	< 2%		> 5%
Eosinophils	< 1%		> 5%
Additional findings:		Curschmann spirals (inspissated mucus/cellular casts)	

muscarinic antagonist, has been described for aerosolized administration in horses and may provide longer acting bronchodilatory action (Art et al. 2003; Hansel et al. 2005).

Anesthetic Considerations

Peri-operative bronchoconstriction and hypoxemia are the main anesthetic concerns associated with anesthesia of a horse with asthma. The degree of how well a horse's clinical signs are controlled is one of the main factors associated with anesthetic risk (Gennaro et al. 2012). Horses with uncontrolled or poorly controlled asthma should have elective procedures postponed until the best possible control is obtained, preferably documented with pulmonary function testing (Kamassai et al. 2020). Pre-anesthetic optimization can be achieved with short-term dose escalation of medications and in urgent or emergency cases, intensive treatment with bronchodilators and steroids within a few hours of anesthesia may be beneficial (Lumb 2019). Regardless of how well the asthma is controlled, systemic steroid pretreatment prior to anesthesia has been recommended in human asthmatics to reduce peri-operative asthma as neither preoperative asthma severity nor duration from last severe episode had any relevance to post-operative asthma attacks (Le et al. 2010).

There are no published guidelines on anesthetizing horses with equine asthma. Following guidelines in humans would suggest that elective procedure should be postponed in horses with uncontrolled or poorly controlled asthma. Pretreatment with systemic steroids has not been investigated in horses and therefore cannot be recommended prophylactically. However, horses on systemic steroids should receive their regularly scheduled dose. Administration of inhaled albuterol just prior to anesthesia should be considered as it has been shown to improve oxygenation in anesthetized horses (see previous section on general considerations). Subsequent administration at the conclusion of anesthesia may also help reduce hypoxemia during recovery. As previously mentioned, ketamine may be helpful in

the management of horses with asthma. In humans, ketamine maintains spontaneous ventilation, bronchodilation, and preservation of the CO_2 curve (Nowacka and Borczyk 2019). Potent airway relaxation and bronchodilation properties of IV ketamine can even prevent the need for intubation in acute asthma attack in children and adults (Sarma 1992; Denmark et al. 2006). However, higher dose of administered ketamine may be necessary for bronchial effects as a low dose constant rate infusion does not improve chronic obstructive pulmonary disease (COPD) airway resistance in long-term ventilated human patients (Nedel et al. 2020). The bronchodilation effect appears to be related to systemic release of endogenous catecholamine. Ketamine appears to have anti-inflammatory effects as well. Interestingly, ketamine can be nebulized in patients with severe asthma and may act locally as an anti-inflammatory as well as have systemic uptake for bronchodilation (Elkoundi et al. 2018). There is little information on the effect of ketamine for use in horses with asthma. However, as ketamine is a common induction agent used in horses, its use in horses with asthma may be beneficial and should probably be included in the anesthetic plan.

Magnesium sulfate relieves bronchoconstriction by inhibition of uptake and release of calcium from bronchial smooth muscle, inhibits mast cell degranulation, and decreases excitability of membranes by decreased acetylcholine release at motor end plates. Infusions are helpful in moderate-to-severe acute asthma in children and may be helpful in horses (Carrié and Anderson 2015).

Maintenance of anesthesia with isoflurane or sevoflurane can also be beneficial in asthma as they rapidly reverse bronchoconstriction (Carrié and Anderson 2015). Desflurane should be avoided as it has been shown to increase airway resistance in children with reactive airways (Von Ungern-Sternberg et al. 2008). However, when first initiating anesthesia with inhalants, additional injectable anesthetic (preferably, ketamine in adult horses) should be available as bronchoconstriction delays anesthetic uptake and therefore a longer time to anesthetic maintenance (Kretzschmar et al. 2016). Similarly, anesthetic elimination is delayed and should be considered during recovery.

Pulse oximetry and arterial blood gas analysis during the anesthetic period is warranted to monitor oxygenation status of horses with asthma and to assess response to therapy.

Oxygen support should continue in the recovery period with insufflation of oxygen. If bronchoconstriction is present in recovery, prolonged recovery from inhalant anesthetics may occur. Provision of longer acting sedatives such as acepromazine during recovery may be necessary to prevent horses from rising while still disoriented from residual inhalant anesthetic and resulting in a poor recovery.

Pleuropneumonia

Pathophysiology

Bacterial infection and associated inflammation of the bronchi and lung parenchyma defines bacterial bronchopneumonia (Raidal 1995; Ainsworth and Hackett 2004; Giguère 2019). Extension of infection to the pleura and pleural space represents the more severe condition of pleuropneumonia. Bacterial bronchopneumonia can be diagnosed in horses of any age, but more common in younger horses (<5 years of age; Sweeney et al. 1991). Transportation is one of the most common causes, especially when postural drainage of airway secretions are prevented through elevated head restraint during transport (Raidal 1995; Reuss and Giguère 2015; Giguère 2019). Other predisposing causes include viral infection (EIV, EHV), strenuous exercise, dysphagia, esophageal obstruction, general anesthesia (see Section 3.7.2), and potentially other factors associated with increased physiologic stress (Bayly 1990; Raidal 1995). Polymicrobic infections are common (Ainsworth and Hackett 2004; Giguère 2019) with identification of anaerobic bacteria often associated with a more guarded prognosis.

Bacterial bronchopneumonia or pleuropneumonia most commonly develop through aspiration of bacteria from the oral cavity or nasopharynx but can also develop secondary to thoracic trauma or tracheobronchial foreign bodies (Bodecek et al. 2011; Giguère 2019). Colonization within the lung becomes possible when the amount of bacteria and oropharyngeal secretions overwhelms normal respiratory defense mechanisms or when predisposing factors have compromised those defense mechanisms (Raidal 1995; Raidal et al. 1997; Ainsworth and Hackett 2004; Giguère 2019). Damage to the airway epithelium, as with viral infection, favors bacterial attachment and diminishes mucociliary clearance of tracheobronchial secretions. In horses, mucociliary clearance is poorly effective against gravity, and bacterial contamination with airway inflammation is detected in horses within several hours of restraint with the head elevated (Racklyeft and Love 1990; Raidal 1995; Raidal et al. 1995). Compromise to pulmonary and systemic immunity that accompanies viral infection, transport, or strenuous exercise, can include diminished surfactant production, increased destruction of alveolar macrophages, and decreased phagocytic and bactericidal function of alveolar macrophages and peripheral blood neutrophils (Bayly 1990; Raidal et al. 2000). Conditions decreasing surfactant or favoring atelectasis (e.g. viral infection, general anesthesia) create an environment favorable for bacterial growth.

Regardless of the cause, bacterial colonization within the lung initiates an inflammatory response involving recruitment of neutrophils and other inflammatory cells and results in damage to the airway epithelium and pulmonary capillary endothelium (Raidal 1995; Giguère 2019). Initially, cellular debris, exudate, and fibrin accumulate within and obstruct the airways. As disease progresses, purulent exudate and necrotic material are deposited within the airways, lung consolidation or abscess formation is noted, and gas exchange can become significantly impaired (Ainsworth and Hackett 2004; Giguère 2019). Extension of inflammation and bacterial infection to the pleura (pleuropneumonia) is possible when

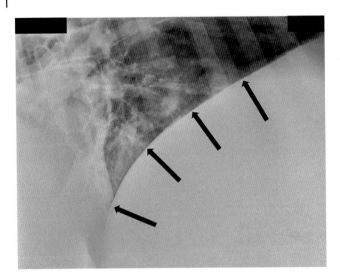

Figure 3.6 A ventrolateral thoracic radiograph of a horse with mild pneumonia. The black arrows indicate the outline of the diaphragm. An alveolar pattern in the ventral lung can be seen caudal to the base of the heart and cranial to the diaphragm.

there is significant parenchymal disease. Pleural effusion initially presents as a sterile exudative process in response to inflammation and increased permeability of the capillaries within the visceral pleura (Ainsworth and Hackett 2004). Bacterial dissemination into the pleural fluid corresponds with disease progression. In response, degenerative neutrophils, bacteria, and cellular debris can be found in the pleural fluid. Fibrin deposition occurs, adhering to pleural and lung surfaces. Fibrin accumulation can be significant, forming loculations within the pleural cavity and rendering areas of lung nonfunctional (Giguère 2019). Pulmonary hemorrhage and pneumothorax secondary to bronchopleural fistulas in areas of necrotic lung are possible with severe disease.

The clinical presentation and prognosis for horses diagnosed with pneumonia depends on severity of disease, early recognition, and timely initiation of appropriate therapy. Tracheobronchial aspirate is an important diagnostic tool in horses with bronchopneumonia. Cytological evaluation, gram stain, and microbial culture with sensitivity should be performed. In horses with pleuropneumonia, this should be paired with analysis of pleural fluid collected via thoracocentesis as differences in culture results can exist between sampling sights. Thoracic imaging (ultrasound and radiography) can be used to assess severity of disease and to guide treatment (Figures 3.6 and 3.7). Hematologic evaluation can be used to assess systemic health. Findings are generally reflective of systemic inflammation and in severe cases coagulopathy or other complications of systemic inflammatory response syndrome (SIRS) may be evident. Administration of broad-spectrum antimicrobials remains the cornerstone of treatment. Standing lateral thoracotomy is often recommended to allow for manual removal of necrotic lung and fibrinous material (Hilton et al. 2010). This procedure is best suited for chronic disease, with walled-off lesions, or in horses where ongoing disease is localized to one hemithorax.

Anesthetic Considerations

General anesthesia is not often performed in horses with pleuropneumonia and should be avoided if at all possible. Standing lateral thoracotomy has been well described for access to the thoracic space in horses (Hilton et al. 2010). Pleural lesions are often walled off with fibrous tissue and there is usually no communication between the hemi-thoraxes due to extensive fibrous tissue formation on the mediastinum. Unilateral pneumothorax is often well tolerated by the standing horse. Standing sedation with detomidine (8–18 µg/kg loading dose,

Figure 3.7 A ventrolateral thoracic radiograph of a horse with severe pneumonia. The black arrows indicate the outline of the diaphragm. An alveolar pattern in the ventral lung can be seen masking the heart and ventral boarder of the diaphragm.

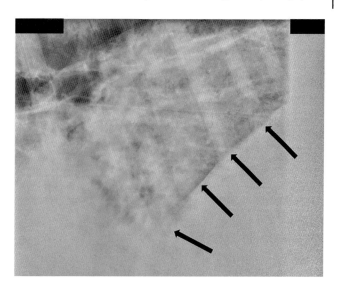

0.3–0.5 µg/kg/min infusion) is effective and renders horses generally unresponsive in stocks. Support for the head may be necessary. Local anesthesia must be utilized to desensitize the surgical incision and rib resection (if necessary). Intercostal perineural block and/or local infiltration of the skin, intercostal muscle, and pleura with mepivacaine or bupivacaine can be performed. The intercostal nerve runs caudal to each rib in a concave depression. Blockade of the intercostal space where the incision will be made as well as two intercostal spaces cranial and caudal may be necessary as there can be extensive overlap of sensory nerve innervation of the intercostal space. Additional analgesia can be provided with butorphanol (17.8 µg/kg loading dose, 0.38 µg/kg/min infusion), lidocaine (0.5 mg/kg loading dose, 40–60 µg/kg/min infusion), or ketamine (0.4–0.8 mg/kg/hour infusion). Supplemental oxygen should be administered via nasal insufflation before and during sedation. Oxygen status can be monitored with pulse oximetry and arterial blood gas analysis. Upon completion of the surgical procedure, horses should be slowly weaned off supplemented oxygen over a gradual period of time (hours to days) by incremental decreases in oxygen flow rates. Oxygen status should be monitored at various time intervals until the horse is deemed to be oxygenating satisfactorily on room air.

General anesthesia may be necessary for horses with very severe or deep lesions or in younger or smaller horses. These horses should be stabilized with supportive care and pleural space drainage prior to anesthesia. Pneumothorax will occur and will require mechanical ventilation. Lung-protective ventilator strategies (i.e. lower tidal volumes, use of PEEP, and higher ventilation rates) may be necessary as damaged alveoli and bronchopleural fistulas may be present. Intensive monitoring of blood pressure and respiratory variables can help guide ventilator settings. Use of analgesic/sedative infusions will help lower the MAC of inhalants and facilitate a smoother recovery. Oxygen support throughout the recovery period is also necessary.

Post-anesthetic Complications Involving the Respiratory System

Obstructive/Negative Pressure Pulmonary Edema

Upper airway obstruction can occur in horses during the recovery period subsequent to extubation. Physical obstruction of the upper airway can occur at the level of the larynx secondary to laryngeal dysfunction, within the nasal passages due to nasal mucosal edema and thickening, or at the opening of the nares secondary to levator nasolabialis and caninus muscle paralysis (Kollias-Baker et al. 1993; Tute et al. 1996; Lukasik et al. 1997). With development of partial or complete upper airway obstruction, pulmonary edema can develop. The pathogenesis of this type of pulmonary edema is thought to results from generation of large intrathoracic negative pressures that occurs as horses attempt to inhale against an obstructed airway (Senior 2005). The increased negative pressure in the thorax causes blood to pool in the pulmonary vasculature with subsequent increased afterload on the heart. Hydrostatic pressure increases causing extravasation of fluid with the development of interstitial and alveolar edema (Lang et al. 1990). Horses develop clinical signs of tachypnea, dyspnea, the presence of pink frothy fluid at the nares and in the mouth, distress, and abnormal lung sounds (Kollias-Baker et al. 1993; Senior 2005). Blood gas analysis may indicate hypoxemia. Immediate and aggressive treatment is warranted upon diagnosis. Rapid administration of anesthetic induction agents may be necessary in distressed horses to administer treatment safely. Some horse may become unconscious secondary to hypoxemia and do not require anesthetic medications. Obtaining a patent airway is of paramount importance and should be the primary goal of intervention/therapy. Endotracheal intubation should be attempted and, if necessary, an endotracheal tube of smaller diameter than what would be used for a horse of that specific size may be easier to insert past the obstruction. If endotracheal intubation fails or is not practical, a tracheostomy should be performed. For horses with paralysis of the muscles of the nares, insertion of cut syringe cases or short length of endotracheal tubes provide stenting of the nasal opening and allows airflow. Nasal hyperemia and edema tend to develop more commonly in horses in dorsal recumbency during anesthesia. Administration of a 0.15%

phenylephrine solution into the nasal passages reduces nasal edema and reduces the requirement of upper airway support by 60% (Lukasik et al. 1997). Once an airway is established, insufflation with oxygen should be made available to combat hypoxemia. Suctioning of the airway to remove edema fluid may be useful in improving gas exchange and decrease the work of breathing (Tute et al. 1996). Administration of furosemide may be useful to decrease pulmonary vascular pressure and edema formation through venodilation and fluid diuresis (Senior 2005). Anti-inflammatory medications such as non-steroidal anti-inflammatory drugs or corticosteroids may be beneficial in reducing pulmonary inflammation and pain. Lower doses of acepromazine can be administered for further vasodilation and sedation of anxious horses. Broad-spectrum antimicrobial agents should also be administered to reduce the development of infections. The mortality rate of horses that develop obstructive pulmonary edema has not been determined and horses can die acutely or develop complications such as pleuropneumonia; however, for horses that survive the initial obstructive episode, with appropriate therapy and correction of the cause of obstruction, full recovery is possible (Kollias-Baker et al. 1993).

Anesthetic Associated Pneumonia

Pneumonia is reported as an anesthetic complication in many species. In human medicine, it represents a significant cause of increased patient morbidity and mortality (Sopena et al. 2005; Russotto et al. 2019). In horses, general anesthesia is recognized as a predisposing cause of bacterial pneumonia (Raphel and Beech 1982; Rainger et al. 2006; Reuss and Giguère 2015; Anderson et al. 2017; Giguère 2019). Unfortunately, limited information exists regarding its true prevalence. In one retrospective study of bacterial pneumonia in 90 horses, recent general anesthesia was identified as a causative factor in 12% of cases

(Raphel and Beech 1982). Proposed causes for the development of pneumonia in horses include aspiration of gastric contents during anesthesia or in recovery, oropharyngeal contamination of lower airways during endotracheal intubation, compromised mucociliary clearance, atelectasis, and impaired pulmonary immune function (Raidal 1995; Ainsworth and Hackett 2004; Rainger et al. 2006; Anderson et al. 2017; Monticelli and Adami 2019; Rossi et al. 2019a,b).

Bacterial contamination of the lower airways and impaired mucociliary clearance can both be associated with endotracheal intubation during anesthesia, particularly if placement of the tube or inflation of the cuff induces trauma or inflammation to the tracheal epithelium. Exposure of the airways to dry gases and increased oxygen concentrations can diminish ciliary clearance by altering viscosity of tracheal mucus or by directly inhibiting ciliary function (Wilkes et al. 2003; Ainsworth and Hackett 2004; Nakagawa et al. 2005). Although evidence is somewhat conflicting, experimental studies in humans and laboratory animals have described direct dose-dependent inhibition of ciliary motility associated with administration of alpha-2 agonists, or volatile anesthetic agents, including sevoflurane and isoflurane (Raphael and Butt 1997; Ledowski et al. 2006; Kesimci et al. 2008). Inhibition of ciliary function not only reduces protection against bacterial contamination in the perianesthetic period, but may also increase susceptibility for post-anesthetic atelectasis. Atelectatic regions may harbor bacteria and provide conditions favorable for bacterial multiplication.

Mechanical ventilation and administration of volatile anesthetic agents can also result in pulmonary inflammation and impaired immune function both intra- and postoperatively (Kalimeris et al. 2011). Independently, these do not cause pneumonia, but in a compromised patient or in the face of other risk factors they may increase the likelihood or severity of disease. Histological evidence of inflammation and changes in BALF cytology and inflammatory mediator expression have been identified in other species in association with both mechanical ventilation and use of volatile anesthetic agents. Specific findings have included impaired pulmonary and systemic antioxidant activity, increased expression of pro-inflammatory mediators, and impaired alveolar macrophage phagocytic and microbicidal activity (Allaouchiche et al. 2001; Hofstetter et al. 2007). These findings are somewhat contradictory as under certain experimental conditions use of sevoflurane has reduced inflammatory mediator expression in ventilated lungs and has demonstrated an immunoprotective effect on alveolar macrophages (De Conno et al. 2009; Vaneker et al. 2009). Investigations into pulmonary inflammation and immunomodulation in anesthetized horses are limited. Clinically relevant changes in BALF cytology or expression of inflammatory mediators in healthy horses anesthetized and mechanically ventilated have not been identified (Ito et al. 2003; Rossi et al. 2019a,b). Whether this differs under clinical conditions is not known.

Anesthetic associate pneumonia is diagnosed in horses that were previously healthy but then develop signs of pneumonia after a recent episode of general anesthesia. Clinical signs include fever, cough, serous or mucopurulent nasal discharge, lethargy, and respiratory pattern changes. Diagnostics include tracheal aspirates for cytology and bacterial culture, thoracic ultrasound, and thoracic radiographs. Treatment includes broad-spectrum antibiotics and anti-inflammatory medications.

Prevention is mainly through prophylactic administration of antibiotics and should be considered for horses that may have compromised respiratory tracts (i.e. young horses in training or older horses with asthma). Additionally, good hygiene and anesthetic equipment maintenance and cleaning should be part of the standard protocol of any equine hospital.

References

Ainsworth, D.M. and Hackett, R.P. (2004). Disorders of the respiratory system. In: *Equine Internal Medicine*, 2e (eds. S.M. Reed, W.M. Bayly and D.C. Sellon), 289–353. Saint Louis, MO: Saunders.

Aleman, M., Nieto, J.E., Benak, J. et al. (2008). Tracheal collapse in American miniature horses: 13 cases (1985–2007). *Journal of the American Veterinary Medical Association* 233 (8): 1302–1306.

Allaouchiche, B., Debon, R., Goudable, J. et al. (2001). Oxidative stress status during exposure to propofol, sevoflurane and desflurane. *Anesthesia and Analgesia* 93 (4): 981–985.

Allen, G.P., Kydd, J.H., Slater, J.D. et al. (2004). Equid herpesvirus 1 and equid herpesvirus 4 infections. In: *Infectious Diseases of Livestock, Vol 2* (eds. J.A.W. Coetzer and R.C. Tustin), 829–859. Newmarket UK: Oxford University Press.

Anderson, S., Wobeser, B., Duke-Novakovski, T. et al. (2017). Pathology in practice: aspiration pneumonia. *Journal of the American Veterinary Medical Association* 251 (4): 409–411.

Andrade, F.S.R.M., Faćo, L.L., Ida, K.K. et al. (2019). Effects of 12 and 17 cm H_2O positive end-expiratory pressure applied after alveolar recruitment maneuver on pulmonary gas exchange and compliance in isoflurane-anesthetized horses. *Veterinary Anaesthesia and Analgesia* 46 (1): 64–73.

Art, T., Anderson, L., Woakes, A.J. et al. (1990). Mechanics of breathing during strenuous exercise in thoroughbred horses. *Respiratory Physiology* 82 (3): 279–294.

Art, T., de Moffarts, B., van Erck, E. et al. (2003). Effects of glycopyrrolate inhalation on pulmonary function in heaves-affected horses in crisis. *Annales de Médecine Vétérinaire* 147 (3): 175–180.

Auckburally, A. and Nyman, G. (2017). Review of hypoxaemia in anesthetized horses: predisposing factors, consequences and management. *Veterinary Anaesthesia and Analgesia* 44 (3): 397–408.

Auer, U., Schramel, J.P., Moens, Y.P. et al. (2019). Monitoring changes in distribution of pulmonary ventilation by functional electrical impedance tomography in anaesthetized ponies. *Veterinary Anaesthesia and Analgesia* 46 (2): 200–208.

Baptiste, K.E., Naylor, J.M., Bailey, J. et al. (2000). A function for guttural pouches in the horse. *Nature* 403 (6768): 382–383.

Baracco, G.J. (2019). Infections caused by group C and G Streptococcus (*Streptococcus dysgalactiae* subsp. *equisimilis* and others): epidemiological and clinical aspects. *Microbiology Spectrum* 7 (2) https://doi.org/10.1128/microbiolspec.GPP3-0016-2018.

Barakzai, S.Z. and Dixon, P.M. (2019). Disorders of the trachea. In: *Large Animal Internal Medicine*, 6e (eds. B.P. Smith, D. Van Metre and N. Pusterla), 625–626. Philadelphia, PA: Elsevier Inc.

Bayly, W.M. (1990). Stress and equine respiratory immunity. *Proceedings American College of Veterinary Internal Medicine* 8: 505.

Beyeler, S.A., Hodges, M.R., and Huxtable, A.G. (2020). Impact of inflammation on developing respiratory control networks: rhythm generation, chemoreception and plasticity. *Respiratory Physiology & Neurobiology* 274: 103357.

Bodecek, S., Jahn, P., Ottova, L. et al. (2011). Pleuropneumonia in two horses caused by a tracheobronchial foreign body. *Equine Veterinary Education* 23: 296–301.

Bond, S., Léguillette, R., Richard, E.A. et al. (2018). Equine asthma: integrative biologic relevance of a recently proposed nomenclature. *Journal of Veterinary Internal Medicine* 32 (6): 2088–2098.

Borges, A.S. and Watanabe, M.J. (2011). Guttural pouch diseases causing neurologic dysfunction in the horse. *The Veterinary Clinics of North America. Equine Practice* 27 (3): 545–572.

Boyle, A.G., Sweeney, C.R., Kristula, M. et al. (2009). Factors associated with likelihood of horses having a high serum *Streptococcus equi*

SeM-specific antibody titer. *Journal of the American Veterinary Medical Association* 235 (8): 973–977.

Boyle, A.G., Timoney, J.F., Newton, J.R. et al. (2018). *Streptococcus equi* infections in horses: guidelines for treatment, control, and prevention of strangles-revised consensus statement. *Journal of Veterinary Internal Medicine* 32 (2): 633–647.

Breeze, R. and Turk, M. (1984). Cellular structure, function and organization in the lower respiratory tract. *Environmental Health Perspectives* 55: 3–24.

Bullone, M. and Lavoie, J.P. (2017). The contribution of oxidative stress and inflamm-aging in human and equine asthma. *Internal Journal of Molecular Sciences* 18 (12): 2612. https://doi.org/10.3390/ijms18122612.

Bullone, M. and Lavoie, J.P. (2020). The equine asthma model of airway remodeling: from a veterinary to a human perspective. *Cell and Tissue Research* 380 (2): 223–236.

Bullone, M., Beauchamp, G., Godbout, M. et al. (2015). Endobronchial ultrasound reliably quantifies airway smooth muscle remodeling in an equine asthma model. *PLoS One* 10 (9): e0136284.

Bullone, M., Joubert, P., Gagné, A. et al. (2018). Bronchoalveolar lavage fluid neutrophilia is associated with the severity of pulmonary lesions during equine asthma exacerbations. *Equine Veterinary Journal* 50 (5): 609–615.

Canning, B.J., Mori, N., and Mazzone, S.B. (2006). Vagal afferent nerves regulating the cough reflex. *Respiratory Physiology & Neurobiology* 152 (3): 223–242.

Carrié, S. and Anderson, T.A. (2015). Volatile anesthetics for status asthmaticus in pediatric patients: a comprehensive review and case series. *Paediatric Anaesthesia* 25 (5): 460–467.

Ceriotti, S., Bullone, M., Leclere, M. et al. (2020). Severe asthma is associated with a remodeling of the pulmonary arteries in horses. *PLoS One* 15 (10): e0239561.

Charlton, C. and Tulleners, E. (1991). Transendoscopic contact neodymium:yttrium aluminum garnet laser excision of tracheal

lesions in two horses. *Journal of the American Veterinary Medical Association* 199 (2): 241–243.

Christmann, U., Livesey, L.C., Taintor, J.S. et al. (2006). Lung surfactant function and composition in neonatal foals and adult horses. *Journal of Veterinary Internal Medicine* 20 (6): 1402–1407.

Christmann, U., Buechner-Maxwell, V.A., Witonsky, S.G. et al. (2009). Role of lung surfactant in respiratory disease: current knowledge in large animal medicine. *Journal of Veterinary Internal Medicine* 23 (2): 227–242.

Cohen, M.M. and Cameron, C.B. (1991). Should you cancel the operation when a child has an upper respiratory tract infection? *Anesthesia and Analgesia* 72 (3): 282–288.

Coleridge, H.M. and Coleridge, J.C.G. (1986). Reflexes evoked from tracheobronchial tree and lungs. In: *Handbook of Physiology, Section 3, Respiration, Volume II, Control of Breathing* (eds. N.S. Chemiack and J.G. Widdicombe), 395–429. Bethesda, MD: American. Physiological Society.

Colles, C.S. and Cook, W.R. (1983). Carotid and cerebral angiography in the horse. *Veterinary Record* 113 (21): 483–489.

Connally, B. and Derksen, F. (1994). Tidal breathing flow-volume loop analysis as a test of pulmonary function in exercising horses. *American Journal of Veterinary Research* 55 (5): 589–594.

Cook, W.R. (1968). The clinical features of guttural pouch mycosis in the horse. *Veterinary Record* 83 (14): 336–345.

Cook, W.R., Campbell, R.S., and Dawson, C. (1968). The pathology and aetiology of guttural pouch mycosis in the horse. *Veterinary Record* 83 (17): 422–428.

Costa, L.R.R., Johnson, J.R., Baur, M.E. et al. (2006). Temporal clinical exacerbation of summer pasture-associated recurrent airway obstruction and relationship with climate and aeroallergens in horses. *American Journal of Veterinary Research* 67 (9): 1635–1642.

Couëtil, L.L., Gallatin, L.L., Blevins, W. et al. (2004). Treatment of tracheal collapse with an intraluminal stent in a miniature horse. *Journal of the American Veterinary Medical Association* 225 (11): 1727–1732.

Couëtil, L.L., Cardwell, J.M., Gerber, V. et al. (2016). Inflammatory airway disease of horses–revised consensus statement. *Journal of Veterinary Internal Medicine* 30 (2): 503–515.

Couëtil, L., Cardwell, J.M., Leguillette, R. et al. (2020). Equine asthma: current understanding and future directions. *Frontiers in Veterinary Science* 7: 450.

Cunningham, D.J.C., Robbins, P.A., and Wolf, C.B. (1986). Integration of respiratory responses to changes in alveolar partial pressures of CO_2, O_2 and pH. In: *Handbook of Physiology, Section 3, Respiration, Volume II, Control of Breathing* (eds. N.S. Cherniak and J.G. Widdicombe), 475–527. Bethesda, MD: American Physiological Society.

Day, T.K., Gaynor, J.S., Muir, W.W. et al. (1995). Blood gas values during intermittent positive pressure ventilation and spontaneous ventilation in 160 anesthetized horses position in lateral or dorsal recumbency. *Veterinary Surgery* 24 (3): 266–276.

De Conno, E., Steurer, M.P., Wittlinger, M. et al. (2009). Anesthetic-induced improvement of the inflammatory response to one-lung ventilation. *Anesthesiology* 110 (6): 1316–1326.

Del Negro, C.A., Funk, G.D., and Feldman, J.L. (2018). Breathing matters. *Nature Reviews. Neuroscience* 19 (6): 351–367.

Dempsey, J.A. and Smith, C.A. (2014). Pathophysiology of human ventilatory control. *European Respiratory Journal* 44 (2): 495–512.

Denmark, T.K., Crane, H.A., and Brown, L. (2006). Ketamine to avoid mechanical ventilation in severe pediatric asthma. *Journal of Emergency Medicine* 30 (2): 163–166.

Derksen, F.J., Olszewski, M.A., Robinson, N.E. et al. (1999). Aerosolized albuterol sulfate used as a bronchodilator in horses with recurrent airway obstruction. *American Journal of Veterinary Research* 60 (6): 689–693.

Diaz-Méndez, A., Viel, L., Hewson, J. et al. (2010). Surveillance of equine respiratory viruses in Ontario. *Canadian Journal of Veterinary Research* 74 (4): 271–278.

Diaz-Méndez, A., Hewson, J., Shewen, P. et al. (2014). Characteristics of respiratory tract disease in horses inoculated with equine rhinitis a virus. *American Journal of Veterinary Research* 75 (2): 169–178.

Dixon, P.M. (1992). Respiratory mucociliary clearance in the horse in health and disease, and its pharmacological modification. *Veterinary Record* 131 (11): 229–235.

Dixon, P.M., Schumacher, J., and Collins, N. (2007). Disorders of the trachea. In: *Equine Respiratory Medicine and Surgery* (eds. B.C. McGorum, P.M. Dixon, N.E. Robinson, et al.), 543–562. Philadelphia, PA: WB Saunders.

Dobesova, O., Schwarz, B., Velde, K. et al. (2012). Guttural pouch mycosis in horses: a retrospective study of 28 cases. *Veterinary Record* 171 (22): 561.

Duffee, L.R., Stefanovski, D., Boston, R.C. et al. (2015). Predictor variables for and complications associated with *Streptococcus equi* subsp *equi* infection in horses. *Journal of the American Veterinary Medical Association* 247 (10): 1161–1168.

Elkoundi, A., Bentalha, A., El Koraichi, A. et al. (2018). Nebulized ketamine to avoid mechanical ventilation in a pediatric patient with severe asthma exacerbation. *American Journal of Emergency Medicine* 36 (4): 734. e3-734.e4.

Feldman, J.L., Mitchell, G.S., and Nattie, E.E. (2003). Breathing: rhythmicity, plasticity, chemosensitivity. *Annual Review of Neuroscience* 26: 239–266.

Feldman, J.L., Del Negro, C.A., and Gray, P.A. (2013). Understanding the rhythm of breathing: so near, yet so far. *Annual Review of Physiology* 75 (1): 423–452.

Ferrari, C.R., Cooley, J., Mujahid, N. et al. (2018). Horses with pasture asthma have airway remodeling that is characteristic of human asthma. *Veterinary Pathology* 55 (1): 144–158.

Freeman, D.E. (2015). Update on disorders and treatment of the guttural pouch. *The Veterinary Clinics of North America. Equine Practice* 31 (1): 63–89.

Freeman, D.E. and Hardy, J. (2012). Guttural Pouch. In: *Equine surgery*, 4e (eds. J.A. Auer and J.A. Stick), 623–642. Philadelphia, PA: WB Saunders.

Freeman, S.L., Bowen, I.M., Bettschart-Wolfensberger, R. et al. (2000). Cardiopulmonary effects of romifidine and detomidine used as premedicants for ketamine/halothane anaestheisa in ponies. *Veterinary Record* 147 (19): 535–539.

Furniss, C., Carstens, A., and Cillers, I. (2007). Eustachian tube diverticulum chondroids and neck abscessation in a case of *Streptococcus equi* subsp. *equi*. *Journal of the South African Veterinary Association* 78 (3): 166–170.

Garcia, A.J., Zanella, S., Kich, H. et al. (2011). Chapter 3 – networks within networks: the neuronal control of breathing. *Progress in Brain Research* 188: 310–350.

Gehr, P., Mwangi, D.K., Ammann, A.A. et al. (1981). Design of the mammalian respiratory system. V. Scaling morphometric pulmonary diffusion capacity to body mass: wild and domestic mammals. *Respiration Physiology* 44 (1): 61–86.

Gennaro, L., Antonello, S., Mattelo, S. et al. (2012). Bronchial asthma. *Current Opinion in Anaesthesiology* 25 (1): 30–37.

Genton, M., Farfan, M., Tesson, C. et al. (2021). Balloon catheter occlusion of the maxillary, internal, and external carotid arteries in standing horses. *Veterinary Surgery* 50 (3): 546–555.

Gerber, V., Robinson, N.E., Luethi, S. et al. (2003). Airway inflammation and mucus in two age groups of asymptomatic well-performing sport horses. *Equine Veterinary Journal* 35 (5): 491–495.

Gerber, V., Tessier, C., and Marti, E. (2015). Genetics of upper and lower airway diseases in the horse. *Equine Veterinary Journal* 47 (4): 390–397.

Giguère, S. (2019). Bacterial pneumonia and pleuropneumonia in adult horses. In: *Large Animal Internal Medicine*, 6e (eds. B.P. Smith, D. Van Metre and N. Pusterla), 526–534. Philadelphia, PA: Elsevier Inc.

Gilkerson, J.R., Bailey, K.E., Diaz-Méndez, A. et al. (2015). Update on viral diseases of the equine respiratory tract. *The Veterinary Clinics of North America. Equine Practice* 31 (1): 91–104.

Goyal, S. and Agrawal, A. (2013). Ketamine in status asthmaticus: a review. *Indian Journal of Critical Care Medicine* 17 (3): 154–161.

Greene, S.A., Thurmon, J.C., Tranquilli, W.J. et al. (1986). Cardiopulmonary effects of continuous intravenous infusion of guaifenesin, ketamine, and xylazine in ponies. *American Journal of Veterinary Research* 47 (11): 2364–2367.

Greet, T.R. (1987). Outcome of treatment in 35 cases of guttural pouch mycosis. *Equine Veterinary Journal* 19 (5): 483–487.

Guyenet, P.G. and Bayliss, D.A. (2015). Neural control of breathing and CO_2 homeostasis. *Neuron* 87 (5): 946–961.

Gy, C., Leclere, M., Vargas, A. et al. (2019). Investigation of blood biomarkers for the diagnosis of mild to moderate asthma in horses. *Journal of Veterinary Internal Medicine* 33 (4): 1789–1795.

Hall, W.J., Douglas, R.G. Jr., Hyde, R.W. et al. (1976). Pulmonary mechanics after uncomplicated influenza A infection. *American Review of Respiratory Disease* 113 (2): 141–148.

Hamlen, H.J., Timoney, J.F., and Bell, R.J. (1994). Epidemiologic and immunologic characteristics of *Streptococcus equi* infection in foals. *Journal of the American Veterinary Medical Association* 204 (5): 768–775.

Hansel, T.T., Neighbour, H., Erin, E.M. et al. (2005). Glycopyrrolate causes prolonged bronchoprotection and bronchodilatation in patients with asthma. *Chest* 128 (4): 1974–1197.

Hazari, M.S. and Farraj, A.K. (2015). Comparative control of respiration. In: *Comparative Biology of the Normal Lung* (ed. R.A. Parent), 245–288. Saint Louis, MO: Elsevier Inc.

Heidmann, P., Tornquist, S.J., Qu, A. et al. (2005). Laboratory measures of hemostasis and fibrinolysis after intravenous administration of epsilon-aminocaproic acid in clinically normal horses and ponies. *American Journal of Veterinary Research* 66 (2): 313–318.

Hilton, H., Aleman, M., Madigan, J. et al. (2010). Standing lateral thoracotomy in horses: indications, complications, and outcomes. *Veterinary Surgery* 39 (7): 847–855.

Hines, M. (2018). Control of breathing. In: *Equine Internal Medicine*, 4e (eds. S.M. Reed, W.M. Bayly and D.C. Sellon), 232–310. St. Louis, MO: Elsevier.

Hirshman, C.A., McCullough, R.E., Cohen, P.J. et al. (1975). Hypoxic ventilator drive in dogs during thiopental, ketamine, or pentobarbital anesthesia. *Anesthesiology* 43 (6): 628–634.

Hockey, C.A., van Zundert, A.A.J., and Paratz, J.D. (2016). Does objective measurement of tracheal tube cuff pressures minimise adverse effects and maintain accurate cuff pressures? A systematic review and meta-analysis. *Anaesthesia and Intensive Care* 44 (5): 560–570.

Hofstetter, C., Boost, K.A., Flondor, M. et al. (2007). Anti-inflammatory effects of sevoflurane and mild hypothermia in endotoxemic rats. *Acta Anaesthesiologica Scandinavica* 51 (7): 893–899.

Holland, M., Snyder, J.R., Steffey, E.P. et al. (1986). Laryngotracheal injury associated with nasotracheal intubation in the horse. *Journal of the American Veterinary Medical Association* 189 (11): 1447–1450.

Hopster, K., Kästner, S.B.B., Rohn, K. et al. (2011). Intermittent positive pressure ventilation with constant positive end-expiratory pressure and alveolar recruitment manoeuvre during inhalation anaesthesia in horses undergoing surgery for colic, and its influence on the early recovery period. *Veterinary Anaesthesia and Analgesia* 38 (3): 169–177.

Hornicke, H., Weber, M., and Schweiker, W. (1987). Pulmonary ventilation in thoroughbred horses at maximum performance. In: *Equine Exercise Physiology*, 2e (eds. J.R. Gillespie and N.E. Robinson), 216–224. Davis, CA: ICEEP Publications.

Hotchkiss, J.W., Reid, S.W.J., and Christley, R.M. (2007). A survey of horse owners in Great Britain regarding horses in their care. Part 1: horse demographic characteristics and management. *Equine Veterinary Journal* 39 (4): 294–300.

Houtsma, A., Bedenice, D., Pusterla, N. et al. (2015). Association between inflammatory airway disease of horses and exposure to respiratory viruses: a case control study. *Multidisciplinary Respiratory Medicine* 10: 33.

Hubbell, J.A.E. and Muir, W.W. (2009). Monitoring anesthesia. In: *Equine Anesthesia Monitoring and Emergency Therapy*, 2e (eds. W.W. Muir and J.A.E. Hubbell), 149–170. St. Louis, MO: Saunders Elsevier.

Ito, S., Hobo, S., and Kasashima, Y. (2003). Bronchoalveolar lavage fluid findings in the atelectatic regions of anesthetized horses. *The Journal of Veterinary Medical Science* 65 (9): 1011–1013.

Jacoby, D.B. and Hirshman, C.A. (1991). General anesthesia in patients with viral respiratory infections: an unsound sleep? *Anesthesiology* 74 (6): 969–972.

Jaspar, N., Mazzarelli, M., Tessier, C. et al. (1983). Effect of ketamine on control of breathing in cats. *Journal of Applied Physiology* 55 (3): 851–859.

Judy, C.E., Chaffin, M.K., and Cohen, N.D. (1999). Empyema of the guttural pouch (auditory tube diverticulum) in horses: 91 cases (1977-1997). *Journal of the American Veterinary Medical Association* 215 (11): 1666–1670.

Kalimeris, K., Christodoulaki, K., Karakitsos, P. et al. (2011). Influence of propofol and volatile anaesthetics on the inflammatory response in the ventilated lung. *Acta*

Anaesthesiologica Scandinavica 55 (6): 740–748.

Kamassai, J.D., Aina, T., Hauser, J.M. (2020). Asthma Anesthesia. StatPearls, https://www.ncbi.nlm.nih.gov/books/NBK537327

Katz, L., Bayly, W.M., Roeder, M. et al. (2000). Effects of training on maximum oxygen consumption of ponies. *American Journal of Veterinary Research* 61 (8): 986–991.

Kerr, C.L. and McDonell, W.N. (2009). Oxygen supplementation and ventilatory support. In: *Equine Anesthesia Monitoring and Emergency Therapy*, 2e (eds. W.W. Muir and J.A.E. Hubbell), 332–352. St. Louis, MO: Saunders Elsevier.

Kesimci, E., Bercin, S., Kutluhan, A. et al. (2008). Volatile anesthetics and mucociliary clearance. *Minerva Anestesiologica* 74 (4): 107–111.

Kollias-Baker, C.A., Pipers, F.S., Heard, D. et al. (1993). Pulmonary edema associated with transient airway obstruction in three horses. *Journal of the American Veterinary Medical Association* 202 (7): 1116–1118.

Koterba, A.M., Kosch, P.C., and Beech, J. (1988). The breathing strategy of the adult horse (*Equus caballus*) at rest. *Journal of Applied Physiology* 64 (1): 337–346.

Koterba, A.M., Wozniak, J.A., and Kosch, P.C. (1995). Changes in breathing pattern in the normal horse at rest up to age one year. *Equine Veterinary Journal* 27 (4): 265–274.

Kretzschmar, M., Kozian, A., Baumgardner, J.E. et al. (2016). Bronchoconstriction induced by inhaled methacholine delays desflurane uptake and elimination in a piglet model. *Respiratory Physiology & Neurobiology* 220: 88–94.

Kydd, J.H., Hannant, D., and Mumford, J.A. (1996). Residence and recruitment of leucocytes to the equine lung after EHV-1 infection. *Veterinary Immunology and Immunopathology* 52 (1–2): 15–26.

Landolt, G.A. (2019). Equine respiratory viruses. In: *Large Animal Internal Medicine*, 6e (eds. B.P. Smith, D. Van Metre and N. Pusterla), 569–578. Philadelphia, PA: Elsevier Inc.

Lang, S.A., Duncan, P.G., Shephard, D.A.E. et al. (1990). Pulmonary oedema associated with airway obstruction. *Canadian Journal of Anaesthesia* 37: 210–218.

Lascola, K.M., Vander Werf, K., Freese, S. et al. (2017) Comparison of jugular and transverse facial venous sinus blood analytes in healthy and critically ill adult horses. *Journal of Veterinary Emergency and Critical Care* 27 (2): 198–205.

Lavoie, J.-P., Bullone, M., Rodrigues, N. et al. (2019). Effect of different doses of inhaled ciclesonide on lung function, clinical signs related to airflow limitation and serum cortisol levels in horses with experimentally induced mild to severe airway obstruction. *Equine Veterinary Journal* 51 (6): 779–786.

Le, K., Yoshizawa, A., Hirano, S. et al. (2010). A survey of perioperative asthmatic attack among patients with bronchial asthma underwent general anesthesia. *Arerugī* 59 (7): 831–838.

Leclere, M., Lavoie-Lamoureux, A., Gélinas-Lymburner, E. et al. (2011). Effect of antigenic exposure on airway smooth muscle remodeling in an equine model of chronic asthma. *American Journal of Respiratory Cell and Molecular Biology* 45 (1): 181–187.

Ledowski, T., Hilmi, S., and Paech, M.J. (2006). Bronchial mucus transport velocity in patients receiving anaesthesia with propofol and morphine or propofol and remifentanil. *Anaesthesia* 61 (8): 747–751.

Lepage, O.M. and Piccot-Crézollet, C. (2005). Transarterial coil embolization in 31 horses (1999–2002) with guttural pouch mycosis: a 2-year follow-up. *Equine Veterinary Journal* 37 (5): 430–434.

Lerche, P. (2015). Anticholinergics. In: *Veterinary Anesthesia and Analgesia, the Fifth Edition of Lumb and Jones* (eds. K.A. Grimm, L.A. Lamont, W.J. Tranquilli, et al.), 178–182. Ames, IA: Wiley.

Li, F., Drummer, H.E., Ficorilli, N. et al. (1997). Identification of noncytopathic equine rhinovirus 1 as a cause of acute febrile respiratory disease in horses. *Journal of Clinical Microbiology* 35 (4): 937–943.

Lopez, A. (2001). Respiratory system, thoracic cavity, and pleura. In: *Thompson's Special Veterinary Pathology* (eds. M. McGavin, W. Carlton and J. Zachary), 125–195. Saint Louis, MO: Mosby.

Lukasik, V.M., Gleed, R.D., Scarlett, J.M. et al. (1997). Intranasal phenylephrine reduces post anesthetic upper airway obstruction in horses. *Equine Veterinary Journal* 29 (3): 236–238.

Lumb, A.B. (2019). Pre-operative respiratory optimisation: an expert review. *Anaesthesia* 74 (supplement 1): 43–48.

Lumb, A.B. and Slinger, R. (2015). Hypoxic pulmonary vasoconstriction. *Anesthesiology* 122 (4): 932–946.

Lynch, S.E., Gilkerson, J.R., Symes, S.J. et al. (2013). Persistence and chronic urinary shedding of the aphthovirus equine rhinitis a virus. *Comparative Immunology, Microbiology and Infections Disease* 36 (1): 95–103.

Mair, T.S. and Lane, J.G. (1990). Tracheal obstructions in two horses and a donkey. *Veterinary Record* 126 (13): 303–304.

Mallicote, M. (2015). Update on *Streptococcus equi* subsp *equi* infections. *Veterinary Clinics of North America. Equine Practice* 31 (1): 27–41.

Mama, K.R., Steffey, E.P., and Pascoe, P.J. (1995). Evaluation of propofol as a general anesthetic for horses. *Veterinary Surgery* 24 (4): 188–194.

Marntell, S. and Nyman, G. (1996). Effects of additional premedication on romifidine and ketamine anaesthesia in horses. *Acta Veterinaria Scandinavica* 37 (3): 315–325.

Marntell, S., Nyman, G., Funkquist, P. et al. (2005). Effects of acepromazine on pulmonary gas exchange and circulation during sedation and dissociative anaesthesia in horses. *Veterinary Anaesthesia and Analgesia* 32 (2): 83–93.

Maxwell, L.K., Bentz, B.G., Gilliam, L.L. et al. (2017). Efficacy of the early administration of valacyclovir hydrochloride for the treatment of neuropathogenic equine herpesvirus type-1 infection in horses. *American Journal of Veterinary Research* 78 (10): 1126–1139.

McLaughlin, R.F., Tyler, W.S., and Canada, R.O. (1961). A study of the subgross pulmonary anatomy in various mammals. *American Journal of Anatomy* 108 (2): 149–165.

Menozzi, A., Pozzoli, C., Poli, E. et al. (2014). Pharmacological characterization of muscarinic receptors in contractions of isolated bronchi in the horse. *Journal of Veterinary Pharmacology and Therapeutics* 37: 325–331.

Moens, Y. (2013). Mechanical ventilation and respiratory mechanics during equine anesthesia. *The Veterinary Clinics of North America. Equine Practice* 29 (1): 51–67.

Monticelli, P. and Adami, C. (2019). Aspiration pneumonitis (Mendelson's syndrome) as a perianaesthethic complication occurring in two horses: a case report. *Equine Veterinary Education* 31 (4): 183–187.

Mosing, M., Rysnik, M., Bardell, D. et al. (2013). Use of continuous positive airway pressure (CPAP) to optimize oxygenation in anaesthetized horses – a clinical study. *Equine Veterinary Journal* 45 (4): 414–418.

Muir, W.W., Skarda, R.T., and Sheehan, W.C. (1978). Cardiopulmonary effects of narcotic agonists and a partial agonist in horses. *American Journal of Veterinary Research* 39 (10): 1632–1635.

Nakagawa, N.K., Franchini, M.L., Driusso, P. et al. (2005). Mucociliary clearance is impaired in acutely ill patients. *Chest* 128 (4): 2772–2777.

Nedel, W., Costa, R., Mendez, G. et al. (2020). Negative results for ketamine use in severe acute bronchospasm: a randomized controlled trial. *Anaesthesiology Intensive Therapy* 52 (3): 215–218.

Newton, J.R., Verheyen, K., Talbot, N.C. et al. (2000). Control of strangles outbreaks by isolation of guttural pouch carriers identified using PCR and culture of *Streptococcus equi*. *Equine Veterinary Journal* 32 (6): 515–526.

Nowacka, A. and Borczyk, M. (2019). Ketamine applications beyond anesthesia – a literature review. *European Journal of Pharmacology* 860: 172547. https://doi.org/10.1016/j.ejphar.2019.172547.

Nyman, G., Marntell, S., Edner, A. et al. (2009). Effect of sedation with detomidine and butorphanol on pulmonary gas exchange in the horse. *Acta Veterinaria Scandinavica* 51 (1): 22.

Ohmura, J., Odano, A., Mudai, K. et al. (2016). Cardiorespiratory and anesthetic effects of combined alfaxalone, butorphanol, and medetomidine in thoroughbred horses. *Journal of Equine Veterinary Science* 27 (1): 7–11.

van Oostrom, H., Schaap, M.W.H., and van Loon, J.P.A.M. (2015). Oxygen supplementation before induction of general anaesthesia in horses. *Equine Veterinary Journal* 49 (1): 130–132.

Pascoe, J. (2019). Guttural pouch diseases. In: *Large Animal Internal Medicine*, 6e (eds. B.P. Smith, D. Van Metre and N. Pusterla), 614–616. Philadelphia, PA: Elsevier Inc.

Pattinson, K.T.S. (2008). Opioids and the control of respiration. *British Journal of Anaesthesia* 100 (6): 747–758.

Perkins, J.D., Schumacher, J., Kelly, G. et al. (2006). Standing surgical removal of inspissated guttural pouch exudate (chondroids) in ten horses. *Veterinary Surgery* 35 (7): 658–662.

Pirie, R.S. (2014). Recurrent airway obstruction: a review. *Equine Veterinary Journal* 46 (3): 276–288.

Pirie, M., Pirie, H.M., Cranston, S. et al. (1990). An ultrastructural study of the equine lower respiratory tract. *Equine Veterinary Journal* 22 (5): 338–342.

Pirie, R.S., Dixon, P.M., and McGorum, B.C. (2003). Endotoxin contamination contributes to the pulmonary inflammatory and functional response to *Aspergillus fumigatus* extract inhalation in heaves horses. *Clinical and Experimental Allergy* 33 (9): 1289–1296.

Pirie, R.S., Couëtil, L.L., Robinson, N.E. et al. (2016). Equine asthma: an appropriate, translational and comprehendible terminology? *Equine Veterinary Journal* 48 (4): 403–405.

Powell, R.J., du Toit, N., Burden, F.A. et al. (2010). Morphological study of tracheal shape in donkeys with and without tracheal obstruction. *Equine Veterinary Journal* 42 (2): 136–141.

Prabhakar, N.R. and Peng, Y. (2017). Oxygen sensing by the carotid body: past and present. *Advances in Experimental Medicine and Biology* 977: 3–8.

Quandt, J.E., Robinson, E.P., Rivers, W.J. et al. (1998). Cardiorespiratory and anesthetic effects of propofol and thiopental in dogs. *American Journal of Veterinary Research* 59 (9): 1137–1143.

Racklyeft, D.J. and Love, D.N. (1990). Influence of head posture on the respiratory tract of healthy horses. *Australian Veterinary Journal* 67 (11): 402–405.

Raidal, S.L. (1995). Equine pleuropneumonia. *British Veterinary Journal* 151 (3): 233–262.

Raidal, S.L., Love, D.N., and Bailey, G.D. (1995). Inflammation and increased numbers of bacteria in the lower respiratory tract of horses within 6 to 12 hours of confinement with the head elevated. *Australian Veterinary Journal* 72 (2): 45–50.

Raidal, S.L., Love, D.N., and Bailey, G.D. (1997). Effect of a single bout of high intensity exercise on lower respiratory tract contamination in the horse. *Australian Veterinary Journal* 75 (4): 293–295.

Raidal, S.L., Love, D.N., Bailey, G.D. et al. (2000). The effect of high intensity exercise on the functional capacity of equine pulmonary alveolar macrophages and BAL-derived lymphocytes. *Research in Veterinary Science* 68 (3): 249–225.

Raidal, S.L., Burnheim, K., Evans, D. et al. (2017). Effects of sedation and salbutamol administration on hyperpnoea and tidal breathing spirometry in healthy horses. *The Veterinary Journal* 222: 22–28.

Rainger, J.E., Hughes, K.J., Kessell, A. et al. (2006). Pleuropneumonia as a sequela of myelography and general anaesthesia in a thoroughbred colt. *Australian Veterinary Journal* 84 (4): 138–140.

Raphael, J.H. and Butt, M.W. (1997). Comparison of isoflurane with propofol on respiratory cilia. *British Journal of Anaesthesia* 79 (4): 473–475.

Raphel, C.F. and Beech, J. (1982). Pleuritis secondary to pneumonia or lung abscessation in 90 horses. *Journal of the American Veterinary Medical Association* 181 (8): 808–810.

Read, J.R., Boston, R.C., Abraham, G. et al. (2012). Effect of prolonged administration of clenbuterol on airway reactivity and sweating in horses with inflammatory airway disease. *American Journal of Veterinary Research* 73 (1): 140–145.

Reuss, S.M. and Giguère, S. (2015). Update on bacterial pneumonia and pleuropneumonia in the adult horse. *The Veterinary Clinics of North America. Equine Practice* 31 (1): 105–120.

Rickards, K.J. and Thiemann, A.K. (2019). Respiratory disorders of the donkey. *The Veterinary Clinics of North America. Equine Practice* 35 (3): 561–573.

Robertson, S.A. and Bailey, J.E. (2002). Aerosolized salbutamol (albuterol) improves PaO_2 in hypoxaemic anaesthetized horses – a prospective clinical trial in 81 horses. *Veterinary Anaesthesia and Analgesia* 29 (4): 212–218.

Robertson, J.T., Muir, W.W., and Sams, R. (1981). Cardiopulmonary effects of butorphanol tartrate in horses. *American Journal of Veterinary Research* 42 (1): 41–44.

Robinson, N.E. and Sorenson, P.R. (1978). Pathophysiology of airway obstruction in horses: a review. *Journal of the American Veterinary Medical Association* 172 (3): 299–303.

Rossi, H., Virtala, A.-M., and Raekallio, M. (2018). Comparison of tracheal wash and bronchoalveolar lavage cytology in 154 horses with and without respiratory signs in a referral hospital over 2009–2015. *Frontiers in Veterinary Science* 5: 61.

Rossi, T.M., Moore, A., O'Sullivan, T.L. et al. (2019a). Equine rhinitis a virus infection at a Standardbred training facility: incidence, clinical signs, and risk factors for clinical disease. *Frontiers in Veterinary Science* 6: 71. https://doi.org/10.3389/fvets.2019.00071.

Rossi, H., Raekallio, M., Määttä, H. et al. (2019b). Effects of general anaesthesia in dorsal recumbency with and without vatinoxan on bronchoalveolar lavage cytology of healthy horses. *The Veterinary Journal* 251: 105352.

Rush, B. and Mair, T. (2004). Noninfectious pulmonary diseases. In: *Equine Respiratory Diseases* (eds. B. Rush and T. Mair), 189–231. Ames, IA: Blackwell Publishing.

Russotto, V., Sabaté, S., and Canct, J. (2019). Development of a prediction model for postoperative pneumonia. *European Journal of Anaesthesiology* 36: 93–104.

Sarma, V.J. (1992). Use of ketamine in acute severe asthma. *Acta Anaesthesiologica Scandinavica* 36 (1): 106–107.

Saulez, M.N., Dzikiti, B., and Voigt, A. (2009). Traumatic perforation of the trachea in two horses caused by orotracheal intubation. *Veterinary Record* 164 (23): 719–722.

Séguin, V., Garon, D., Lemauviel-Lavenant, S. et al. (2012). How to improve the hygienic quality of forages for horse feeding. *Journal of the Science of Food and Agriculture* 92 (4): 975–986.

Senior, M. (2005). Post-anaesthetic pulmonary oedema in horses: a review. *Veterinary Anaesthesia and Analgesia* 32: 193–200.

Soliman, M.G., Brindle, G.F., and Kuster, G. (1975). Response to hypercapnia under ketamine anaesthesia. *Canadian Anaesthetists' Society Journal* 22 (4): 486–494.

Sopena, N. and Sabrià, M., Neunos 2000 Study Group (2005). Multicenter study of hospital-acquired pneumonia in non-ICU patients. *Chest* 127 (1): 213–219.

Steffey, E.P., Kelly, A.B., Farver, T.B. et al. (1985). Cardiovascular and respiratory effects of acetylpromazine and xylazine on halothane anesthetized horses. *Journal of Veterinary Pharmacology and Therapeutics* 8 (3): 290–302.

Steiger, R.R. and Williams, M.A. (2000). Granulomatous tracheitis caused by *Conidiobolus coronatus* in a horse. *Journal of Veterinary Internal Medicine* 14 (3): 311–314.

Sweeney, C.R., Whitlock, R.H., Meirs, D.A. et al. (1987). Complications associated with *Streptococcus equi* infection on a horse farm. *Journal of the American Veterinary Medical Association* 191 (11): 1446–1448.

Sweeney, C.R., Holcombe, S.J., Barningham, S.C. et al. (1991). Aerobic and anaerobic isolates from horses with pneumonia or pleuropneumonia and antimicrobial susceptibility patterns of aerobes. *Journal of the American Veterinary Medical Association* 198 (5): 839–842.

Tilley, P., Sales Luis, J.P., and Branco Ferreira, M. (2012). Correlation and discriminant analysis between clinical, endoscopic, thoracic X-ray and bronchoalveolar lavage fluid cytology scores, for staging horses with recurrent airway obstruction (RAO). *Research in Veterinary Science* 93 (2): 1006–1014.

Timoney, J.F. and Kumar, P. (2008). Early pathogenesis of equine *Streptococcus equi* infection (strangles). *Equine Veterinary Journal* 40 (7): 637–642.

Timoney, J.F., Suther, P., Velineni, S. et al. (2014). The antiphagocytic activity of SeM of *Streptococcus equi* requires capsule. *Journal of Equine Science* 25 (2): 53–56.

Tomasic, M., Mann, L.S., and Soma, L.R. (1997). Effects of sedation, anesthesia, and endotracheal intubation on respiratory mechanics in adult horses. *American Journal of Veterinary Research* 58 (6): 641–646.

Touzot-Jourde, G., Stedman, N.L., and Trim, C.M. (2005). The effect of two endotracheal tube cuff inflation pressure on liquid aspiration and tracheal wall damage in horses. *Veterinary Anaesthesia and Analgesia* 32 (1): 23–29.

Trim, C.M. (2015). Endotracheal intubation in the horse – are complications really rare? *Equine Veterinary Education* 27 (4): 176–178.

Tute, A.S., Wilkins, P.A., Gleed, R.D. et al. (1996). Negative pressure pulmonary edema as a post-anesthetic complication associated with upper airway obstruction in a horse. *Veterinary Surgery* 25 (6): 519–523.

Tyagi, R.P., Arnold, J.P., Usenik, E.A. et al. (1964). Effects of thiopental sodium (pentothal sodium) anesthesia on the horse. *The Cornell Veterinarian* 54: 584–602.

Tyler, W.S., Gillespie, J.R., and Nowell, J.A. (1971). Modern functional morphology of the equine lung. *Equine Veterinary Journal* 3 (3): 84–94.

Vaneker, M., Santosa, J.P., Heunks, L.M. et al. (2009). Isoflurane attenuates pulmonary interleukin-1beta and systemic tumor necrosis factor-alpha following mechanical ventilation in healthy mice. *Acta Anaesthesiologica Scandinavica* 53 (6): 742–748.

Von Ungern-Sternberg, B.S., Saudan, S., Petak, F. et al. (2008). Desflurane but not sevoflurane impairs airway and respiratory tissue mechanics in children with susceptible airways. *Anesthesiology* 108 (2): 216–224.

Waller, A.S. (2014). New perspectives for the diagnosis, control, treatment, and prevention of strangles in horses. *The Veterinary Clinics of North America. Equine Practice* 30 (3): 591–607.

Wasko, A.J., Barkema, H.W., Nicol, J. et al. (2011). Evaluation of a risk-screening questionnaire to detect equine lung inflammation: results of a large field study. *Equine Veterinary Journal* 43 (2): 145–152.

Watkins, A.R. and Parente, E.J. (2018). Salpingopharyngeal fistula as a treatment for guttural pouch mycosis in seven horses. *Equine Veterinary Journal* 50 (6): 781–786.

West, J.B. (2011). Mechanics of Breathing. In: *Respiratory Physiology – the Essentials*, 9e,

95–122. Baltimore, MD: Lippincott, Williams & Wilkins.

Widdicombe, J. (2006). Reflexes from the lungs and airways: historical perspective. *Journal of Applied Physiology* 101 (2): 628–634.

Wiklund, M., Kellgren, M., Wulcan, S. et al. (2020). Effects of pulsed inhaled nitric oxide on arterial oxygenation during mechanical ventilation in anaesthetised horses undergoing elective arthroscopy or emergency colic surgery. *Equine Veterinary Journal* 52 (1): 76–82.

Wilkes, A.R., Raj, N., and Hall, J.E. (2003). Adverse airway events during brief nasal inhalations of volatile anaesthetics: the effect of humidity and repeated exposure on incidence in volunteers preselected by response to desflurane. *Anaesthesia* 58 (3): 207–216.

Willoughby, R., Ecker, G., McKee, S. et al. (1992). The effects of equine rhinovirus, influenza virus and herpesvirus infection on tracheal clearance rate in horses. *Canadian Journal of Veterinary Research* 56 (2): 115–121.

Wilson, W.D. (1993). Equine influenza. *The Veterinary Clinics of North America. Equine Practice* 9 (2): 257–282.

Wood, J.L.N., Newton, J.R., Chanter, N. et al. (2005). Association between respiratory disease and bacterial and viral infections in British racehorses association between respiratory disease and bacterial and viral infections in British racehorses. *Journal of Clinical Microbiology* 43 (1): 120–126.

Yamanaka, T. and Sadikot, R.T. (2013). Opioid effect of lungs. *Respirology* 18: 255–262.

Yu, M.F., Wang, Z.W., Robinson, N.E. et al. (1994). Modulation of bronchial smooth muscle function in horses with heaves. *Journal of Applied Physiology* 77 (5): 2149–2154.

4

Anesthetic Management for Surgery of the Respiratory Tract

Klaus Hopster[1] and Eileen Hackett[2]

[1] *Department of Clinical Studies, School of Veterinary Medicine, University of Pennsylvania, 382 West Street Road, Kennett Square, PA, 19348, USA*
[2] *Department of Clinical Sciences, College of Veterinary Medicine, Cornell University, 930 Campus Road, Ithaca, NY, 14853, USA*

Introduction

Maintaining respiratory system function is critical to safe anesthetic management. Hence, surgery of the respiratory tract adds challenges and necessitates cooperation between the surgical and anesthetic team especially when managing horses with pre-existing respiratory disease. Sedation and anesthesia may further impair respiratory system function, and thoughtful selection of protocols, careful application, and monitoring are imperative.

Pre-procedural Evaluation

Horses undergoing surgery of the respiratory system have often undergone extensive examination prior to admission. Clinical signs of respiratory disorders are varied, and range in extremes from fulminant respiratory distress to minor performance limiting wind issues. Prior to planning a sedation and anesthetic operative protocol, it is important to consider the history, signalment, physical examination parameters, and diagnostic information available.

Upper airway obstruction is typically accompanied by increased airflow turbulence and breathing sounds, in addition to bradypneic breathing patterns. Static disorders that contribute to upper airway obstruction include subepiglottic or nasopharyngeal cysts, nasal septum enlargement, nasal edema, arytenoid chondritis, epiglottitis, and tracheal stenosis. Static disorders are generally identified with flexible endoscopy or via radiographic examination. Conditions that contribute to increased inspiratory negative pressure and dynamic airway collapse include recurrent laryngeal neuropathy, laryngeal dysplasia, epiglottic retroversion, nasopharyngeal collapse, and tracheal collapse. Identification of dynamic disorders often requires exercising endoscopic examination.

Assessments of the lower airway for pulmonary and pleural space conditions typically begin with cardiopulmonary auscultation and rebreathing examination. Resting tachypnea or an altered respiratory pattern, especially one associated with increased abdominal effort, could signify lung disease. Diagnostics could include tracheal wash, bronchoalveolar lavage, thoracic ultrasonography, and thoracic radiographs. Arterial blood gas analysis is an important diagnostic element when altered pulmonary function is suspected. Diaphragmatic integrity can be assessed with thoracic ultrasound or radiography. A lung biopsy could be considered if interstitial pulmonary disease is identified.

Anatomical and Physiological Considerations

In addition to the primary gas exchange functions of the respiratory system, thermoregulation, local immunity, filtration of inhaled gases, and protection of the respiratory tract from aspiration of swallowed substances are important (David and Marshall 2012). Anatomically and physiologically, the respiratory system can be divided into gas conduction and gas exchanging segments (Weibel 2017). The upper airways of the horse, including the nasopharynx, trachea, bronchi, and bronchioles, facilitate gas conduction into the lungs. In the lungs, gas exchange is dependent on alveolar ventilation, pulmonary perfusion, and gaseous diffusion (Petersson and Glenny 2014). The diaphragm and intercostal muscles provide force needed for ventilation. The pumping action of these respiratory muscles results in large pressure changes in the airway. On inhalation, pressures are negative, resulting in movement of air from outside the nares to inside the lungs (Nason et al. 2012). On exhalation, pressure in the upper airway becomes positive, driving the air out of the lungs against the atmospheric pressure. In certain upper airway regions, rigid support by bone or cartilage is incompatible with other functions, such as swallowing. The larynx and pharynx are therefore supported by upper airway dilator muscles. On inhalation, these muscles begin to contract just before the diaphragm contracts and remain active during inhalation for the purpose of opening and stiffening the airway before sub-atmospheric pressure is created (Parente 2018). When functioning, these muscles provide appropriate tension to prevent dynamic collapse of tissues during inhalation. Most sedatives, including alpha-2-agonists, and most general anesthetics, cause a certain degree of muscle relaxation (Manneveau et al. 2018). This decrease in muscle tone leads to a smaller, more compliant, airway conduction system, resulting in a reduction of airflow and an increase in respiratory work (Petersson and Glenny 2014).

Upper airway impedance is further affected by head and neck position. In resting horses, a neutral head position results in an angle between the head and neck $>100°$. Reducing this angle can increase the work of breathing due to an increase in impedance (Parente 2018). When horses maintain a low head position, as with sedation, resulting nasal edema and narrowing of the nasal passage could further increase airway impedance. Multiple strategies have been developed to overcome the increase in impedance resulting from decreased upper airway diameter during sedation and anesthesia. In some circumstances, endotracheal intubation or tracheotomy could be necessary (Mahmood and Wahidi 2016). Positive pressure ventilation can help reduce the work of breathing, and delivering helium gas mixtures can reduce turbulent flow and airway resistance, improving ventilation and gas exchange. Numerous studies suggest that people with lower airway obstruction benefit from helium gas mixtures during mechanical ventilation (Truebel et al. 2019).

Diffusion is the primary mode of gas transport in lung capillaries and due to differences in diffusion efficiency among gases, hypoxemia is often recognized prior to hypoventilation (Spaeth and Friedlander 1967). In amenable non-intubated or standing equids with recognized hypoxemia, intranasal or mask supplementation with flow-by oxygen can be attempted. Flow-by oxygen supplementation efficacy has been evaluated in horses and foals. Healthy foals experience a dose-dependent increase in inspired oxygen fraction and arterial oxygen partial pressure with nasal cannula insufflation (Wong et al. 2010). Similar increases in inspired oxygen fraction and arterial oxygen partial pressure have been observed in healthy horses and those with lung disease during nasal cannula insufflation (Wilson et al. 2006). A short duration of intranasal oxygen supplementation prior to induction of general anesthesia has been shown to moderately increase arterial oxygenation measured immediately after induction in adult horses undergoing elective surgery (van Oostrom et al. 2017).

Multiple lower airway disorders, such as pulmonary edema, acute respiratory distress syndrome, and bacterial or viral pneumonia, can lead to ventilation-perfusion and diffusion impairments that affect pulmonary gas exchange (Mellor and Beausoleil 2017). As respiratory function is frequently depressed with most sedative and anesthetic agents, co-existing respiratory diseases can impair function even further (Auckburally and Nyman 2017). Most sedatives and tranquilizers like acepromazine and alpha-2-agonists have some, although often minimal, respiratory depressant effects that may be potentiated by other opioid or anesthetic drugs. Alpha-2-agonists have been shown to impair pulmonary perfusion and arterial oxygenation, and increase pulmonary shunting in standing, sedated, and anesthetized horses (Marntell et al. 2005). These detrimental effects can be partially limited by adding acepromazine to the sedation protocol, which has been shown to subsequently improve pulmonary perfusion (Marntell et al. 2005). General anesthesia and changes induced by positioning in lateral or dorsal recumbency also contribute to an impairment of ventilation and perfusion matching, leading to worsening respiratory function especially in patients with co-existing respiratory disease (Hopster et al. 2017a,b).

Sedation for Standing Upper Airway Surgeries

Upper respiratory surgery performed in the standing sedated horse is common and represents a special challenge. The horse must be sufficiently sedated to tolerate the surgical manipulation but must also maintain a safe standing position without significant compromise to breathing. The length and complexity of the surgical procedure often dictates whether sedation is administered as a bolus or variable rate infusion. Sedation is primarily achieved via administration of alpha-2-agonists. Combination of alpha-2-agonists with opioid agents results in synergistic sedative and analgesic effects (Corletto et al. 2005). The authors recommend placing a jugular catheter prior to surgery, which allows for repeated dosing or infusions, in addition to providing venous access if complications are encountered.

Local anesthesia of the surgical site is often necessary prior to surgery in the standing, sedated horse. Common methods of local anesthetic delivery in equine airway surgery include topical mucosal splash blocks, local infiltration, and regional perineural injection. Local anesthetics should be applied approximately 5–10 minutes prior to the surgical procedures.

Tracheotomy/Tracheostomy

As tracheotomy is typically a short procedure, horses are typically sedated with a single intravenous bolus of xylazine, detomidine, or romifidine. This may be combined with morphine (e.g. 0.05 mg/kg) or butorphanol (e.g. 0.02 mg/kg) to take advantage of the sedative and analgesic synergy of alpha-2-agonists and opioids. This combined approach could inhibit the superficial hypersensitivity associated with alpha-2-agonists and decrease tracheal sensitivity due to opioid mediated cough-suppression, resulting in improved patient compliance during tracheal manipulation (Kamei et al. 1989). Low dosages of opioids are recommended when being used for sedation enhancement as these drugs can lead to excitement and mild headshaking and bobbing in horses (Dönselmann Im Sande et al. 2017) which could make these procedures challenging. Local anesthetic application for tracheotomy and tracheostomy is typically achieved via subcutaneous infiltration of 3–4 ml lidocaine (2%) per 100 kg bwt. Local anesthetic can be injected directly along ventral midline in the region of planned tracheotomy, or in a U-shaped infiltration cranial and lateral to the surgical site. When the tracheotomy is done prior to performing surgery under anesthesia as for example an arytenoidectomy, the endotracheal tube can be introduced through this site prior to anesthetic induction to maintain control of the airway and facilitate mechanical ventilation during recumbency (Figure 4.1). Note that the size of the endotracheal tube may be of a smaller diameter than an orotracheal tube increasing resistance and work of breathing in the spontaneously breathing horse.

In horses with life-threatening acute upper airway obstruction, emergency tracheotomy

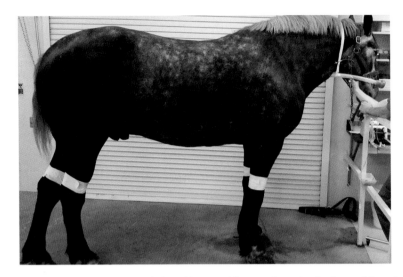

Figure 4.1 This photograph depicts a draft breed horse with an endotracheal tube positioned via tracheotomy prior to induction of anesthesia. Pre-placement of the endotracheal tube simplifies connection to the rebreathing circuit during surgical positioning.

may be required for treatment. In some cases, surgical preparation and local anesthesia is forgone in the interest of immediate control of the airway. For this reason, we often clip, prepare, and inject local anesthetic in horses in which development of upper airway obstruction is a concern (e.g. prior to recovery following sinus surgery). We have also found it helpful to have a tracheotomy kit, including a scalpel and tracheotomy tube, hung on the stall of horses considered to be at risk for upper airway obstruction, as this can save time and confusion. If a horse has collapsed as a result of airway obstruction, insertion of a nasal or oral endotracheal tube could be lifesaving and potentially more rapid than surgical intervention. In this instance, if multiple personnel are present, and it is determined interventions can be achieved safely, one person could intubate while another could begin the tracheotomy.

Intraluminal Nasopharyngeal and Laryngeal Procedures

Multiple surgical upper airway procedures are performed in the standing horse with flexible endoscopic guidance (Hawkins and Andrews-Jones 2001) using specially designed scissors,

hooked knives, electrocautery loops, or where appropriate lasers. Examples of these procedures include epiglottic entrapment correction, subepiglottic cyst removal, ventriculectomy, ventriculocordectomy, auditory tube diverticulotomy, and nasopharyngeal mass removal. Sedation may be performed as previously mentioned. Local anesthetic can be applied as a mucosal splash block by injecting via the endoscopic working channel under visual control, ensuring the area of planned excision is well coated (Figure 4.2). Topical local anesthetic can be delivered to this region without endoscopic control via a nasopharyngeal catheter inserted to the level of the medial ocular canthus (Colbath et al. 2017). Swallowing during nasopharyngeal administration was shown to be important for distribution of the topical agent.

Prosthetic Laryngoplasty

Because of the length and complexity of the prosthetic laryngoplasty in the standing horse, sedation with a variable rate infusion of alpha-2-agonist is recommended. This can be preceded by an initial intravenous bolus. For example, detomidine (up to 10 µg/kg) as a bolus may be followed by an infusion ranging from 0.2 to

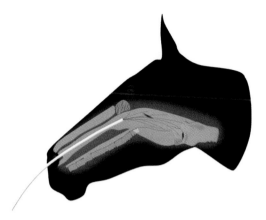

Figure 4.2 Nasopharyngeal topical local anesthetic application. A catheter is inserted to the level of the medial ocular canthus and local anesthetic is injected to facilitate topical mucosal anesthesia. If the anesthetic is injected via a flexible endoscopic working channel, it is possible to specifically target the application with visual control. *Source:* Illustration provided by Kelsea A. Ericksen, DVM, MS.

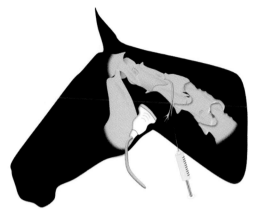

Figure 4.3 Cervical plexus local anesthetic injection provides regional anesthesia of the superficial structures over the larynx and upper neck. Ultrasound guidance is used to identify the cervical plexus prior to injection. *Source:* Illustration provided by Kelsea A. Ericksen, DVM, MS.

0.6 μg/kg/min. If necessary, based on the horse's behavior, additional intravenous detomidine bolus (e.g. 5 μg/kg) can be administered during the procedure or the infusion rate can be adjusted for the desired sedation. An intravenous morphine bolus (0.03–0.1 mg/kg) can be administered early in the procedure to augment operative analgesia.

A variety of techniques have been utilized for local anesthetic application with prosthetic laryngoplasty in the standing horse. A dual approach utilizes surgical site infiltration with local anesthetic in combination with a topical laryngeal mucosal splash block (Figure 4.2). Infiltration of the surgical site can be performed with a ring or line block immediately ventral to the linguofacial vein and injection or topical sponge application of local anesthetic prior to needle passage through the dorsal cricoid cartilage and muscular process of the arytenoid cartilage (Rossignol et al. 2015). Recently this dual approach has been compared in horses undergoing prosthetic laryngoplasty to ultrasound-guided cervical plexus injection (Figure 4.3) combined with a subcutaneous line block immediately ventral to the

linguofacial vein (Campoy et al. 2018). Investigators found that infiltration of the cervical plexus region provided similar block quality but improved surgical field conditions relative to tissue edema and landmark identification (Campoy et al. 2018). As described by Campoy et al., an ultrasound transducer is positioned midway between the body of the second cervical vertebrae, caudal to the parotid gland and ventral to the omotransversarius muscle. The ventral branch of the second cervical spinal nerve (C2) is identified. A 20-gauge 9 cm Tuohy needle is then advanced toward the intermuscular plane between the cleidomastoideus and the longus capitis muscles. Once the tip of the needle is located in the proximity of C2, approximately 8–10 ml of local anesthetic per 100 kg bwt. is injected.

General Anesthesia for Airway Surgery

Airway surgery is commonly performed under general anesthesia and the decision to do so is often related to the type of surgery, preference of the surgeon, and health, breed, and demeanor of the horse. The risk of fatal complications related to general anesthesia is <1% for elective surgical procedures in horses; therefore, with careful preparation and planning, performance of surgery requiring general anesthesia is considered to be associated with a low risk of attendant anesthetic complications (Johnston et al. 2002).

Laryngeal Tie-Forward

Surgical laryngeal advancement (laryngeal tie-forward) is performed for dorsal displacement of the soft palate, dysphagia, and other disorders associated with laryngeal descent (Woodie et al. 2005; Ortved et al. 2010; Virgin et al. 2016). Orotracheal intubation is appropriate, as the surgical procedure does not require penetration of the airway or luminal endoscopic guidance. The surgery is performed in dorsal recumbency with the head supported. Prior to securing the sutures, the head must be lifted by an assistant such that the head and neck are angled at approximately 90° (Woodie et al. 2005). After the laryngeal advancement sutures are secured, the head should be supported in a moderately flexed position for the remainder of the procedure, and care should be taken not to radically extend the head and neck during movement to anesthetic recovery. The anesthetist and surgeon should discuss whether placement of the arterial line in the facial artery will interfere with the surgical field. Particular attention to the endotracheal tube must also be paid during repositioning to ensure its positioning in the airway and patency. Luminal airway hemorrhage is possible if the ventricle is penetrated during suture passage.

Sternothyroideus Myectomy/Tenectomy

Myectomy/tenectomy of the sternothyroideus insertion is a relatively short procedure that can be performed under injectable general anesthesia. After sufficient sedation, an intravenous bolus of ketamine (2.2 mg/kg) can be used to induce anesthesia. Combining this induction agent with a muscle relaxant drug such as guaifenesin (80 mg/kg) or midazolam (0.05 mg/kg) is recommended to reduce laryngeal reflexes and improve the surgical conditions. Orotracheal intubation should be performed to secure and maintain the airway and facilitate supplementation of oxygen or use of an inhaled agent if needed.

Cleft Palate Repair

Cleft palate is an uncommon congenital condition in horses, affecting palatal structure and function. This deformity results from failure of the lateral palatine processes to fuse during embryonic development. Foals with cleft palate often have difficulty nursing and swallowing, with a higher risk of aspiration and subsequent pneumonia. Prognosis following surgical correction depends on the size and location of the cleft, with early repair considered an important factor in successful outcomes. Because cleft palate repair is often pursued in neonates with some degree of aspiration pneumonia, supplementation of oxygen via nasal catheter prior to induction is recommended due to the positive effects on arterial oxygen partial pressure (van Oostrom et al. 2017). Continuous pulse oximetry with intermittent arterial blood gas assessment of oxygenation is recommended. Nasotracheal intubation will facilitate improved surgical access to the oral cavity. The relatively small nasal tube diameter can however result in an increase in airway resistance; therefore, breathing pattern and effort should be monitored closely, especially in foals breathing spontaneously. If the foal is cardiovascularly stable, mechanical ventilation may be instituted. Esophagostomy tube placement may be elected for peri-operative management and patient support. During recovery, the foal should continue to receive oxygen and necessary support until ambulatory.

Prosthetic Laryngoplasty

In horses, recurrent laryngeal neuropathy is a common upper airway disorder resulting in altered upper airway dynamics, where degenerative axonopathy of the recurrent laryngeal nerve leads to cricoarytenoideus dorsalis muscle atrophy and subsequent collapse of the arytenoid cartilage and associated vocal fold (Krueger et al. 2019). Prosthetic laryngoplasty is pursued to maintain moderate arytenoid abduction. This procedure is often combined with ventriculectomy or ventriculocordectomy, which can be performed during the same sedative (as noted previously) or anesthetic episode. Following routine sedation and induction protocols, general anesthesia can be maintained with either total intravenous anesthesia (TIVA) or volatile anesthetics. Endotracheal intubation is recommended regardless of the strategy selected. Endotracheal tube insertion can be more difficult due to loss of arytenoid abduction resulting in narrowing of the rima glottidis. To minimize trauma and facilitate the surgeon working around the tube without extubation, a smaller lumen endotracheal tube may be selected. Positive pressure ventilation may be used to overcome the increased resistance and work of breathing. On occasion, a surgeon may wish to temporarily extubate the horse while an endoscope is passed into the trachea to visualize the lumen (to ensure no luminal suture is evident) and degree of abduction of the arytenoid. The anesthetist should be prepared to administer injectable medications to maintain anesthesia and provide oxygen until re-intubation is possible.

If a ventriculocordectomy is conducted with a surgical laser during the anesthetic episode, the fraction of inspired oxygen should be maintained at ≤30% (Lampotang et al. 2005). Higher fractions of oxygen delivered via endotracheal tube located adjacent to the laser surgical site increase the risk of fire and thermal injuries (Jones et al. 2019). To accommodate these recommendations, horses anesthetized using TIVA may be allowed to breathe room air during the laser surgery. For horses administered volatile anesthetics, strategies to maintain a low fraction of inspired oxygen include delivering the anesthetic with medical air, an air and oxygen mixture, or a helium and oxygen mixture. Helium and oxygen mixtures are preferred in human medicine due to their superior laminar flow characteristics (Papamoschou 1995). However, a recent study performed in horses indicated that there are no clinically relevant differences in lung compliance or oxygenation when comparing room air to helium oxygen mixtures (Varner et al. 2019).

Surgical Arterial Occlusion for Guttural Pouch Mycosis

Sedation and anesthesia of horses with guttural pouch mycosis is often complicated by recent acute blood loss history and increased risk of repeat hemorrhage. Pre-anesthetic blood transfusion is generally considered necessary in horses with a packed cell volume <20–25% during acute hemorrhage and with blood lactate concentrations ≥4 mmol/l following fluid resuscitation (Mudge 2014). Use caution when administering alpha-2-agonists as they will decrease cardiac output and increase blood pressure, possibly resulting in clot disruption and additional hemorrhage risk (Wagner et al. 1991). Regional changes in blood flow dynamics can be avoided by maintaining a neutral head position in the sedated horse, or well above the level of the heart, and this may lessen risk of hemorrhage. During anesthesia, mean arterial blood pressure targets of 60–65 mmHg for brief periods may help reduce bleeding, but this type of management must be balanced with risk for myopathy that is clearly linked to hypotension in horses. (Grandy et al. 1987). Hypertension should be avoided to increase surgical success by minimizing risk of hemorrhage, as well as the impact on successful ligation, occlusion, or coil placement. Surgical ligation of guttural pouch arteries occluded by blood clot can illicit hemorrhage or embolism, which can impact the brain and special senses; therefore, careful monitoring during the anesthetic and post anesthetic recovery period is essential. These animals can have either seizure-like behaviors or severely reduced mental status and visual impairment during the recovery and early post-operative period. Human safety considerations must be paramount if neurological or visual deficits are suspected.

Ceratohyoidectomy

Temporohyoid osteoarthropathy results in ankylosis and microfracture, with facial nerve paralysis and vestibular syndrome as common sequelae (Oliver and Hardy 2015). This disorder can be unilateral or bilateral and is typically confirmed with guttural pouch endoscopic or computed tomographic examination (Hilton et al. 2009). Ceratohyoidectomy removes the connection between the stylohyoid and basihyoid bones of the hyoid apparatus, decreasing cycling pressure on the arthritic temporohyoid joint and subsequent pain and inflammation. Applying minimal tension to the tongue during endotracheal intubation and instrumentation can lessen hyoid support injury, especially in horses with bilateral disease. Because of facial nerve deficits and subsequent ocular injury, temporary tarsorrhaphy or other procedures may be required during the anesthetic episode, which could necessitate a change in patient positioning. Lubrication and protection of the eye(s) into the recovery period is recommended. Hemorrhage encountered intraoperatively has led to hematoma formation and external compression resulting in acute upper airway obstruction following extubation (Oliver and Hardy 2015). Ataxia and other vestibular deficits can also create notable challenges during anesthetic recovery, and again caution is advised when intervening to ensure personnel safety.

Thoracotomy

A variety of equine conditions require a thoracotomy. These disorders include pleuropneumonia, lung abscessation/foreign body penetration, diaphragmatic hernia, or neoplastic disease, in particular granular cell tumor resection. In horses with pleuropneumonia, thoracotomy or thoracostomy are pursued to establish drainage, assess prognosis, or for adhesiolysis, tissue plasminogen activator administration, or pleural lavage.

Horses undergoing thoracic surgery have a higher risk of hypoxemia because of the interaction of general anesthesia, required recumbency, atelectasis and ventilation-perfusion mismatch (Rehder and Sessler 1973). Increasingly, thoracotomy procedures have been replaced by thoracoscopy (Lewis et al. 1992). Advantages of thoracoscopy over thoracotomy are the lower degree of invasiveness and therefore lesser nociceptive stimulation during, and lower degrees of pain after the procedure. Hemodynamic parameters should be closely monitored, in addition to evaluation of arterial blood gas parameters at regular intervals to investigate ventilation and gas exchange. In most cases, controlled ventilation is required to maintain lung function and gas exchange. Atelectasis and ventilation-perfusion mismatch can be reduced by applying positive end-expiratory pressure (Hopster et al. 2011). However, this technique, particularly when using positive end expiratory pressure (PEEP) of 15 cm H_2O or higher, can reduce preload and contribute to decreases in cardiac output (Hopster et al. 2017a,b). Therefore, intraoperative monitoring of cardiovascular parameters, including blood pressure, is critical.

Surgery of the lung often requires independent lung ventilation, with only the unoperated lung ventilated during the procedure. This can be conducted by using a double-lumen endotracheal tube, which can be positioned in the trachea following induction of general anesthesia. However, large double-lumen tubes are not available and therefore this might only be an option for small ponies and foals. Correct positioning of the double-lumen endotracheal tube is confirmed with bronchoscopy. Alternatively, in large and adult horses, an endotracheal blocker system can be created by combining a standard endotracheal tube and a commercially available bronchoalveolar catheter (Gozalo-Marcilla et al. 2012). Following induction, the bronchoalveolar catheter is advanced into the bronchus of the affected lung with endoscopic guidance. The bronchoalveolar catheter balloon can then be inflated and deflated to block ventilation, hence allowing ventilation of one or both lungs as indicated throughout the procedure. Single lumen tubes may be placed endobronchially via a tracheotomy, but do not allow for support of the contralateral lung.

Summary

Sedation and anesthetic management of horses with respiratory disease requiring surgical intervention requires communication between surgery and anesthesia personnel. All personnel should be familiar with relevant history, examination findings, diagnostic information, and unique procedural requirements prior to protocol development. Use of analgesics and sedatives can minimize patient stress, but these can worsen respiratory difficulty. Hence it is important to have necessary equipment to provide support to the animal and facilitate delivery of oxygen and support of breathing when needed. Preparing treatment and barn areas with emergency drug access, tracheotomy and endotracheal intubation supplies will ensure that critical materials are on hand in case of respiratory emergency.

References

Auckburally, A. and Nyman, G. (2017). Review of hypoxaemia in anaesthetized horses: predisposing factors, consequences and management. *Veterinary Anaesthesia and Analgesia* 44(3): 397–408.

Campoy, L., Morris, T.B., Ducharme, N.G. et al. (2018). Unilateral cervical plexus block for prosthetic laryngoplasty in the standing horse. *Equine Veterinary Journal* 50(6): 727–732.

Colbath, A.C., Valdes-Martinez, A., Leise, B.S., and Hackett, E.S. (2017). Evaluation of two methods for topical application of contrast medium to the pharyngeal and laryngeal region of horses. *American Journal of Veterinary Research* 78(9): 1098–1103.

Corletto, F., Raisis, A.A., and Brearley, J.C. (2005). Comparison of morphine and butorphanol as pre-anaesthetic agents in combination with romifidine for field castration in ponies. *Veterinary Anaesthesia and Analgesia* 32(1): 16–22.

David, E.A. and Marshall, M.B. (2012). Physiologic evaluation of lung resection candidates. *Thoracic Surgery Clinics* 22 (1): 47–54, vi.

Dönselmann Im Sande, P., Hopster, K., and Kästner, S. (2017). Effects of morphine, butorphanol and levomethadone in different doses on thermal nociceptive thresholds in horses. *Tierärztliche Praxis. Ausgabe G, Grosstiere/Nutztiere* 45(2): 98–106.

Gozalo-Marcilla, M., Schauvliege, S., Torfs, S. et al. (2012). An alternative for one lung ventilation in an adult horse requiring thoracotomy. *Vlaams Diergeneeskd Tijdschr* 81: 98–101.

Grandy, J.L., Steffey, E.P., Hodgson, D.S., and Woliner, M.J. (1987). Arterial hypotension and the development of postanesthetic myopathy in halothane-anesthetized horses. *American Journal of Veterinary Research* 48(2): 192–197.

Hawkins, J.F. and Andrews-Jones, L. (2001). Neodymium:yttrium aluminum garnet laser ventriculocordectomy in standing horses. *American Journal of Veterinary Research* 62(4): 531–537.

Hilton, H., Puchalski, S.M., and Aleman, M. (2009). The computed tomographic appearance of equine temporohyoid osteoarthropathy. *Veterinary Radiology & Ultrasound* 50(2): 151–156.

Hopster, K., Kastner, S.B., Rohn, K., and Ohnesorge, B. (2011). Intermittent positive pressure ventilation with constant positive end-expiratory pressure and alveolar recruitment manoeuvre during inhalation anaesthesia in horses undergoing surgery for colic, and its influence on the early recovery period. *Veterinary Anaesthesia and Analgesia* 38(3): 169–177.

Hopster, K., Rohn, K., Ohnesorge, B., and Kastner, S.B.R. (2017a). Controlled mechanical ventilation with constant positive end-expiratory pressure and alveolar recruitment manoeuvres during anaesthesia in laterally or dorsally recumbent horses. *Veterinary Anaesthesia and Analgesia* 44(1): 121–126.

Hopster, K., Wogatzki, A., Geburek, F. et al. (2017b). Effects of positive end-expiratory pressure titration on intestinal oxygenation and perfusion in isoflurane anaesthetised horses. *Equine Veterinary Journal* 49(2): 250–256.

Johnston, G.M., Eastment, J.K., Wood, J., and Taylor, P.M. (2002). The confidential enquiry into perioperative equine fatalities (CEPEF): mortality results of phases 1 and 2. *Veterinary Anaesthesia and Analgesia* 29(4): 159–170.

Jones, T.S., Black, I.H., Robinson, T.N., and Jones, E.L. (2019). Operating room fires. *Anesthesiology* https://doi.org/10.1097/ ALN. 0000000000002598.

Kamei, J., Mori, T., Ogawa, M., and Kasuya, Y. (1989). Subsensitivity to the cough-depressant effects of opioid and nonopioid antitussives in morphine-dependent rats: relationship to central serotonin function. *Pharmacology, Biochemistry, and Behavior* 34(3): 595–598.

Krueger, C.R., Lewis, R.D., McIlwraith, C.W. et al. (2019). A retrospective cohort study of racing performance in quarter horses undergoing prosthetic laryngoplasty for treatment of recurrent laryngeal neuropathy. *Journal of the American Veterinary Medical Association* 254(4): 496–500.

Lampotang, S., Gravenstein, N., Paulus, D.A., and Gravenstein, D. (2005). Reducing the

incidence of surgical fires: supplying nasal cannulae with sub-100% O_2 gas mixtures from anesthesia machines. *Anesthesia and Analgesia* 101(5): 1407–1412.

Lewis, R.J., Caccavale, R.J., Sisler, G.E., and Mackenzie, J.W. (1992). One hundred consecutive patients undergoing video-assisted thoracic operations. *The Annals of Thoracic Surgery* 54(3): 421–426.

Mahmood, K. and Wahidi, M.M. (2016). The changing role for tracheostomy in patients requiring mechanical ventilation. *Clinics in Chest Medicine* 37(4): 741–751.

Manneveau, G., Lecallard, J., Thorin, C. et al. (2018). Comparison of morphological changes and tactile sensitivity of the pharynx and larynx between four standing sedative and analgesic protocols in eight adult healthy horses. *Veterinary Anaesthesia and Analgesia* 45(4): 477–486.

Marntell, S., Nyman, G., Funkquist, P., and Hedenstierna, G. (2005). Effects of acepromazine on pulmonary gas exchange and circulation during sedation and dissociative anaesthesia in horses. *Veterinary Anaesthesia and Analgesia* 32(2): 83–93.

Mellor, D.J. and Beausoleil, N.J. (2017). Equine welfare during exercise: an evaluation of breathing, breathlessness and bridles. *Animals (Basel)* 7(6).

Mudge, M.C. (2014). Acute hemorrhage and blood transfusions in horses. *The Veterinary Clinics of North America. Equine Practice* 30(2): 427–436, ix.

Nason, L.K., Walker, C.M., McNeeley, M.F. et al. (2012). Imaging of the diaphragm: anatomy and function. *Radiographics* 32(2): E51–E70.

Oliver, S.T. and Hardy, J. (2015). Ceratohyoidectomy for treatment of equine temporohyoid osteoarthropathy (15 cases). *The Canadian Veterinary Journal* 56(4): 382–386.

Ortved, K.F., Cheetham, J., Mitchell, L.M., and Ducharme, N.G. (2010). Successful treatment of persistent dorsal displacement of the soft palate and evaluation of laryngohyoid position in 15 racehorses. *Equine Veterinary Journal* 42(1): 23–29.

Papamoschou, D. (1995). Theoretical validation of the respiratory benefits of helium-oxygen mixtures. *Respiration Physiology* 99(1): 183–190.

Parente, E.J. (2018). Upper airway conditions affecting the equine athlete. *The Veterinary Clinics of North America. Equine Practice* 34(2): 427–441.

Petersson, J. and Glenny, R.W. (2014). Gas exchange and ventilation-perfusion relationships in the lung. *The European Respiratory Journal* 44(4): 1023–1041.

Rehder, K. and Sessler, A.D. (1973). Function of each lung in spontaneously breathing man anesthetized with thiopental-meperidine. *Anesthesiology* 38(4): 320–327.

Rossignol, F., Vitte, A., Boening, J. et al. (2015). Laryngoplasty in standing horses. *Veterinary Surgery* 44(3): 341–347.

Spaeth, E.E. and Friedlander, S.K. (1967). The diffusion of oxygen, carbon dioxide, and inert gas in flowing blood. *Biophysical Journal* 7(6): 827–851.

Truebel, H., Wuester, S., Boehme, P. et al. (2019). A proof-of-concept trial of HELIOX with different fractions of helium in a human study modeling upper airway obstruction. *European Journal of Applied Physiology* 119(5): 1253–1260.

Van Oostrom, H., Schaap, M.W., and van Loon, J.P. (2017). Oxygen supplementation before induction of general anaesthesia in horses. *Equine Veterinary Journal* 49(1): 130–132.

Varner, K.M., Hopster, K., and Driessen, B. (2019). Efficacy of alveolar recruitment in dorsally recumbent horses: a comparison of different types of inert gas components as inspired fresh gas. *American Journal of Veterinary Research* 80(7): 631–636.

Virgin, J.E., Holcombe, S.J., Caron, J.P. et al. (2016). Laryngeal advancement surgery improves swallowing function in a reversible equine dysphagia model. *Equine Veterinary Journal* 48(3): 362–367.

Wagner, A.E., Muir, W.W. 3rd, and Hinchcliff, K.W. (1991). Cardiovascular effects of xylazine and detomidine in horses. *American Journal of Veterinary Research* 52(5): 651–657.

Weibel, E.R. (2017). Lung morphometry: the link between structure and function. *Cell and Tissue Research* 367(3): 413–426.

Wilson, D.V., Schott, H.C. 2nd, Robinson, N.E. et al. (2006). Response to nasopharyngeal oxygen administration in horses with lung disease. *Equine Veterinary Journal* 38(3): 219–223.

Wong, D.M., Alcott, C.J., Wang, C. et al. (2010). Physiologic effects of nasopharyngeal administration of supplemental oxygen at various flow rates in healthy neonatal foals. *American Journal of Veterinary Research* 71(9): 1081–1088.

Woodie, J.B., Ducharme, N.G., Kanter, P. et al. (2005). Surgical advancement of the larynx (laryngeal tie-forward) as a treatment for dorsal displacement of the soft palate in horses: a prospective study 2001–2004. *Equine Veterinary Journal* 37(5): 418–423.

5

Anesthetic Management for Interventional Cardiac Procedures

Stephanie Keating and Ryan Fries

Department of Veterinary Clinical Medicine, College of Veterinary Medicine, University of Illinois, 1008 West Hazelwood Drive, Urbana, IL, 61802, USA

Introduction

While there are many similarities in cardiovascular physiology and pathophysiology among mammalian species, the unique aspects of equine anatomy, temperament, pharmacodynamics, and pharmacokinetics result in markedly different anesthetic practices between horses and other domestic species. These differences limit the range of anesthetic and cardiovascular agents that are administered to horses, as well as the applicability of anesthetic methodologies reported in other species. An additional challenge is the paucity of literature evaluating anesthetic management of horses with many different cardiovascular conditions. Despite these limitations, knowledge of the underlying pathophysiology allows for targeted goals for key cardiovascular parameters, including heart rate, systemic vascular resistance (SVR), pulmonary vascular resistance (PVR), contractility, preload, and arrhythmias. Ultimately, anesthetizing a horse with cardiovascular disease should be performed with a solid understanding of the underlying pathophysiology and cardiovascular goals, while acknowledging the considerations specific to equine anesthesia.

Cardiovascular Physiology

Horses possess a four-chambered heart identical in function and anatomical layout with other mammals (Budras et al. 2012). In addition to mechanical pumping, the heart has inherent electrical properties that allow generation and propagation of action potentials through the cells. In the normal horse, spontaneous depolarization of the sinus node initiates an action potential within the right atrium. Conduction travels throughout both atria and the atrioventricular (AV) node. Subsequently the action potential enters the specialized conduction tissue, known as the His-Purkinje system. This network is distributed extensively throughout both ventricles and penetrates the entire thickness of the walls. Once excited there is nearly simultaneous activation of both ventricles resulting in mechanical contraction and pumping of blood (Hamlin and Smith 1965). Specific arrhythmias and their consequences related to anesthesia will be discussed later in this chapter.

The cardiac cycle is divided into ventricular systole and diastole. Mechanical ventricular systole begins immediately after the QRS complex, with contraction of the ventricular myocardium and closure of the AV valves. Pressure within the ventricles rises rapidly, without forward movement of blood (isovolumetric contraction), until the pressures exceed the aorta and pulmonary artery pressures causing the semilunar valves to open and blood to flow into their respective circulations. Blood flow peaks during the first third of ejection, after which time flow slowly decreases until ejection stops and the semilunar valves abruptly close marking the end of ventricular systole. Ventricular diastole begins at semilunar valve closure. The ventricular pressures, which have been declining due to relaxation of the myocytes, continue to decline rapidly during early diastole, but ventricular volume remains unchanged because all cardiac valves are closed (isovolumetric relaxation). Once ventricular pressure drops below atrial pressure, the AV valves open and blood passively moves from the atria to ventricles resulting in rapid filling of the ventricles. Temporarily the atrial and ventricular pressures equilibrate resulting in minimal or no changes in ventricular pressure or volume (diastasis). Finally, atrial contraction recreates an AV pressure gradient that produces augmented ventricular filling. In healthy resting horses, atrial systole has minimal effects on ventricular filling and cardiac performance. However, the absence of atrial contraction or loss of AV synchrony on exercising and anesthetized horses can have considerable effects on cardiac performance. A complete review of cardiovascular physiology is beyond the scope of this chapter, and readers are directed to medical physiology textbooks for more information.

Hemodynamic Variables in Normal, Standing Horses

Variable	Value	Unit
Heart rate	26–50	beats/min
Central venous pressure	5–10	mmHg

Variable	Value	Unit
RV end-diastolic pressure	10–20	mmHg
RV end-systolic pressure	40–60	mmHg
Pulmonary artery systolic pressure	35–45	mmHg
Mean pulmonary artery pressure	25–30	mmHg
Pulmonary artery diastolic pressure	20–25	mmHg
Pulmonary capillary wedge pressure	13–15	mmHg
LV end-diastolic pressure	12–24	mmHg
LV end-systolic pressure	110–130	mmHg
Cardiac output	30–40	l/min
Cardiac index	60–80	ml/min/kg

Cardiovascular Effects of Common Anesthetic, Analgesic, and Sedative Agents

Alpha-2 Adrenergic Agonists

Alpha-2 adrenergic agonists are the class of drug most widely used to provide profound, reliable sedation in mature horses for preanesthetic sedation and general restraint, and include xylazine, detomidine, romifidine, dexmedetomidine, and medetomidine. Their sedative effects are accompanied by marked cardiovascular changes mediated both centrally and peripherally. Peripheral activation of alpha receptors on the vasculature increases both systemic and pulmonary vascular resistance. Peripheral reflexes and a reduction in sympathetic outflow result in a decrease in heart rate, contractility, stroke volume, and cardiac output (Wagner et al. 1991; Yamashita et al. 2000; Freeman et al. 2002). Changes in blood pressure are variable, but are classically characterized by an initial increase followed by a decrease back to or below baseline values, although mean arterial pressure remains above 80 mmHg following alpha-2 administration in conscious, healthy horses (Yamashita et al. 2000). These physiologic changes have the potential to worsen valvular insufficiency in horses and should be considered (Buhl et al. 2007). Second-degree atrioventricular block is also common following administration (Yamashita et al. 2000). The duration and degree of cardiovascular effects are influenced by the specific alpha-2 agonist administered, dose, and route of administration, with detomidine having the most marked and longest lasting effects (Wagner et al. 1991; Bryant et al. 1996; Yamashita et al. 2000).

Acepromazine

Acepromazine is the primary phenothiazine used in horses, providing mild sedation for approximately 6–12 hours depending on the dose and route of administration (Parry et al. 1982). The predominant cardiovascular effect is a reduction in vascular tone and blood pressure mediated by alpha-1 antagonism on the vasculature. Reductions in blood pressure are dose dependent and prolonged (Muir et al. 1979; Parry et al. 1982; Leise et al. 2007). Heart rate generally does not significantly change following administration, but can be highly variable with increases noted in individuals with lower blood pressure, likely due to the baroreflex (Muir et al. 1979; Parry et al. 1982; Marroum et al. 1994; Buhl et al. 2007). Despite changes in vascular tone, left ventricular internal diameter (an indicator of preload), fractional shortening and other cardiac indices remain unchanged in healthy horses (Buhl et al. 2007).

Opioids

The administration of opioid alone to healthy, pain-free horses results in increases in heart rate, blood pressure, and cardiac index, without significant changes in stroke volume or SVR (Muir et al. 1978, Skarda and Muir 2003, Carregaro et al. 2006, Figueiredo et al. 2012). This is thought to be the result of increased sympathetic

outflow accompanied by central excitatory effects, and is observed with a range of agents, including morphine, fentanyl, hydromorphone, buprenorphine, and butorphanol (Kamerling et al. 1985; Skarda and Muir 2003; Carregaro et al. 2006; Figueiredo et al. 2012; Reed et al. 2019). These affects may not be present when administered to painful horses, are minimal to absent when opioids are co-administered with alpha-2 adrenergic agonists or during inhalant anesthesia, which may be due to the suppression of central excitement and sympathetic outflow (Clarke and Paton 1988; Solano et al. 2009; Hofmeister et al. 2008).

Benzodiazepines

Benzodiazepines are commonly administered for the co-induction of anesthesia and as part of total intravenous anesthesia protocols in horses. Benzodiazepines provide anesthetic benefits as centrally acting muscle relaxants with minimal cardiovascular effects. Even when administered above clinically recommended doses, diazepam did not result in any significant change in heart rate, blood pressure, or cardiac output (Muir et al. 1982).

Guaifenesin (GG)

Guaifenesin is a centrally acting muscle relaxant, and is used similarly to benzodiazepines as an anesthetic adjunct in equine anesthesia. The administration of GG alone at doses that cause recumbency does not significantly affect heart rate, right atrial pressure, pulmonary artery pressure, or cardiac output, but does reduce arterial blood pressure (Hubbell et al. 1980). However, cardiovascular function was not significantly different in horses receiving either GG or diazepam in conjunction with xylazine and ketamine, to induce anesthesia (Brock and Hildebrand 1990). In addition to use as a co-induction agent, GG has demonstrated cardiovascular advantages when combined with other agents to provide partial or total intravenous anesthesia compared to inhalant alone (Taylor et al. 1998; Yamashita et al. 2002).

Ketamine

Ketamine is an N-methyl-D-aspartate (NMDA) antagonist that provides analgesia and dissociative anesthetic effects. In horses, ketamine is routinely administered as an induction agent, and incorporated into partial and total intravenous anesthesia protocols. The cardiovascular effects of ketamine are variable depending on the dose, concurrent administration of other drugs, and physiologic status. In healthy dogs and humans, the administration of ketamine alone results in sympathetic stimulation with dose-dependent increases in heart rate, cardiac output, arterial blood pressure, and coronary blood flow, which is met by increases in myocardial oxygen demand (Folts et al. 1975; Johnstone 1976). However, when administered to patients with compromised sympathetic outflow, the direct myocardial depression of ketamine predominates resulting in a reduction in ventricular contractility, cardiac output, and systemic blood pressure (Waxman et al. 1980; Christ et al. 1997). While the cardiovascular effects of a ketamine bolus alone have not been evaluated in horses, a favorable cardiovascular profile of ketamine was demonstrated in healthy anesthetized horses, with the infusion of ketamine resulting in higher heart rates and cardiac output compared to concurrent xylazine and ketamine infusions (Mama et al. 2005). Additionally, the administration of a ketamine infusion at 0.4 and 0.8 mg/kg/h in horses did not significantly affect heart rate or mean blood pressure until an infusion duration of six hours when mild decreases were noted (Fielding et al. 2006).

Propofol

The use of propofol alone to induce anesthesia in horses is associated with excitatory signs and elevated heart rate and blood pressure, and is not recommended (Mama et al. 1995). However, when propofol is administered following premedication with alpha-2 agonists, changes in heart rate and blood pressure are minimal following induction (Nolan and Hall 1985; Matthews et al. 1999). The cardiovascular effects of propofol total intravenous anesthesia following premedication with an alpha-2 adrenergic agonist are also minimal, with no significant changes in heart rate, SVR, systemic blood pressure, cardiac output, or stroke volume or just mild decreases in blood pressure reported in horses undergoing anesthesia without surgical stimulation (Nolan and Hall 1985; Umar et al. 2007). In equine surgical patients, the combination of propofol with other agents, including alpha-2 agonists, results in clinically acceptable heart rates and blood pressures (Aguiar et al. 1993; Matthews et al. 1999; Bettschart-Wolfensberger et al. 2005).

Lidocaine

In addition to the administration of lidocaine for its local anesthetic and antiarrhythmic effects, lidocaine can also be administered intravenously as an analgesic and anesthetic adjunct during general anesthesia or for analgesia in conscious horses (Robertson et al. 2005). When administered alone to conscious horses, lidocaine does not alter heart rate or blood pressure and electrocardiogram (ECG) values remain within clinically normal values, even when administered at supraclinical doses (Meyer et al. 2001). Although the cardiovascular effects are minimal in conscious horses, lidocaine does not improve cardiovascular performance in sevoflurane-anesthetized horses despite a reduction in minimum alveolar concentration (MAC) (Wagner et al. 2011).

Inhalant Anesthetics

The cardiovascular effects of the currently administered inhaled anesthetics, isoflurane, sevoflurane, and desflurane are characterized by dose-dependent reductions in systemic blood pressure, cardiac output, and stroke volume (Steffey et al. 1987; Steffey et al. 2005; Wagner et al. 2011). While isoflurane and sevoflurane have similar cardiovascular effects in horses (Grosenbaugh and Muir 1998), cardiac output is better preserved with desflurane when delivered at clinically administered concentrations (Steffey et al. 2005).

Dose-dependent respiratory depression is an additional consideration with these agents, with intermittent positive pressure ventilation resulting in further cardiovascular depression (Steffey et al. 2005).

Pre-anesthetic Cardiac Evaluation

Physical Examination

Auscultation is the principal means to evaluate the equine heart (Bonagura 1990). Auscultation alone can diagnose mitral and tricuspid regurgitation with 53% (Naylor et al. 2001) to 100% (Young and Wood 2000) specificity, making auscultation an essential part of the pre-anesthetic evaluation in horses. Before a diagnosis of a murmur can be made, it is first necessary to identify normal heart sounds. In all horses, the first two heart sounds (S1 and S2) are audible at the level of the apex beat. S1 corresponds to closure of the AV valves at the beginning of systole, while S2 corresponds to closure of the semilunar valves at the end of systole. Diastolic heart sounds are heard in Thoroughbred-type horses and less commonly in ponies and other smaller horses. There are two diastolic heart sounds, early rapid ventricular filling (S3), and atrial contraction (S4). Murmurs heard between the first two heart sounds are classified as systolic, while murmurs that occur between S3 and S4 are classified as diastolic. Murmurs should be classified based on location (e.g. left apex, left base), intensity grade 1–6 (Levine and Harvey 1950), and timing: systolic, diastolic, or continuous (Littlewort 1962). Specific murmurs will be discussed in detail for each cardiac disease described in this chapter. In addition to normal heart sounds and murmur detection, auscultation is the primary means of detecting any dysrhythmias. Simply, the horse's heart rate should be obtained and the rhythm characterized (regular, regularly irregular, or irregularly irregular). The normal adult horse has a sinus heart rate of 28–44 bpm at rest with a regular rhythm, while foals and neonates have average heart rates of 70–80 bpm (Patteson 1996). Once a dysrhythmia has been detected, further evaluation with an ECG is indicated.

Most horses with mild-to-moderate heart disease are subclinical, requiring precise auscultation and palpation to detect heart disease. However, some horses may present with symptoms of heart failure (HF). Clinical signs of HF can be attributed to a combination of reduced cardiac output and increased ventricular filling pressures. Depending on the etiology of the cardiac disease, clinical signs may include: tachycardia, weight loss, weakness, exercise intolerance, pale mucous membranes, weak arterial pulses, ataxia, syncope, tachypnea, dyspnea, nasal discharge, coughing, jugular pulsation, distention of peripheral veins, and peripheral edema of the ventral thoracic, limbs, or prepuce (Marr 2010a). Any horse with these clinical signs should be evaluated fully for cardiac disease, including echocardiography, thoracic radiographs, electrocardiography, and if available direct measurement of pulmonary artery and pulmonary capillary wedge pressure. Elective anesthetic procedures should be avoided or postponed and stabilization therapy administered prior to any necessary anesthetic procedure is required.

Electrocardiogram

An ECG is required to definitively diagnose any dysrhythmia. In horses, dysrhythmias can be associated with a wide range of cardiac and noncardiac diseases, including: valvular disease (Reef et al. 1998), congenital defects, pericardial disease (Reef 1993), myocarditis (Diana et al. 2007), myocardial ischemia (Dickinson et al. 1996), toxicosis (Alleman et al. 2007; Doonan et al. 1989), myocardial neoplasia (Delesalle et al. 2002), hypoxia, electrolyte disturbances (Maxon-Sage et al. 1998), autonomic tone (Bright and Hellyer 2002), septicemia (Dolente et al. 2000), endotoxemia (Cornick et al. 1990), and various drugs (Reimer et al. 1992). An important diagnostic goal in horses with dysrhythmias is to identify any contributing cardiac or noncardiac disease. The relative risks associated with anesthesia will be determined by the underlying etiology of the arrhythmia, the hemodynamic consequences of the arrhythmia, and the ability to maintain normal heart rhythm during an anesthetic procedure. Proper position of electrodes for an ECG and specific anesthetic considerations for specific dysrhythmias are described elsewhere in this chapter.

Echocardiogram

Echocardiography encompasses a number of specific imaging techniques. The two-dimensional echocardiogram is used to identify lesions of the heart and great vessels, assess myocardial function, and provide a template for guiding contrast echocardiography, color-coded Doppler echocardiography, and spectral Doppler studies. M-mode echocardiography is used to measure cardiac size and ventricular function and can be combined with contrast or color-coded Doppler studies for accurate timing of flow events. Pulsed wave and continuous wave Doppler echocardiography display the direction and velocity of red blood cells within the heart and circulation. Continuous wave Doppler studies are used to calculate pressure gradients in the circulation. Any of the Doppler techniques can be used to identify abnormal or high velocity flow responsible for pathologic heart murmurs. Each Doppler format is complementary to the others: color-coded Doppler can pinpoint regions of abnormal flow; and continuous wave Doppler quantifies the maximum velocities of blood flow across cardiac lesions. Echocardiographic studies are very useful for the diagnosis and assessment of horses with cardiac murmurs, arrhythmias, or poor exercise performance. A number of cardiac disorders can be evaluated by echocardiography, including: cardiac malformation, valvular heart disease, cardiomyopathy, bacterial endocarditis, pericardial effusion, and congestive HF (Bonagura and Blissitt 1995). When combined with a careful clinical examination, exercise evaluation, and results of ECG, the echocardiogram provides the best overall clinical assessment of the equine heart.

Cardiovascular Monitoring

Monitoring the cardiovascular system during anesthesia is critical to promptly identify cardiovascular complications allowing appropriate goal-directed therapies. The American College of Veterinary Anesthesia and Analgesia (ACVAA) guidelines for anesthesia in horses recommend minimum monitoring techniques, including digital pulse palpation, and evaluation of capillary refill time and mucous membrane color in all patients, with additional ECG and arterial blood pressure monitoring if indicated.

Blood Pressure

Palpation of peripheral arteries is a rapid and qualitative method of assessing arterial blood pressure. The pulse pressure difference (systolic – diastolic arterial pressure) is evaluated by assessing how forceful the pulse feels (i.e.: how bounding or palpable the pulse is), while blood pressure can be gauged by how much digital pressure is required to occlude the pulse. Accessible sites for peripheral pulse palpation include the facial, transverse facial, greater palatine, metatarsal, digital, and coccygeal arteries.

Direct blood pressure measurement is the most accurate technique and is strongly recommended in horses undergoing inhalational anesthesia. This technique requires the catheterization of a peripheral artery – most commonly the facial, transverse facial, and metatarsal arteries – which is connected to a transducer via a noncompliant fluid line. The pulse pressure waves are then converted to an electrical signal and displayed on the monitor as a pulse pressure waveform with measured systolic and diastolic pressures and a continuously calculated mean blood pressure. An alternative method is to connect the peripheral arterial catheter to an aneroid manometer to provide an ongoing measurement of mean blood pressure. The placement of the aneroid manometer or transducer should be at the level of the right atrium. While this technique provides the most accurate and rapid blood pressure measurement, there are disadvantages and considerations: arterial catheterization may not always be possible, complications can occur (i.e.: hematomas, thromboembolism, infection), catheterization creates a risk of inadvertent intra-arterial drug administration, and accuracy can be reduced by mechanical factors that create under- or overdamping of the system.

Non-invasive blood pressure measurement techniques are possible in foals and mature horses, and include the Doppler flow method and oscillometric method. The accuracy of oscillometric blood pressure readings in anesthetized adult horses is variable and influenced by the specific monitor, cuff size, cuff site, position of the horse and whether the horse is hyper-, hypo-, or normotensive (Hatz et al. 2015; Heliczer et al. 2016; Tearney et al. 2016; Yamaoka et al. 2017). Furthermore, interpretation of study findings are confounded by comparison of oscillometric and direct blood pressure readings from different anatomical locations. While oscillometric monitors may offer the benefit of following blood pressure trends in mature horses, relying on oscillometric derived values to provide guidance on when to institute or discontinue hemodynamic therapies should be considered carefully. In foals, oscillometric readings are also variable based on the monitor used, cuff site, and hemodynamic status, but agreement with invasive blood pressure readings is generally acceptable (Nout et al. 2002; Giguère et al. 2005).

ECG

Monitoring the ECG of the anesthetized horse provides information about heart rate and rhythm. Due to the extensive Purkinje system throughout the equine myocardium, simultaneous electrical activity within the left and right ventricular myocardium cancel each other out leaving the electrical activity within the interventricular septum and parts of the left ventricular free wall creating the vectors detectable on a surface ECG. Due to the electrical activity within the equine heart and its orientation within the thorax, cardiac rhythm is often evaluated in lead 1 using a base-apex orientation, as opposed to the frontal plane orientation in humans and small animals. This requires placement of the left forelimb electrode (black) at the level of the apex on the left side of the thorax, with the right forelimb electrode (white) at the top of the right scapular spine, and the left hind limb (red) electrode placed at variable locations distant to the heart. These differences result in equine ECG morphology that has unique characteristics that differ from small animals. Specifically, the P wave may be simple positive, bifid, or biphasic, with a predominantly negative deflection of the QRS complex, and a T wave that is variable in size and orientation (Figure 5.1).

Cardiac Output

Cardiac output is not routinely measured in clinical equine patients due to expense, practicality, and potential invasiveness, but provides a better measure of hemodynamic status than heart rate, blood pressure, and hematologic values. Various cardiac output measurement techniques have been evaluated in horses and foals.

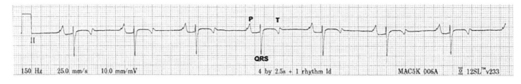

Figure 5.1 Normal ECG of the horse.

Indicator dilution techniques include transcardiac or transpulmonary thermodilution, lithium dilution, and ultrasound dilution techniques. Dilution techniques require the administration of an indicator substance into the venous circulation or right atrium and subsequent measurement of the indicator substance distal to the heart to determine flow based on versions of the Stewart-Hamilton equation. These methods are intermittent and the most invasive, but are considered the most accurate in equine patients (Linton et al. 2000, Shih et al. 2009a). Both thermodilution and lithium dilution techniques can be used to calibrate pulse waveform analysis methods, which provide a beat-by-beat determination of cardiac output (Shih et al. 2009a,b). The indirect Fick principle can also be used to determine cardiac output in foals non-invasively using the partial carbon dioxide rebreathing method (Valverde et al. 2007). While this technique is limited to use in foals and very small equine patients, it correlates well with lithium dilution measurements and provides a clinically practical option for cardiac output measurement. Imaging techniques, such as magnetic resonance imaging (MRI) and echocardiography are other possible techniques for evaluating cardiac output in equine patients, but require expertise in interpretation (Young et al. 1996). More comprehensive reviews of cardiac output monitoring techniques in equine patients have been previously published (Corley et al. 2003; Shih 2013). While capnography is not a substitute for cardiac output monitoring, changes in end-tidal CO_2 during stable ventilation may be reflective of changes in pulmonary perfusion and thus cardiac output, and can be helpful to trend during periods of cardiovascular change.

Hypotension

Systemic blood pressure is not a surrogate measure of tissue perfusion; however, hypotension can reflect low perfusion states and is associated with an increased risk of myopathy and other potential complications (Grandy et al. 1987; Johnston et al. 2002). Blood pressure monitoring is particularly important in horses undergoing inhalational anesthesia, in hemodynamically unstable patients, and in those at risk of cardiovascular complications. By identifying hypotension early, appropriate cardiovascular supportive therapies can be implemented with the goal of minimizing morbidity and mortality. The primary factors that determine arterial blood pressure are cardiac output and SVR. Cardiac output is determined by heart rate and stroke volume, while stroke volume is determined by preload, afterload, and contractility.

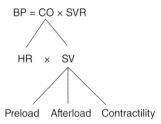

Thus, hypotension may be due to bradycardia, decreased vascular tone, decreased preload, poor contractility, or a combination of these factors. *Hypotension* is often defined as a mean arterial blood pressure below 60 mmHg in anesthetized dogs (Ruffato et al. 2015). While there is no such consensus reported in equine patients, maintaining a mean arterial blood pressure of at least 70 mmHg reduces the incidence of myopathy in mature halothane-anesthetized horses, with neonatal foals generally tolerating lower blood pressures (Grandy et al. 1987).

Treatment should be directed at correcting the underlying cause of hypotension. *Bradycardia*, typically defined as a heart rate below 26 beats/minute in mature horses, is a common finding in horses that are physically fit and following administration of alpha-2 adrenergic agonists. While anticholinergics effectively elevate heart rate, their administration to hypotensive and bradycardic equine patients should be considered carefully due to resulting reductions in gastrointestinal motility, but is often warranted with heart rates below 20 beats/minute.

Reductions in vascular tone can often be improved by decreasing the end-tidal concentration of inhalational anesthetic administered, which may require the use of partial or total intravenous anesthetic techniques to maintain appropriate anesthetic depth. Vasoactive agents, such as phenylephrine, can also be administered with the goal of improving vascular tone; however, they should be used judiciously as excessive increases in vascular tone may increase blood pressure at the expense of tissue perfusion (Dancker et al. 2018).

A reduction in preload due to deficits in circulating volume or inadequate venous return is a common source of hypotension in horses undergoing anesthesia for colic surgery and other emergent procedures. Correcting volume deficits prior to anesthesia is ideal, but not always possible. Pre-existing deficits and ongoing fluid losses should be replaced with a balanced electrolyte solution, with or without the addition of hypertonic saline, synthetic colloids, or blood products depending on the nature and severity of fluid losses, and the presence of other systemic diseases. In some cases of abdominal distention, dorsal recumbency will result in caval compression and dramatically reduce venous return. While fluid therapy can help improve preload in these instances, the most immediately effective treatment is often a change in position or abdominal decompression.

Myocardial depression and compromised contractility can be caused by a number of factors, including the administration of inhalational anesthetics. Positive inotropes can effectively improve contractility and elevate blood pressure. Dobutamine is commonly infused to increase contractility in anesthetized horses due to its selectively for beta receptors. The slow infusion of calcium is also indicated to improve contractility if ionized calcium is marginal or low. Other agents with inotropic activity, such as dopamine,

norepinephrine, and ephedrine, affect both contractility and vascular tone, and can be used when both are compromised (Dancker et al. 2018).

Common Drugs Used to Treat Hypotension in Anesthetized Equine Patients

Drug	Mechanism of action	Dose	Possible adverse effects
Atropine	Muscarinic receptor antagonist	0.01–0.02 mg/kg IV	Tachycardia Reduced GI motility
Glycopyrrolate	Muscarinic receptor antagonist	0.002–0.005 mg/kg IV	Tachycardia Reduced GI motility
23% Calcium gluconate	Increases intracellular calcium in cardiomyocytes	0.2–0.4 ml/kg IV over 15 minutes	Bradycardia when administered rapidly IV
Dobutamine	Beta receptor agonist	0.5–5 ug/kg/ min IV	Brady- or tachycardia Atrial or ventricular arrhythmias
Dopamine	Alpha, beta, and dopamine receptor agonist	0.5–5 ug/kg/ min IV	Tachycardia Atrial or ventricular arrhythmias
Norepinephrine	Alpha and beta receptor agonist	0.1–1.0 ug/ kg/min IV	Atrioventricular block Possible atrial or ventricular arrhythmias
Ephedrine	Direct beta receptor agonist, stimulates norepinephrine release from nerve terminals for alpha and beta stimulation	0.02–0.1 mg/kg IV	Variable change in heart rate, tachyphylaxis

Congenital Cardiac Conditions in Horses

Patent Ductus Arteriosus (PDA)

Pathophysiology

The ductus arteriosus is an essential part of normal fetal circulation between the aorta and pulmonary artery. Persistence of the ductus arteriosus after birth with left-to-right shunting causes volume overload of the left atrium and ventricle, which leads to remodeling in the form of eccentric hypertrophy (dilatation) predisposing patients to the development of congestive HF (Buchanan 2001). Patent ductus arteriosus (PDA) occurs infrequently in horses, either alone or in combination with other artery defects (Huston et al. 1977). Auscultation findings in a foal with a PDA reveal a loud, continuous, left basilar murmur, and hyperkinetic arterial pulse quality with a rapid rise and decline (Fregin 1982). In most foals, physiologic closure of the PDA occurs within 16 hours post-partum; however, trivial flow through the PDA has been identified in foals up to a week of age and rarely in adult horses (Hare 1931). Echocardiography can be used to definitively diagnose a PDA and assess the severity of myocardial changes. Foals with PDAs may develop signs of congestive HF within the first few weeks post-partum or may reach maturity before signs develop. Rarely, PDAs can result in pulmonary hypertension resulting in a reversal of flow through the PDA causing systemic hypoxia. Primary closure of a PDA in a horse has not been reported (Figure 5.2).

Anesthetic Considerations and Management

Anesthetic considerations for foals with a PDA vary depending on the size of the communication as well as the presence of other congenital abnormalities and secondary cardiac changes. The majority of foals undergoing anesthesia in the first week of life will have a PDA in varying states of closure. In healthy neonatal foals, there is a degree of hemodynamic compromise under isoflurane anesthesia, characterized by a decrease in heart rate and cardiac index, with minimal changes in pulmonary and SVR, and only mildly reduced blood pressure compared with the conscious state (Lombard et al. 1984; Craig et al. 2007). These changes are expected due to age-related cardiovascular physiology alone, and the contribution of PDA on cardiovascular performance is unquantified. Regardless, cardiovascular sparing protocols should still be selected in neonatal foals, with benzodiazepines providing better hemodynamic performance than alpha-2 agonists, particularly in foals under two weeks of age (Kerr et al. 2009).

Figure 5.2 Echocardiographic image of a PDA in foal.

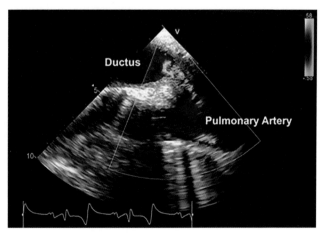

Pathological or persistent PDA rarely occurs as a sole condition in foals, and is typically part of a complex congenital defect. When persistent PDA presents in isolation, anesthetic goals should include: maintaining heart rate in upper normal range, maintaining vascular tone and avoiding decreases in blood pressure (particularly diastolic), preserving or increasing contractility with dobutamine or other positive inotropes depending on the presence of HF or hypotension, and maintaining sufficient preload without volume excess. Alpha-2 agonists should be avoided when typical left-to-right shunting is present within the PDA as the increase in afterload will increase the fraction of blood diverted from systemic circulation, and bradycardia will further compromise cardiac output. Acepromazine and high concentrations of inhalational anesthetics reduce SVR, and in the presence of high PVR, have the potential to create or worsen right-to-left shunting in addition to increasing the incidence of hypotension. Benzodiazepines and opioids are ideal agents for premedication in foals with PDA resulting in few cardiovascular changes. Induction agents should be titrated carefully to minimize any unwanted cardiovascular effects, and include ketamine used alone or in combination with propofol or alfaxalone. While the cardiovascular and endocrine effects of etomidate have not yet been evaluated in foals, the cardiovascular stability provided by this agent may justify its use in foals with HF despite reductions in steroidogenesis. Maintenance of anesthesia should focus on minimizing inhalational anesthetic requirements. Total intravenous anesthesia using propofol and opioid infusions has been used during canine PDA surgery (Musk and Flaherty 2007), and may also be a suitable option in foals; however, it is unknown if this approach offers cardiovascular advantages in foals with PDA. Supportive therapy should be provided as needed, including judicious manual ventilation and fluid therapy, as well as the administration of positive inotropes and vasoactive drugs in order to optimize cardiovascular performance.

Atrial Septal Defects (ASD)

Pathophysiology

Atrial septation is a complex process occurring during embryologic development of the fetus (Kittleson and Kienle 1998). If septation is interrupted, defects within the atrial septum can arise. The size and location of the defect can vary, and, with it, the degree and direction of shunting. In the absence of right heart pressure overload, flow through an atrial septal defect (ASD) will move from the left atrium to the right atrium. Subsequently, extra blood volume will pass through the right ventricle and pulmonary circulation resulting in right ventricular dilatation and increased hydrostatic pressure in the pulmonary vasculature. Foals with a large ASD are at risk for right-sided HF, pulmonary edema, and pulmonary hypertension. A large ASD can create an audible, left basilar, systolic heart murmur associated with physiologically increased pulmonic flow velocities. Most ASDs in foals are clinically insignificant, although atrial fibrillation (AF) and progressive HF has been reported (Taylor et al. 1991) (Figure 5.3).

Anesthetic Considerations and Management

Similar to PDA, a patent foramen ovale (PFO) is a normal finding in neonatal foals, in contrast to a persistent ASD, alone or in combination as a complex congenital defect. The expected cardiovascular performance under anesthesia and associated risk for these conditions depend largely on the size of the defect, the presence of other defects, and the direction of shunting. Hemodynamic goals during anesthesia include: maintaining heart rate at normal conscious values, avoiding extremes in SVR and PVR, preserving or increasing contractility depending on the pre-existing degree of dysfunction, ensuring preload without overload, and being prepared for arrhythmias. These goals closely parallel those for PDA (see above) and share the same anesthetic recommendations, most notably, sedating foals with benzodiazepines and opioids, titrating

Figure 5.3 Echocardiographic image of an ASD in a foal.

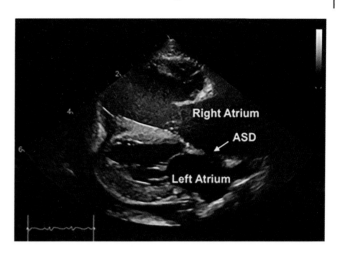

induction agents to effect in neonatal foals to minimize reductions in SVR, and minimizing inhalational anesthetic requirements. The use of alpha-2 adrenergic agonists may be required in older foals, in which case intramuscular (IM) administration and dose reduction can reduce the cardiovascular impact of these agents. The most important goal for the anesthetic management of isolated ASD is the balance between SVR and PVR. In the more likely scenario of left-to-right shunting, SVR should be maintained to preserve systemic blood pressure. Extremes in both should be avoided, as systemic hypertension will increase left-to-right shunt, increase right ventricular workload, and promote the development of pulmonary hypertension, and hypotension creates the potential for the development of right-to-left shunting and subsequent hypoxemia. Due to the direct connection between the atria, iatrogenic air emboli entering the systemic circulation are a risk with ASD, particularly in the presence of right-to-left shunting, and all fluid lines and injectable agents should have air bubbles removed.

Ventricular Septal Defects (VSD)

Pathophysiology

Ventricular septal defects (VSD) are the most common congenital defect in horses (Lombard

et al. 1983). While most VSDs are an isolated defect, they can also be a component of other congenital heart defects (Marr 2010b). The location of a VSD can vary, most commonly they are found in the membranous portion of the left ventricular outflow tract (subarterial) and less commonly in the membranous portion of the right ventricular outflow tract (subpulmonic) or muscular interventricular septum. The size of the defect will determine the relative hemodynamic significance of the shunting. In the absence of right ventricular pressure overload, flow through a VSD will move from the left ventricle to the right ventricle. Subsequently, extra blood volume will pass immediately into the pulmonary circulation, left atrium, and ultimately back to the left ventricle. This left-to-right shunting results in an increased hydrostatic pressure in the pulmonary vasculature, left atrial, and left ventricular dilatation. A common sequalae of large, subarterial VSDs is aortic insufficiency (AI) which may further contribute to volume overload of the left ventricle (Reef and Spencer 1987). Auscultation of a horse with a VSD will reveal a loud, systolic murmur with a point of maximal intensity over the right fourth intercostal space. If significant AI is concurrently present, a diastolic murmur will be present over aortic valve area in the left basilar fourth intercostal space (Reef and Spencer 1987). Generally, loud, right-sided systolic murmurs are associated with

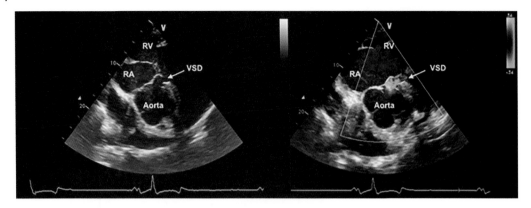

Figure 5.4 Echocardiographic image of a horse with a membranous VSD.

small VSDs; however, any horses with a loud murmur should have an echocardiogram performed. Echocardiography can definitively diagnose the location and size of the defect, maximum velocity across the shunt, and assess the severity of myocardial changes (Reef 1995) (Figure 5.4).

Anesthetic Considerations and Management

The range in severity of VSD in horses will have a notable impact on their cardiovascular performance under anesthesia. Given the similarities in pathology, the anesthetic goals for VSD are similar to that for ASD; however, the potential for larger pressure gradient and shunting carries greater consequence. Hemodynamic goals during anesthesia for VSD include: maintaining heart rate at normal values, avoiding extremes in both SVR and PVR, preserving or increasing contractility depending on the preexisting degree of dysfunction, and being prepared to treat arrhythmias. Similar to ASD, the most important anesthetic goal is managing the balance between SVR and PVR. Shunt is often left-to-right-sided favoring mild reductions in SVR, which can be readily achieved during inhalational anesthesia. Care should still be taken to minimize inhalational anesthetic requirements to prevent dramatic reductions in SVR that could create right-to-left shunting. Successful anesthesia and recovery has been reported for a stallion with clinical signs of cardiac disease attributable to VSD, comprised of pre-anesthetic sedation using romifidine and butorphanol, anesthetic induction with ketamine, propofol, and diazepam, and maintenance with isoflurane and infusions of ketamine, propofol, and fentanyl (Michlik et al. 2014). As with any intracardiac shunt, care should be taken to minimize the risk of air emboli.

Tetralogy of Fallot (TOF)

Pathophysiology

Tetralogy of Fallot (TOF), occasionally seen in foals, is a complex cardiac congenital abnormality comprised of four defects: a large VSD, pulmonic stenosis, dextroposition (overriding) of the aorta, and right ventricular hypertrophy (Houe et al. 1996). As a result of right ventricular pressure overload, foals with TOF develop right-to-left shunting of blood and systemic hypoxemia. Auscultation typically reveals a systolic, left basilar murmur associated with pulmonic stenosis. Clinical signs may include stunted growth, exercise intolerance, and cyanosis. As a consequence of systemic hypoxemia, a compensatory increase in red blood cell production can lead to polycythemia. Echocardiography is used to definitively diagnose TOF, and contrast echocardiography, using agitated saline, can allow for visualization of right-to-left shunting across the VSD. Most foals with TOF die or are euthanized early in life due

Figure 5.5 Echocardiographic image of a foal with Tetralogy of Fallot.

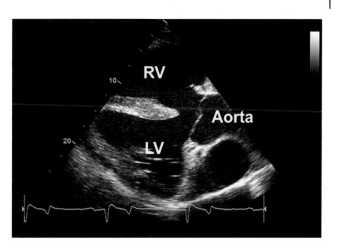

to the severity of their clinical signs, with rare cases of foals surviving into adulthood (Gesell and Brandes 2006) (Figure 5.5).

Anesthetic Considerations and Management

Anesthesia is rarely pursued in foals with TOF due to a poor prognosis and high anesthetic risk (Schmitz et al. 2008). If anesthesia is elected in foals or horses with less severe disease, anesthetic management should be directed at reducing right-to-left shunting, while maintaining sufficient cardiac output. Anesthetic goals include: maintaining heart rate, maintaining or increasing SVR, preventing increases in PVR, avoiding excessive contractility, and increasing preload.

The severity of the shunt is determined by the pressure gradient between the right and left ventricles and depends on the degree of right ventricular outflow tract obstruction, the size of the VSD, as well as SVR and PVR. While right ventricular outflow obstruction affects right ventricular pressure more than PVR, elevations in PVR should still be minimized by avoiding hypoxemia, hypercapnia, and acidosis, as well as avoiding elevations in airway pressure caused by high tidal volumes and high positive end-expiratory pressure during manual ventilation. Systemic hypotension and reductions in SVR should also be avoided by excluding or minimizing the use of vasodilatory agents. A hypoxemic episode in the absence of respiratory

changes may indicate right-to-left shunting due to reductions in SVR, and can be detected using pulse oximetry and evaluating mucous membrane color. If right-to-left shunting occurs, it can be treated by increasing SVR with the judicious use of phenylephrine.

Other causes of hypotension include reductions in contractility or inadequate preload. Excessive contractility should be avoided in patients with TOF due to increased myocardial oxygen consumption of the hypertrophied right ventricle, as well as an increased risk for dynamic right ventricular outflow tract obstruction and potential shunt exacerbation. If poor contractility is a suspected cause of hypotension, dobutamine can be titrated carefully while monitoring the patient for signs of shunting. Ensuring adequate preload is also important due to the reduced compliance of the right ventricle and the importance of maintaining patency of the right ventricular outflow tract. Unlike left-sided cardiac conditions, fluids should be administered generously in patients with TOF to provide full right ventricular preload, optimize cardiac output, and minimize right-to-left shunt. A fluid bolus may also be helpful in resolving acute episodes of right-to-left shunt if dynamic collapse of the right ventricular outflow tract is a contributing etiology. Premedication in equine patients with TOF can include alpha-2 agonists and opioids, and in the case of foals, benzodiazepines.

Acepromazine causes dose-dependent reductions in SVR and is contraindicated, worsening right-to-left shunt. Ketamine maintains SVR and is the ideal agent for anesthetic induction in equine patients with TOF. While co-induction agents can be administered, benzodiazepines are preferred over propofol, due to better preservation of vascular tone. Inhalational anesthetics are often used to maintain anesthesia in human patients with TOF (Rajput et al. 2014), and should be administered at the lowest possible concentration using MAC reducing techniques, such as locoregional anesthesia and partial intravenous anesthetic techniques, such as infusions of ketamine or dexmedetomidine (Hiscox 2012; Rajput et al. 2014). An additional consideration is the potential for systemic air embolism if air bubbles are administered intravenously, and extra precautions should be made to check fluid lines, injectable drugs, and flush for bubbles before IV administration.

Acquired Cardiac Conditions in Horses

Aortic Insufficiency

Pathophysiology

AI is the most common form of valvular pathology in middle-aged and older horses (Bishop et al. 1966). The etiology of AI is degenerative, nodular, fibrous thickening of the aortic valve leaflets. Less commonly, AI can be the result of infective endocarditis and as previously mentioned associated with congenital heart diseases. Affected leaflets develop mechanical failure, leading to prolapse of the valves and ultimately decreased coaptation allowing for regurgitant flow during valve closure (Else and Holmes 1972). The prevalence of AI is difficult to determine; the disease is more common in older horses, and reports on prevalence based on audible murmurs range from 5.5 to 8.7% (Stevens et al. 2009 and Holmes et al. 1986); however, the true

prevalence is likely greater. AI can lead to volume overload of the left ventricle, dilatation, and in rare cases cardiac failure. In middle-aged horses with mild-to-moderate AI, there is minimal impact on quality of life. The disease process is slowly progress and most horses can continue their riding and work for several years after diagnosis. It should be noted, however, some horses develop ventricular dysrhythmias as a result of AI, and younger horses and those with a more rapid progression of disease must be considered differently. Auscultation of a horse with AI reveals a diastolic, decrescendo murmur with a point of maximum intensity over the left heart base in the fifth intercostal space. The murmur quality and intensity can be variable and has been reported to sound musical or creaking in some cases. Superior to auscultation, examination of the arterial pulse quality is an excellent guide to the severity of AI. Severe AI significantly lowers systemic diastolic blood pressure as a result of diastolic runoff of blood through the aortic valve leaflets. This drop in diastolic pressure increases the pulse pressure difference between systole and diastole resulting in hyperkinetic arterial pulses (Horn 2002). As such, the arterial pulses quality increases as the severity of AI increases. Echocardiography can readily identify AI via color Doppler, and two-dimensional and M-mode echocardiography are useful in assessing the degree of volume overload. Additionally, assessment of myocardial function is of particular importance in horses with AI prior to undergoing anesthesia. As previously mentioned, horses with moderate-to-severe AI are at higher risk for developing ventricular dysrhythmias (Horn 2002). Ambulatory and exercising ECGs are recommended as part of the diagnostics evaluation in cases of horses with AI prior to anesthesia (Figure 5.6).

Anesthetic Considerations and Management

Due to the prevalence of AI and the absence of a detectable murmur in many cases, the majority of equine anesthetists likely anesthetize

Figure 5.6 Echocardiographic image of a horse with aortic insufficiency.

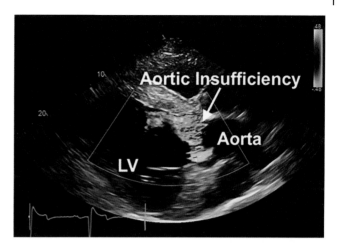

many horses with mild AI unknowingly and uneventfully. While anesthesia in horses with more advanced AI has not been evaluated compared to horses without cardiac pathology, conscious horses with more advanced AI have lower diastolic blood pressure than those with mild disease, and hypotension would be expected during inhalational anesthesia in these patients. In light of this and the underlying pathophysiology, ideal hemodynamic goals for horses with AI include: maintain HR and minimize bradycardia, balance changes in SVR to minimize resistance to forward flow without causing hypotension or reductions in diastolic blood pressure that compromise cardiac perfusion, preserve or increase contractility depending on the stage of the disease, ensure adequate preload, and anticipate ventricular arrhythmias in more severe cases. One of the most important considerations is maintaining heart rate at the high end of normal to minimize time for regurgitation; however, this goal can be challenging in horses given the reliance for alpha-2 adrenergic agonists to provide effective pre-anesthetic sedation. Intramuscular administration of a longer lasting alpha-2 agonist, such as detomidine, can minimize reductions in heart rate compared to IV administration while still providing effective sedation (Mama et al. 2009), and prevent or reduce the dosing requirements for intravenous alpha-2 agonist administration prior to

anesthesia. Correcting fluid deficits prior to anesthesia is also important to ensure sufficient preload and left ventricular end-diastolic pressure in patients with AI, although caution must be taken to avoid overload and the development of pulmonary edema. Positive inotropes, such as dobutamine, will increase contractility with a dilated left ventricle and increase cardiac output, and are preferred over strictly vasoconstricting agents for the management of hypotension as unbalanced increases in afterload can worsen the regurgitant fraction and cause reductions in heart rate, and disproportionately compromise flow despite successfully elevating blood pressure.

Mitral Regurgitation

Pathophysiology

Mitral regurgitation (MR) is the second most common valvular pathology in horses and is most often the result of a degenerative process (Miller and Bonagura 1985). Uncommonly, MR may be the result of infective endocarditis, neoplasia, non-septic valvulitis, or congenital valvular dysplasia (Reef et al. 1998). Similar to AI, affected mitral valve leaflets develop mechanical failure, leading to prolapse of the valves and ultimately decreased coaptation allowing for regurgitant flow during valve closure. Chronic MR leads to volume overload of the left atrium and ventricle leading to dilatation and increased end-diastolic pressure. Subsequently, this can lead to increased pulmonary venous pressure and left-sided congestive HF. Pulmonary hypertension, AF, ventricular dysrhythmias, and sudden death are other possible sequalae (Reef et al. 1998). MR and associated murmurs are present in 2.9–3.5% of clinically healthy horses (Patteson and Cripps 1993). The prevalence is much higher in racing Thoroughbreds (7–18%) and highest for hurdlers (19%) and steeplechasers (23%) (Young et al. 2008). Auscultation of a horse with MR reveals a loud, apical, systolic murmur with a point of maximal intensity over the left fifth intercostal space. The grade or intensity of the murmur is positively correlated with severity of disease in most cases, and any horse with a ≥ grade 3/6 murmur warrants further evaluation including echocardiography and electrocardiography. Color Doppler echocardiography can assess the size and direction of regurgitation and, coupled with two-dimensional echocardiography, left atrial and ventricular dilatation and myocardial function can be quantified. Prognosis for horses with MR is negatively correlated with disease severity. While many horses with MR can live a normal lifespan, prognostic information gained from the echocardiogram and ECG (left atrial size, left ventricular function, pulmonary artery dilatation, AF, ventricular dysrhythmias) can help determine the relative risk for each patient. Echocardiography and electrocardiography are recommended for all horses with MR prior to undergoing anesthesia (Figure 5.7).

Anesthetic Considerations and Management

Mitral insufficiency is common, and presents a range of anesthetic risk, depending on the severity of the condition. Hemodynamic goals during anesthesia include: maintaining a high normal heart rate, minimizing SVR while preserving blood pressure, avoiding large increases in PVR, preserving or increasing contractility, ensuring preload while preventing overload, and being ready to treat both supraventricular and ventricular arrhythmias. The most important goals are to prevent bradycardia, as it reduces cardiac output and causes a greater left ventricular end-diastolic volume which worsens the regurgitant fraction, and to facilitate forward blood flow by preventing excessive increases in SVR. These goals can be difficult to achieve, given the reliance on alpha-2 adrenergic agonists in equine anesthesia, but adverse effects can be minimized through IM administration, dose reduction, and judicious use of acepromazine in patients that do not have severe disease. While reductions in SVR facilitate forward blood flow, the vasodilatory effects of inhalational anesthetics may induce hypotension, and MAC reducing strategies, such as locoregional anesthetic techniques and MAC reducing infusions, such as ketamine,

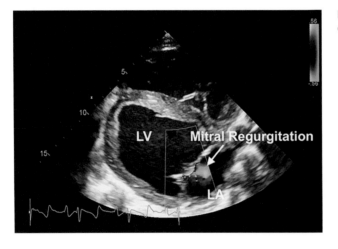

Figure 5.7 Echocardiographic image of a horse with mitral regurgitation.

are helpful to improve cardiovascular performance. Cardiac rhythm should be monitored closely, given the potential for AF, as well as atrial arrhythmias and ventricular arrhythmias, and dysrhythmias should be treated if warranted (see Section Disturbances in Conduction, Rhythm, and Rate).

Disturbances in Conduction, Rhythm, and Rate

Sinus Bradycardia

Pathophysiology

The normal resting heart rate in horses is reported to be between 22 and 50 bpm (Hilwig 1977; McGuirk and Muir 1985; Patteson 1996; Radostits et al. 2002). Sinus bradycardia in horses is characterized by a sustained heart rate < 24 bpm. Normal heart rate is controlled by a balance between the sympathetic and parasympathetic efferent activities. Sinus bradycardia is believed to be a preponderance of parasympathetic activity (vagally mediated) in normal horses (Bonagura and Miller 1986). Sinus bradycardia often occurs with other dysrhythmias, including: sinus arrhythmia, sinoatrial block, second-degree AV block, sinus arrest, and rarely high-grade second- or third-degree AV block. Sinus bradycardia can develop as a result of cardiac and noncardiac diseases, including: extreme fitness, myocardial dysfunction, electrolyte disturbances, increased intracranial pressure, and hypothyroidism. Sinus bradycardia should disappear with a decrease in parasympathetic tone, easily induced with exercise or excitement. Rarely, vagolytic drugs (glycopyrrolate or atropine) need to be administered to abolish sinus bradycardia in normal horses.

Anesthetic Considerations and Management

When mild-to-moderate bradycardia occurs during anesthesia as a result of cardiovascular fitness in athletic horses or as an expected result of alpha-2 adrenergic agonist administration, and arterial blood pressure is considered acceptable, treatment is not indicated. When bradycardia is marked, accompanied by hypotension, or there are long sinus pauses with the threat of sinus arrest, treatment is warranted and selected based on the underlying etiology. Vagally mediated bradycardia resulting from the trigeminovagal (oculocardiac) reflex, traction on abdominal viscera, or other physiologic causes, can be treated with intravenous anticholinergic administration (glycopyrrolate or atropine), and may be coupled with other means of stimulating sympathetic activity of the heart, including reducing anesthetic depth when appropriate and administering cardiac sympathomimetic agents, such as dobutamine. Due to the reduction in gastrointestinal motility and the potential for colic following anticholinergic administration in horses (Donnellan et al. 2013), their use is generally reserved for situations where bradycardia is causing marked decreases in cardiovascular performance. Bradycardia induced by hyperkalemia is best treated by addressing the hyperkalemia itself through the administration of intravenous crystalloids, dextrose, and insulin. When bradycardia is due to elevated intracranial pressure and accompanied by elevated systemic blood pressure, treatment is directed at reducing intracranial pressure through the IV administration of mannitol and/or hypertonic saline and dexamethasone, by reducing inhalational anesthetics as much as possible, and by tightly controlling $PaCO_2$ within the low-normal physiologic range.

Atrioventricular Block

Pathophysiology

Atrioventricular block (AVB) can be divided into two groups: physiologic AVB and advanced or pathologic AVB. As described in sinus bradycardia section, high vagal tone and athletic fitness can lower resting heart rate and physiologically prolong conduction through the AV node (first-degree AVB) or intermittently block conduction through the AV node (second-degree AVB). Physiologic AVB is the most common vagally mediated arrhythmia in normal horses, and second-degree AVB has been reported to be detected in >40% of healthy horses during 24-hour Holter monitoring (Reef and Marr 2010). The frequency of blocked beats is usually regular and can range upward from one in every three beats. Importantly, the number of blocked P waves in succession is usually one and as more P waves are blocked successively, the degree of AVB advances. Pathologic AVB is characterized by frequent intermittent conduction block (high-grade second-degree AVB) or completely conduction block (third-degree AVB). High-grade or advanced second-degree AVB can be caused by electrolyte imbalances, drug toxicity, or AV nodal disease (Bonagura and Miller 1986). Affected horses will have slow heart rates, and ECG will reveal normal QRS complexes with near normal P-R intervals with frequency P waves not followed by a QRS complex. Different from vagally mediated second-degree AVB, high-grade second-degree AVB will often have multiple P waves in succession without conduction. Treatment should be based on the probable etiology, and anesthesia should be delayed until the arrhythmia is corrected. Complete or third-degree AVB is a rare occurrence in horses and is typically associated with inflammation or degeneration of the AV node (Reef et al. 1986). Less commonly, third-degree AVB (Reef et al. 1986) has be associated with electrolyte or metabolic abnormalities (Whitton and Trim 1985),

congenital heart block (Pibarot et al. 1993), lymphoma (Sugiyama et al. 2008), and rattlesnake envenomation (Lawler et al. 2008). Third-degree AVB results in severe bradycardia, decreased cardiac output, and affected horses typically have severe exercise intolerance and occasionally syncope. The ECG reveals regular P waves that are not followed by a QRS complexes and QRS complexes that are widened and regularly spaced. There is no association between the P waves and the QRS escape complexes. Treatment for third-degree AVB is required immediately and if the underlying causes cannot be corrected as in the case of envenomation or inflammation, a permanent transvenous pacemaker should be placed (Reef et al. 1986). Anesthesia should be avoided in horses with third-degree AVB. Prior to inducing anesthesia for a permanent pacemaker, a transvenous temporary pacemaker should be used. Specific discussion regarding temporary and permanent pacing is discussed later in this chapter (Figures 5.8–5.10).

Anesthetic Considerations and Management

As a normal finding due to high resting vagal tone, first- and second-degree AV block are expected in many horses undergoing anesthesia and do not require treatment. When AV block becomes high grade and impairs heart rate and blood pressure, treatment is similar to vagally mediated bradycardia, and is comprised largely of anticholinergic administration (see the preceding text). The infusion of dopamine may resolve AV block that is partially or nonresponsive to

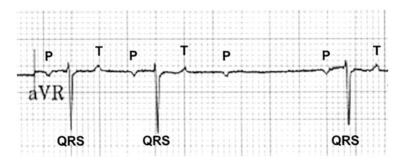

Figure 5.8 Electrocardiogram of second-degree AV block type I in a horse.

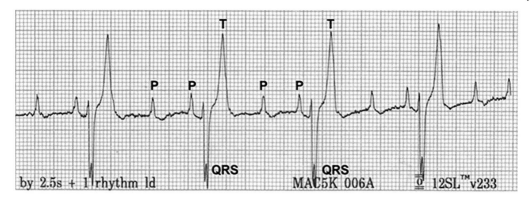

Figure 5.9 Electrocardiogram of second-degree AV block type II in a horse.

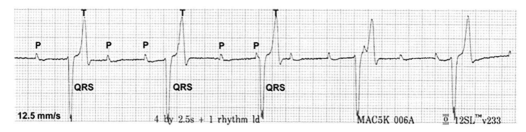

Figure 5.10 Electrocardiogram of third-degree AV block in a horse.

anticholinergic administration (Whitton and Trim 1985; Lawler et al. 2008), but carries the risk of considerable tachycardia with over-administration. Corticosteroids may also be administered due to the possibility of an inflammatory etiology of AV nodal disturbances. High-grade second-degree AV block or third-degree AV block that is nonresponsive to pharmaceutical intervention is uncommon to discover under anesthesia and may require the placement of a temporary pacemaker in order to maintain adequate cardiovascular performance under anesthesia.

Sinus Tachycardia

Pathophysiology

Sinus tachycardia in horses can be defined as a sinus rhythm with a sustained heart rate of >50 bpm. While not all sinus tachycardias are sustained, they are the result of a systemic underlying cause that if not addressed will result in continuation of the tachycardia. Sinus tachycardia is typically the result of a preponderance of the sympathetic tone and may be caused by pain, fear, excitement, fever, shock, hemorrhage, colic, catecholamine administration, hyperthyroidism, and electrolyte abnormalities (McGuirk and Muir 1985). Treatment with anti-arrhythmic drugs is not necessary, as addressing these primary conditions typically results in a return to normal sinus rate. These conditions should be addressed prior to anesthesia if possible, and evaluation of heart structure and function may be indicated, as rapid heart rate is the compensatory mechanism for decreased cardiac output.

Anesthetic Considerations and Management

Sinus tachycardia is uncommon in the healthy anesthetized horse, as heart rate often remains within the normal range even at light planes of anesthesia and with surgical stimulation. When it does occur, it is most commonly due to pre-existing elevations in sympathetic tone prior to anesthesia from pain and/or volume depletion, as can be seen in some horses undergoing colic surgery. Iatrogenic causes should also be considered, as the administration of sympathomimetic agents can also cause dramatic increases in sinus rate. Treatment of sinus tachycardia during anesthesia should focus on addressing the primary cause and may include fluid therapy, administration of analgesic agents, and/or reduction in dobutamine in the case of over-administration.

Supraventricular Arrhythmias

Pathophysiology

Supraventricular arrhythmias are any ectopic depolarizations originating in the atria before SA nodal discharge (Miller and Bonagura 1985). These ectopic depolarizations can occur as a single beat (supraventricular premature complex, SVPC) or in groups; 2 = couplet, 3 = triplet, ≥ = supraventricular tachycardia (SVT). The presence of frequent SVPC or SVT may indicate myocardial disease, and further evaluation of the cardiac structure and function is warranted. A specific type of SVT common in horses is AF. AF can develop in healthy horses with structurally normal hearts. AF is more common in racehorses older than four years, and many cases of AF develop during racing and stop spontaneously (Holmes et al. 1986; Ohmura et al. 2003). However, AF can also be related to atrial enlargement secondary to acquired or congenital heart disease. As such, evaluation of cardiac structure and function is recommended in horses presenting with AF. The ECG reveals an irregular R-R interval with no discernable P waves. A rapid fibrillating baseline reveals small fine or large course "f" waves. The treatment for AF should be based on the underlying cause and etiology of the AF. In cases of electrolyte abnormalities, particularly hypokalemia and hypomagnesemia, replacement is recommended. Horses with little or no structural heart disease are candidates for pharmacological or electrical cardioversion. The decision should be determined by the attending clinician. In horses with significant structural heart changes, pharmacological rate control is advised (Figure 5.11).

Anesthetic Considerations and Management

Horses with AF or flutter may not have notable changes in overall ventricular rate and systemic blood pressure compared to healthy horses undergoing anesthesia, and thus, treatment may not be warranted during the peri-anesthetic period. If treatment is desired, horses can undergo oral antiarrhythmic therapy or transvenous electrical cardioversion (TVEC) (see the following text). Acute treatment of anesthetized horses experiencing SVT due to AF with a high ventricular response rate or other supraventricular ectopic activity should be directed toward rate control. While clinical studies have not identified a first-line therapy, procainamide, propranolol, or amiodarone may be administered to reduce ventricular rate. While quinidine is routinely used for oral pharmacologic cardioversion in conscious horses, its vagolytic effect may increase heart rate further (Muir et al. 1990), and intravenous administration should be avoided in horses with notable tachycardia during anesthesia.

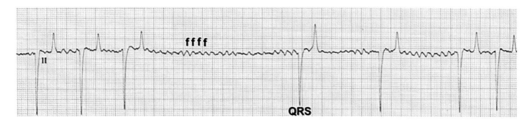

Figure 5.11 Electrocardiogram of atrial fibrillation in a horse.

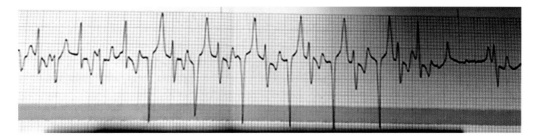

Figure 5.12 Electrocardiogram of multiform ventricular tachycardia in a horse.

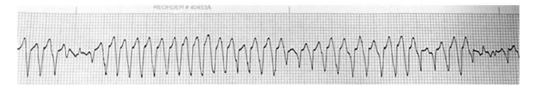

Figure 5.13 Electrocardiogram of sustained ventricular tachycardia in a horse.

Ventricular Arrhythmias

Pathophysiology

Ventricular premature complexes (VPC) are ectopic depolarizations that arise within the ventricular myocardium (Bonagura and Miller 1985). As with SVPC, these ectopic depolarizations can occur as a single beat (VPC) or in groups; 2 = couplet, 3 = triplet, ≥ 4 = ventricular tachycardia (VT). Potential causes for VPCs including: myocardial inflammation, degeneration, necrosis or fibrosis, electrolyte abnormalities, hypoxia, endotoxemia, and HF (Miller and Bonagura 1985; Reimer et al. 1992). Treatment should be focused on addressing these underlying etiologies. The ECG reveals wide, bizarre QRS complexes with no associated P wave that occurs at a rate faster than underlying sinus rhythm. The VPC QRS complexes may all appear uniform (monomorphic) or it may have multiple morphologies (polymorphic). Polymorphic VPCs are associated with increased electrical inhomogeneity and instability and thus an increased risk for developing fatal ventricular arrhythmias. Additionally, horses with very fast VPCs displaying R on T phenomenon are at increased risk for developing ventricular fibrillation. Treatment for rare single VPCs is not always warranted; however, fast, complex, frequent, or sustained VPCs should be addressed immediately as these rhythms are risk factors for spontaneous ventricular fibrillation and sudden death. Horses with VPCs detected prior to anesthesia should have a full evaluation, including an echocardiogram (Figures 5.12 and 5.13).

Anesthetic Considerations and Management

Isolated ventricular arrhythmias and VT are typically seen in anesthetized horses with endotoxemia or septic shock, which is often due to intestinal compromise or rupture. Occasional ventricular arrhythmias may not require specific treatment; however, VT (particularly with wide QRS complexes), polymorphic ventricular arrhythmias, R on T phenomenon, and torsade de pointes may deteriorate into ventricular fibrillation and death, and require prompt treatment. Lidocaine is commonly used as a first-line antiarrhythmic for VT, while magnesium is the preferred choice for torsade de pointes. Other therapeutic options that can be used as adjunctive antiarrhythmics include other sodium channel blockers (procainamide, propafenone, quinidine), beta blockers (propranolol), and potassium channel blockers (amiodarone). Selection of adjunctive or second-to-third-line agents depends largely on available clinical data in horses, as well as familiarity, availability, and cost. It should be noted that all antiarrhythmic agents can have proarrhythmogenic effects, and the ECG should be monitored continuously during administration.

Antiarrhythmic drugs for use in equine patients

Drug	Mechanism of action	Dose	Possible adverse effects
Lidocaine	Na$^+$ channel blocker	0.5 mg/kg IV increments, up to 1.5 mg/kg Higher doses are well tolerated in anesthetized patients	Central nervous system (CNS) disturbances (excitement, seizures), twitching with higher doses and rapid administration
Procainamide	Na$^+$ channel blocker	0.5–1 mg/kg increments IV, up to 20 mg/kg	Hypotension, CNS or GI disturbances
Propafenone	Na$^+$ channel blocker	0.5–1 mg/kg IV	CNS or GI disturbances, bronchospasm
Quinidine gluconate	Na$^+$ channel blocker	0.5–2 mg/kg IV	CNS disturbances, hypotension, nasal edema, laminitis, GI disturbances
Propranolol	Beta blocker	0.05–0.15 mg/kg IV	Bradycardia, bronchoconstriction
Amiodarone	K$^+$ channel blocker	5–7 mg/kg slow IV	Hind limb weakness, depression, GI disturbances, hepatopathy
Magnesium	Ca^{2+} channel blocking activity, Membrane threshold stabilization via Na$^+$/K$^+$ ATPase activation	2–6 mg/kg slow IV increments, up to 50 mg/kg	Hypotension

Cardiac Procedures

Transvenous Electrical Cardioversion (TVEC)

Procedure

Both external (transthoracic) and interval (transvenous) electrical cardioversion for lone AF has been described in horses (Frye et al. 2002; Kimberly et al. 2005; De Clercq et al. 2008). However, because of the size of horses and the energy required to depolarize the myocardial, transthoracic cardioversion is largely unsuccessful and has been supplanted by TVEC. Briefly, TVEC is performed by utilizing two open lumen cardioversion electrocatheters via a jugular approach. Using echocardiography to guide the positioning of the catheters, one catheter is positioned in the left pulmonary artery and one catheter is positioned just above the cranial margin of the tricuspid valve in the ventral right atrium. Thoracic radiographs are obtained to confirm proper position of the electrode catheters prior to inducing anesthesia. Cardioversion is then attempted using synchronized, biphasic shocks at increasing levels every two to three minutes, until cardioversion is achieved or a maximum of 300 J is applied. Cardioversion of AF to sinus rhythm using this method is very successful with conversion rates of >98% achieved in some reports (Kimberly et al. 2005).

Anesthetic Considerations and Management

AF in horses free of structural heart disease is not a contraindication to general anesthesia. While the previously described cardiac indices may be altered, heart rate and systemic blood pressures are similar between anesthetized ASA 1 equine patients and those with lone AF, and generally fall within the expected range for healthy anesthetized horses (Muir and McGuirk 1984; Costa-Farré et al. 2006; Bellei et al. 2007; Schauvliege et al. 2009). Following successful conversion and return to sinus rhythm, stroke index and cardiac index are reported to rapidly increase, accompanied by a mild reduction in systolic blood pressure

(Schauvliege et al. 2009). While complications appear to be infrequent, third-degree AVB has been reported in a single horse following shock administration, which required temporary right ventricular pacing (van Loon et al. 2005).

Because cardiovascular function is generally stable, anesthetic protocols used in horses undergoing TVEC do not differ markedly from protocols used for other elective procedures. Sedation is required during cardiac catheter placement and prior to the induction of general anesthesia, and is achieved with the administration of infusions or boluses of various alpha-2 agonists (xylazine, romifidine, dexmedetomidine, detomidine) with or without an opioid (Bellei et al. 2007; Schauvliege et al. 2009; Marly-Voquer et al. 2016). Anesthetic induction is performed using ketamine with or without a benzodiazepine or guaifenesin, followed by isoflurane or sevoflurane to maintain general anesthesia (Bellei et al. 2007, Schauvliege et al. 2009). A continuous rate infusion of dexmedetomidine has also been administered during anesthesia in horses undergoing TVEC resulting in stable cardiovascular performance (Marly-Voquer et al. 2016). Positive inotropic agents, such as dobutamine, are discontinued at least five minutes prior to shock administration due to the excitatory effect on the myocardium and the arrhythmogenic potential of these agents; however, no adverse effects have been reported with their use (Bellei et al. 2007, Schauvliege et al. 2009, Marly-Voquer et al. 2016). Lidocaine causes a dose-dependent increase in the defibrillation threshold (requiring more energy to defibrillate) in many species. While this effect is less with biphasic shock administration (Ujhelyi et al. 1995), as is used with equine TVEC, systemic lidocaine administration should be avoided to facilitate conversion at the lowest possible energy level.

Standard monitoring, including direct blood pressure monitoring, pulse oximetry, ECG, and capnography, are recommended, as well as conventional ventilation and fluid support. Careful attention should be paid to the security and position of the cardiac catheters to avoid displacement with the transition to recumbency and while positioning the horse during the procedure. Strong muscular contractions associated with shock administration should be anticipated, requiring appropriate support from an inflatable mattress or pad, intermittent repositioning throughout the procedure, and checking the patient for potential disconnections from the anesthesia circuit and monitoring equipment.

Pacemaker Implantation

Procedure

Pacemaker implantation is an uncommon procedure in horses. Indications for a pacemaker are conditions that result in severe bradydysrhythmia: third-degree AVB, high-grade second-degree AVB, and sick sinus syndrome. The decision to place a permanent pacemaker is multifactorial and the type (epicardial vs. endocardial) and location (atrial, ventricular, or dual chamber) of permanent pacing should be determined based on the underlying dysrhythmia. In horses, successful placement of epicardial and transvenous pacemakers have been described. The type of pacemaker procedure will largely dictate the anesthetic considerations required. At our institution, all animals regardless of pacemaker placement have a temporary pacing lead placed prior to sedation or anesthesia.

Anesthetic Considerations and Management

Both epicardial and transvenous pacemaker implantation techniques require placement of a temporary pacing lead via the jugular vein prior to implantation of the permanent pacemaker. While experimental studies have sedated healthy horses with alpha-2 agonists and opioids to facilitate placement of temporary pacing leads (van Loon et al. 2000, 2001), alternations in autonomic tone associated with sedative and opioid administration have the potential to worsen bradyarrhythmias, and should be avoided in clinical patients prior to temporary pacing. Instead, infiltration of local anesthetic over the catheterization site alone can facilitate placement and increase patient comfort.

Epicardial pacemaker placement is invasive, requiring general anesthesia and surgical implantation via lateral thoracotomy. While this has been performed successfully in equine patients (Pibarot et al. 1993), transvenous pacemaker implantation is considerably less invasive and can be performed under standing sedation, removing many of the risks associated with general anesthesia.

The jugular and cephalic veins have both been proposed as insertion sites for transvenous permanent pacing leads, with the pacemaker inserted in a subcutaneous pocket at the level of the pectoral muscle (van Loon et al. 2001, 2002). Infusions or boluses of alpha-2 agonists and opioids, combined with infiltration of local anesthetics, provide effective sedation and analgesia for the procedure once temporary pacing is ensured.

References

Aguiar, A.J.A., Hussni, C.A., Luna, S.P.L. et al. (1993). Propofol compared with propofol/guaifenesin after detomidine premedication for equine surgery. *Veterinary Anaesthesia and Analgesia* 20 (1): 26–28.

Alleman, M., Magdesian, K.G., Peterson, T.S. et al. (2007). Salinomycin toxicosis in horses. *Journal of the American Veterinary Medical Association* 230: 1822–1826.

Bellei, M.H., Kerr, C., McGurrin, M.K. et al. (2007). Management and complications of anesthesia for transvenous electrical cardioversion of atrial fibrillation in horses: 62 cases (2002–2006). *Journal of the American Medical Association* 231 (8): 1225–1230.

Bettschart-Wolfensberger, R., Kalchofner, K., Neges, K. et al. (2005). Total intravenous anaesthesia in horses using medetomidine and propofol. *Veterinary Anaesthesia and Analgesia* 32 (6): 348–354.

Bishop, S., Cole, C.R., and Smetzer, D.L. (1966). Functional and morphologic pathology of equine aortic insufficiency. *Pathologia Veterinaria* 3: 137–158.

Bonagura, J.D. (1990). Clinical evaluation and management of heart disease. *Equine Veterinary Education* 2: 31–37.

Bonagura, J.D. and Blissitt, K.J. (1995). Echocardiography. *Equine Veterinary Journal* 19: 5–17.

Bonagura, J.D. and Miller, M.S. (1985). Junctional and ventricular arrhythmias. *Journal of Equine Veterinary Science* 5: 347–350.

Bonagura, J.D. and Miller, M.S. (1986). Common conduction disturbances. *Journal of Equine Veterinary Science* 6: 23–25.

Bright, J.M. and Hellyer, P. (2002). ECG of the month. Atrial fibrillation. *Journal of the American Veterinary Medical Association* 221 (7): 942–943.

Brock, N. and Hildebrand, S.V. (1990). A comparison of xylazine-diazepam-ketamine and xylazine-guaifenesin-ketamine in equine anesthesia. *Veterinary Surgery* 19 (6): 468–474.

Bryant, C.E., Clarke, K.W., and Thompson, J. (1996). Cardiopulmonary effects of medetomidine in sheep and in ponies. *Research in Veterinary Science* 60 (3): 267–271.

Buchanan, J.W. (2001). Patent ductus arteriosus morphology, pathogenesis, types and treatments. *Journal of Veterinary Cardiology* 3 (7): 7–16.

Budras, K.D., Sack, W.O., and Röck, S. (2012). *Anatomy of the Horse*, 6e, 54–57. Schluetersche Germany: Thieme.

Buhl, R., ErsbØll, A.K., Larsen, N.H. et al. (2007). The effects of detomidine, romifidine or acepromazine on echocardiographic measurements and cardiac function in normal horses. *Veterinary Anaesthesia and Analgesia* 34 (1): 1–8.

Carregaro, A.B., Teixeira-Neto, F.J., Beier, S.L. et al. (2006). Cardiopulmonary effects of buprenorphine in horses. *American Journal of Veterinary Research* 67 (10): 1675–1680.

Christ, G., Mundigler, G., Merhaut, C. et al. (1997). Adverse cardiovascular effects of ketamine infusion in patients with catecholamine-dependent heart failure. *Anaesthesia and Intensive Care* 25 (3): 255–259.

Clarke, K.W. and Paton, B.S. (1988). Combined use of detomidine with opiates in the horse. *Equine Veterinary Journal* 20 (5): 331–334.

Corley, K.T., Donaldson, L.L., Durando, M.M. et al. (2003). Cardiac output technologies with special reference to the horse. *Journal of Veterinary Internal Medicine* 17 (3): 262–272.

Cornick, J.L., Hartsfield, S.M., and Miller, M. (1990). ECG of the month. Premature ventricular complexes in an anesthetized colt. *Journal of the American Veterinary Medical Association* 196 (3): 420–422.

Costa-Farré, C., García-Martínez, A., Segura, D. et al. (2006). Anesthesia case of the month. *Journal of the American Veterinary Medical Association* 229 (12): 1859–1961.

Craig, C.A., Haskins, S.C., Hildebrand, S.V. et al. (2007). The cardiopulmonary effects of dobutamine and norepinephrine in isoflurane-anesthetized foals. *Veterinary Anaesthesia and Analgesia* 34 (6): 377–387.

Dancker, C., Hopster, K., Rohn, K. et al. (2018). Effects of dobutamine, dopamine, phenylephrine and noradrenaline on systemic haemodynamics and intestinal perfusion in isoflurane anaesthetised horses. *Equine Veterinary Journal* 50 (1): 104–110.

De Clercq, D., van Loon, G., and Schauvliege, S.T. (2008). Transvenous electrical cardioversion of atrial fibrillation in six horses using custom made cardioversion catheters. *Veterinary Journal* 177 (2): 198–204.

Delesalle, C., van Loon, G., Nollet, H. et al. (2002). Tumor-induced ventricular arrhythmia in a horse. *Journal of Veterinary Internal Medicine* 16: 612–617.

Diana, A., Guglielmini, C., Candini, D. et al. (2007). Cardiac arrhythmias associated with piroplasmosis in the horse: a case report. *Veterinary Journal* 174: 193–195.

Dickinson, C.E., Traub-Dargatz, J.L., Dargatz, D.A. et al. (1996). Rattlesnake venom poisoning in horses: 32 cases (1973–1993). *Journal of the American Veterinary Medical Association* 208: 1866–1871.

Dolente, B.A., Seco, O.M., and Lewis, M.L. (2000). Streptococcal toxic shock in a horse. *Journal of the American Veterinary Medical Association* 217 (1): 64–67.

Donnellan, C.M., Page, P.C., Nurton, J.P. et al. (2013). Comparison of glycopyrrolate and atropine in ameliorating the adverse effects of imidocarb dipropionate in horses. *Equine Veterinary Journal* 45 (5): 625–629.

Doonan, G., Brown, C.M., Mullaney, T.P. et al. (1989). Monensin poisoning in horses. *Canadian Veterinary Journal* 30: 165–169.

Else, R. and Holmes, J.R. (1972). Cardiac pathology in the horse. 2. Microscopic pathology. *Equine Veterinary Journal* 16: 125–135.

Fielding, C.L., Brumbaugh, G.W., Matthews, N.S. et al. (2006). Pharmacokinetics and clinical effects of a subanesthetic continuous rate infusion of ketamine in awake horses. *American Journal of Veterinary Research* 67: 1484–1490.

Figueiredo, J.P., Muir, W.W., and Sams, R. (2012). Cardiorespiratory, gastrointestinal, and analgesic effects of morphine sulfate in conscious healthy horses. *American Journal of Veterinary Research* 73 (6): 799–808.

Folts, J.D., Afonso, S., and Rowe, G.G. (1975). Systemic and coronary haemodynamic effects of ketamine in intact anaesthetized and unanaesthetized dogs. *British Journal of Anaesthesia* 47 (6): 686–694.

Freeman, S.L., Bowen, I.M., Bettschart-Wolfensberger, R. et al. (2002). Cardiovascular effects of romifidine in the standing horse. *Research of Veterinary Science* 72 (2): 123–129.

Fregin, G.F. (1982). The cardiovascular system. In: *Equine Medicine and Surgery*, 3e (eds. R.A. Mansmann, E.S. McAllister and P.W. Pratt), 645–704. Santa Barbara, CA, USA: *American Veterinary Publications*.

Frye, M.A., Selders, C.G., Mama, K.R. et al. (2002). Use of biphasic electrical cardioversion for treatment of idiopathic atrial fibrillation in two horses. *Journal of the American Veterinary Medical Association* 220 (7): 1039–1045.

Gesell, S. and Brandes, K. (2006). Tetralogy of Fallot in a 7-year-old gelding. *Veterinářství* 22: 427–430.

Giguère, S., Knowles, H.A., Valverde, A. et al. (2005). Accuracy of indirect measurement of blood pressure in neonatal foals. *Journal of Veterinary Internal Medicine* 19 (4): 571–576.

Grandy, J.L., Steffey, E.P., Hodgson, D.S. et al. (1987). Arterial hypotension and the development of postanesthetic myopathy in halothane-anesthetized horses. *American Journal of Veterinary Research* 48 (2): 192–197.

Grosenbaugh, D.A. and Muir, W.W. (1998). Cardiorespiratory effects of sevoflurane, isoflurane, and halothane anesthesia in horses. *American Journal of Veterinary Research* 59 (1): 101–106.

Hamlin, R.L. and Smith, C.R. (1965). Categorization of common domestic mammals based upon their ventricular activation process. *Annals of the New York Academy of Sciences* 127 (1): 195–203.

Hare, T. (1931). A patent ductus arteriosus in an aged horse. *The Journal of Pathology and Bacteriology* 84: 124.

Hatz, L.A., Hartnack, S., Kümmerle, J. et al. (2015). A study of measurement of noninvasive blood pressure with the oscillometric device, sentinel, in isoflurane-anaesthetized horses. *Veterinary Anaesthesia and Analgesia* 42 (4): 369–376.

Heliczer, N., Lorello, O., Casoni, D. et al. (2016). Accuracy and precision of noninvasive blood pressure in normo-, hyper-, and hypotensive standing and anesthetized adult horses. *Journal of Veterinary Internal Medicine* 30 (3): 866–872.

Hilwig, R.W. (1977). Cardiac arrhythmias in the horse. *Journal of the American Veterinary Medical Association* 170: 153–163.

Hiscox, K.L. (2012). Dexmedetomidine infusion as an adjunct anesthetic for tetralogy of fallot repair during a pediatric cardiac mission trip in Jamaica: a case report. *American Association of Nurse Anesthetists* 80 (5): 385–391.

Hofmeister, E.H., Mackey, E.B., and Trim, C.M. (2008). Effect of butorphanol administration on cardiovascular parameters in isoflurane-anesthetized horses – a retrospective clinical evaluation. *Veterinary Anaesthesia and Analgesia* 35 (1): 38–44.

Holmes, J.R., Henigan, M., Williams, R.B. et al. (1986). Paroxysmal atrial fibrillation in racehorses. *Equine Veterinary Journal* 18: 37–42.

Horn, J. (2002). *Sympathetic Nervous Control of Cardiac Function and its role in Equine Heart Disease*. Royal Veterinary College University of London.

Houe, H., Koch, J., and Bindseil, E. (1996). Tetralogy of Fallot in horses. *Dansk Veterinaertidsskrift* 79 (2): 43–45.

Hubbell, J.A., Muir, W.W., and Sams, R.A. (1980). Guaifenesin: cardiopulmonary effects and plasma concentrations in horses. *American Journal of Veterinary Research* 41 (11): 1751–1755.

Huston, R., Saperstein, G., and Leipold, H.W. (1977). Congenital defects in foals. *Journal of Equine Medicine and Surgery* 1: 146–161.

Johnston, G.M., Eastment, J.K., Wood, J.L.N. et al. (2002). The confidential enquiry into perioperative equine fatalities (CEPEF): mortality results of phases 1 and 2. *Veterinary Anaesthesia and Analgesia* 29 (4): 159–170.

Johnstone, M. (1976). The cardiovascular effects of ketamine in man. *Anesthesia* 31 (7): 873–882.

Kamerling, S.G., DeQuick, D.J., Weckman, T.J. et al. (1985). Dose-related effects of fentanyl on autonomic and behavioral responses in performance horses. *General Pharmacology* 16 (3): 253–258.

Kerr, C.L., Bouré, L.P., Pearce, S.G. et al. (2009). Cardiopulmonary effects of diazepam-ketamine-isoflurane or xylazine-ketamine-isoflurane during abdominal surgery in foals. *American Journal of Veterinary Research* 70 (5): 574–580.

Kimberly, M., McGurrin, J., Physick-Sheard, P.W., and Kenney, D.G. (2005). How to perform transvenous electrical cardioversion in horses with atrial fibrillation. *Journal of Veterinary Cardiology* 7: 109–119.

Kittleson, M.D. and Kienle, R.D. (eds.) (1998). Cardiac embryology. In: *Small Animal Cardiovascular Medicine*, 1e. St. Louis, MO, USA: Mosby.

Lawler, J.B., Frye, M.A., Ehrhart, E.J. et al. (2008). Third-degree Atrioventricular block in a horse secondary to rattlesnake envenomation. *Journal of Veterinary Internal Medicine* 22 (2): 486–490.

Leise, B.S., Fugler, L.A., Stokes, A.M. et al. (2007). Effects of intramuscular administration of acepromazine on palmar digital blood flow, palmar digital arterial pressure, transverse facial arterial pressure, and packed cell volume in clinically healthy, conscious horses. *Veterinary Surgery* 36 (8): 717–723.

Levine, S.A. and Harvey, W.P. (1950). *Clinical Examination of the Heart*, 51. Philadelphia: WB Saunders.

Linton, R.A., Young, L.E., Marlin, D.J. et al. (2000). Cardiac output measured by lithium dilution, thermodilution, and transesophageal Doppler echocardiography in anesthetized horses. *American Journal of Veterinary Research* 61 (7): 731–737.

Littlewort, M.C.G. (1962). The clinical auscultation of the equine heart. *The Veterinary Record* 74: 1247–1159.

Lombard, C., Scarratt, W.K., and Ruergelt, C.D. (1983). Ventricular septal defects in the horse. *Journal of the American Veterinary Medical Association* 167 (1): 562–565.

Lombard, C.W., Evans, M., Martin, L. et al. (1984). Blood pressure, electrocardiogram and echocardiogram measurements in the growing pony foal. *Equine Veterinary Journal* 16 (4): 342–347.

van Loon, G., Tavernier, R., Duytschaever, M. et al. (2000). Pacing induced atrial fibrillation in a pony. *The Canadian Journal of Veterinary Research* 64 (4): 254–258.

van Loon, G., Fonteyne, W., Rottiers, H. et al. (2001). Dual-chamber pacemaker implantation via the cephalic vein in healthy equids. *Journal of Veterinary Internal Medicine* 15 (6): 564–571.

van Loon, G., Fonteyne, W., Rottiers, H. et al. (2002). Implantation of a dual-chamber, rate-adaptive pacemaker in a horse with suspected sick sinus syndrome. *Veterinary Record* 151 (18): 541–545.

van Loon, G., De Clercq, D., Tavernier, R. et al. (2005). Transient complete atrioventricular block following transvenous electrical cardioversion of atrial fibrillation in a horse. *The Veterinary Journal* 170 (1): 124–127.

Mama, K.R., Steffey, E.P., and Pascoe, P.J. (1995). Evaluation of propofol as a general anesthetic for horses. *Veterinary Surgery* 24 (2): 188–194.

Mama, K.R., Wagner, A.E., Steffey, E.P. et al. (2005). Evaluation of xylazine and ketamine for total intravenous anesthesia in horses. *American Journal of Veterinary Research* 66 (6): 1002–1007.

Mama, K.R., Grimsrud, K., Snell, T. et al. (2009). Plasma concentrations, behavioural and physiological effects following intravenous and intramuscular detomidine in horses. *Equine Veterinary Journal* 41 (8): 772–777.

Marly-Voquer, C., Schwarzwald, C.C., and Bettschart-Wolfensberger, R. (2016). The use of dexmedetomidine continuous rate infusion for horses undergoing transvenous electrical cardioversion – a case series. *Canadian Veterinary Journal* 57 (1): 70–75.

Marr, C. (2010a). *Heart Failure, in Cardiology of the Horse*, 2e, 239–252. Edinburgh: WB Saunders.

Marr, C. (2010b). Cardiac murmurs: congenital heart disease. In: *Cardiology of the Horse*, 2e, 193–205. Edinburgh: WB Saunders.

Marroum, P.J., Webb, A.I., Aeschbacher, G. et al. (1994). Pharmacokinetics and pharmacodynamics of acepromazine in horses. *American Journal of Veterinary Research* 55 (10): 1428–1433.

Matthews, N.S., Hartsfield, S.M., Hague, B. et al. (1999). Detomidine-propofol anesthesia for abdominal surgery in horses. *Veterinary Surgery* 28 (3): 196–201.

Maxon-Sage, A., Parente, E.J., Beech, J. et al. (1998). Effect of high-intensity exercise on atrial blood gas tensions and upper airway and cardiac function in clinically normal quarter horses and horses with heterozygous and homozygous for hyperkalemic periodic paralysis. *American Journal of Veterinary Research* 59: 615–618.

McGuirk, S.M. and Muir, W.W. (1985). Diagnosis and treatment of cardiac arrhythmias. *The Veterinary Clinics of North America. Equine Practice* 1: 353–370.

Meyer, G.A., Lin, H.C., Hanson, R.R. et al. (2001). Effects of intravenous lidocaine overdose on cardiac electrical activity and blood pressure in the horse. *Equine Veterinary Journal* 33 (5): 434–437.

Michlik, K.M., Biazik, A.K., Henklewski, R.Z. et al. (2014). Quadricuspid aortic valve and a ventricular septal defect in a horse. *BMC Veterinary Research* 30: 10142. https://doi.org/10.1186/1746-6148-10-142.

Miller, M. and Bonagura, J.D. (1985). Atrial arrhythmias. *Journal of Equine Veterinary Science* 5: 300–303.

Muir, W.W. and McGuirk, S.M. (1984). Hemodynamics before and after conversion of atrial fibrillation to normal sinus rhythm in horses. *Journal of the American Veterinary Medical Association* 184 (8): 965–970.

Muir, W.W., Skarda, R.T., and Sheehan, W. (1978). Cardiopulmonary effects of narcotic agonists and a partial agonist in horses. *American Journal of Veterinary Research* 39 (10): 1632–1635.

Muir, W.W., Skarda, R.T., and Sheehan, W. (1979). Hemodynamic and respiratory effects of a xylazine-acetylpromazine drug combination in horses. *American Journal of Veterinary Research* 40 (11): 1518–1522.

Muir, W.W., Sams, R.A., Huffman, R.H. et al. (1982). Pharmacodynamic and pharmacokinetic properties of diazepam in horses. *American Journal of Veterinary Research* 43 (10): 1756–1762.

Muir, W.W., Reed, S.M., and McGuirk, S.M. (1990). Treatment of atrial fibrillation in horses by intravenous administration of quinidine. *Journal of the American Veterinary Medical Association* 197 (12): 1607–1610.

Musk, G.C. and Flaherty, D.A. (2007). Target-controlled infusion of propofol combined with variable rate infusion of remifentanil for anaesthesia of a dog with patent ductus arteriosus. *Veterinary Anaesthesia and Analgesia* 34 (5): 359–364.

Naylor, J.M., Yadernuck, L.M., and Oharr, J.W. (2001). An assessment of the ability of diplomates, practitioners, and students to describe and interpret recording of heart murmurs and arrhythmia. *Journal of Veterinary Internal Medicine* 15: 507–515.

Nolan, A.M. and Hall, L.W. (1985). Total intravenous anaesthesia in the horse with propofol. *Equine Veterinary Journal* 17 (5): 394–398.

Nout, Y.S., Corley, K.T., Donaldson, L.L. et al. (2002). Indirect oscillometric and direct blood pressure measurements in anesthetized and conscious neonatal foals. *Journal of Veterinary Emergency and Critical Care* 12: 75–80.

Ohmura, H., Hiraga, A., Takahashi, T. et al. (2003). Risk factors for atrial fibrillation during racing in slow-finishing horses. *Journal of the American Veterinary Medical Association* 223: 84–88.

Parry, B.W., Anderson, G.A., and Gay, C.C. (1982). Hypotension in the horse induced by acepromazine maleate. *Australian Veterinary Journal* 59 (5): 148–152.

Patteson, M. (1996). *Equine Cardiology*. Oxford, UK: Blackwell Science Ltd.

Patteson, M.W. and Cripps, P.J. (1993). A survey of cardiac auscultatory findings in horses. *Equine Veterinary Journal* 25 (5): 409–415.

Pibarot, P., Vrins, A., Salmon, Y. et al. (1993). Implantation of a programmable atrioventricular pacemaker in a donkey with complete atrioventricular block and syncope. *Equine Veterinary Journal* 25 (3): 248–251.

Radostits, O.M., Mayhew, I.G.J., and Houston, D.M. (2002). *Veterinary Clinical Examination and Diagnosis*, 104. London, UK: W.B. Saunders.

Rajput, R.S., Das, S., Makhija, N. et al. (2014). Efficacy of dexmedetomidine for the control of junctional ectopic tachycardia after repair of tetralogy of Fallot. *Annals of Pediatric Cardiology* 7 (3): 167–172.

Reed, R., Barletta, M., Mitchell, K. et al. (2019). The pharmacokinetics and pharmacodynamics of intravenous hydromorphone in horses. *Veterinary Anaesthesia and Analgesia* 46 (3): 395–404.

Reef, V.B. (1993). Pericardial and myocardial disease. In: *The Horse: Diseases and Clinical Management*, 185–197. Edinburgh: Churchill Livingstone.

Reef, V.B. (1995). Evaluation of ventricular septal defect in horses using two-dimensional and Doppler echocardiography. *Equine Veterinary Journal* 19: 86–95.

Reef, V.B. and Marr, C.M. (2010). Dysrhythmias: assessment and medical management. In: *Cardiology of the Horse*, 2e (ed. C.M. Marr), 159–178. Edinburgh: W.B. Saunders.

Reef, V.B. and Spencer, P.A. (1987). Echocardiographic evaluation of equine aortic insufficiency. *American Journal of Veterinary Research* 48 (6): 904–909.

Reef, V.B., Clark, E.S., and Oliver, J.A. (1986). Implantation of a permanent transvenous pacing catheter in a horse with complete heart block and syncope. *Journal of the American Veterinary Medical Association* 189: 449–452.

Reef, V.B., Bain, F.T., and Spencer, P.A. (1998). Severe mitral regurgitation in horses: clinical, echocardiographic and pathologic findings. *Equine Veterinary Journal* 30: 18–27.

Reimer, J.M., Reef, V.B., and Sweeney, R.W. (1992). Ventricular arrhythmias in horses: 21 cases (1984–1989). *Journal of the American Veterinary Medical Association* 201: 1237–1243.

Robertson, S.A., Sanchez, L.C., Merritt, A.M. et al. (2005). Effect of systemic lidocaine on visceral and somatic nociception in conscious horses. *Equine Veterinary Journal* 37 (2): 122–127.

Ruffato, M., Novello, L., and Clark, L. (2015). What is the definition of intraoperative hypotension in dogs? Results from a survey of diplomates of the ACVAA and ECVAA. *Veterinary Anaesthesia and Analgesia* 42 (1): 55–64.

Schauvliege, S., van Loon, G., De Clercq, D. et al. (2009). Cardiovascular responses to transvenous electrical cardioversion of atrial fibrillation in anaesthetized horses. *Veterinary Anaesthesia and Analgesia* 36 (4): 341–351.

Schmitz, R.R., Klaus, C., and Grabner, A. (2008). Detailed echocardiographic findings in a newborn foal with tetralogy of Fallot. *Equine Veterinary Education* 20 (6): 298–303.

Shih, A. (2013). Cardiac output monitoring in horses. *The Veterinary Clinics of North America. Equine Practice* 29 (1): 155–167.

Shih, A.C., Giguère, S., Sanchez, L.C. et al. (2009a). Determination of cardiac output in neonatal foals by ultrasound velocity dilution and its comparison to the lithium dilution method. *Journal of Veterinary Emergency and Critical Care* 19 (5): 438–443.

Shih, A.C., Giguère, S., Sanchez, L.C. et al. (2009b). Determination of cardiac output in anesthetized neonatal foals by use of two pulse wave analysis methods. *American*

Journal of Veterinary Research 70 (3): 334–339.

Skarda, R.T. and Muir, W.W. 3rd. (2003). Comparison of electroacupuncture and butorphanol on respiratory and cardiovascular effects and rectal pain threshold after controlled rectal distention in mares. *American Journal of Veterinary Research* 64 (2): 137–144.

Solano, A.M., Valverde, A., Desrochers, A. et al. (2009). Behavioural and cardiorespiratory effects of a constant rate infusion of medetomidine and morphine for sedation during standing laparoscopy in horses. *Equine Veterinary Journal* 41 (2): 153–159.

Steffey, E.P., Dunlop, C.I., Farver, T.B. et al. (1987). Cardiovascular and respiratory measurements in awake and isoflurane-anesthetized horses. *American Journal of Veterinary Research* 48 (1): 7–12.

Steffey, E.P., Woliner, M.J., Puschner, B. et al. (2005). Effects of desflurane and mode of ventilation on cardiovascular and respiratory functions and clinicopathologic variables in horses. *American Journal of Veterinary Research* 66 (4): 669–677.

Stevens, K.B., Marr, C.M., Horn, J.N. et al. (2009). Effect of left-sided valvular regurgitation on mortality and causes of death among a population of middle-aged and older horses. *Veterinary Record* 164 (1): 6–10.

Sugiyama, A., Takeuchi, T., Salmon, Y. et al. (2008). Mediastinal lymphoma with complete atrioventricular block in a horse. *The Journal of Veterinary Medical Science* 70: 1101–1105.

Taylor, F.G., Wotton, P.R., Hillyer, M.H. et al. (1991). Atrial septal defect and atrial fibrillation in a foal. *The Veterinary Record* 128: 80–81.

Taylor, P.M., Kirby, J.J., Shrimpton, D.J. et al. (1998). Cardiovascular effects of surgical castration during anaesthesia maintained with halothane or infusion of detomidine, ketamine and guaifenesin in ponies. *Equine Veterinary Journal* 30 (4): 304–309.

Tearney, C.C., Guedes, A.G., and Brosnan, R.J. (2016). Equivalence between invasive and

oscillometric blood pressures at different anatomic locations in healthy normotensive anaesthetised horses. *Equine Veterinary Journal* 48 (3): 357–361.

Ujhelyi, M.R., Schnur, M., Frede, T. et al. (1995). Differential effects of lidocaine on defibrillation threshold with monophasic versus biphasic shock waveforms. *Circulation* 92 (6): 1644–1650.

Umar, M.A., Yamashita, K., Kushiro, T. et al. (2007). Evaluation of cardiovascular effects of total intravenous anesthesia with propofol or a combination of ketamine-medetomidine-propofol in horses. *American Journal of Veterinary Research* 68 (2): 121–127.

Valverde, A., Giguère, S., Morey, T.E. et al. (2007). Comparison of noninvasive cardiac output measured by use of partial carbon dioxide rebreathing or the lithium dilution method in anesthetized foals. *American Journal of Veterinary Research* 68 (2): 141–147.

Wagner, A.E., Muir, W.W. 3rd, and Hinchcliff, K.W. (1991). Cardiovascular effects of xylazine and detomidine in horses. *American Journal of Veterinary Research* 52: 651–657.

Wagner, A.E., Mama, K.R., Steffey, E.P. et al. (2011). Comparison of the cardiovascular effects of equipotent anesthetic doses of sevoflurane alone and sevoflurane plus an intravenous infusion of lidocaine in horses. *American Journal of Veterinary Research* 72 (4): 452–460.

Waxman, K., Shoemaker, W.C., and Lippmann, M. (1980). Cardiovascular effects of anesthetic induction with ketamine. *Anesthesia and Analgesia* 59 (5): 355–358.

Whitton, D.L. and Trim, C.M. (1985). Use of dopamine hydrochloride during general anesthesia in the treatment of advanced atrioventricular heart block in four foals. *Journal of the American Veterinary Medical Association* 187 (12): 1357–1361.

Yamaoka, T.T., Flaherty, D., Pawson, P. et al. (2017). Comparison of arterial blood pressure measurements obtained invasively or oscillometrically using a Datex S/5 compact monitor in anaesthetised adult horses. *Veterinary Anesthesia and Analgesia* 44 (3): 492–501.

Yamashita, K., Tsubakishita, S., Futaoka, S. et al. (2000). Cardiovascular effects of medetomidine, detomidine, and xylazine in horses. *Journal of Veterinary Medical Science* 62 (10): 1025–1032.

Yamashita, K., Muir, W.W., Tsubakishita, S. et al. (2002). Infusion of guaifenesin, ketamine, and medetomidine in combination with inhalation of sevoflurane versus inhalation of sevoflurane alone for anesthesia of horses. *Journal of the American Veterinary Medical Association* 221 (8): 1150–1155.

Young, L.E. and Wood, J.L.N. (2000). The effects of age and training on murmurs and atrioventricular valvular regurgitation in your Thoroughbreds. *Equine Veterinary Journal* 32: 195–199.

Young, L.E., Blissitt, K.J., Bartram, D.H. et al. (1996). Measurement of cardiac output by transesophageal Doppler echocardiography in anaesthetized horses: comparison with thermodilution. *British Journal of Anaesthesia* 77 (6): 773–780.

Young, L.E., Rogers, K., and Wood, J.L. (2008). Heart murmurs and valvular regurgitation in thoroughbred racehorses: epidemiology and associations with athletic performance. *Journal of Veterinary Internal Medicine* 22 (2): 418–426.

6

Anesthetic Management for Medical and Surgical Neurologic Conditions

Marlis Rezende and Jeremiah Easley

Department of Clinical Sciences, College of Veterinary Medicine and Biomedical Sciences, Colorado State University, 300 West Drake Road, Fort Collins, CO, 80523, USA

Introduction

This chapter aims to review anesthetic considerations for the management of surgical and diagnostic procedures in the neurologic equine patient as well as the short-term management of neurologic conditions that may develop in the post-anesthetic period. Increasing advancements in knowledge and imaging capabilities and the resulting expanded diagnostic and surgical options provide evolving challenges for the anesthetist. Willingness to explore these options in horses that may have previously been euthanized in combination with longer and more complex procedures increases the potential for complications significantly. An understanding of central nervous system physiology and pathophysiology and procedure-specific complications and their management is therefore important. Communication between the diagnostic imaging, surgical, and anesthetic teams is key to ensure that positioning considerations (and needed positioning aids), surgical/anesthesia time, potential for blood loss, intracranial pressure (ICP) management, analgesia, recovery method, and any other unique challenges have been discussed prior to anesthesia.

General Considerations

Common causes of neurologic presentation in horses include developmental disorders (cervical vertebral malformation/instability), trauma to the brain or spinal cord, and infectious diseases (West Nile virus, equine protozoal myeloencephalitis, equine herpes myeloencephalopathy). Other diseases such as neoplasia, abscessation, vestibular, and cerebellar disease, as well as pharmacological or environmental toxicities may also be seen. Seizures may be observed concurrently or due to unexplained causes. Severity of other clinical signs can range from mild ataxia to recumbency and abnormal mentation, which further challenge anesthetic management.

Anesthetic management for the neurologic horse should focus on maintaining adequate cerebral perfusion pressures (CPPs), avoiding increased ICPs, minimizing ataxia and seizure activity, and managing other body systems (e.g. minimize myopathy) to maximize a favorable outcome. In addition to a detailed neurological evaluation, pre-anesthetic assessment should include history, signalment, physical examination, and other diagnostic information available. Of particular interest to the anesthetist is the horse's mentation, degree of ataxia, age, temperament, and ability to lie down and get back up, as this will help plan for anesthesia induction and recovery. For example, one might avoid or minimize sedation in an ataxic horse until it is positioned in the induction area to avoid worsening the ataxia with resulting immobility or inadvertent recumbency. If the horse is unable to stand, safely inducing anesthesia in the stall or trailer and the logistics of transporting the anesthetized animal to the imaging or operating room (i.e. cart, forklift) need to be outlined in advance. Availability of experienced personnel, method of transportation, and the ability to oxygenate and ventilate the horse during transport (using a demand valve or portable anesthesia machine) are important considerations; these should similarly be considered for recovery from anesthesia for a horse that is severely ataxic and has difficulty or is not capable of rising without assistance. Ideally, a padded stall set-up for neurologic horses should be available and additional tools such as a sling or lift support (i.e. Anderson Sling, UC Davis Large Animal Lift) may be needed for the most severely affected animals. Less severely affected animals with documented ability to lay down and rise on their own often do well with less assistance.

Anesthetic Management for Conditions Affecting the Brain

When anesthetizing horses where brain trauma, neoplasia, inflammation, or abscessation is suspected, minimizing increases in ICP and maintaining CPPs is paramount. The brain has limited capacity for expansion within the calvarium, and an increase in tissue mass (from edema, abscessation, or tumor growth) will require a reduction of cerebral blood flow (CBF) and cerebrospinal fluid (CSF) in order to maintain ICP within normal values. As intracranial compliance is exceeded, ICP raises rapidly. Since CPP is determined by the difference

between mean arterial pressure (MAP) and ICP ($CPP = MAP - ICP$), an increase in ICP will compromise CBF and CPP, leading to potential cerebral hypoxia and ischemia. In addition, elevated ICPs may lead to cerebral herniation and death (Drummond and Patel 2010).

Preventing increases in ICP or reducing ICP in cases where it is already elevated is a critical aspect in the anesthetic management of conditions affecting the brain. Brain tissue and the CSF can only be influenced by invasive procedures (removal of tumor mass, drainage of a subdural or extradural hematoma, CSF drainage from the cerebral ventricle), tissue edema can be addressed with the use of steroids and diuretics (discussed later in the chapter), but from an anesthesia perspective, CBF is where the most rapid changes can be achieved and therefore is typically the focus of management.

The venous side of the cerebral circulation is mostly passive, and venous drainage can be improved by maintaining the head and neck areas at a higher level than the heart, and by avoiding any compression or obstruction of the neck vessels. While head position has shown to have minimal effect in ICP of healthy awake standing horses (Brosnan et al. 2002a), it is particularly significant in anesthetized horses, where cerebral autoregulation may be disrupted and changes in hydrostatic gradients between the brain and the heart as a result of changing head position can significantly influence ICP (Brosnan et al. 2002b). Both dorsal and lateral recumbency were shown to cause intracranial hypertension in anesthetized horses, with dorsal recumbency causing the highest levels of intracranial hypertension (independent of head position) (Brosnan et al. 2002b). Therefore, when possible, lateral recumbency is favored during anesthesia of cases with suspected intracranial disease or trauma and special attention should be given to head and neck position. While intermittent positive pressure ventilation (IPPV) is routinely required to avoid hypoxemia and maintain carbon dioxide (CO_2) levels within normal limits (as discussed later in the chapter), the use of high positive end-expiratory pressure (PEEP) should be avoided (Muench et al. 2005; Drummond and Patel 2010; Chen et al. 2019) as increases in central venous or intrathoracic pressures are associated with decreased cerebral venous drainage. High intrathoracic pressures also lead to a reduction in venous return, cardiac output, and MAPs, which in turn may impact the arterial side of the cerebral circulation, as discussed in the following text.

The arterial side of cerebral circulation represented by CBF is regulated by myogenic (autoregulation), chemical (cerebral metabolic rate [CMR], $PaCO_2$, and PaO_2), and neurogenic factors (Patel and Drummond 2010). In humans, CBF remains relatively constant for MAPs between 65 and 150 mmHg due to cerebral autoregulation (Lassen 1959; Drummond 1997; Rangel-Castilla et al. 2008). When blood pressures fall below or rise above this range, CBF becomes directly dependent on systemic blood pressure. Cerebral autoregulation can be disrupted by intracranial disease/trauma and by anesthesia. Inhalant anesthetics have a dose-dependent effect in cerebral autoregulation. With concentrations below the minimum alveolar concentration (1 MAC), cerebral autoregulation is maintained, but when concentrations rise above 1 MAC, cerebral vasodilation occurs, resulting in increase in CBF and cerebral volume. The pressure ranges that support autoregulation in the horse are not known, but autoregulation disruption by the effects of inhalant anesthetics at concentrations above 1 MAC have been shown (Brosnan et al. 2002b; Brosnan et al. 2003b). While ICP values in standing, awake horses are similar to what is described for other healthy animals (Brosnan et al. 2002a), that is not the case in laterally recumbent, isoflurane-anesthetized horses (Brosnan et al. 2002b; Brosnan et al. 2003a,b). The significant intracranial hypertension described in isoflurane-anesthetized horses suggests that horses are at a much higher risk of inadequate CPP and cerebral ischemia (Brosnan et al. 2002b). Inotropes and vasopressors, such as dobutamine, ephedrine, norepinephrine, and phenylephrine, do not have a direct effect on the cerebral circulation, but their effect on the systemic arterial pressure during anesthesia can help support CPP (Steiner et al. 2004).

CMR, $PaCO_2$, and PaO_2 further influence CBF. CMR is directly coupled with CBF and a decrease in CMR leads to a decrease in CBF. Reduction in brain function (as during sleep), with most anesthetic drugs (with the exception of ketamine and nitrous oxide) and hypothermia all lead to a decrease in CMR and CBF. Conversely, seizure activity is associated with significant increases in CMR and CBF (Madsen and Vorstrup 1991; Theodore et al. 1996).

CBF is very responsive to changes in $PaCO_2$, particularly within the 25–70 mmHg range. This is due to changes in cerebral pH caused by CO_2. As $PaCO_2$ rises, cerebral pH decreases, leading to cerebral vasodilation and increase in CBF (mediated in part by nitric oxide and prostaglandins). This is of particular concern during inhalant anesthesia, where CBF may be already increased. It is therefore important to control ventilation and maintain $PaCO_2$ levels at mid-to-lower end of the normal range (provided that appropriate MAP can be maintained). Hyperventilation (hypocapnia) should be avoided and limited to emergent situations where intracranial hypertension is severe and the risk of herniation is imminent. This is because while the response to changes in $PaCO_2$ is rapid, it is not sustained. Over a period of six to eight hours, cerebral pH starts to normalize and CBF returns to pre-hyperventilation levels despite a high systemic arterial pH as bicarbonate is removed from the CSF and out across the blood brain barrier. Because the changes in CO_2 occur much faster than this equilibration process, if a patient has been hyperventilated for an extended period of time, acute normalization of CO_2 levels should be avoided as it could result in significant CSF acidosis and an acute increase in CBF and ICP. Hypoxemia, or a PaO_2 below 60 mmHg, also causes cerebral vasodilation leading to an increase in CBF (but not CMR) and should be avoided. Intranasal oxygen insufflation during induction and the use of a demand valve to supplement oxygen and support ventilation during transport to and from the operating room or computed tomography (CT)/magnetic resonance imaging (MRI) unit is recommended as is monitoring of PaO_2 and $PaCO_2$ during anesthesia. While a pulse oximeter and capnograph could be used in addition to arterial blood gases, it is important to remember that those monitoring modalities may not be as accurate in the horse. Pulse oximetry tends to underestimate hemoglobin saturation levels while the $ET\text{-}PaCO_2$ differences can be as high as 15 mmHg in horses with normal lung function (Koenig et al. 2003).

Most injectable anesthetics, sedatives, and analgesic agents preserve cerebral autoregulation, decrease CMR and CBF, and do not increase ICP (Patel and Drummond 2010). Sedation of neurologic horses is routinely performed with alpha-2 agonists as they provide reliable sedation, analgesia and help improve induction quality and reduce anesthetic requirements (Hubbell et al. 2010). Short-acting alpha-2 agonists, such as xylazine or dexmedetomidine, may be preferred to minimize duration of ataxia and cardiovascular effects. Opioids can be added to augment sedation. While effects are not well documented in horses, certain intravenous opioids (e.g. morphine and meperidine) have the potential to release histamine, which is a cerebral vasodilator and may cause an increase in CBF and CBV (Schregel et al. 1994). Hence, if utilized, slow administration is recommended. The use of acepromazine in patients with a history of seizures or undergoing procedures that can facilitate seizures (i.e. myelogram) remains controversial and is typically avoided. While there is no data in horses, phenothiazine tranquilizers have been historically associated with facilitation of seizure activity in humans (Shaw 1959; Logothetis 1967). A retrospective study in dogs with a history of seizures that received acepromazine did not show any evidence of epileptogenic activity (Tobias et al. 2006). Similarly, a study that evaluated the use of acepromazine as part of the premedication of dogs undergoing myelography reported no increase in seizure incidence when compared to dogs that did not receive acepromazine (Drynan et al. 2012). Acepromazine can however cause hypotension (Parry et al. 1982) and should be avoided in hypovolemic or systemically compromised horses.

Before being removed from the US market, thiopental used to be the preferred induction agent for horses with neurologic disease. While propofol is currently the induction agent of choice in small animals (and young foals) at risk of increased ICP, its use as an induction agent in the adult horse is limited as induction quality is not as good, and is associated with excitement, myoclonus, and paddling (Mama et al. 1995, 1996). However, induction quality can be significantly improved with the addition of guaifenesin. A guaifenesin-propofol combination as described by Brosnan et al. (2011) can be used when intracranial hypertension is suspected. Ketamine is associated with increases in CMR and CBF; however, studies in humans indicate that when combined with other drugs such as benzodiazepines or propofol, the adverse effects on ICP are mostly eliminated (Strebel et al. 1995; Sakai et al. 2000). The combination of ketamine and propofol is an acceptable option and may have the benefit of better recovery quality then when ketamine is combined to a benzodiazepine (Wagner et al. 2002; Jarrett et al. 2018).

Maintenance of general anesthesia typically requires inhalant anesthetics. As described previously, inhalant anesthetics (isoflurane, sevoflurane, and desflurane) can disrupt cerebral autoregulation and cause dose-dependent vasodilation at concentrations higher than 1 MAC. Therefore, it is recommended to avoid inhalant concentrations higher than 1 MAC if possible. A partial intravenous anesthesia technique may be considered such as the adjunctive use of propofol and/or dexmedetomidine continuous infusions to help reduce the inhalant anesthetic requirement (Marcilla et al. 2012; Villalba et al. 2014; Sacks et al. 2017; Tokushige et al. 2018). While there is no horse specific data regarding the effects of these anesthetic combinations on ICP and CPP, the use of dexmedetomidine infusions has been described in dogs undergoing craniotomies (Tayari and Bell 2019; Marquez-Grados et al. 2020) and dexmedetomidine has been shown to inhibit the cerebrovascular dilation induced by isoflurane and sevoflurane in dogs (Ohata et al. 1999). Arterial blood gases and direct arterial blood pressures should be continuously monitored, and hypercapnia, hypoxemia, and hypotension should be prevented. The occurrence of Cushing's response (hypertension and bradycardia) is a classical sign of severe intracranial hypertension and high risk of brain herniation in humans and in dogs (Doba and Reis 1972; Fodstad et al. 2006; Platt et al. 2001), but it has not been well described in the horse.

Additional strategies to reduce brain tissue edema and prevent secondary brain injury are also mostly based on data from human and small animal medicine. Early effective correction of hypotension is recommended. Fluid therapy should aim to maintain normovolemia and avoid reduction of serum osmolarity (Magdesian 2000; Pinto et al. 2006; Farrokh et al. 2019). Isotonic fluids such as Lactated Ringers (LRS) or normal saline are routinely used. LRS is slightly less osmolar than plasma but does not seem to negatively impact serum osmolality at typical rates. Normal saline may lead to hyperchloremic metabolic acidosis and if large volumes are required to re-establish normovolemia, one may alternate saline and LRS to minimize this effect (Farrokh et al. 2019).

Osmotic diuretics are extensively used to reduce the volume of intra and extracellular fluid compartments in the brain as well as decrease the hematocrit and blood viscosity via plasma expansion (Knapp 2005). Early administration of osmotic diuretics, such as mannitol, is a cornerstone of intracranial hypertension

management in humans (Carney et al. 2017; Farrokh et al. 2019), small animals (Sande and West 2010; DiFazio and Fletcher 2013), and horses (Feary et al. 2007) as it is fast acting and effective. Hypertonic saline is an alternative to mannitol as both seem to be equally effective in humans (Gu et al. 2019; Chen et al. 2020), with a recent study suggesting that hypertonic saline may have a more sustained effect on ICP (Shi et al. 2020). Hypertonic saline may be more practical to administer in the horse and have the additional benefit of improving circulating blood volume and perfusion in hypovolemic patients with intracranial hypertension (Fielding and Magdesian 2010; Mangat et al. 2020). It is also less likely to create dehydration and hypovolemia as its diuretic effect is not as pronounced. Also, the efficacy of mannitol, but not hypertonic saline, decreases with repeated dosing, which has encouraged studies in humans evaluating the potential use of hypertonic saline as a continuous infusion with promising results (Asehnoune et al. 2017; Mangat 2018). Electrolyte, acid–base status, and serum osmolality should be carefully monitored during osmotic diuretic therapy (Feary et al. 2007; Hoehne et al. 2021). Hypertonic saline tends to increase both sodium and chloride plasma levels and can lead to hyperchloremic metabolic acidosis, which in turn may have negative renal effects (Schmall et al. 1990; Fielding and Magdesian 2010; Sigmon et al. 2020). Although specific studies have not been performed in the horse, recommendations based on the human literature suggest that serum sodium concentrations above 155 mmol/l and serum osmolality above 320 mOsm/l should generally be avoided (Adelson et al. 2003; Fielding and Magdesian 2010; Alshayeb et al. 2011). Excessive brain cell shrinkage and development of hypernatremic encephalopathy are typical concerns in human and small animal medicine (Adrogue and Madias 2000; Guillaumin and DiBartola 2017), although this is not well documented in the horse (Mayhew 2009; Collins et al. 2018). Cases of refractory intracranial hypertension in humans seem to respond to hypertonic saline (Gu et al. 2019).

A combination of osmotic and loop diuretics (mannitol and furosemide) is sometimes used, with the idea that mannitol would create the osmotic gradient resulting in fluid being pulled out of the parenchyma into the intravascular space and furosemide would then remove the excess fluid from the intravascular space via diuresis, helping maintain the osmotic gradient (Todd et al. 2006). Furosemide, by inhibiting chloride channels may also slow down the normal volume-restoring mechanism of neurons and glia, which regulates cell volume (Staub et al. 1994). Care should be taken to avoid dehydration and hypovolemia. There is some concern with the use of mannitol and other osmotic diuretics when intracranial bleeding is suspected as it may cause an increase in the intracerebral hemorrhage volume (Aminmansour et al. 2017). While the use of mannitol in patients with large intracranial hematomas has been described (Dastur and Yu 2017), other studies have shown that mannitol does not seem to be effective in reducing hemorrhage volume after a stroke and does not improve outcome (Wang et al. 2015).

The beneficial effects of using steroids to reduce brain tissue edema and increase blood brain barrier permeability in patients with brain tumors is well described in humans (Miller et al. 1977; Yeung et al. 1994; Wilkinson et al. 2006). Dexamethasone remains the mainstay of treatment of tumor edema (Shapiro et al. 1990; Dietrich et al. 2011) although other glucocorticoids such as prednisone, prednisolone, and methylprednisolone are also used (Dietrich et al. 2011). The recommendation is that, whenever possible, steroid therapy should be started 48 hours prior to anesthesia (although beneficial effects can be noticed within 24 hours) and be continued during anesthesia (Miller and Leech 1975; Miller et al. 1977; Bell et al. 1987). High doses of glucocorticoids were frequently used in the treatment of acute brain or spinal cord injuries in horses (Feary et al. 2007). While there may be a benefit in the neurological outcome of acute spinal cord injuries (Bracken et al. 1990; Bracken et al. 1992), the use of steroids in the treatment of traumatic brain injury in humans is not recommended as controlled trials have shown no benefit and even potential deleterious effects (Edwards et al. 2005). Based on this information and potential for side effects (e.g. laminitis) its use in the horse with head trauma is not currently recommended.

Dimethyl sulfoxide (DMSO) has been historically used as part of the treatment for traumatic brain and spinal cord injuries in horses (Reed 2007). The rationale for its use is based on the drug's anti-inflammatory and possible antioxidant properties (de la Torre et al. 1975; Rucker et al. 1981; Shi et al. 2001), but there are no studies evaluating if it is effective. Vitamin E and C have also been used for their antioxidant effects, but no evidence of benefit is available.

Anesthetic Considerations for Conditions Affecting the Neck

Suspected cervical vertebral stenotic myelopathy (CVSM) is likely the most common equine neurologic presentation for which anesthesia is required. A definitive CVSM diagnosis depends on myelography (and more recently a combination of myelography and computed tomography) to identify the exact location(s) of spinal cord compression (van Biervliet et al. 2004; Kristoffersen et al. 2014). This is particularly important if ventral cervical stabilization will be surgically attempted. Some lesions may be dynamic and are only seen when the neck is flexed (Kühnle et al. 2018). Several complications have been associated following myelography and include transient worsening of ataxia, delayed recovery from anesthesia, seizures, blindness, hyperesthesia, depression, fever, anaphylaxis, neuropathy, and myopathy (Stowater et al. 1978; Nyland et al. 1980; Mullen et al. 2015). Adverse reactions with different degrees of severity were reported in one-third of the horses anesthetized for myelography in a multi-center study, but only 2% of those required euthanasia (Mullen et al. 2015).

The severity of the horse's neurologic status is an important consideration for the anesthetist as previously discussed. A higher grade of ataxia (grade 4) at presentation has been associated with an increased incidence of severe complications and deterioration of neurologic status post-myelogram, while in less severe cases (grade 3 or less) the worsening of ataxia was typically transient (24–48 hours) and unlikely to affect outcome (Hubbell et al. 1988). A recent multi-center study (Mullen et al. 2015) reported worsening of the neurologic status post-myelogram in 25% of the study horses, but was not able to establish a correlation between the severity of neurologic status pre-myelogram and an increased risk of adverse reactions.

Myelography is a relatively short procedure (typically less than one hour), but technical difficulties or additional imaging such as computed tomography can significantly increase anesthetic time and further impact recovery time and quality (Voulgaris and Hofmeister 2009; Clark-Price 2013). Due to limited padding and the required positioning during the myelogram, a prolonged anesthetic time may increase the risk of myopathies and neuropathies (Johnston et al. 2004).

Administration of contrast solution into the CSF may significantly expand its volume and increase ICP. Typically, this is minimized by removal of a similar amount of CSF immediately prior to contrast administration and by administering the contrast slowly. Many of the complications associated with myelography seem to be related to the contrast media used; iohexol is preferred as it is associated with fewer adverse reactions than metrizamide (Widmer et al. 1998).

Induction of anesthesia is typically performed with ketamine combined with a benzodiazepine (midazolam or diazepam) or propofol. The ketamine-propofol combination has been shown to provide better recovery quality than ketamine-midazolam after a short period of general anesthesia (Jarrett et al. 2018). The decreased ataxia associated with this induction protocol may be particularly beneficial in neurologic horses after myelography. If the myelography can be completed in less than one hour, injectable agents may be used for maintenance of anesthesia. A combination of guaifenesin, ketamine, and xylazine (GKX) is commonly used. If guaifenesin is not available, it can be replaced with midazolam (Aarnes et al. 2018). For procedures >1 hour, inhalant anesthesia is preferred to avoid drug accumulation resulting in ataxia and prolonged recovery.

The jugular catheter is usually placed in the upper side to avoid being displaced during procedural positioning. It should be placed as low as possible on the neck as to not be occluded when the neck is flexed during the myelogram. (Figure 6.1) With the extreme position changes of the neck (Figures 6.2 and 6.3a,b), the endotracheal tube may also become bent or obstructed (Figure 6.4). Monitoring of the capnograph and changes in the sound of the ventilator (with certain machines if being used) will alert the anesthetist prior to this being observed on the radiographs. When inhalant anesthesia is used, direct arterial pressures should be continuously monitored. The arterial catheter is generally placed in the metatarsal artery to minimize interference with positioning during myelography and maintain accuracy. Dobutamine continuous infusion should be used as needed to maintain MAPs above 70 mmHg, and the upper limbs should be supported (Figure 6.5).

During recovery, the horse should be placed in a padded recovery stall and positioned with the head elevated to help move the contrast away from the brain and potentially reduce the risk of seizures. Midazolam or diazepam should be easily accessible in case of need. Dependent limbs should be moved forward to minimize any nerve pressure. Additional sedation may be administered, depending on the duration of the procedure and the degree of ataxia of the horse. Usually, a low dose of

Figure 6.1 Image depicts cervical radiographic image obtained during cervical myelography where a kinked jugular catheter is observed. Source: Courtesy of Dr. Marlis Rezende.

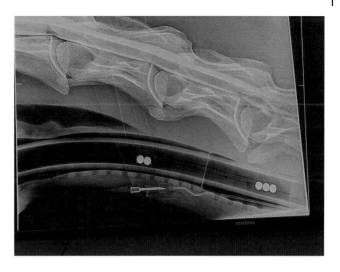

romifidine or dexmedetomidine is preferred. Romifidine has been shown to provide better recovery quality than xylazine at equipotent doses (Woodhouse et al. 2013) and has been the drug of choice for post-anesthetic sedation, particularly as it tends to cause less ataxia. A recent clinical study comparing equipotent doses of romifidine and dexmedetomidine reported that no differences in recovery quality were observed between drugs (Hector et al. 2020). Therefore, either one would be

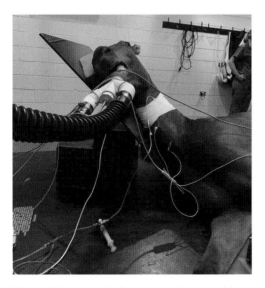

Figure 6.2 Image depicts elevated neck position during cervical myelography. Source: Courtesy of Dr. Marlis Rezende.

appropriate if additional sedation is needed. Administration of anti-inflammatory drugs such as flunixin meglumine may also be indicated to mitigate pain and inflammation. Horses anesthetized for longer periods of time and the ones with more severe ataxia may benefit from assistance (head and tail ropes or manual tail support) while the less compromised usually do well if left undisturbed.

In order to improve the neurological status in cases of CVSM, ventral cervical stabilization is often required. Pending the experience of the surgical team, this can be a challenging and complex surgical procedure, carrying an increased anesthetic risk. Positioning of the horse for surgery should be well thought out, with the horse in dorsal recumbency and the neck well supported as per the preference of the surgeon. Particular attention should be placed in preventing overextension of the head. Laryngeal paralysis is a well-known complication associated with the ventral cervical approach (McCoy et al. 1984), and there is a high risk for upper airway obstruction in recovery and the immediate post-operative period. Upper airway endoscopy has been recommended to evaluate laryngeal function prior to anesthesia and surgery and may be repeated in the post-operative period. Inhaled anesthetics with low solubility coefficients (sevoflurane, desflurane) when available are

(a) (b)

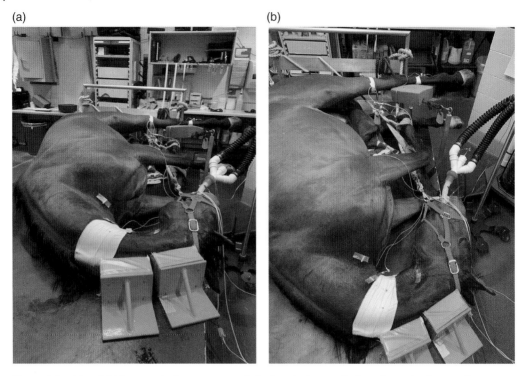

Figure 6.3 (a) and (b) Images depict extreme neck flexion during cervical myelography. Source: Courtesy of Dr. Marlis Rezende.

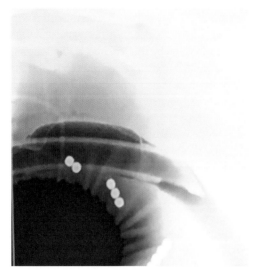

Figure 6.4 Image depicts obstruction of the open end of the endotracheal tube during cervical myelography. Source: Courtesy of Dr. Morgan Oakleaf.

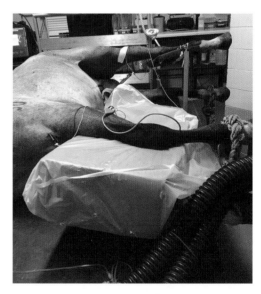

Figure 6.5 Image depicts supported limbs during cervical myelography. Note the arterial catheter in the upper hind limb. Source: Courtesy of Dr Marlis Rezende.

preferred to speed drug elimination at the end of the procedure to minimize their effects on the recovery phase. The jugular catheter should be placed away from the surgical site or sites. Pending the procedure duration, a urinary catheter may be placed to keep the bladder empty and help reduce stimulation of a distended bladder in recovery.

Pain management is another important consideration in these procedures. A non-steroidal anti-inflammatory drug should be administered in the preoperative period. A partial intravenous anesthetic technique is typically used with an alpha-2 agonist continuous infusion such as dex/medetomidine being administered as an adjunct to inhalant anesthesia. Benefits of the dex/medetomidine infusion include intraoperative analgesia, reduction of anesthetic requirement (lower inhalant concentrations) and modulation of recovery. While lidocaine and ketamine infusions may also be used in addition to dexmedetomidine in the intraoperative period, it is important that these infusions are discontinued early to avoid potential adverse effects of the drugs in recovery such as weakness, ataxia, and excitation (Bettschart-Wolfensberger and Larenza 2007). A single dose of a pure mu opioid (morphine, methadone, or hydromorphone) may also be administered at the end of the surgical procedure to provide additional analgesia in the recovery period. The use of head and tail ropes can be controversial as there is concern with the head rope putting additional force and strain on the neck. However, it can be used safely by experienced personnel. Direct assistance at the head using a halter, and manual assistance on the tail may be used instead.

Additional sedation (low dose romifidine or dexmedetomidine) may be administered in recovery when the horse is breathing spontaneously. In high-risk patients, a propofol-xylazine combination can be used to further modulate recovery quality from inhalant anesthesia using a technique described elsewhere (Steffey et al. 2009a,b). In some cases, a sling recovery may also be considered. Regardless of recovery

assistance, tools to support breathing should be available (e.g. demand valve) as respiratory depression is possible. A diluted phenylephrine solution may be sprayed in the horse's nasal passages once the horse is placed in the recovery stall and if necessary, once standing (prior to extubation where the endotracheal tube is left in place during the recovery period) to decrease nasal congestion and facilitate airway movement. Induction drugs should be readily available during extubation in case airway obstruction occurs and the horse has to be rapidly re-anesthetized. Excitable horses may benefit from a low dose of acepromazine once standing and prior to returning to the stall.

Neurectomy and Neuroma Formation

Plantar or palmar digital neurectomy is a last resort treatment to alleviate pain from chronic foot problems (affections of the navicular apparatus, distal deep digital flexor tendon, etc.) when conservative therapy is unsuccessful. It is a palliative treatment as it does not address the underlying disease process causing the discomfort, and it is also not a permanent solution, as the nerves tend to regrow over time (Gutierrez-Nibeyro et al. 2018).

When nerves are severed, the proximal nerve portion will attempt to reach the distal one by growing multiple axons in a disorganized fashion. Unorganized bundles of nerve fibers, Schwann cells, collagen, fibroblasts, myofibroblasts, and capillaries can give origin to neuromas (Devor 2013). Not all neuromas are painful and the mechanism as to why some become painful is not well understood, but may involve changes in the characteristics and distribution of sodium and potassium channels in the axons, leading to ectopic activity (Devor 1983; England et al. 1998). Constant irritation of the nerve endings from frequent movement or mechanical compression may also contribute to the development of painful neuromas. The reported incidence of painful neuroma formation after surgical neurectomy ranges from 4% to 25%

(Fubini et al. 1988; Jackman et al. 1993; Dabareiner et al. 1997; Maher et al. 2008) and is one of the main concerns associated with these procedures (Said et al. 1984; Jackman et al. 1993; Maher et al. 2008; Gutierrez-Nibeyro et al. 2015).

Intraoperative perineural infiltration of the palmar/plantar nerves with local anesthetics is common practice in neurectomies with both standing sedation and general anesthesia (Matthews et al. 2003; Maher et al. 2008; Gutierrez-Nibeyro et al. 2015). A combination of an alpha-2 agonist and an opioid are typically used for standing sedation. If inhalant anesthesia is used, dexmedetomidine, ketamine, or lidocaine continuous infusions may be added to help reduce anesthetic requirement and provide additional analgesia. A nonsteroidal anti-inflammatory (phenylbutazone) should be administered prior to surgery and continued in the post-operative period (Maher et al. 2008). Post-operative care should also include compression bandaging of the surgical site, initial strict stall confinement until sutures are removed, followed by limited hand-walking and small paddock confinement to minimize movement at the surgical site until the tissue inflammation is resolved (Matthews et al. 2003; Maher et al. 2008). In horses that develop post-surgical painful neuromas, a second procedure with neuroma resection seems to offer a good prognosis (Matthews et al. 2003).

Post-Anesthetic Neurologic Conditions: Peripheral Neuropathies, Myelomalacia, and Cerebral Necrosis

Peripheral neuropathies/myopathies are well recognized as potential complications in the post-anesthetic period (Wagner 2008; Dugdale and Taylor 2016). They can be difficult to differentiate, as with both pathologies, the horse is typically unable or unwilling to bear weight in the affected limb(s). Unlike myopathies, neuropathies are typically not painful, and are not associated with hardened, swollen muscles, myoglobinuria, or marked increases in serum muscle enzyme activity (Dyson et al. 1988). However, a myopathy may develop concurrently to a neuropathy or following a neuropathy due to prolonged recumbency or over-use of the weight-bearing limb (Dyson et al. 1988; Franci et al. 2006; Oosterlinck et al. 2013).

Neuropathies are typically a result of inadequate padding and positioning of the horse, resulting in excessive pressure on the affected nerve (Dyson et al. 1988; Franci et al. 2006). Increasing body mass and anesthetic duration seem to be predisposing factors. Horses undergoing MRI, particularly of the proximal pelvic limbs, may be at a higher risk (Franci et al. 2006; Moreno et al. 2020), likely due to limited padding and the special positioning often required to achieve proximal limb images.

Facial, radial, and femoral nerve paralysis has been reported in the post-anesthetic period (Dyson et al. 1988; Wagner 2008; Oosterlinck et al. 2013; Mirra et al. 2018; Moreno et al. 2020). Facial nerve paralysis is often associated with procedures performed in lateral recumbency, particularly ones involving the head, where inappropriate padding is used or added pressure is placed on the head (Wagner 2008). The halter can also cause pressure injury to the facial nerve and should not be kept in place during anesthesia. During rope-assisted recoveries, the halter should be very well padded or placed over a padded recovery helmet. Facial nerve paralysis is typically characterized by a one-sided droop of the lip and nose, although the ear and the eyelid on the affected side may also be affected if the facial nerve injury is more proximal and affects the auricular and palpebral nerves.

Radial nerve paralysis is also associated with inappropriate positioning of the horse during lateral recumbency. The dependent forelimb should be pulled forward to reduce pressure on the radial nerve and the upper limb should be supported at approximately chest width (to help minimize the occurrence of a triceps myopathy). The dependent limb should be padded to support the shoulder and elbow and avoid undue pressure on the nerves from the edge of the padding. Radial nerve paralysis is characterized by a dropped elbow and inability to extend the forelimb. (Figure 6.6) In these cases, it is important to rule out other conditions that may have a similar presentation such as an olecranon fracture or triceps myopathy (Wagner 2008). If radial nerve paralysis is diagnosed, the horse should be placed in a splint bandage to keep the carpus in flexion to allow the horse to bear weight on the affected limb.

Post-anesthetic neuropathies of the pelvic limb are rare and typically involve the femoral or sciatic nerves (Dugdale and Taylor 2016). Femoral nerve paralysis is characterized by the inability to extend the stifle, which also results in the flexion of the hock and fetlock (Dyson et al. 1988). In the cases reported in the literature (Dyson et al. 1988; Mirra et al. 2018; Moreno et al. 2020), an obvious cause was not clearly identified, although in the most recent

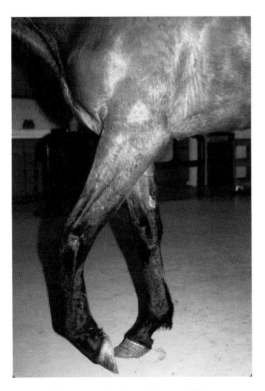

Figure 6.6 Image depicts a dropped elbow as may be observed with radial nerve paralysis. Source: Courtesy of R. Reid Hanson, DVM, DACVS, DACVECC.

report (Moreno et al. 2020), it seems likely associated with the traction placed on the affected limb in order to acquire the desired images in the MRI unit. Traction applied to the limb may result in increased tension of the nerve fibers causing compression of the axons and leading to an ischemic injury, which is described in humans (Abel et al. 2018; Sunderland 1990; Fowler et al. 2001). This mechanism is likely to be at least in part associated with neuropathies of the non-dependent limb (Dyson et al. 1988; Oosterlinck et al. 2013; Mirra et al. 2018; Moreno et al. 2020). In addition, if the non-dependent limb is not well supported, increases in compartmental and venous pressures may occur and contribute to regional ischemia of the nerve and muscles despite adequate systemic pressures (Young and Taylor 1993; Moreno et al. 2020).

The importance of adequate padding and positioning (dependent limbs pulled forward and non-dependent limbs supported and maintained in parallel with the dependent limb) is now well recognized, and the incidence of severe neuropathy is rare. In most cases, when injury is not severe, horses recover with supportive care, although it may take days to several weeks. The use of anti-inflammatory drugs (non-steroidal anti-inflammatories, corticosteroids, and DMSO) have been suggested to reduce nerve edema, as well as using a splint to support the affected limb. In horses that are unable to stand, sling support should be considered (Mirra et al. 2018).

Post-anesthetic myelopathy or myelomalacia is a rare anesthetic complication that seems to most commonly affect young (6–24 months), fast growing, draft, or large breed horses undergoing general anesthesia in dorsal recumbency (Schatzmann et al. 1979; Blakemore et al. 1984; Brearley et al. 1986; Lerche et al. 1993; Joubert et al. 2005; van Loon et al. 2010; Ragle et al. 2011), albeit cases have been reported in other breeds (Quarterhorse, Appaloosa, Thoroughbred, Connemara) (Zink 1985; Yovich et al. 1986; Wan et al. 1994; Lam et al. 1995; Raidal et al. 1997) and recumbencies (Raidal et al. 1997). Anesthesia duration does not seem to be a factor as the majority of the reported cases were short procedures (Ragle et al. 2011). The typical clinical signs include an inability to stand or move the pelvic limbs during recovery, with horses often achieving a "dog sitting" position but being unable to rise on the hind limbs (Lerche et al. 1993; Joubert et al. 2005). In some cases, the horses had a slow recovery and were able to initially stand, but their neurologic condition deteriorated, and they became recumbent hours after recovery (Zink 1985; Brearley et al. 1986; Raidal et al. 1997). Lack of deep pain, tail tone, or anal reflex was noted in the majority of the cases (Ragle et al. 2011). In all reported cases, horses were euthanized due to neurologic deterioration despite various treatments, and evidence of spinal cord damage was confirmed with necropsy and histopathology. Typical pathology includes variable degrees of myelomalacia and hemorrhage (particularly of the gray matter) anywhere from the caudal cervical to the lumbosacral spinal cord (Trim 1997; Joubert et al. 2005; Ragle et al. 2011). The etiology of this condition remains unclear, but the lesions are suggestive of compromised oxygenation of the spinal cord resulting in congestion and ischemic poliomyelopathy. The mechanisms causing the lack of spinal cord oxygenation are unknown, but it has been speculated that it may be due to a poorly developed blood supply or individual variations in spinal cord microcirculation (Schatzmann et al. 1979). Venous congestion (from dorsal recumbency potentially impairing venous return) coupled with a reduced cardiac output and arterial blood pressure, as often seen during inhalant anesthesia, has also been suggested (Schatzmann et al. 1979; Blakemore et al. 1984; Yovich et al. 1986). A subclinical deficiency of vitamin E has also been proposed as a cause for this condition (Stolk and Gruys 1995). Vitamin E deficiency may destabilize biological membranes of the spinal cord, making it more susceptible to hypoxic damage. Degenerative changes of the *nucleus cuneatus accessorius*, which is consistent with vitamin E deficiency, were described in a report of nine cases (Stolk and Gruys 1995). Due to our lack of understanding of this anesthetic complication, no preventive measures or definitive treatment can be recommended at this time (Ragle et al. 2011).

Post-anesthetic cerebral necrosis is another extremely rare complication associated with general anesthesia. The lesions observed are suggestive of cerebral ischemia (Summers et al. 1995; Spadavecchia et al. 2001; McKay et al. 2002), although the mechanism is not well understood. Intracranial hypertension has been shown to occur in healthy anesthetized horses in both dorsal and lateral recumbency (Brosnan et al. 2002b). This may place horses at a higher risk of decreased CPP and cerebral ischemia if intraoperative hypotension and hypercapnia were to occur (Brosnan et al. 2003b). Periods of significant hypoxemia could also predispose to cerebral necrosis. However, in several reported cases, anesthesia was uneventful, leading to speculation that a pre-existing but non-clinical and microscopic brain lesions could be involved (Spadavecchia et al. 2001). Clinical signs include abnormal behaviors such as pacing, head pressing, myoclonus, and seizures. Bilateral blindness has also been reported (Summers et al. 1995, Spadavecchia et al. 2001, McKay et al. 2002). Symptoms may start as early as the anesthetic recovery period (Spadavecchia et al. 2001) or develop as late as two to seven days post-anesthesia (Summers et al. 1995). Maintenance of adequate MAPs, ventilation, and oxygenation during anesthesia may further reduce the risk of this complication.

Summary

Anesthetic management of the neurologic horse can be challenging and requires a good understanding of the central nervous system physiology and pathophysiology. Careful patient evaluation is recommended. Communication between the diagnostic, surgical, and anesthesia teams is important to set expectations, discuss anticipated complications and potential interventions such that all necessary supplies, equipment, and facilities are readily available. Special attention should be dedicated to the recovery period, ensuring that experienced personnel and any specialized equipment, such as lifts and slings, are on hand in case the horse needs assistance to stand. A tracheostomy set should be readily available as for example when cervical stabilization procedures are performed.

References

Aarnes, T.K., Lerche, P., Bednarski, R.M., and Hubbell, J.A.E. (2018). Total intravenous anesthesia using a midazolam-ketamine-xylazine infusion in horses: 46 cases (2011–2014). *The Canadian Veterinary Journal* 59 (5): 500–504.

Abel, N.A., Januszewski, J., Vivas, A.C., and Uribe, J.S. (2018). Femoral nerve and lumbar plexus injury after minimally invasive lateral retroperitoneal transpsoas approach: electrodiagnostic prognostic indicators and a roadmap to recovery. *Neurosurgical Review* 41: 457–464.

Adelson, P.D., Bratton, S.L., Carney, N.A. et al. (2003). Guidelines for the acute medical management of severe traumatic brain injury in infants, children, and adolescents. *Pediatric Critical Care Medicine* 4 (suppl): S1–S75.

Adrogue, H.J. and Madias, N.E. (2000). Hypernatremia. *The New England Journal of Medicine* 342 (20): 1493–1499.

Alshayeb, H.M., Showkat, A., Babar, F. et al. (2011). Severe hypernatremia correction rate and mortality in hospitalized patients. *The American Journal of the Medical Sciences* 341 (5): 356–360.

Aminmansour, B., Tabesh, H., Rezvani, M., and Poorjafari, H. (2017). Effects of mannitol 20% on outcomes in nontraumatic intracerebral hemorrhage. *Advanced Biomedical Research* 6: 75.

Asehnoune, K., Lasocki, S., Seguin, P. et al. (2017). Association between continuous hyperosmolar therapy and survival in patients with traumatic brain injury – a multicentre prospective cohort study and systematic review. *Critical Care* 21 (1): 328.

Bell, B.A., Smith, M.A., Kean, D.M. et al. (1987). Brain water measured by magnetic resonance imaging. Correlation with direct estimation and changes after mannitol and dexamethasone. *Lancet* 1 (8524): 66–69.

Bettschart-Wolfensberger, R. and Larenza, M.P. (2007). Balanced anesthesia in the equine. *Clin Tech in Equine Pract.* 6: 104–110.

van Biervliet, J., Scrivani, P.V., Divers, T.J. et al. (2004). Evaluation of decision criteria for detection of spinal cord compression based on cervical myelography in horses: 38 cases (1981–2001). *Equine Veterinary Journal* 36 (1): 14–20.

Blakemore, W.F., Jefferies, A., White, R.A. et al. (1984). Spinal cord malacia following general anaesthesia in the horse. *The Veterinary Record* 114 (23): 569–570.

Bracken, M.B., Shepard, M.J., Collins, W.F. et al. (1990). A randomized, controlled trial of methylprednisolone or naloxone in the treatment of acute spinal-cord injury. Results of the second national acute spinal cord injury study. *The New England Journal of Medicine* 322 (20): 1405–1411.

Bracken, M.B., Shepard, M.J., Collins, W.F. Jr. et al. (1992). Methylprednisolone or naloxone treatment after acute spinal cord injury: 1-year follow-up data. Results of the second national acute spinal cord injury study. *Journal of Neurosurgery* 76 (1): 23–31.

Brearley, J.C., Jones, R.S., Kelly, D.F., and Cox, J.E. (1986). Spinal cord degeneration following general anaesthesia in a Shire horse. *Equine Veterinary Journal* 18 (3): 222–224.

Brosnan, R.J., LeCouteur, R.A., Steffey, E.P. et al. (2002a). Direct measurement of intracranial pressure in adult horses. *American Journal of Veterinary Research* 63 (9): 1252–1256.

Brosnan, R.J., Steffey, E.P., LeCouteur, R.A. et al. (2002b). Effects of body position on intracranial and cerebral perfusion pressures in isoflurane=anesthetized horses. *Journal of Applied Physiology* 92: 2542–2546.

Brosnan, R.J., Steffey, E.P., LeCouteur, R.A. et al. (2003a). Effects of duration of isoflurane anesthesia and mode of ventilation on intracranial and cerebral perfusion pressures in horses. *American Journal of Veterinary Research* 64 (11): 1444–1448.

Brosnan, R.J., Steffey, E.P., LeCouteur, R.A. et al. (2003b). Effects of ventilation and isoflurane end-tidal concentration on intracranial pressure and cerebral perfusion pressures in horses. *American Journal of Veterinary Research* 64 (1): 21–25.

Brosnan, R.J., Steffey, E.P., Escobar, A. et al. (2011). Anesthetic induction with guaifenesin and propofol in adult horses. *American Journal of Veterinary Research* 72 (12): 1569–1575.

Carney, N., Totten, A.M., O'Reilly, C. et al. (2017). Guidelines for the management of severe traumatic brain injury, fourth edition. *Neurosurgery* 80 (1): 6–15.

Chen, H., Menon, D.K., and Kavanagh, B.P. (2019). Impact of altered airway pressure on intracranial pressure, perfusion, and oxygenation: a narrative review. *Critical Care Medicine* 47 (2): 254–263.

Chen, H., Song, Z., and Dennis, J.A. (2020). Hypertonic saline versus other intracranial pressure-lowering agents for people with acute traumatic brain injury. *Cochrane Database of Systematic Reviews* 1 (1): CD010904.

Clark-Price, S.C. (2013). Recovery of horses from anesthesia. *The Veterinary Clinics of North America. Equine Practice* 29 (1): 223–242.

Collins, N.M., Carrick, J.B., Russell, C.M., and Axon, J.E. (2018). Hypernatremia in 39 hospitalized foals: clinical findings, primary diagnosis and outcome. *Australian Veterinary Journal* 96 (10): 385–389.

Dabareiner, R.M., White, N.A., and Sullins, K.E. (1997). Comparison of current techniques for palmar digital neurectomy in horses. *AAEP Proceedings* 47: 231–232.

Dastur, C.K. and Yu, W. (2017). Current management of spontaneous intracerebral haemorrhage. *Stroke and Vascular Neurology* 2 (1): 21–29.

Devor, M. (1983). Potassium channels moderate ectopic excitability of nerve-end neuromas in rats. *Neuroscience Letters* 40 (2): 181–186.

Devor, M. (2013). Neuropathic pain: pathophysiological response of nerves to injury. In: *Wall and Melzack's Textbook of Pain*, 6e (eds. S.B. McMahon, M. Koltzenburg, I. Tracey and D.C. Turk), 861–888. Philadelphia: Elsevier Saunders.

Dietrich, J., Rao, K., Pastorino, S., and Kesari, S. (2011). Corticosteroids in brain cancer patients: benefits and pitfalls. *Expert Review of Clinical Pharmacology* 4 (2): 233–242.

DiFazio, J. and Fletcher, D.J. (2013). Updates in the management of the small animal patient with neurologic trauma. *The Veterinary Clinics of North America. Small Animal Practice* 43 (4): 915–940.

Doba, N. and Reis, D.J. (1972). Localization within the lower brainstem of a receptive area mediating the pressor response to increased intracranial pressure (the Cushing response). *Brain Research* 47 (2): 487–491.

Drummond, J.C. (1997). The lower limit of autoregulation: time to revise our thinking? *Anesthesiology* 86 (6): 1431–1433.

Drummond, J.C. and Patel, P.M. (2010). Neurosurgical anesthesia. In: *Miller's Anesthesia*, 7e (eds. R.D. Miller, L.I. Eriksson, L.A. Fleisher, et al.), 2045–2087. Philadelphia: Churchill Livingstone/Elsevier.

Drynan, E.A., Gray, P., and Raisis, A.L. (2012). Incidence of seizures associated with the use of acepromazine in dogs undergoing myelography. *Journal of Veterinary Emergency and Critical Care* 22 (2): 262–266.

Dugdale, A.H. and Taylor, P.M. (2016). Equine anaesthesia-associated mortality: where are we now? *Veterinary Anaesthesia and Analgesia* 43 (3): 242–255.

Dyson, S., Taylor, P., and Whitwell, K. (1988). Femoral nerve paralysis after general anaesthesia. *Equine Veterinary Journal* 20 (5): 376–380.

Edwards, P., Arango, M., Balica, L. et al. (2005). Final results of MRC CRASH, a randomised placebo-controlled trial of intravenous corticosteroid in adults with head injury-outcomes at 6 months. *Lancet* 365 (9475): 1957–1959.

England, J.D., Happel, L.T., Liu, Z.P. et al. (1998). Abnormal distributions of potassium channels in human neuromas. *Neuroscience Letters* 255 (1): 37–40.

Farrokh, S., Cho, S.M., and Suarez, J.I. (2019). Fluids and hyperosmolar agents in neurocritical care: an update. *Current Opinion in Critical Care* 25 (2): 105–109.

Feary, D.J., Magdesian, K.G., Aleman, M.A., and Rhodes, D.M. (2007). Traumatic brain injury in horses: 34 cases (1994–2004). *Journal of the American Veterinary Medical Association* 231 (2): 259–66. doi: 10.2460/javma.231.2.259. PMID: 17630894.

Fielding, C.L. and Magdesian, K.G. (2010). Review of the use of hypertonic saline in equine practice. *AAEP Proceedings* 56: 270–273.

Fodstad, H., Kelly, P.J., and Buchfelder, M. (2006). History of the Cushing reflex. *Neurosurgery* 59 (5): 1132–1137.

Fowler, S.S., Leonetti, J.P., Banich, J.C. et al. (2001). Duration of neuronal stretch correlates with functional loss. *Otolaryngology and Head and Neck Surgery* 124: 641–644.

Franci, P., Leece, E.A., and Brearley, J.C. (2006). Post anaesthetic myopathy/neuropathy in horses undergoing magnetic resonance imaging compared to horses undergoing surgery. *Equine Veterinary Journal* 38 (6): 497–501.

Fubini, S.L., Cummings, J.F., and Todhunter, R.J. (1988). The use of intraneural doxorubicin in association with palmar digital neurectomy in 28 horses. *Veterinary Surgery* 17 (6): 346–349.

Gu, J., Huang, H., Huang, Y. et al. (2019). Hypertonic saline or mannitol for treating elevated intracranial pressure in traumatic brain injury: a meta-analysis of randomized controlled trials. *Neurosurgical Review* 42 (2): 499–509.

Guillaumin, J. and DiBartola, S.P. (2017). A quick reference on hypernatremia. *The Veterinary Clinics of North America. Small Animal Practice* 47 (2): 209–212.

Gutierrez-Nibeyro, S.D., Werpy, N.M., White, N.A. 2nd et al. (2015). Outcome of palmar/plantar digital neurectomy in horses with foot pain evaluated with magnetic resonance imaging: 50 cases (2005–2011). *Equine Veterinary Journal* 47 (2): 160–164.

Gutierrez-Nibeyro, S.D., McCoy, A.M., and Selberg, K.T. (2018). Recent advances in conservative and surgical treatment options of common equine foot problems. *Veterinary Journal* 237: 9–15.

Hector, R.C., Rezende, M.L., Mama, K.R., and Hess, A.M. (2020). Recovery quality following a single post-anaesthetic dose of dexmedetomidine or romifidine in sevoflurane anaesthetised horses. *Equine Veterinary Journal* 52 (5): 685–691.

Hoehne, S.N., Yozova, I.D., Vidondo, B., and Adamik, K.N. (2021). Comparison of the effects of 7.2% hypertonic saline and 20% mannitol on electrolyte and acid-base variables in dogs with suspected intracranial hypertension. *Journal of Veterinary Internal Medicine* 35 (1): 341–351.

Hubbell, J.A., Reed, S.M., Myer, C.W., and Muir, W.W. (1988). Sequelae of myelography in the horse. *Equine Veterinary Journal* 20 (6): 438–440.

Hubbell, J.A., Saville, W.J., and Bednarski, R.M. (2010). The use of sedatives, analgesic and anesthetic drugs in the horse: an electronic survey of members of the American Association of Equine Practitioners (AAEP). *Equine Veterinary Journal* 42 (6): 487–493.

Jackman, B.R., Baxter, G.M., Doran, R.E. et al. (1993). Palmar digital neurectomy in horses 57 cases (1984–1990). *Veterinary Surgery* 22 (4): 285–288.

Jarrett, M.A., Bailey, K.M., Messenger, K.M. et al. (2018). Recovery of horses from general anesthesia after induction with propofol and ketamine versus midazolam and ketamine. *Journal of the American Veterinary Medical Association* 253 (1): 101–107.

Johnston, G.M., Eastment, J.K., Taylor, P.M., and Wood, J.L.N. (2004). Is isoflurane safer than halothane in equine anaesthesia? Results from a prospective multicentre randomised controlled trial. *Equine Veterinary Journal* 36: 64–71.

Joubert, K.E., Duncan, N., and Murray, S.E. (2005). Post-anesthetic myelomalacia in a horse. *Journal of the South African Veterinary Association* 76 (1): 36–39.

Knapp, J.M. (2005). Hyperosmolar therapy in the treatment of severe head injury in children: mannitol and hypertonic saline. *AACN Clinical Issues* 16 (2): 199–211.

Koenig, J., McDonel, W., and Valverde, A. (2003). Accuracy of pulse oximetry and capnography in healthy and compromised horses during spontaneous and controlled ventilation. *Canadian Journal of Veterinary Research* 67 (3): 169–174.

Kristoffersen, M., Puchalski, S., Skog, S., and Lindegaard, C. (2014). Cervical computed tomography (CT) and CT myelography in live horses: 16 cases. *Equine Veterinary Journal* 46: 11–11.

Kühnle, C., Fürst, A.E., Ranninger, E. et al. (2018). Outcome of ventral fusion of two or three cervical vertebrae with a locking compression plate for the treatment of cervical stenotic myelopathy in eight horses. *Veterinary and Comparative Orthopaedics and Traumatology* 31 (5): 356–363.

Lam, K.H., Smyth, J.B., Clarke, K., and Platt, D. (1995). Acute spinal cord degeneration following general anaesthesia in a young pony. *The Veterinary Record* 136 (13): 329–330.

Lassen, N.A. (1959). Cerebral blood flow and oxygen consumption in man. *Physiological Reviews* 39: 183–238.

Lerche, E., Laverty, S., Blais, D. et al. (1993). Hemorrhagic myelomalacia following general anesthesia in a horse. *The Cornell Veterinarian* 83 (4): 267–273.

Logothetis, J. (1967). Spontaneous epileptic seizures and electroencephalographic changes in the course of phenothiazine therapy. *Neurology* 17 (9): 869–877.

van Loon, J.P., Meertens, N.M., van Oldruitenborgh-Oosterbaan, M.M., and van Dijk, R. (2010). Post-anaesthetic myelopathy in a 3-year-old Friesian gelding. *Tijdschrift voor Diergeneeskunde* 135 (7): 272–277.

Madsen, P.L. and Vorstrup, S. (1991). Cerebral blood flow and metabolism during sleep. *Cerebrovascular and Brain Metabolism Reviews* 3 (4): 281–296.

Magdesian, K.G. (2000). Traumatic brain and spinal cord injury in horses, in *proceedings*. In: *4th Annu UC Davis SVECCS Symp*, 137–141.

Maher, O., Davis, D.M., Drake, C. et al. (2008). Pull-through technique for palmar digital neurectomy: forty-one horses (1998–2004). *Veterinary Surgery* 37: 87–93.

Mama, K.R., Steffey, E.P., and Pascoe, P. (1995). Evaluation of propofol as a general anesthetic for horses. *Veterinary Surgery* 24 (2): 188–194.

Mama, K.R., Steffey, E.P., and Pascoe, P. (1996). Evaluation of propofol for general anesthesia in premedicated horses. *American Journal of Veterinary Research* 57 (4): 512–515.

Mangat, H.S. (2018). Hypertonic saline infusion for treating intracranial hypertension after severe traumatic brain injury. *Critical Care* 22 (1): 37.

Mangat, H.S., Wu, X., Gerber, L.M. et al. (2020). Hypertonic saline is superior to mannitol for the combined effect on intracranial pressure and cerebral perfusion pressure burdens in patients with severe traumatic brain injury. *Neurosurgery* 86 (2): 221–230.

Marcilla, M.G., Schauvliege, S., Segaert, S. et al. (2012). Influence of a constant rate infusion of dexmedetomidine on cardiopulmonary function and recovery quality in isoflurane anesthetized horses. *Veterinary Anaesthesia and Analgesia* 39 (1): 49–58.

Marquez-Grados, F., Vettorato, E., and Corletto, F. (2020). Sevoflurane with opioid or dexmedetomidine infusions in dogs undergoing intracranial surgery: a retrospective observational study. *Journal of Veterinary Science* 21 (1): e8.

Matthews, S., Dart, A.J., and Dowling, B.A. (2003). Palmar digital neurectomy in 24 horses using the guillotine technique. *Australian Veterinary Journal* 81 (7): 402–405.

Mayhew, I.G. (2009). Toxic diseases. In: *Large Animal Neurology*, 2e (ed. I.G. Mayhew), 321–359. West Sussex: Willey-Blackwell.

McCoy, D.J., Shires, P.K., and Beadle, R. (1984). Ventral approach for stabilization of atlantoaxial subluxation secondary to odontoid fracture in a foal. *Journal of the American Veterinary Medical Association* 185 (5): 545–549.

McKay, J.S., Forest, T.W., Senior, M. et al. (2002). Postanaesthetic cerebral necrosis in five horses. *The Veterinary Record* 150 (3): 70–74.

Miller, J.D. and Leech, P. (1975). Effects of mannitol and steroid therapy on intracranial volume-pressure relationships in patients. *Journal of Neurosurgery* 42 (3): 274–281.

Miller, J.D., Sakalas, R., Ward, J.D. et al. (1977). Methylprednisolone treatment in patients with brain tumors. *Neurosurgery* 1 (2): 114–117.

Mirra, A., Klopfenstein Bregger, M.D., and Levionnois, O.L. (2018). Suspicion of postanesthetic femoral paralysis of the non-dependent limb in a horse. *Frontiers in Veterinary Science* 7: 5–12.

Moreno, K.L., Scallan, E.M., Friedeck, W.O., and Simon, B.T. (2020). Transient pelvic limb neuropathy following proximal metatarsal and tarsal magnetic resonance imaging in seven horses. *Equine Veterinary Journal* 52: 359–363.

Muench, E., Bauhuf, C., Roth, H. et al. (2005). Effects of positive end-expiratory pressure on regional cerebral blood flow, intracranial pressure, and brain tissue oxygenation. *Critical Care Medicine* 33 (10): 2367–2372.

Mullen, K.R., Furness, M.C., Johnson, A.L. et al. (2015). Adverse reactions in horses that underwent general anesthesia and cervical myelography. *Journal of Veterinary Internal Medicine* 29 (3): 954–960.

Nyland, T.G., Blythe, L.L., Pool, R.R. et al. (1980). Metrizamide myelography in the horse: clinical, radiographic, and pathologic changes. *American Journal of Veterinary Research* 41 (2): 204–211.

Ohata, H., Lida, H., Dohi, S., and Watanabe, Y. (1999). Intravenous dexmedetomidine inhibits cerebrovascular dilation induced by isoflurane and sevoflurane in dogs. *Anesthesia and Analgesia* 89 (2): 370–377.

Oosterlinck, M., Schauvliege, S., Martens, A., and Pille, F. (2013). Postanesthetic neuropathy/myopathy in the nondependent forelimb in 4 horses. *Journal of Equine Veterinary Science* 33: 996–999.

Parry, B.W., Anderson, G.A., and Gay, C.C. (1982). Hypotension in the horse induced by acepromazine maleate. *Australian Veterinary Journal* 59 (5): 148–152.

Patel, P.M. and Drummond, J.C. (2010). Cerebral physiology and the effects of anesthetic drugs. In: *Miller's Anesthesia*, 7e (eds. R.D. Miller, L.I. Eriksson, L.A. Fleisher, et al.), 305–339. Philadelphia: Churchill Livingstone/Elsevier.

Pinto, F.C., Capone-Neto, A., Prist, R. et al. (2006). Volume replacement with lactated Ringer's or 3% hypertonic saline solution during combined experimental hemorrhagic shock and traumatic brain injury. *The Journal of Trauma* 60 (4): 758–763.

Platt, S.R., Radaelli, S.T., and McDonnell, J.J. (2001). The prognostic value of the modified Glasgow coma scale in head trauma in dogs. *Journal of Veterinary Internal Medicine* 15 (6): 581–584.

Ragle, C., Baetge, C., Yiannikouris, S. et al. (2011). Development of equine post anaesthetic myelopathy: thirty cases (1979–2010). *Equine Veterinary Education* 23: 630–635.

Raidal, S.R., Raidal, S.L., Richards, R.B. et al. (1997). Acute paraplegia in a thoroughbred racehorse after general anaesthesia. *Australian Veterinary Journal* 75 (3): 178–179.

Rangel-Castilla, L., Gasco, J., Nauta, H.J.W. et al. (2008). Cerebral pressure autoregulation in traumatic brain injury. *Neurosurgical Focus* 25 (4): E7.

Reed, S.M. (2007). Head trauma: a neurologic emergency. *Equine Veterinary Education (AE)*: 365–367.

Rucker, N.C., Lumb, W.V., and Scott, R.J. (1981). Combined pharmacologic and surgical treatments for acute spinal cord trauma. *American Journal of Veterinary Research* 42 (7): 1138–1142.

Sacks, M., Ringer, S.K., Bischofberger, A.S. et al. (2017). Clinical comparison of dexmedetomidine and medetomidine for isoflurane balanced anaesthesia in horses. *Veterinary Anaesthesia and Analgesia* 44 (5): 1128–1138.

Said, A.H., Khamis, Y., Mahfouz, M.F., and Hegazy, A. (1984). Clinicopathological studies on neurectomy in equids. *Equine Veterinary Journal* 16 (5): 442–446.

Sakai, K., Cho, S., Fukusaki, M. et al. (2000). The effects of propofol with and without ketamine on human cerebral blood flow velocity. *Anesthesia and Analgesia* 90 (2): 377–382.

Sande, A. and West, C. (2010). Traumatic brain injury: a review of pathophysiology and management. *Journal of Veterinary Emergency and Critical Care* 20 (2): 177–190.

Schatzmann, U., Meister, V., and Fankhauser, R. (1979). Acute hematomyelia after prolonged dorsal recumbency in the horse. *Schweizer Archiv für Tierheilkunde* 121 (3): 149–155.

Schmall, L.M., Muir, W.W., and Robertson, J.T. (1990). Haematological, serum electrolyte and blood gas effects of small volume hypertonic saline in experimentally induced haemorrhagic shock. *Equine Veterinary Journal* 22 (4): 278–283.

Schregel, W., Weyerer, W., and Cunitz, G. (1994). Opioids, cerebral circulation and intracranial pressure. *Der Anaesthesist* 43 (7): 421–430.

Shapiro, W.R., Hiesiger, E.M., Cooney, G.A. et al. (1990). Temporal effects of dexamethasone on blood-to-brain and blood-to-tumor transport of 14C-alpha-aminoisobutyric acid in rat C6 glioma. *Journal of Neuro-Oncology* 8 (3): 197–204.

Shaw, E.B. (1959). Phenothiazine tranquilizers as a cause of severe seizures. *Pediatrics* 23 (3): 485–492.

Shi, R., Qiao, X., Emerson, N., and Malcom, A. (2001). Dimethylsulfoxide enhances CNS neuronal plasma membrane resealing after injury in low temperature or low calcium. *Journal of Neurocytology* 30: 829–839.

Shi, J., Tan, L., Jing, Y., and Hu, L. (2020). Hypertonic saline and mannitol in patients with traumatic brain injury: a systematic and meta-analysis. *Medicine* 99 (35): e21655.

Sigmon, J., May, C.C., Bryant, A. et al. (2020). Assessment of acute kidney injury in neurologically injured patients receiving hypertonic sodium chloride: does chloride load matter? *The Annals of Pharmacotherapy* 54 (6): 541–546.

Spadavecchia, C., Jaggy, A., Fatzer, R., and Schatzmann, U. (2001). Postanaesthetic cerebral necrosis in a horse. *Equine Veterinary Journal* 33 (6): 621–624.

Staub, F., Stoffel, M., Berger, S. et al. (1994). Treatment of vasogenic brain edema with the novel cl⁻ transport inhibitor torasemide. *Journal of Neurotrauma* 11 (6): 679–690.

Steffey, E.P., Brosnan, R.J., Galuppo, L.D. et al. (2009a). Use of propofol-xylazine and the Anderson sling suspension system for recovery of horses from desflurane anesthesia. *Veterinary Surgery* 38 (8): 927–933.

Steffey, E.P., Mama, K.R., Brosnan, R.J. et al. (2009b). Effect of administration of propofol and xylazine hydrochloride on recovery of horses after four hours of anesthesia with desflurane. *American Journal of Veterinary Research* 70 (8): 956–963.

Steiner, L.A., Johnston, A.J., Czosnyka, M. et al. (2004). Direct comparison of cerebrovascular effects of norepinephrine and dopamine in head-injured patients. *Critical Care Medicine* 32 (4): 1049–1054.

Stolk, P.W.T. and Gruys, E. (1995). Thoracolumbar myelomalacia following general anesthesia in the horse. *Journal of Veterinary Anaesthesia* 22: 37.

Stowater, J.L., Kneller, S.K., and Froehlich, P.S. (1978). Metrizamide myelography in two horses. *Veterinary Medicine, Small Animal Clinician* 73 (2): 177–183.

Strebel, S., Kaufmann, M., Maitre, L., and Schaefer, H.G. (1995). Effects of ketamine on cerebral blood flow velocity in humans. Influence of pretreatment with midazolam or esmolol. *Anaesthesia* 50 (3): 223–228.

Summers, B.A., Cummings, J.F., and deLahunta, A. (1995). *Veterinary Neuropathology*, 241–242. St Louis, Missouri: Mosby Year Book Inc.

Sunderland, S. (1990). The anatomy and physiology of nerve injury. *Muscle & Nerve* 13: 771–784.

Tayari, H. and Bell, A. (2019). Dexmedetomidine infusion as a perioperative adjuvant in a dog undergoing craniotomy. *Veterinary Record Case Reports* 7: 1–6.

Theodore, W.H., Balish, M., Leiderman, D. et al. (1996). Effect of seizures on cerebral blood flow measured with 15O-H2O and positron emission tomography. *Epilepsia* 37 (8): 796–802.

Tobias, K.M., Marioni-Henry, K., and Wagner, R. (2006). A retrospective study on the use of acepromazine maleate in dogs with seizures. *Journal of the American Animal Hospital Association* 42 (4): 283–289.

Todd, M.M., Cutkomp, J., and Brian, J.E. (2006). Influence of mannitol and furosemide, alone and in combination, on brain water content after fluid percussion injury. *Anesthesiology* 105 (6): 1176–1181.

Tokushige, H., Okano, A., Arima, D. et al. (2018). Clinical effects of constant rate infusions of medetomidine-propofol combined with sevoflurane anesthesia in thoroughbred racehorses undergoing arthroscopy surgery. *Acta Veterinaria Scandinavica* 60 (1): 71.

de la Torre, J.C., Kawanaga, H.M., Johnson, C.M. et al. (1975). Dimethyl sulfoxide in central nervous system trauma. *Annals of the New York Academy of Sciences* 243: 362–389.

Trim, C.M. (1997). Postanesthetic hemorrhagic myelopathy or myelomalacia. *The Veterinary Clinics of North America. Equine Practice* 13 (1): 73–77.

Villalba, M., Santiago, I., and Gomez de Segura, I.A. (2014). Effects of a constant rate infusion of medetomidine-propofol on isoflurane minimum alveolar concentrations in horses. *Veterinary Journal* 202 (2): 329–333.

Voulgaris, D.A. and Hofmeister, E.H. (2009). Multivariate analysis of factors associated with post-anesthetic times to standing in isoflurane-anesthetized horses: 381 cases. *Veterinary Anaesthesia and Analgesia* 36 (5): 414–420.

Wagner, A.E. (2008). Complications in equine anesthesia. *The Veterinary Clinics of North America. Equine Practice* 24 (3): 735–752.

Wagner, A.E., Mama, K.R., Steffey, E.P. et al. (2002). Behavioral responses following eight anesthetic induction protocols in horses. *Veterinary Anaesthesia and Analgesia* 29 (4): 207–211.

Wan, P.Y., Latimer, F.G., Silva-Krott, I., and Goble, D. (1994). Hematomyelia in a colt: a post anesthesia/surgery complication. *Journal of Equine Veterinary Science* 14: 495–497.

Wang, X., Arima, H., Yang, J. et al. (2015). Mannitol and outcome in intracerebral hemorrhage: propensity score and multivariable intensive blood pressure reduction in acute cerebral hemorrhage trial 2 results. *Stroke* 46 (10): 2762–2767.

Widmer, W.R., Blevins, W.E., Jakovljevic, S. et al. (1998). A prospective clinical trial comparing metrizamide and iohexol for equine myelography. *Veterinary Radiology & Ultrasound* 39 (2): 106–109.

Wilkinson, I.D., Jellineck, D.A., Levy, D. et al. (2006). Dexamethasone and enhancing solitary cerebral mass lesions: alterations in perfusion and blood-tumor barrier kinetics shown by magnetic resonance imaging. *Neurosurgery* 58 (4): 640–646.

Woodhouse, K.J., Brosnan, R.J., Nguyen, K.Q. et al. (2013). Effects of postanesthetic sedation with romifidine or xylazine on quality of recovery from isoflurane anesthesia in horses. *Journal of the American Veterinary Medical Association* 242 (4): 533–539.

Yeung, W.T., Lee, T.Y., Del Maestro, R.F. et al. (1994). Effect of steroids on iopamidol blood-brain transfer constant and plasma volume in brain tumors measured with X-ray computed tomography. *Journal of Neuro-Oncology* 18 (1): 53–60.

Young, S.S. and Taylor, P.M. (1993). Factors influencing the outcome of equine anaesthesia: a review of 1,314 cases. *Equine Veterinary Journal* 25 (2): 147–151.

Yovich, J.V., LeCouteur, R.A., Stashak, T.S. et al. (1986). Postanesthetic hemorrhagic myelopathy in a horse. *Journal of the American Veterinary Medical Association* 188 (3): 300–301.

Zink, M.C. (1985). Postanesthetic poliomyelomalacia in a horse. *The Canadian Veterinary Journal* 26 (9): 275–277.

7

Anesthetic Management for Orthopedic Conditions

Tom Yarbrough[1] and Eugene Steffey[2,3]

[1] *Dubai Equine Hospital, 2 Street # 22A, Za'abeelZa'abeel 2, Dubai, UAE*
[2] *Department of Surgical and Radiological Sciences, School of Veterinary Medicine, University of California, Davis, One Garrod Drive, CA, 95616, USA*
[3] *Department of Clinical Sciences, College of Veterinary Medicine and Biomedical Science, Colorado State University, 300 West Drake Road, Fort Collins, CO, 80523, USA*

Introduction

Orthopedic conditions of horses frequently necessitate veterinary medical care. Further, musculoskeletal injuries are likely the most common cause of catastrophic injury. Horses scheduled for orthopedic procedures encompass a broad range of conditions impacting on successful anesthetic management. Consider as examples the day-old foal whose limb has been stepped on by its mare and presents with a compound femoral fracture, as opposed to a 10-week-foal presented for management of angular limb deformity. Other examples of the broad diversity of patients include adult horses that present with trauma-related limb injuries where accompanying conditions (e.g. hemorrhage) may substantially impact on anesthetic management or the elderly brood mare with a facial fracture and comorbid conditions as for example chronic laminitis. In this chapter, the authors will focus on circumstances included in, and impacting on, the development of an appropriate *individualized* anesthetic plan for the presented patient. Pre-, peri-, and immediate post-operative conditions with potential to impact successful procedural outcome are discussed as are complications associated with specific anesthetic and orthopedic procedures commonly conducted on horses. Discussion will focus on evidence-based information but author opinion will be included and when done so will be identified as such. The overriding goal will be to provide guidance on principles of anesthetic management for equine patients undergoing orthopedic-related procedures and not focus on technical aspects of anesthetic care, particularly with regard to regional anesthesia, which we consider beyond the scope of this chapter. We will tend to focus on more complex, perhaps less routine orthopedic management circumstances in an attempt to minimize duplication of information common to other forms of patient presentation and available elsewhere in this textbook. By following this approach, our hope is that skills of anesthetic management will improve over the broader base of practice represented by readers regardless of geographic location, horse breed, and/or work-type.

Special Considerations

The Patient

While there may be important geographical/regional differences in equine patients and an individual veterinarian or equine clinical establishment may focus on a particular patient type, in the broadest sense equine patients considered for orthopedic- procedures span groupings according to age, gender, breed (including consideration of physical size, body build, and demeanor), life-stage, use, and degree of physical activity and fitness. For example, they include mini-horses, donkeys, race/performance horses, mules, and draft horses; they may be domesticated or not (e.g. feral, and zoological-based). This chapter will focus on systemically healthy foals and physically active (athletic) adult horses such as, Thoroughbred racehorses, working Quarter horses, performing Warmbloods, and endurance-focused Arabians. Developmental deformities at various stages and degrees are most commonly observed in foals and yearlings while exercise-related acute or chronic joint, ligament, tendon, or bony conditions of the appendicular skeleton are most often seen in adults.

At times, adult horses are engaged in sport or work-performance disciplines that result in extreme degrees of physical exertion immediately prior to injury and the need for emergency intervention (e.g. break down in a flat race). In such cases, decisions require heightened awareness of altered physiological and pharmacological impacts on anesthetic and surgical management

A smaller subgroup of both foals and adult horses may be presented with joint infections or a localized infection occurring as a result of orthopedic trauma especially of long bones, e.g. limb fractures (closed or compounded). Other health-related confounders may accompany such orthopedic considerations and should be considered when developing an anesthetic plan.

Individuals of a still smaller group of aged adult horses are presented for diagnostic and/or surgical management in an attempt to preserve quality of life and/or to support breeding or other very specific owner interests. The degree of individual patient health may vary widely but often is at an extreme stage of chronic orthopedic disease or malfunction necessitating special care as for example assistance with mobility and chronic pain management.

Finally, horses of any age may present for surgical management of fractures or bony displacement.

Environment of Patient Care

Along with aforementioned patient considerations, the environment available for the care of equine patients with orthopedic deformities and injuries has an undeniable influence on the *individualized plan* for anesthetic management, health care personnel, and the facilities being most prominent in this regard, but geographic and/or extremes of climatic considerations may also be a factor.

For purposes of this discussion, health care personnel are identified as primary care providers, i.e. licensed veterinarians, and allied and supportive care personnel that may include both licensed and unlicensed animal nurses and/or animal health technicians with and without advanced training or experience either with handling horses and/or providing anesthesia-related care.

For purpose of highlighting focused clinical knowledge and experience, primary care providers may be identified in one or both of the species and clinical specialty focus groupings. Each grouping is further defined in Table 7.1. which also relates providers to practice facilities. Obviously, in comparison to the large multi-provider equine hospital-based facilities, casual providers would be expected to have less focused knowledge and experience regarding a breath of equine orthopedic conditions and would not have the facilities to successfully manage them. Such expectations also apply to management plans for both general anesthetic and anesthetic recovery.

Table 7.1 Categorization of primary care personnel and facilities.

Species focus	Practice-type examples
Non-equine/casual	Mixed practice or small animal focus with casual equine interest/involvement
Equine general practice	Mostly pleasure horse practice
Equine sports medicine	Racetrack or other performance-related practice focus

Veterinarian Credentials and Facilities	Examples
Not boarded commonly in ambulatory or general practice	Little or no formal advanced credentials[a] in surgery or anesthesia
Boarded surgeon[a]	
Solo practitioner	ACVS[b] credentials in solo or small group practice
Multi-staffed equine referral hospital[a]	
Private	Multi-staffed ACVS[b], and/or likely other, credentialed specialty veterinarians
University-based	Multi-staffed ACVS[b], and other credentialed specialty veterinarians

[a] Frequently including surgeons of different but aligned focus and involvement of anesthesia boarded (American or European College of Veterinary Anesthesia and Analgesia, ACVAA, ECVAA) professional providers or others with equine-focused advanced training in anesthetic management.

[b] Diplomate, American (or European) College of Veterinary Surgeons (ACVS, ECVS): Equine focus.

Before leaving this topic, it is important to note that especially in relation to major and/or uncommon orthopedic procedures, specialist anesthesia providers and/or equine surgeons may be called to travel to distant (often unfamiliar) facilities to collaborate (with potentially unfamiliar health care personnel) and assist in the operative care of a patient. In such circumstances and in support of optimal outcome, unique patient considerations and specialized procedural needs of the consultant(s) along with facility capabilities should be discussed by the primary professional health care team prior to (if possible) the arrival of consultant specialists.

Patient Positioning for Orthopedic Care and Associated Choice of Anesthetic Technique

Orthopedic interventions may be performed in standing and recumbent patients using regional and/or general anesthesia. Orthopedic procedures performed in sedated standing equine patients are increasing in both number and diversity (Auer 2012; Honnas 1991; Madron et al. 2013; Modesto et al. 2015; O'Brien and Hunt 2014; Payne and Compston 2012; Russell and Maclean 2006; Sullins 1991). This development is due to the clear advantages of minimizing patient risk of general anesthesia and recumbency (including transition to and from recumbency), and cost of care. Disadvantages of standing surgery relate to patient, personnel, and facility safety, and potential impact on surgical technique. While some of these procedures can be quite challenging to both anesthetist and surgeon, improvements in drugs, knowledge, and skill (both anesthesia and surgically related), and improved physical facilities have meaningfully supported such change. Regardless, not surprisingly success in this type of patient management is heavily dependent upon careful patient selection and health provider knowledge and skill.

General anesthesia remains most commonly used for extensive orthopedic procedures in the horse. While general anesthesia-induced recumbency reduces incidence of physical injury to health care providers and facilitates surgery-related procedural accuracy, it is a patient risk modifier due to the impact of recumbency (including improper positioning), and drug action on normal physiological (especially circulatory, respiratory, and GI) function and perhaps most importantly, the need for the patient to transition to standing posture in a smooth and atraumatic manner.

Induction of general anesthesia, especially for less routine orthopedic procedures, requires careful a priori planning by the anesthesia/surgical team. Ideally, the entire team is present at the time of induction to facilitate and/or observe the patient's response to the environment and drugs administered. Induction

experiences differ widely and are markedly influenced by facilities and clinician preferences and in this regard, we hasten to share our opinion. While more discussion on pharmacology considerations of general anesthetic induction will follow, Table 7.2 provides an overview of physical techniques of transitioning the patient from standing to recumbency. Without question, the tilt-table and sling techniques in Figures 7.1 and 7.2 (Category II techniques, Table 7.2) offer the most control in body positioning but at a significant economic cost and requirement for personnel knowledge/familiarity and skill. Indeed, the authors consider Category I techniques usually ill-suited for less routine, technically involved orthopedic surgical procedures (e.g. long bone fractures) and lack of such conditions is strong reason, if possible, for referral to facilities that include such patient management possibilities. If on the other hand and all things considered, a Category II technique is not possible or perhaps

Table 7.2 Physical techniques of equine transitioning from awake standing to anesthetized recumbent positioning for orthopedic procedures.

Category I: Recumbent positioning occurs in association with induction of general anesthesia

A. Unguided – little human physical involvement

B. Guided – various degrees of physical involvement

   i. Human physical effort

     a) Considerations

       1) Least controlled of guided patient transitioning techniques

       2) Use under field or enclosed but expansive conditions

       3) Use with smaller stature, manageable animal, e.g. foal, mini-horse, small horse breeds

       4) Knowledgeable, skilled, physically abled persons required for a team effort

       5) Facilities/immediate vicinity impacts animal/personnel safety

       6) Clearly the most potential for physical injury to both patient and closely involved humans

   ii. Rope controlled, head and tail management

     a) Circumstance

       1) Free standing – field condition

       2) Within physical enclosure, e.g. large recovery stall

         a) Wall used

         b) Wall *not* used

   iii. Squeeze door/wall

Category II: Recumbent positioning occurs during or following induction of general anesthesia

A. Tilt-table

B. Sling

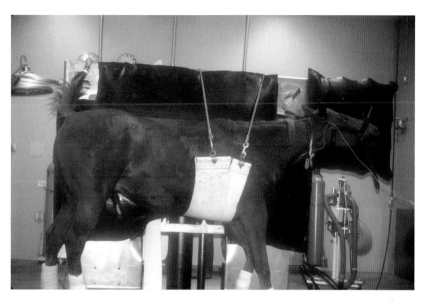

Figure 7.1   Image of a horse being anesthetized using a tilt-table.

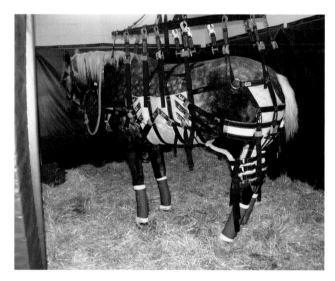

Figure 7.2   Image demonstrating use of a sling to support the horse during anesthesia induction or recovery.

situation-undesirable, the head/tail technique (Category I) is often the technique of choice. For example, with the patient's head and tail secured with ropes, the fractured limb is positioned against the wall. Then as anesthetic induction proceeds and the patient begins to show signs of drug-induced relaxation, attendants should attempt to keep the patient's head elevated while pulling the body into lateral recumbency. Such management should result in less strain at the limb fracture site. This is in contrast, for example, of using a squeeze door/wall for induction of a hind limb long bone fracture where a likely assumed sternal posture on induction will cause inappropriate greater stress at the fracture site.

Before leaving discussion of positional changes, it is important to note that successful fracture repair requires free access to the affected limb and in some cases the ability to apply traction for fracture reduction. These requirements may affect strategic management of anesthetic monitoring (e.g. blood pressure, electrocardiographic and/or muscle twitch monitoring) and may add variability of procedure-induced noxious stimulation, both impacting anesthetic management. Operative limb positioning and immobility should also be addressed. either by physical (e.g. rope) and/or pharmacological (e.g. analgesics, neuromuscular blocking drugs) means.

The magnitude of circulatory and respiratory dysfunction associated with general anesthesia is of special note during dorsal recumbency and time in this posture contributes further complication risk and as a result encourages further thought in the planning process (Muir and Hubbell 2008). For example, dorsal recumbency likely will increase the magnitude of lung ventilation/perfusion imbalance associated with general anesthesia and in unmitigated circumstances likely reduce the magnitude of arterial oxygenation (Muir and Hubbell 2008). It will also likely increase blood volume within both the calvarium and spinal canal which in turn increases local pressure, and potential for reduced regional blood flow and associated reduced tissue perfusion (Brosnan et al. 2002, 2003, 2008, 2011; Steffey 2008; Steffey et al. 2015). Conversely, blood flow to the lower portions of the limbs and feet may be reduced, perhaps to a harmful degree, as a result of dorsal body positioning with limbs a variable height above heart level and/or as a result of placement of a tourniquet.

Anesthetic Management

Choice of Anesthetic Technique

For most types of orthopedic surgery in foals and adults, techniques of anesthetic management follow age-related techniques commonly applied to patients admitted for non-orthopedic (except perhaps gastrointestinal related) surgical procedures performed by the practice. The details of anesthetic management of foals may be found elsewhere (Chapter 13) in this textbook, and their care in most cases would be similar to that of other non-gastrointestinal surgery. An example of a circumstance likely requiring some modification is a long bone fracture proximal to the carpus or hock in which significant associated hemorrhage has occurred

Adult horses with serious orthopedic trauma including long bone fracture and "breakdown" injuries are often "mentally" and physically stressed and may show signs of substantial pain. As a result, confounding drugs may be "on board" at time of presentation and influence especially the early course anesthetic management. Alternatively, some patients may have not been previously treated and especially under climatically challenging conditions present recumbent and in shock. These circumstances require heightened attention to peri-operative monitoring, analgesic and fluid therapy, and management of anesthetic recovery.

In a perfect world, anesthesia technique selection is a collaborative decision between the anesthesia staff's analysis of the situation and animal risk, and the surgical staff's needs relative to safety, surgical skill and knowledge, considerations for outcome, and financial implications. It is the opinion of the authors that the "donation of staff body parts" in an effort to mitigate financial responsibility should no longer enter the decision process within the context of this topic. The most important factors guiding decisions are the needs of the patient-client pair, and the health care team's ability to optimize those needs within the knowledge, and skill-set of the team assembled and available facilities. Collectively, this informs the "individualized" management plan.

Standing surgical intervention is a technique that should be in the repertoire of any clinical practice (private and university-based) providing orthopedic surgical care. The technique should be strongly considered as an option in cases where recovery is a concern due to fracture configuration, patient limitations, or facility and equipment limitations. Once the option for standing intervention is considered the best path for success, a few steps should be taken to increase the likelihood of success. The patient should be brought to the surgical area and lightly sedated. The limb should be clipped and a gross scrub performed under the influence of this light sedation to assess the animal's response to mild stimulation in the area of the fracture and noise that will be present during the procedure. If the patient appears to remain a good candidate, then the operative region should be desensitized. This next step again allows the team to determine if the horse's responses to more moderately painful stimuli are still acceptable to consider them a standing surgical candidate. Information on local and regional analgesic drugs and techniques appropriate for orthopedic procedures may be found elsewhere.

Inhalation anesthesia with injectable adjuvants is often the technique of choice although for some relative short, particularly secondary procedures (e.g. cast change) total intravenous anesthesia may be an appropriate alternative. Variations to the relatively straightforward inhalation anesthetic maintenance format relate largely to circumstances such as: (i) use of local or regional anesthesia in conjunction with general anesthesia to reduce anesthetic requirement and/or use of peri-operative analgesia specific to the horse's orthopedic problem, (ii) patient and/or orthopedic complaint-specific post-anesthetic recovery considerations, and (iii) anticipated surgical needs for prolonged general anesthesia, immobility, and recumbency, e.g. long bone fracture, or less familiar surgical procedures.

Choice of Anesthetic Drugs

Drugs that form the basis for general anesthesia are commonly grouped according to administration technique, i.e. injectable and inhalation. Drugs administered by injection are further categorized according to the route by which they are given as for example local or regional as opposed to systemic. Bolus intravenous injection and/or continuous rate (intravenous) infusion (i.e. CRI) are most common, but intramuscular or subcutaneous routes may also be employed under specific conditions.

With the commercial loss of ultrashort-acting barbiturates to much of the world, the two most common drugs used for injectable anesthesia of equines are ketamine and propofol. These drugs are typically administered after an alpha-2 adrenergic drug such as xylazine or detomidine (Table 7.3) to minimize undesirable effects. A benzodiazepine or guaifenesin may be additionally used with these agents to further enhance a smooth transition to recumbency and reduce the dose of other medications. Isoflurane, sevoflurane, and desflurane are inhalation anesthetics currently available for equine anesthesia (halothane is at best regionally limited).

Globally and pending availability and cost, there are many "preferred" drug and drug dose combinations that may be used in the anesthetic management of horses with orthopedic conditions. However, as the purpose of this chapter is not to provide in-depth pharmacologic review of drugs important to the present subject, readers are referred elsewhere for further information (Carruthers et al. 2018; Grimm et al. 2015; Miller 2018; Muir and Hubbell 2008; Riviere and Papich 2018). In considering drug selection, readers of a broadly circulated text such as these must recognize that although consideration of drug classes from which specific drugs are selected is conducted on the basis of both drug and specific patient characteristics, this is also heavily influenced by clinician training and experience, as well as regional drug availability and cost, i.e. although the knowledge may be global, the drug may not be.

Monitoring Requirements for Major Orthopedic Surgery

Contemporary monitoring of otherwise healthy patients during general anesthetic management for routine or uncomplicated

Table 7.3 Drugs used for supplemental peri-operative analgesia/reduction in anesthetic requirement.

Drug group	Drug Action	Action			Undesirable actions	Comments
		Mode	Site[b]	Drugs[a]		
Non-steroidal Anti-inflammatory (NSAID)		Inhibit (COX enzymes) inflammation; decrease transduction of noxious stimulation	P (C)	Phenylbutazone Flunixin meglumine Firocoxib Others	Dose/condition-related GI and renal side effects	Weak (relative) analgesia, used in multi-modal analgesic plan for especially post-anesthetic care.
Local anesthetic		Bind to Na$^+$ channels thereby blocking Na$^+$ currents and reduce neural impulses	P & C	Lidocaine Mepivacaine Bupivacaine	Dose-related CNS excitation/ convulsions and potential cardiovascular collapse for some drugs with IV use	Systemic lidocaine administered as a cri[c] as part of a multi-modal plan
Opioid	Agonist	Binds especially to Mu receptor	P & C	Morphine Fentanyl Methadone Others	Broadly inconsistent, dose-related: CNS excitation depression of respiration GI morbidity	Wide variation of effect with both joint and systemic use; seemingly more consistent effect with epidural. Direct receptor antagonist available.
	Agonist/ Antagonist or Partial Agonist	Varying affinity for Mu receptor with agonist or antagonist properties. Some with affinity for Kappa receptor (agonist)	C	Butorphanol (Mu antagonist K agonist) Buprenorphine (partial Mu agonist)		Wide variation in effect from none to excitation, usually used in combination with α_2 agonist
α_2-adrenergic agonist		Binds to α_2-adrenergic receptors	C (P)	Xylazine Detomidine Romifidine Medetomidine Dexmedetomidine		Most potent analgesic action for horse with major pain but profound sedative actions accompany. Epidural use may also add to central sedation. **Direct** (central and peripheral) receptor antagonists available.
Dissociative anesthetic		Non-competitive antagonism of NMDA receptors	C	Ketamine		CRI[c] for central supplementary use at sub-anesthetic doses. CNS excitation with higher doses possible in absence of accompanying sedative drugs.

[a] Prominent for equine-focused use.
[b] Site of action – P = peripheral; C = central.
[c] cri = continuous rate infusion.

orthopedic surgery lasting up to about 2–3 hours generally focuses on common clinical signs of anesthesia along with more in-depth observations of circulatory and respiratory function (Muir and Hubbell 2008). Hemodynamic monitoring usually at the least includes regular observation and recording (at least every five minutes) of heart rate and rhythm (electrocardiogram), palpation of a peripheral pulse and at least indirect measurement of systemic arterial blood pressure; direct blood pressure monitoring is strongly recommended for inhaled anesthetic maintained recumbency lasting more than 30–45 minutes. Respiratory (or mechanical ventilation) rate is similarly quantitated and recorded, and subjective observations are made of breathing rhythm (spontaneous ventilation) and depth. Serial observations of body temperature are informative, and pulse oximetry and monitoring of inspired and end-expired anesthetic gas and carbon dioxide are desirable and indeed, routine in many private- and most university-based referral equine hospitals.

Additional monitoring considerations accompany management of more complex operations and/or prolonged anesthetic management. Periodic electrolyte, and selected additional analyte (e.g. lactate, glucose, PCV, total protein [TP] concentration, and arterial acid–base status) analyses are strongly suggested. Early monitoring of these parameters is suggested in animals with known predispositions to abnormalities as a result of their breed, medical history, or pre-anesthetic work-up. Neuromuscular blockade (muscle relaxation) may be an important aspect of management in which case use of a peripheral nerve stimulator and observations of associated muscle responses would be added along with mechanical ventilation. Mechanical ventilation with or without use of muscle relaxants mandates monitoring direct (as opposed to indirectly measured) arterial blood pressure as well as respiratory gases ideally in both breath and arterial blood samples. Catheterization of the urinary bladder should also be a standard accompaniment of prolonged anesthesia to facilitate bladder emptying and periodic monitoring of both urine volume and character. If alpha-2 adrenergic drugs (which increase urine output substantively) are administered during anesthesia maintenance, bladder catheterization is advocated even for shorter procedures to reduce bladder volume and avoid potential influence of bladder distension on recovery from anesthesia.

Peri-anesthetic Analgesia (Table 7.3)

Analgesic drugs should be routinely administered to orthopedic patients. They may be given immediately before, during, and/or immediately following anesthesia. Regardless the timing, they are administered to better insure optimal operative conditions in both the standing and recumbent patient and facilitate patient comfort in the anesthetic and immediate post-anesthetic recovery period. Their actions supplement analgesia provided by the primary anesthetic technique and/or provide anesthetic sparing effects which in turn, usually lessen anesthetic-related depression of vital organ function.

Drugs of particular interest are classified according to their chemical structure, mode, and site of action and/or their function. For simplicity and purposes of this chapter, we will group drugs of analgesic interest into two major categories, i.e. those administered for a specific site effect like local or regional analgesia or those administered systemically for action on the peripheral or central nervous system. This classification is not rigid as some drugs may be used in different circumstances for either or both purposes, e.g. local anesthetics.

Locally Used Analgesics

Local anesthetic agents (e.g. lidocaine, mepivacaine, bupivacaine) are used for local injection and blocking of a single nerve or nerve groups to provide local or regional analgesia of varying duration (Carpenter and Byron 2015).

Motor nerve blockade may accompany such administration and the influence of this on recovery deserves consideration. Lidocaine may also be deposited within the epidural space to produce regional analgesia. However, accompanying motor block limits this use except perhaps in special circumstances with foals. More commonly considered for epidural injection are alpha-2 and opioid drugs such as detomidine and morphine. Intra-articular medication also may be appropriate in some circumstances with proper consideration of potential for chondrotoxicity (Yarbrough 2002). Regional limb perfusion with local anesthetic medications is increasingly common for management of distal limb pain (Colbath et al. 2016). Some drugs more commonly administered systemically may also be used for local analgesia and are briefly highlighted in the subsequent text.

Systemic Use Analgesics

Table 7.3 summarizes drugs used to supplement peri-operative analgesia and reduced general anesthetic requirement. Readers are referred to other recent reviews for specific pharmacological background information on this present topic (Bettschart-Wolfensberger 2015; Knych 2015; KuKanich and Wiese 2015; KuKanich and Papich 2018; Mama and Contino 2015; Mason 2004; Sellon 2015).

Not surprisingly, there are many factors that impact on appropriate selection of analgesic drugs and the route of their administration to supplemental peri-operative anesthetic management. Unfortunately, drugs available for horses are limited and all have dose-/time-related disadvantages especially when considering the recumbent horse with skeletal issues must ultimately return to standing posture with the ability to ambulate at least to a limited degree. Consequently, an important question is how long do we want the drug action to persist? On the one hand, analgesic action into the post-anesthetic period is a good thing. However, if considerable sedation or ataxia accompanies the analgesia into the immediate post-anesthetic phase of management (e.g. alpha-2 agonist or another supplement like ketamine or lidocaine), the smooth uncomplicated transition to a standing posture may be compromised because of, for example, an inopportune stumble during an attempt to stand. Similarly, CNS excitation (as may accompany high dose opioid and ketamine use) may be equally devastating due to an increase in anesthetic requirement and peri-anesthetic arousal or exaggerated vigor in the early post-anesthetic period causing a stormy traumatic recovery from anesthesia. This highlights not only the importance of pharmacodynamic action of peri-anesthetic drug selection but also knowledge of its pharmacokinetics. Unfortunately, such decisions are further impacted by the patient's economic value and medico-legal considerations. The proposed message is not one of all or nothing, but to encourage careful, knowledge-based decision making in support of ideal operative conditions.

Peri-anesthetic Physiological and Pharmacological Supportive Care

Cardiovascular

Intravenous fluid administration is of core importance in the peri-operative period to prevent dehydration at a time when the patient is unable to accomplish this basic need. Its focused goal during anesthetic management is to maintain an adequate circulating blood volume and prevent inadequate tissue perfusion. This basic tenant is true for orthopedic and non-orthopedic patients alike. A review of the physiology, pharmacology, and clinical practice of IV fluid and electrolyte administration in equine patients is beyond the scope of this chapter and the reader is referred elsewhere for general reviews of this subject (Grimm et al. 2015; Muir and Hubbell 2008). However, a few key points are worthy of brief note specifically in relation to the orthopedic patient.

Clinical evidence to guide peri-operative fluid therapy is in general lacking and especially so for equine patients. Accordingly, the usual therapeutic approach is to seek a balance between inadequate fluid administration as evidenced, for example, by arterial hypotension, decreased urine volume, and increasing PCV and PP concentration, and adverse effects of fluid (and possibly its constituents) excess. Beyond the general, commonly applied IV fluid administration guideline of 5–10 ml/kg of balanced crystalloid solution (e.g. lactated Ringer's solution), individually based modifications are appropriate. Added consideration is given to patient-specific circumstances as, for example, the presenting week-old foal with orthopedic trauma unable to ambulate and regularly nurse for the past 24–36 hours and so may present with a low blood glucose, or the extreme case of orthopedic trauma of an endurance horse near the end of a competitive ride under hot climatic conditions where electrolyte aberrations may be observed. The influence of drugs such as xylazine and detomidine which promote increases in urine volume in normal **and** dehydrated horses should also be considered and compensated for. (Nunez et al. 2004; Thurmon et al. 1984; Watson et al. 2002).

When modifications in anesthetic and adjuvant drug doses, and fluid administration are insufficient to correct arterial hypotension in a timely manner, cardiotonic or inotropic (e.g. dobutamine or dopamine) and/or vasoactive (e.g. phenylephrine) drugs or those with mixed effects (e.g. ephedrine, norepinephrine) are often administered. While again the techniques of their individual use is beyond the scope of this chapter and interested readers are referred elsewhere (Fantoni et al. 2013; Grandy et al. 1989; Grimm et al. 2015; Muir and Hubbell 2008; Schauvliege and Gasthuys 2013; Trim 1991), it is important to highlight that of the drugs mentioned, ephedrine may increase anesthetic requirement (Steffey and Eger II 1975). It is also worthwhile to note that duration of isoflurane inhalation anesthesia beyond about two hours often reduces need of active blood pressure support beyond considerations of anesthetic dose and adequacy of fluid therapy in

otherwise healthy horses during orthopedic surgery (*supra vida*) (Steffey et al. 1987).

Respiratory

General anesthesia depresses respiratory system function, increases P_aCO_2, and reduces the efficiency of arterial oxygenation (P_aO_2) compared to awake standing, unmedicated conditions. The magnitude of effect is related to anesthetic agent/technique, drug, dose, body position, and anesthetic duration, and is usually greater in horses compared to an equipotent anesthetic level and other similar conditions in other commonly anesthetized patients including (but not limited to) dogs, cats, and humans (Steffey 2008; Steffey et al. 2015). Accordingly, except for relatively short/minor orthopedic procedures (e.g. cast change, hardware removal), mechanical ventilation (i.e. intermittent positive pressure ventilation) is usually a component of contemporary management of general anesthesia in especially adult horses. Conditions of mechanical ventilation (e.g. frequency of breathing, peak inspiratory pressure, presence or absence of positive end-expired pressure) vary widely and should be individualized to specifically monitored patient conditions (i.e. objective measures of arterial oxygen delivery including hemodynamic function, and carbon dioxide removal) and keeping in mind the overriding goal is to maintain adequacy of oxygen delivery to vital organs. Indeed in this regard, the authors commonly regulate ventilation in favor of mild hypercapnia (i.e. P_aCO_2 of 50–55 mmHg) especially in support of less mechanical suppression of cardiovascular function which often accompanies mechanical ventilation to an end-point of normo-, or even more so, hypo-capnia.

Other Supportive Measures

Use of a neuromuscular blocking drug (i.e. peripheral acting muscle relaxant such as atracurium) as an adjuvant to general anesthesia can provide certain advantages in overall anesthetic management for some of the more involved orthopedic surgical procedures (e.g. long bone fractures above the carpus or fetlock). Muscle relaxants produce skeletal muscle paralysis by interrupting neuromuscular connectivity that normally results in muscle contraction. Accordingly, in some circumstances muscle paralysis may provide conditions for better surgical exposure and/or facilitate, for example, upper limb fracture reduction and repair or spinal surgery. Skeletal muscle relaxation may also be achieved by regional anesthesia or high doses of inhalation anesthetics. However, use of neuromuscular blocking drugs with general anesthesia provide desirable conditions at reduced anesthetic doses which in turn usually spares cardiovascular function. Of course, there are disadvantages of muscle relaxant use including the necessity for mechanical ventilation as a result of paralysis of the respiratory apparatus skeletal muscle. In addition, in the authors' opinion, their use mandates active monitoring of neuromuscular function (e.g. use of a peripheral nerve stimulator) and the concurrent use of analgesic and amnesic drugs. These considerations increase procedural complexity (including knowledge-based) and cost of anesthetic management (drug and equipment related). Indeed, management complexity extends into the immediate post-anesthetic period in that inadequate reversal (passive and active) of paralysis confounds recovery from anesthesia and a patient's smooth transition to a standing posture.

Body Temperature

Changes in body temperature are common during general anesthesia but are not beyond concern during standing procedures associated with prolonged sedation, immobility and extremes of environmental (geographical and operating room) conditions. While an athletic horse presented shortly after injury may arrive in a hyperthermic state, peri-operative hyperthermia is an infrequently reported concern (Aleman et al. 2005; Cornick et al. 1994; Koblin 1992; Waldron-Mease and Rosenberg 1979), except perhaps in the extreme case of prolonged

general anesthesia (Steffey et al. 1993) On the other hand, an anesthesia-related decrease in body temperature is common during all forms of equine surgery. Low operating room temperature, patient sweating, excessive anesthetic dose, and mechanical ventilation may add to other body temperature modifying conditions during surgery. Accordingly, monitoring peri-operative temperature changes may be of special concern in circumstances such as managing the neonatal foal (increased ratio of body surface area to body mass and immature corrective responsiveness), prolonged general anesthesia, and extremes of ambient temperature accompanying anesthetic and immediate post-anesthetic management. In particular, hypothermia may potentiate actions of anesthetic drugs (through reduced anesthetic requirements), contribute to cardiovascular dysfunction (including increased incidence of cardiac dysrhythmias), cause coagulopathies, reduce tissue oxygen availability, and result in shivering (with an associated increased oxygen tissue requirements). Active management strategies during anesthesia include controlling water temperature in water beds used to position recumbent horses, forced air blankets, reduction of anesthetic dose, and use of assisted or spontaneous (vs completely controlled) ventilation where not otherwise contraindicated. Such management practices are important considerations and when appropriate, applied. However, in our experience in many cases (and particularly in relation to climatic conditions) they largely reduce any continued fall of body temperature rather than return the adult horse to normothermia. Hence it can be beneficial to provide external heat well into the recovery period where possible.

Additional special care considerations may accompany prolonged anesthesia and recumbency and as previously mentioned include urinary bladder catheterization and serial volume measurement, and evaluation of PCV and PP concentration. Patient-specific considerations may also include, for example, serial plasma electrolyte concentrations (especially potassium) in, for example, some families of the Quarter Horse breed (Bowling et al. 1996; Meyer et al. 1999; Naylor 1997; Waldridge et al. 1996).

Complications of Orthopedic Surgery

Prolonged Anesthesia and Recumbency

Most hospital-based orthopedic procedures are clinically familiar and when general anesthesia is required, such management is usually an hour or less in duration. However, when primary caregiver familiarity with a condition is reduced, the severity of the condition is increased, and/or special diagnostic procedures (e.g. CT, MRI) are also performed immediately before surgery, duration of required anesthetic management is increased and a 3–6 hour anesthetic term is not unusual for repair of a long bone fracture or other complex orthopedic conditions in an adult horse managed in private or university based specialized equine surgery referral centers.

Prolonged anesthetic management potentially impacts successful patient outcome in a number of important ways especially under less-than-ideal management circumstances. For example, major body tissue (e.g. skeletal muscle) and organ (e.g. intestinal, hepatic, and renal) dysfunction may be a resultant complication as has been highlighted in numerous clinical (Johnston 2004; Johnston et al. 1995; Little et al. 2001; Senior et al. 2004) and laboratory (summarized elsewhere; Steffey 2008; Steffey et al. 2015) investigations. Increasing duration of general anesthesia contributes to prolonged anesthetic elimination and recovery and may contribute to a poor transition from a recumbent to a standing posture. Increasing anesthesia time at least with volatile anesthetics influences the magnitude of cardiovascular performance. For example, both arterial blood pressure and cardiac output increase with time during prolonged constant-dose inhalation anesthesia

(summarized elsewhere; Steffey 2008; Steffey et al. 2015). If unrecognized or misinterpreted, this could further confound peri-anesthetic management.

Post-anesthetic recognition of myopathy/neuropathy remains an anesthetic complication worthy of concern. Though prolonged anesthetic duration is not in itself the cause of this post-anesthetic complication, duration of anesthesia and recumbency contributes to its incidence (Richey et al. 1990). Halothane, one of the early "modern" inhalation anesthetics, was clinically introduced for human patients in the late 1950s and its use with equine patients followed shortly thereafter. Its introduction and the emerging specialization of veterinary anesthesia in academic-focused veterinary hospitals in the 1960s provided an environment for rapidly expanding the breadth and depth of major orthopedic-focused procedures in horses. However, associated with this advancement came post-anesthetic complications rarely before confronted, because equine surgical patients were not previously subjected to prolonged recumbency and immobility which was easily facilitated by inhalation anesthesia. This combined with early, rudimentary physiological monitoring and limited concern for anesthesia associated limb positioning fostered complications such as post-anesthetic myopathy (commonly referred to as "myositis") and neuropathy, complications related to time-dependent associated tissue deficiencies in oxygen delivery (Grandy et al. 1987). Improved knowledge regarding the etiology of anesthesia associated myopathy and neuropathy, advances in monitoring techniques during general anesthesia, and aggressive treatment of systemic arterial hypotension (suggestive of reduced regional blood flow) and respiratory depression have all markedly reduced the incidence of post-anesthetic myopathy and neuropathy. Regardless, vigilance remains a necessity in preventing such devastating complications impacting post-anesthetic recovery.

Surgical (and correspondingly anesthetic) duration may also contribute to an increased likelihood of surgical sepsis. Tissue trauma and exposure of deep structures in and of itself has been shown to increase bacterial adhesion and cause infection. Procedures that take longer are generally more involved and frequently require more intense implants and result in more tissue trauma. The risk of sepsis caused by anesthesia is more likely where there is exacerbation of mild pulmonary infection resulting from exercise or transportation prior to anesthesia. If are pneumonia or pleuritis results, the subsequent increased overall bacterial load can contribute to systemic septicemia.

Note that while much of the focus has been on the recumbent horse, unanticipated and prolonged sedation and waning of regional anesthesia may also modify outcomes when surgery is performed in standing horses.

Tourniquet Use

Tourniquets are commonly applied to the limbs of adult horses to temporarily reduce local blood flow and provide a nearly or complete bloodless surgical field and in turn better operating conditions. Usually, they are placed below the carpus or tarsus, but occasionally they may be placed higher on the limb. Principles (e.g. inflation pressure and duration) and techniques of application (e.g. Esmarch) were largely adapted from physician use in human orthopedic surgery. More recently, tourniquets have been also used to facilitate intravenous regional limb perfusion (IVRLP) of prophylactic and therapeutic drugs (e.g. antibiotics, local anesthetics) for horses undergoing orthopedic procedures (Alkabes et al. 2011; Levine et al. 2010; Rubio-Martinez et al. 2012).

Despite benefits, tourniquet use has disadvantages. Many of the disadvantages associated with use in human patients (Urban 2015) are nonexistent or are of only minor concern with horses (Scott et al. 1979) because, excepting for upper limb use in foals or adults, little skeletal muscle (i.e. active metabolizing tissue) distal to the cuff is involved. Accordingly, local effects associated with reduced regional blood flow and associated muscle ischemia (i.e.

cellular death with acidosis and tissue necrosis) is of limited clinical concern but qualitatively tourniquet-related complications remain important. These include discomfort and pain (nociceptive input) especially accompanying prolonged application, arterial hypertension and direct neural damage in (Copland et al. 1989; Sandler and Scott 1980).

Other Considerations

Peripheral nerve and/or muscle damage may occur peri-operatively and be recognized first at the time of recovery (Dodman et al. 1988; Duke et al. 2006; Forbes 1976; Gleed 1996; Klein 1979; Trim and Mason 1973; White II 1982). The damage is frequently related to localized (neuronal and/or skeletal muscle) hypoxia due to improper positioning, local tissue compression, and reduced tissue oxygen delivery that may or may not also be related to insufficient systemic hemodynamics (Grandy et al. 1987). Improper body/limb positioning and/or padding are common root causes though improper and especially prolonged tourniquet use may also be a source of nerve injury. Often with aggressive supportive care, the condition resolves over the course of four to seven days with little or no residual effect. However, in the worst-case scenario, loss of function is permanent.

There are a number of considerations of little or no reported incidence in equine patients that remain of prominent concern with anesthetic management of human orthopedic surgery patients. For example, complications from deep vein thrombosis and associated thromboembolic events, as well as air and fat embolism remain of significant concern for morbidity and mortality during and following some orthopedic surgeries in human patients (Urban 2015). However, the authors' clinical experience and mostly absent (though not completely; Jones et al. 1988) reporting of similar species-specific documentation in the veterinary medical literature suggests such etiologically related complications are at best rare in equine orthopedic patients. Regardless, we include this brief mention to encourage consideration during the design and implementation of anesthetic plans for horses admitted for procedures involving bones with for example large marrow cavities.

Gastrointestinal issues are a fairly common complication in orthopedic patients. The most common forms are post-operative diarrhea and functional or mechanical obstructions. The formation of diarrhea seems most common in horses where surgery is delayed for a prolonged period after injury and the animal is subjected to a long period of stress. This prolonged stress also seems to be a factor when surgery has failed to mitigate the pain of the injury. Obstructions may be more challenging to diagnose and hence treat in the early post-operative period. Contributing factors may include both a reduced training exercise and change in diet as for example a decrease in grains and increase in roughage. Perioperative analgesic medications may also mask early signs of discomfort. In horses where the complicating issues are related to the large colon feed restrictions, fluid therapy, and administration of mineral oil generally resolve the problem. Cecal obstructions however can be more challenging to diagnose early and treat medically. In these horses, aggressive and protracted feed retraction is required and even then some of these horses may ultimately require surgical intervention. Finally, reduced GI motility or frank ileus may be pharmacologically induced by drugs administered during anesthetic management (e.g. higher dose opioid or alpha-2 agonist than individually appropriate).

Immediate Post-anesthetic Considerations

Recovery from General Anesthesia

For most, particularly adult equine patients, recovery from general anesthesia and recumbency is a potentially life-altering (perhaps even life-ending) event beyond the specific outcome of surgery. This is of particular concern in relation to many post-surgical orthopedic issues that include pre-existing tendon, joint, and/or bony instabilities. Although heavily influenced by their large size and general (often breed, gender, age, and training related) demeanor, there are many other modifiers (e.g. environmental/facility and pharmacological conditions) influencing anesthetic recovery outcome, and interested readers are directed elsewhere in this text and beyond for a more in-depth general review of this subject (Clark-Price 2018; Grimm et al. 2015; Heath 1973; Herthel 1996; Hubbell 1999, 2005; Keegan and Coursin 2009; Muir and Hubbell 2008).

Horse recovery from orthopedic surgery is either facilitative or non-facilitative meaning there is some active mechanical and/or pharmacological intervention to modify the individual horse's recovery behavior or not. In contemporary times, excepting for horses emerging from sedation and local or regional anesthesia supporting standing surgical conditions, orthopedic surgical patients emerging from general anesthesia and recumbent positioning have some degree of intervention ranging from supplemental post-anesthetic sedation to more complex pharmacological intervention and often physical/mechanical assistance (Table 7.4). Indeed, elaborate purposely designed facilities that go beyond simple recovery stalls with added wall and floor padding including the support sling and pool are no longer an unusual extreme in referral-based equine hospitals. Such facility considerations coupled with introduction of new drugs and in particular investigative development of recovery focused-techniques have contributed improvements in the incidence of successful return to productive athletic and non-athletic lifestyles by even the most severely injured orthopedic patients.

Immediate Post-anesthetic Sedation and Analgesia

Drugs administered at the end of surgery to attempt to facilitate a smooth anesthetic recovery are usually selected from tranquilizer,

Table 7.4 Techniques of post-anesthetic recovery for orthopedic surgery.

Minimal/limited physical assistance *OR* physically unassisted		
Technique	**Common circumstances of use**	**Comments/aids to success**
Without recovery-specific drug administration or intervention	Field, or circumstances of no or very limited control, e.g. feral equids	A priori considerations regarding recovery environment helpful to success
With minimal recovery-specific drug administration[a]	Field or limited hospital facilities and/or personnel experience	

Physical *and* technique-related pharmacologically assisted[b]		
Technique	**Common circumstances of use**	**Comments/aids to success**
Padded dedicated recovery stall with hands-on and/or head and tail rope assistance (Steffey et al. 2009a)	Likely overall most used; techniques especially specific to geographic region and veterinarian/hospital clinical practice	Horse behavior knowledge desirable; at least moderate physical strength helpful for especially hands-on technique
Thick pad with head and tail rope assistance	Patients of intermediate concern of complicated recovery or for owner-directed economic reasons accompanying heightened concern	Horse behavior knowledge desirable; at least moderate physical strength helpful
Air-inflatable bed (Hodgson et al. 1996; Ray-Miller et al. 2006)	Patients of intermediate concern for a complicated recovery or for owner-directed economic reasons accompanying heightened concern	Horse behavior knowledge desirable; at least moderate physical strength helpful
Tilt-surgery table (Elmas et al. 2007)	Patients of intermediate and heightened concern for a complicated recovery	Both horse behavior knowledge and at least moderate physical strength helpful. Equipment related experience necessary
Sling (Steffey et al. 2009b; Taylor et al. 2005)	Patients of intermediate and heightened concern of complicated recovery	Horse behavior and sling application knowledge and skill very important and at least moderate physical strength helpful. Equipment related experience necessary
Water/pool (Sullivan et al. 2002; Tidwell et al. 2002)	Patients of heightened concern of complicated recovery	Horse behavior and water facilities-related knowledge and skill extremely important and at least moderate physical strength helpful. Equipment related experience necessary

[a] Examples of published drug technique-related information broadly applicable to both unassisted and uncomplicated assisted recovery Aarnes et al. (2014), Guedes et al. (2017), Hedges et al. (2014), Bauquier and Kona-Boun (2011), Matthews et al. (1998), Santos et al. (2003), Wagner et al. (2008), Wagner et al. (2012), Steffey et al. (2009a).
[b] Listed in order of facility design and personnel interactive complexity (i.e. overhead costs). References noted with each sub-category.

alpha-2 adrenergic agonist and/or opioid drug classes. Actual drug (and drug dose) selection, whether used in isolation or in combination is based on individual patient considerations. For example, following general anesthesia for a relatively minor orthopedic procedure or perhaps a cast change, a small intravenous dose (e.g. 0.005–0.01 mg/kg) of acepromazine might be appropriate to allay "emergence apprehension" in especially a young, minimally schooled adult horse. On the other hand, horses recovering from more invasive surgery and associated pain of high intensity would likely benefit from an alpha-2 agonist. Drug dose is however likely to be lower than that administered as a preanesthetic or to produce standing immobilization. Use of opioids either alone or in addition to alpha-2 agonist drugs may also be considered during recovery from anesthesia but their use tends to be more controversial due to their dose related side effects (including possible excitement and gastrointestinal stasis). Clinician experience and both horse behavior (so excitement is minimized) and environmental circumstances should be considered. The principle guiding present authors is "first do no harm," i.e. if medications are administered in the time window between the end of anesthesia and the patient's standing do so with just cause and at a dose not likely to question of the impact on uncoordinated or early attempts to stand which might result in complications and accompanying medico-legal considerations.

Pharmacological techniques of assisted recovery are also individualized to the techniques of physically assisting transition to standing. Space limitation does not allow for individual review of the various methods highlighted in Table 7.4 and accordingly readers are encouraged to review original descriptive/investigative reports and published reviews on this subject some of which are referenced in Table 7.4.

A requirement of multiple general anesthetic events is predictably associated with some orthopedic problems (e.g. long bone fractures and pastern arthrodesis) presented for surgical repair and commonly relate to frequent limb-cast changes. Our personal opinion from long time experience and supported by published reports (Platt et al. 2018; Valverde et al. 2013) is that the quality of recovery from anesthesia with most of these patients, regardless of the technique initially applied, rapidly improves with consecutive anesthetic episodes. However, an exception to this observation is the patient requiring one or two general anesthesia (e.g. cast application, further diagnostic work) in short time span prior to the actual surgical intervention.

Specific Patient/Surgical Considerations

Long Bone Fracture

The presence of microfracturing and multiple site fractures occur in some cases. A large portion of orthopedic patients are athletes that perform in disciplines where stress fractures are a common occurrence. A complete examination to assess any other fractures present in the patient is almost always beyond the practicality of the presenting problem. Regardless of whether additional confounders are known or not, all efforts should be made to minimize the amount of operative/anesthesia time with the goal of improving chances of a smooth, uncomplicated post-anesthetic transition to standing. In cases of multiple broken bones in the same or multiple limbs, the management intensity is amplified by the potential need to change patient positioning during anesthesia. Need for bilateral casts or heavy bandages can further add to challenges in recovery and highlights the importance of a team effort by all to maximize the chance of a successful patient outcome.

Cast Pain

With clinical experience in placing casts, acute cast pain is rarely a consideration. However, anxiety related to the cast (especially when the entire limb is involved) or circumstances where the pain of the fracture has not been markedly reduced with surgical intervention may occur and sedation or analgesia may be needed in the recovery and post-recovery period. Pending the temperament of the horse and circumstances of the fracture, preoperative placement of a splint or cast to improve the animal's tolerance and familiarity is sometimes recommended. Occasionally, if the horse's anxiety results in physiological changes such as sweating, increased heart rate, respiratory rate, and/or body temperature, that cannot be controlled with medication, if possible the cast should be removed to provide relief. Evaluation and support of the non-surgical limbs is also important and knowledge of the horse's temperament and adaptability preoperatively may help guide intervention.

Summary

Orthopedic conditions requiring anesthesia of horses represent a broad range of circumstances from simple to complex. Most conditions encountered in clinical practice are relatively routine in contemporary equine surgical practice. Accordingly, there is usually little need for major divergence from common principles and techniques of equine anesthetic management. However, as circumstances become more complex (e.g. individual horse complexity, environmental conditions, nature, and degree of orthopedic injury) successful *individualized* care is predicated on thoughtful preparation, skillful management, and availability of appropriate facilities and personnel. This review attempts to focus on principles of anesthetic and operative care of patients with complex orthopedic conditions.

References

Aarnes, T.K., Bednarski, R.M., Bertone, A.L. et al. (2014). Recovery from desflurane anesthesia in horses with and without post-anesthetic xylazine. *Canadian Journal of Veterinary Research* 78(2): 103–109.

Aleman, M., Brosnan, R.J., Williams, D.C. et al. (2005). Malignant hyperthermia in a horse anesthetized with halothane. *Journal of Veterinary Internal Medicine* 19: 363–367.

Alkabes, S.B., Adams, S.B., Moore, G.E., and Alkabes, K.C. (2011). Comparison of two tourniquets and determination of amikacin sulfate concentrations after metacarpophalangeal joint lavage performed simultaneously with intravenous regional limb perfusion in horses. *American Journal of Veterinary Research* 72(5): 613–619.

Auer, J.A. (2012). Angular limb deformities. In: *Equine surgery*, 4e (eds. J.A. Auer and J.A. Stick), 1201–1220. St Louis: Saunders Elsevier.

Bauquier, S.H. and Kona-Boun, J.-J. (2011). Comparison of the effects of xylazine and romifidine administered perioperatively on the recovery of anesthetized horses. *Canadian Veterinary Journal* 52(9): 987–993.

Bettschart-Wolfensberger, R. (2015). Horses. In: *Veterinary Anesthesia and Analgesia*, 5e (eds. K.A. Grimm, L.A. Lamont, W.J. Tranquilli, et al.), 857–866. Ames: Wiley Blackwell.

Bowling, A.T., Byrns, G., and Spier, S. (1996). Evidence for a single pedigree source of the hyperkalemic periodic paralysis susceptibility gene in quarter horses. *Animal Genetics* 27(4): 279–281.

Brosnan, R.J., Steffey, E.P., LeCouteur, R.A. et al. (2002). Effects of body position on intracranial and cerebral perfusion pressures in isoflurane-anesthetized horses. *Journal of Applied Physiology* 92: 2542–2546.

Brosnan, R.J., Steffey, E.P., LeCouteur, R.A. et al. (2003). Effects of duration of isoflurane anesthesia and mode of ventilation on intracranial and cerebral perfusion pressures in horses. *American Journal of Veterinary Research* 64(11): 1444–1448.

Brosnan, R.J., Esteller-Vico, A., Steffey, E.P. et al. (2008). Effects of head-down positioning on regional central nervous system perfusion in isoflurane-anesthetized horses. *American Journal of Veterinary Research* 69(6): 737–743.

Brosnan, R.J., Steffey, E.P., LeCouteur, R.A. et al. (2011). Effects of isoflurane anesthesia on cerebrovascular autoregulation in horses. *American Journal of Veterinary Research* 72(1): 18–24.

Carpenter, R.E. and Byron, C.R. (2015). Equine local anesthetic and analgesic techniques. In: *Veterinary Anesthesia and Analgesia*, 5e (eds. K.A. Grimm, L.A. Lamont, W.J. Tranquilli, et al.), 886–911. Ames: Wiley Blackwell.

Carruthers, S.G., Hoffman, B.B., Melmon, K.L., and Nierenberg, D.W. (eds.) (2018). *Melmon and Morrelli's Clinical Pharmacology: Basic Principles in Therapeutics*, 4e. New York: McGraw-Hill Companies, Inc.

Clark-Price, S. (2018). Recovery of horses from anesthesia. *Veterinary Clinics of North America: Equine Practice* 29: 223–242.

Colbath, A.C., Wittenburg, L.A., Gold, J.R. et al. (2016). The effects of Mepivacaine hydrochloride on antimicrobial activity and mechanical nociceptive threshold during amikacin sulfate regional limb perfusion in the horse. *Veterinary Surgery* 45: 798–803.

Copland, V.S., Hildebrand, S.V., Hill, T. III et al. (1989). Blood pressure response to tourniquet use in anesthetized horses. *Journal of the American Veterinary Medical Association* 195(8): 1097–1103.

Cornick, J.L., Seahorn, T.L., and Hartsfield, S.M. (1994). Hyperthermia during isoflurane anaesthesia in a horse with suspected hyperkalaemic periodic paralysis. *Equine Veterinary Journal* 26: 511–514.

Dodman, N.H., Williams, R., Court, M.H., and Norman, W.M. (1988). Postanesthetic hind limb adductor myopathy in five horses. *Journal of the American Veterinary Medical Association* 193(1): 83–87.

Duke, T., Filzek, U., Read, M.R. et al. (2006). Clinical observations surrounding an increased incidence of postanesthetic myopathy in halothane-anesthetized horses. *Veterinary Anaesthesia and Analgesia* 33(2): 122–127.

Elmas, C.R., Cruz, A.M., and Kerr, C.L. (2007). Tilt table recovery of horses after orthopedic surgery: fifty-four cases (1994–2005). *Veterinary Surgery* 36: 252–258.

Fantoni, D.T., Marchioni, G.G., Ida, K.K. et al. (2013). Effect of ephedrine and phenylephrine on cardiopulmonary parameters in horses undergoing elective surgery. *Veterinary Anaesthesia and Analgesia* 40(4): 367–374.

Forbes, J.R.S. (1976). Postoperative lameness after the use of halothane as a general anaesthetic in horses. *Australian Veterinary Journal* 52 244-.

Gleed, R.D. (1996). Postanesthetic myopathy. In: *Equine Fracture Repair* (ed. A.J. Nixon), 343–349. Philadelphia: W.B. Saunders Co.

Grandy, J.L., Steffey, E.P., Hodgson, D.S., and Woliner, M.J. (1987). Arterial hypotension and the development of postanesthetic myopathy in halothane-anesthetized horses. *American Journal of Veterinary Research* 48: 192–197.

Grandy, J.L., Hodgson, D.S., Dunlop, C.I. et al. (1989). Cardiopulmonary effects of ephedrine in halothane-anesthetized horses. *Journal of Veterinary Pharmacology and Therapeutics* 12: 389–396.

Grimm, K.A., Lamont, L.A., Tranquilli, W.J. et al. (eds.) (2015). *Veterinary Anesthesia and Analgesia*, 5e. Ames: John Wiley & Sons, Inc.

Guedes, A.G.P., Tearney, C.C., Cenani, A. et al. (2017). Comparison between the effects of postanesthetic xylazine and dexmedetomidine on characteristics of recovery from sevoflurane anesthesia in horses. *Veterinary Anaesthesia and Analgesia* 44(2): 273–280.

Heath, R.B. (1973). Anesthetic management and recovery of large orthopedic patients. *Veterinary Clinics of North America: Equine Practice* 3(1): 127–135.

Hedges, A.R., Pypendop, B.H., Shilo, Y. et al. (2014). Impact of the blood sampling site on time-concentration drug profiles following intravenous or buccal drug administration. *Journal of Veterinary Pharmacology and Therapeutics* 37(2): 145–150.

Herthel, D.J. (1996). Systems for recovery from anesthesia. In: *Equine Fracture Repair* (ed. A.J. Nixon), 339–342. Philadelphia: W.B. Saunders Co.

Hodgson, D.S., Dunlop, C.I., McMurphy, R.M., and Chapman, P.L. (1996). Anesthetic recovery in horses using a rapidly deflating air pillow. *Veterinary Surgery* 25: 182.

Honnas, C.M. (1991). Standing surgical procedures of the foot. *Veterinary Clinics of North America: Equine Practice* 7(3): 395–722.

Hubbell, J.A.E. (1999). Recovery from anaesthesia in horses. *Equine Veterinary Education* 11(3): 160–167.

Hubbell, J.A.E. (2005). Recovery from anaesthesia in horses. *Equine Veterinary Education* 7: 45–52.

Johnston, G.M. (2004). Findings from the CEPEF epidemiological studies into equine perioperative complications. *Proceedings of the American Association of Equine Practitioners* 50: 281–286.

Johnston, G.M., Taylor, P.M., Holmes, M.A., and Wood, J.L.N. (1995). Confidential enquiry of perioperative equine fatalities (CEPEF-1): preliminary results. *Equine Veterinary Journal* 27(3): 193–200.

Jones, R.S., Payne-Johnson, C.E., and Seymour, C.J. (1988). Pulmonary micro-embolism following orthopaedic surgery in a thoroughbred gelding. *Equine Veterinary Journal* 20(5): 382–384.

Keegan, M.T. and Coursin, D.B. (2009). Evidence in evolution: glycemic control in the ICU. *American Society of Anesthesiologists Newsletter* 73(9): 14–15.

Klein, L. (1979). A review of 50 cases of postoperative myopathy in the horse - intrinsic and management factors affecting risk. *Proceedings of the American Association of Equine Practitioners* 24: 89–94.

Knych, H.K. (2015). Analgesic pharmacology. In: *Robinson's Current Therapy in Equine Medicine*, 7e (eds. K.A. Sprayberry and N.E. Robinson), 55–57. St Louis: Elsevier.

Koblin, D.D. (1992). Characteristics and implications of desflurane metabolism and toxicity. *Anesthesia & Analgesia* 75: S10–S16.

KuKanich, B. and Papich, M.G. (2018). Opioid analgesic drugs. In: *Veterinary Pharmacology and Therapeutics*, 10e (eds. J.E. Riviere and M.G. Papich), 281–323. Hoboken: Wiley Blackwell.

KuKanich, B. and Wiese, A.J. (2015). Opioids. In: *Veterinary Anesthesia and Analgesia*, 5e (eds. K.A. Grimm, L.A. Lamont, W.J. Tranquilli, et al.), 207–226. Ames: Wiley Blackwell.

Levine, D.G., Epstein, K.L., Ahern, B.J., and Richardson, D.W. (2010). Efficacy of three tourniquet types for intravenous antimicrobial regional limb perfusion in standing horses. *Veterinary Surgery* 39(8): 1021–1024.

Little, D., Redding, W.R., and Blikslager, A.T. (2001). Risk factors for reduced postoperative fecal output in horses: 37 cases (1997-1998). *Journal of the American Veterinary Medical Association* 218(3): 414–420.

Madron, M., Caston, S., and Kersh, K. (2013). Placement of bone screws in a standing horse for treatment of a fracture of the greater tubercle of the humerus. *Equine Veterinary Education* 25: 381–385.

Mama, K.R. and Contino, E.K. (2015). Postoperative pain control. In: *Robinson's Current Therapy in Equine Medicine*, 7e (eds. K.A. Sprayberry and N.E. Robinson), 60–62. St Louis: Elsevier.

Mason, D.E. (2004). Anesthetics, tranquillizers and opioid analgesics. In: *Equine Clinical Pharmacology* (eds. J.J. Bertone and L.J.I. Horspool), 267–309. New York: Saunders.

Matthews, N.S., Hartsfield, S.M., Mercer, D. et al. (1998). Recovery from sevoflurane anesthesia in horses: comparison to isoflurane and effect of postmedication with xylazine. *Veterinary Surgery* 27(5): 480–485.

Meyer, T.S., Fedde, M.R., Cox, J.H., and Erickson, H.H. (1999). Hyperkalaemic periodic paralysis in horses: a review. *Equine Veterinary Journal* 31(5): 362–367.

Miller, R.D. (ed.) (2018). *Miller's Anesthesia*, 8e. Philadelphia: Elsevier Saunders.

Modesto, R.B., Rodgerson, D.H., Masciarelli, A.E., and Spirito, M. (2015). Standing placement of transphyseal screw in the distal radius in 8 thoroughbred yearlings. *Canadian Veterinary Journal* 56: 605–609.

Muir, W.W. and Hubbell, J.A. (eds.) (2008). *Equine Anesthesia, Monitoring and Emergency Therapy*, 2e. St Louis: Saunders/Elsevier.

Naylor, J.M. (1997). Hyperkalemic periodic paralysis. *Veterinary Clinics of North America: Equine Practice* 13(1): 129–144.

Nunez, E., Steffey, E.P., Ocampo, L. et al. (2004). Effects of a$_2$-adrenergic receptor agonists on urine production in horses deprived of food and water. *American Journal of Veterinary Research* 65(10): 1342–1346.

O'Brien, T. and Hunt, R.J. (2014). Recent advances in standing equine orthopedic surgery. *Veterinary Clinics of North America: Equine Practice* 30: 221–237.

Payne, R.J. and Compston, P.C. (2012). Short- and long-term results following standing fracture repair in 34 horses. *Equine Veterinary Journal* 44: 721–725.

Platt, J.P., Simon, B.T., Coleman, M. et al. (2018). The effects of multiple anaesthetic episodes on equine recovery quality. *Equine Veterinary Journal* 50: 111–116.

Ray-Miller, W.M., Hodgson, D.S., McMurphy, R.M., and Chapman, P.L. (2006). Comparison of recoveries from anesthesia of horses placed on a rapidly inflating-deflating air pillow or the floor of a padded stall. *Journal of the American Veterinary Medical Association* 229: 711–716.

Richey, M.T., Holland, M.S., McGrath, C.J. et al. (1990). Equine post-anesthetic lameness: a retrospective study. *Veterinary Surgery* 19(5): 392–397.

Riviere, J.E. and Papich, M.G. (eds.) (2018). *Veterinary Pharmacology and Therapeutics*, 10e. Hoboken: John Wiley & Sons, Inc.

Rubio-Martinez, L.M., Elmas, C.R., Black, B., and Monteith, G. (2012). Clinical use of antimicrobial regional limb perfusion in horses: 174 cases (1999-2009). *Journal of the American Veterinary Medical Association* 241 (12): 1650–1658.

Russell, T.M. and Maclean, A.A. (2006). Standing surgical repair of propagating metacarpal and metatarsal condylar fractures in racehorses. *Equine Veterinary Journal* 38(5): 423–427.

Sandler, G.A. and Scott, E.A. (1980). Vascular responses in equine thoracic limb during and after pneumatic tourniquet application. *American Journal of Veterinary Research* 41: 648–649.

Santos, M., Fuente, M., Garcia-Iturralde, P. et al. (2003). Effects of alpha-2 adrenoceptor agonists during recovery from isoflurane anaesthesia in horses. *Equine Veterinary Journal* 35 (2): 170–175.

Schauvliege, S. and Gasthuys, F. (2013). Drugs for cardiovascular support in anesthetized horses. *Veterinary Clinics of North America: Equine Practice* 29: 19–49.

Scott, E.A., Reibold, T.W., Lamar, A.M. et al. (1979). Effect of pneumatic tourniquet application to the distal extremities of the horse: blood gas, serum electrolyte, osmolality and hematologic alterations. *American Journal of Veterinary Research* 40: 1078–1081.

Sellon, D. (2015). Pain management in the trauma patient. In: *Robinson's Current Therapy in Equine Medicine*, 7e (eds. K.A. Sprayberry and N.E. Robinson), 6–10. St Louis: Elsevier.

Senior, J.M., Pinchbeck, G.L., Dugdale, A.H.A., and Clegg, P.D. (2004). Retrospective study of the risk factors and prevalence of colic in horses after orthopaedic surgery. *Veterinary Record* 155: 321–325.

Steffey, E.P. (2008). Inhalation anesthetics and gases. In: *Equine Anesthesia, Monitoring, and Emergency Therapy*, 2e (eds. W.W. Muir and J.A.E. Hubbell), 288–314. St Louis: Saunders/Elsevier.

Steffey, E.P. and Eger, E.I. II (1975). The effect of seven vasopressors on halothane MAC in dogs. *British Journal of Anaesthesia* 47: 435–438.

Steffey, E.P., Hodgson, D.S., Dunlop, C.I. et al. (1987). Cardiopulmonary function during 5 hours of constant-dose isoflurane in laterally recumbent, spontaneously breathing horses.

Journal of Veterinary Pharmacology and Therapeutics 10: 290–297.

Steffey, E.P., Dunlop, C.I., Cullen, L.K. et al. (1993). Circulatory and respiratory responses of spontaneously breathing, laterally recumbent horses to 12 hours of halothane anesthesia. *American Journal of Veterinary Research* 54: 929–936.

Steffey, E.P., Mama, K.R., Brosnan, R.J. et al. (2009a). Effect of administration of propofol and xylazine hydrochloride on recovery of horses after four hours of anesthesia with desflurane. *American Journal of Veterinary Research* 70(8): 956–963.

Steffey, E.P., Brosnan, R.J., Galuppo, L.D. et al. (2009b). Use of propofol-xylazine and the Anderson sling suspension system for recovery of horses from desflurane anesthesia. *Veterinary Surgery* 38: 927–933.

Steffey, E.P., Mama, K.R., and Brosnan, R.J. (2015). Inhalation anesthetics. In: *Veterinary Anesthesia and Analgesia*, 5e (eds. K.A. Grimm, L.A. Lamont, W.J. Tranquilli, et al.), 297–331. Ames: Wiley Blackwell.

Sullins, K.E. (1991). Standing musculoskeletal surgery. *Veterinary Clinics of North America: Equine Practice* 7(3): 685–694.

Sullivan, E.K., Klein, L.V., Richardson, D.W. et al. (2002). Use of a pool-raft system for recovery of horses from general anesthesia: 393 horses (1984–2000). *Journal of the American Veterinary Medical Association* 221 (7): 1014–1018.

Taylor, E.L., Galuppo, L.D., Steffey, E.P. et al. (2005). Use of the Anderson sling suspension system for recovery of horses from general anesthesia. *Veterinary Surgery* 34: 559–564.

Thurmon, J.C., Steffey, E.P., Zinkl, J.G. et al. (1984). Xylazine causes transient dose-related hyperglycemia and increased urine volumes in mares. *American Journal of Veterinary Research* 45(2): 224–227.

Tidwell, S.A., Schneider, R.K., Ragle, C.A. et al. (2002). Use of a hydro-pool system to recovery horses after general anesthesia: 60 cases. *Veterinary Surgery* 31: 455–461.

Trim, C.M. (1991). Inotropic agents and vasopressors in equine anesthesia. *Compendium on Continuing Education for the Practicing Veterinarian* 13: 118–121.

Trim, C.M. and Mason, J. (1973). Post-anaesthetic forelimb lameness in horses. *Equine Veterinary Journal* 5(2): 71–76.

Urban, M.K. (2015). Anesthesia for orthopedic surgery. In: *Miller's Anesthesia*, 8e (ed. R.D. Miller), 2386–2406. Philadelphia: Elsevier Saunders.

Valverde, A., Black, B., Cribb, N.C. et al. (2013). Assessment of unassisted recovery from repeated general isoflurane anesthesia in horses following post-anesthetic administration of xylazine or acepromazine or a combination of xylazine and ketamine. *Veterinary Anaesthesia and Analgesia* 40(1): 3–12.

Wagner, A.E., Mama, K.R., Steffey, E.P., and Hellyer, P.W. (2008). A comparison of equine recovery characteristics after isoflurane or isoflurane followed by a xylazine-ketamine infusion. *Veterinary Anaesthesia and Analgesia* 35(2): 154–160.

Wagner, A.E., Mama, K.R., Steffey, E.P., and Hellyer, P.W. (2012). Evaluation of infusions of xylazine with ketamine or propofol to modulate recovery following sevoflurane anesthesia in horses. *American Journal of Veterinary Research* 73(3): 346–352.

Waldridge, B.M., Lin, H.-C., and Purohit, R.C. (1996). Anesthetic management of horses with hyperkalemic periodic paralysis. *Compendium on Continuing Education for the Practicing Veterinarian* 18: 1030–1039.

Waldron-Mease, E. and Rosenberg, H. (1979). Postanesthetic myositis in the horse associated with in vitro malignant hyperthermia susceptibility. *Veterinary Science Communications* 3: 45–50.

Watson, Z.E., Steffey, E.P., Van Hoogmoed, L.M., and Snyder, J.R. (2002). Effect of general anesthesia and minor surgical trauma on urine and serum measurements in horses. *American Journal of Veterinary Research* 63(7): 1061–1065.

White, N.A. II (1982). Postanesthetic recumbency myopathy in horses. *Compendium on Continuing Education for the Practicing Veterinarian* 4(2): S44–S50.

Yarbrough, T. (2002). Intraarticular medication. In: *Equine Clinical Pharmacology* (eds. J.J. Bertone and L.J.I. Horspool), 121–134. New York: Saunders.

8

Anesthetic Management for Muscular Conditions

Erica McKenzie[1] and Stuart Clark-Price[2]

[1] Department of Clinical Sciences, Carlson College of Veterinary Medicine, Oregon State University, 700 SW 30th Street, Corvallis, OR, 97331, USA
[2] Department of Clinical Sciences, College of Veterinary Medicine, Auburn University, 1220 Wire Road, Auburn, AL, 36849, USA

Introduction

Anesthesia of adult horses and foals with pre-existing muscular disorders is likely commonly practiced since clinical signs are often subtle, inhibiting recognition in advance of the procedure. The incidence of neuromuscular complications related to general anesthesia of horses has continued to decline as practices have evolved and greater understanding of equine muscular disorders is achieved (Bidwell et al. 2004, Bidwell et al. 2007; Senior et al. 2007; Dugdale and Taylor 2016; Valberg 2018). However, general anesthesia retains the potential to cause substantial primary muscle or peripheral nerve damage in horses, and may trigger clinical disease in a proportion of horses with pre-existing muscular disorders. Minimizing the potential for harm relies on thorough pre-anesthesia assessment of equine patients, attention to specific features relevant to the muscular and nervous systems during anesthesia, and careful post-anesthesia monitoring and management of complications.

Muscle Physiology

Muscle is a large and metabolically active tissue in the horse, comprising between 40 and 55% of body mass, and receiving as much as 80% of cardiac output during intense exercise activity (Piercy and Rivero 2012; Poole and Erickson 2011). The vast majority of the horse's muscle mass is located in the back and upper limbs, which facilitates speed and power (Kearns et al. 2002). This distribution makes horses considerably more vulnerable to neuromuscular injury during anesthesia, since some degree of compression of dependent muscle tissue and potentially peripheral nerves is likely to occur in typical recumbency positions. Total muscle mass and distribution of mass can vary considerably between different breeds, which also likely influences individual vulnerability to disease and clinical manifestation of disease. For example, Quarter Horses typically have considerably greater muscle mass in the hindquarter region than do comparable light breeds such as Arabians (Crook et al. 2008, 2010). Draft horses have proportionately less muscle than Thoroughbreds and Quarter horses; however, their much larger total body mass likely increases their risk of neuromuscular complications during general anesthesia (Gleed and Short 1980; Kearns et al. 2002; Rothenbuhler et al. 2006).

Over 90% of muscle tissue is composed of myofibers, with the remainder comprised of

Equine Anesthesia and Co-Existing Disease, First Edition. Stuart Clark-Price and Khursheed Mama.

specialized connective tissues, vessels, and nerves. Horses have a considerably higher proportion of fast twitch muscle fibers compared to other species with this fiber type representing more than 90% of muscle fiber populations in Thoroughbreds and Quarter horses, and ≥75% in other breeds (Piercy and Rivero 2012; Valberg 2014). Fast twitch fibers are located more superficially in the musculature, with type I, slow twitch fibers located deeper in the tissue to support the constant activity of postural maintenance. Muscle fibers are grouped into motor units, each of which consists of a single alpha motor neuron and the multiple fibers innervated by that neuron. A single motor neuron might service over a thousand individual fibers distributed among many different fascicles in the muscle; however, all fibers within that motor unit will be of a similar type. The number of motor units that are activated at one time is the key determinant of the force that the muscle will ultimately produce (Piercy and Rivero 2012; Valberg 2014).

The majority of the internal environment of the muscle cell consists of organized bundles of overlapping contractile filaments that are arranged longitudinally into repeating units, referred to as sarcomeres. Individual sarcomeres are demarcated at each end by Z-disks, which appear ultrastructurally as dense perpendicular striations. Emerging work indicates that Z-disks are not inert and simple anchoring structures, but large and complicated arrays of different proteins with important roles in cell structure and signaling (Luther 2009). Between the Z-disks, each sarcomere contains longitudinally oriented actin filaments anchored at each disk and extending from each disk toward the center of the cell, with their associated proteins including tropomyosin and troponins C, T, and I in contact along their length. Actin filaments overlap with centrally located and thicker bipolar myosin filaments, the globular heads of which are oriented toward each Z-disk. Contraction occurs when calcium ions bind to troponin C which subsequently interacts with troponin I

to resolve its inhibitory effect, resulting in exposure of myosin binding sites on actin. Cyclical binding of the many myosin heads to actin filaments brings the actin filaments in toward the center of the sarcomere from each end, resulting in shortening of the sarcomere (Cooper 2000; Lodish et al. 2000; Valberg 2014).

Contraction of skeletal muscle commences with a nervous impulse, which must be converted to mechanical action (excitation-contraction coupling). Depolarization of the motor neuron releases acetylcholine into the synaptic cleft, which binds reversibly to the motor end plate via nicotinic acetylcholine receptors, inducing depolarization of the sarcolemma. The electrical signal propagates internally into the myofiber along extensive invaginations of the sarcolemma, the T-tubules. Depolarization of the tubules results in conformational change in their membrane-associated voltage sensors, the dihydropyridine receptors. This subsequently invokes a change in conformation of the closely apposed calcium release receptors, also known as ryanodine receptors, which occur as the *RYR1* isoform in skeletal muscle. Rapid release of a large number of calcium ions into the sarcoplasm massively increases the calcium concentration around the myofilaments, encouraging binding of calcium to troponin C and subsequent events promoting contraction. Relaxation is achieved via active transport of calcium ions back into the SR via the activity of the SR calcium ATPase enzyme. (Cooper 2000; Lodish et al. 2000; Valberg 2014).

Effects of Commonly Used Anesthetic/Analgesic Medications on Equine Skeletal Muscle

Many of the anesthetic, analgesic, and adjunct medications used during anesthesia of horses have direct or indirect effects on skeletal muscle. There is relatively limited information regarding the effects of these drugs on contractile mechanics or myocyte metabolism in horses. Most studies have focused on responses to halothane, and have usually examined *in vitro* systems (Hildebrand et al. 1990; Beech et al. 1993; Lentz et al. 1999a, b; Raisis et al. 2000; Edner et al. 2005). Investigations have commonly focused on the impact of drugs on perfusion of muscle tissue because of the association of hypoperfusion with muscle damage in anesthetized horses, attributed to factors including large muscle mass and hypotension creating particular risk to dependent musculature (Trim and Mason 1973; Grandy et al. 1987; Serteyn et al. 1988; Lindsay et al. 1989; Raisis et al. 2000; Raisis 2005). The effects of individual drugs used in premedication, induction, maintenance, and as adjunct therapies on the muscular system are described below.

Premedication and Adjunctive Agents

α2-Adrenergic Receptor Agonists

The α2-adrenergic receptor agonist agents, encompassing xylazine, detomidine, romifidine, medetomidine, and dexmedetomidine, are frequently utilized in standing sedation of horses for examination and diagnostic purposes, for analgesia, and as premedications prior to general anesthesia. In addition to sedative and analgesic effects, these drugs can provide muscle relaxation via centrally mediated effects. Muscle relaxation may arise from depressant effects on the locus coeruleus neurons in the brain resulting in disfacilitation of spinal reflexes (Palmeri and Wiesendanger 1990). The cardiovascular side effects of α2-adrenergic receptor agonists are well described and include vasoconstriction followed by vasodilation, bradycardia, and decreased cardiac output (Bettschart-Wolfensberger 2015). In combination, these effects can reduce blood flow to skeletal muscle in standing and anesthetized horses (Hennig et al. 1995; Raisis 2005). This can promote anaerobic metabolism within

affected muscle tissue during anesthesia, and may increase vulnerability of skeletal muscle to continued insult after anesthetic recovery (Edner et al. 2002).

Phenothiazines

Phenothiazine use in horses is largely limited to acepromazine. Acepromazine provides minor sedation with some muscle relaxation and is commonly used as a sedative prior to equine anesthesia and during anesthetic recovery. However, as a potent alpha antagonist, acepromazine can provoke profound vasodilation and decrease blood pressure and perfusion. Conversely, at moderate dosages, acepromazine may improve arterial oxygen tension and systemic perfusion, particularly in anesthetic plans that utilize α2-adrenergic receptor agonists in healthy horses, and may therefore preserve or promote muscle perfusion (Marntell et al. 2005). Interestingly, a large-scale study of anesthetized horses reported a reduced risk of mortality when acepromazine was utilized as a sole premedication agent. However, there is no evidence that this beneficial effect related to preservation of perfusion in skeletal muscle, and other mechanisms are more likely responsible (Johnston et al. 2002; Auckburally and Flaherty 2009a). Nonetheless, acepromazine can cause a substantial decrement in blood pressure, which should be taken into account when other exacerbating factors for hypotension are expected.

Opioids

There is little available data on the effect of opioid medications on intrinsic skeletal muscle function in horses. Butorphanol, an agonist–antagonist opioid had no effect on ex-vivo equine esophageal skeletal muscle response to electrical stimulation and was thought to not interfere with *in vivo* contractile mechanisms (Wooldridge et al. 2002).

Benzodiazepines

Benzodiazepines likely have little to no direct effect on skeletal muscle perfusion or metabolism. However, they have potent muscle relaxant properties that are centrally mediated through enhancing the inhibitory effects of gamma-aminobutyric acid (GABA) at the GABA$_A$ receptor, making them beneficial in reducing spasticity in combinations with ketamine (Olkkola and Ahonen 2008). Diazepam and midazolam represent the most commonly utilized benzodiazepine agents in horses. Administration at high doses can promote weakness, fasciculations, ataxia, and recumbency, even in the absence of sedation, and the potential for synergistic effects with other relaxant agents should also be considered (Muir et al. 1982; Hubbell et al. 2013).

Guaifenesin (Glyceryl Guaiacolate)

Guaifenesin is a centrally acting muscle relaxant used as an adjunct agent during equine anesthesia for sedation and relaxant properties. However, excessive or repeated dosing can lead to toxic effects manifesting as extensor muscle spasm or rigidity (Funk 1973). Although not completely understood, the central effects of guaifenesin appear to be mediated through inhibition of the N-methyl-D-aspartate receptor (Keshavarz et al. 2013).

Anticholinergics

The use of anticholinergic agents in horses under anesthesia is controversial, mainly because of their potential to induce gastrointestinal stasis and subsequent colic (Teixeira Neto et al. 2004). The authors could find no reports on the direct effect of atropine or glycopyrrolate on skeletal muscle in horses; however, glycopyrrolate improved cardiac output, arterial blood pressure, and tissue oxygen delivery during halothane anesthesia and xylazine infusion in horses (Teixeira Neto et al. 2004), suggesting implications for muscle resilience under anesthesia.

Dobutamine

Dobutamine is currently considered the sympathomimetic agent of choice for the treatment of hypotension during anesthesia in horses. Its primary action is mediated via agonist activity at the beta-1 receptor, increasing cardiac contractility and cardiac output. Dobutamine increases peripheral oxygen delivery and increased femoral artery blood flow when mean arterial pressure approached 80 mmHg in horses (Schier et al. 2016). In contrast, dopamine, norepinephrine, and phenylephrine have more variable effects on cardiac output, vascular resistance, and peripheral perfusion (Dancker et al. 2018). Dobutamine therefore appears to be the agent of choice for improvement of cardiac output in anesthetized horses that are hypotensive. However, it should be noted that increased femoral artery flow has not been definitively proven to translate to improved muscle tissue perfusion at the microvascular level in anesthetized horses (Raisis et al. 2000).

Induction Agents

Dissociatives

The dissociative anesthetic ketamine is the most commonly used induction agent utilized in equine anesthesia, and disrupts communication between the limbic and thalamocortical systems (Reich and Silvay 1989). The result of this action is to induce a cataleptic-like state that manifests as muscle spasticity, rigidity, and even unconscious spontaneous movement (Berry 2015). For this reason, medications with muscle relaxant properties are frequently co-administered with ketamine. These include α2-adrenergic receptor agonists, benzodiazepines, and guaifenesin (Nowrouzian et al. 1981; Fisher 1984; Matthews et al. 1991; Vien and Chhabra 2017). In regard to muscular perfusion, ketamine is generally accepted to maintain or increase cardiovascular function in horses, and in a rabbit model of hemorrhage, ketamine maintained skeletal muscle capillary perfusion more effectively than pentobarbital or propofol, suggesting possible benefit in hemorrhaging patients (Gustafsson et al. 1995; Gozalo-Marcilla et al. 2014).

Propofol

Propofol is being progressively utilized in equine anesthesia. It is not useful as a sole induction agent in adult horses; however, when combined with other agents such as ketamine, it can replace benzodiazepines for sedation and muscle relaxation (Wagner et al. 2002; Posner et al. 2013). If used as a sole maintenance agent in horses, propofol infusion decreases cardiac contractility and systemic vascular resistance in a dose-dependent manner (Nolan and Hall 1985; Oku et al. 2006) which may impair skeletal muscle perfusion during anesthesia. However, when infused in combination with ketamine it creates minimal cardiovascular depression and appears to have limited impact on skeletal muscle perfusion in horses (Mama et al. 1996; Edner et al. 2002; Umar et al. 2015). In humans, prolonged propofol infusion has resulted in "propofol infusion syndrome" in a small number of patients, characterized by metabolic acidosis, cardiac electrical abnormalities, cardiac and/or renal failure, hyperkalemia, hepatomegaly, hyperlipidemia, and rhabdomyolysis (Krajčová et al. 2018). This is thought to occur through an adverse effect on mitochondrial function of skeletal muscle and is considered a propofol-related bioenergetics failure. Although this condition has not been described in veterinary patients, long-term propofol infusion in animals with skeletal muscle dysfunction should be performed with caution. Furthermore, propofol may enhance the potency of nondepolarizing neuromuscular blocking agents such as rocuronium (Stäuble et al. 2015).

Alfaxalone

Alfaxalone is a neuroactive steroid anesthetic, and its action is mediated via the $GABA_A$ receptor. Although the pharmacokinetics of alfaxalone have been studied in horses, and it has been utilized in intravenous combinations for brief surgical procedures in this species, there is minimal information available regarding its effects on equine musculature (Goodwin et al. 2011; Goodwin et al. 2013; Aoki et al. 2017). However, there is a higher probability of muscle tremors at induction and more prolonged recovery time when alfaxalone is utilized for induction of horses compared to ketamine, which could have implications for muscular health and post-anesthesia serum muscle enzyme activity (Keates et al. 2012; Wakuno et al. 2017).

Maintenance Agents

Volatile Anesthetics

The volatile anesthetic agents currently used most commonly in horses are isoflurane and sevoflurane. Isoflurane has largely replaced halothane as the standard inhalant used for general anesthesia in horses because of reduced cardiovascular depression. Specifically, horses anesthetized with isoflurane have higher heart rate, cardiac output and cardiac index, greater oxygen delivery, aortic blood flow velocity, and femoral arterial and venous blood flow, and lower systemic vascular resistance compared to horses anesthetized with halothane (Steffey and Howland 1980; Raisis et al. 2000; Durongphongtorn et al. 2006). Sevoflurane appears to be very similar to isoflurane in regard to cardiopulmonary function (Steffey et al. 2005). Anesthesia with isoflurane also improves intramuscular blood flow compared to halothane (Lee et al. 1998). However, muscle blood flow is still decreased compared to that in nonanesthetized horses, and decreases as the minimum alveolar concentration (MAC) of isoflurane is increased (Goetz et al. 1989). Furthermore, there is no evidence in a large-scale study that the risk of equine anesthesia associated myopathy is less with isoflurane compared with halothane (Johnston et al. 2004). However, reducing cardiovascular depression via inhalant agent selection, and preventing hypoxemia and maintaining mean blood pressure above 70 mmHg might prevent or reduce muscle damage during anesthesia and into the recovery period (Grandy et al. 1987; Duke et al. 2006; Portier et al. 2009).

Specific Neuromuscular Disorders of Horses

Equine Anesthesia Associated Myopathy

Equine anesthesia associated myopathy (EAAM) is the most common muscular complication of general anesthesia in horses. Previously implicated in more than 7% of equine peri-anesthetic deaths in a large study in the 1990s (Johnston et al. 2002), the transition to newer inhalant agents combined with greater recognition and control of potential precipitating factors appears to have resulted in a substantial decline in clinical cases (Dugdale and Taylor 2016). More recent studies report prevalences of 0.76% and 1.7% for clinical disease (Johnston et al. 2004; Franci et al. 2006), though higher prevalences are reported in special procedures including magnetic resonance imaging (2.3%) and transvenous electrical cardioversion (9.2%) for undefined reasons (Franci et al. 2006; Bellei et al. 2007). It is likely that subclinical muscle damage is also a common occurrence in anesthetized horses. In a study by one of the authors of a Quarter horse dominant group of 116 horses undergoing general anesthesia at four different institutions between 2008 and 2010, 6% of studied horses had serum creatine kinase (CK) activities exceeding 5000 U/l within 24 hours after anesthesia without clinical signs of EAAM (McKenzie, unpublished data). A total of 50% of horses had post-anesthesia serum CK activities exceeding 1000 U/l, a value which was used as a benchmark for EAAM in a commonly cited study (Duke et al. 2006). Muscle and/or nerve damage is also suggested to increase the probability of traumatic fractures in horses in recovery, which is regarded as the greatest cause of recovery mortality (Friend 1981; Johnston et al. 2004; Dugdale and Taylor 2016).

Predisposing factors that contribute to neuromuscular damage under or after anesthesia include inadequate padding of vulnerable body regions, long duration of anesthesia and/or anesthetic recovery, inappropriate positioning of limbs, hypotension, and potentially hypoxemia (Dugdale and Taylor 2016; Ayala et al. 2009; Young 2005). Large body mass is likely also a factor, and 6% of draft horses undergoing upper airway surgery were reported to develop neuromuscular complications related to anesthesia (Kraus et al. 2003). A history of fitness, recent exertion, or exertional rhabdomyolysis (ER) is also linked to anesthesia-related muscle damage in horses (Hildebrand et al. 1990; Klein 1978; Aleman et al. 2009, Auckburally and Flaherty 2009a, McKenzie, unpublished data). In a large study of over 8000 horses, procedures lasting greater than 90 minutes were associated with a tenfold increase in risk of myopathy, and lateral recumbency was also associated with greatly increased risk (Johnston et al. 2004). An association of EAAM with hypotension has been made in several studies, leading to the recommendation for mean arterial blood pressure (MAP) to be maintained at or above 70 mmHg, which might not prevent myopathy but which might decrease clinical severity (Grandy et al. 1987; Duke et al. 2006; Young 2005). Though commonly accepted, the validity of this specific recommendation is unclear, since it was based on a small number of horses in one institution, and was not verified by large-scale assessment across multiple institutions (Johnston et al. 2004). Furthermore, severe EAAM has been reported in horses with optimal blood pressure status, suggesting that maintenance of blood pressure cannot reliably prevent EAAM, particularly if other precipitating factors are present (Short and White 1978; Johnston et al. 2004; Ayala et al. 2009).

Clinical manifestations of EAAM most frequently involve dependent muscle groups including the quadriceps, triceps, and masseter muscles in laterally positioned animals or the gluteal and longissimus dorsi muscles in dorsally positioned animals (Clark-Price et al. 2012). The adductor muscles can be compromised in dorsally positioned horses in spite of their non-dependent position, possibly due to constriction of the medial circumflex femoral artery (Dodman et al. 1988). Anecdotal reports of horses developing EAAM in other dependent and non-dependent muscle groups emphasize the limited understanding of the pathophysiology of this disorder.

Clinical signs consistent with EAAM are most likely to become evident during recovery or in the hours afterward. Whether single or multiple muscles are involved, affected horses display combinations of prolonged recumbency, violent or difficult recovery with repeated attempts to rise, weakness or reduced weight bearing on one or more limbs, fasciculations, distress, myoglobinuria, and sweating, with pain, swelling, and firmness of the affected muscle groups (Friend 1981; Dodman et al. 1988; Ayala et al. 2009; Clark-Price et al. 2012). A dropped position of the elbow can reflect triceps muscle damage with or without accompanying radial nerve paralysis (Figure 8.1), and crouching or weakness of the hind limbs can reflect damage to large muscles and/or nerves in these regions. Neuropathy related to anesthesia has been suggested to be minimally painful despite obvious dysfunction of the affected limb, with minimally deranged serum CK values (Coumbe 2005; Auckburally and Flaherty 2009a). However, horses may become frantic from an inability to utilize a limb and may manifest behavioral signs that can be confused with pain (e.g. tachycardia, sweating, frenetic movement). Mixed neuropathy and myopathy syndromes are possible and

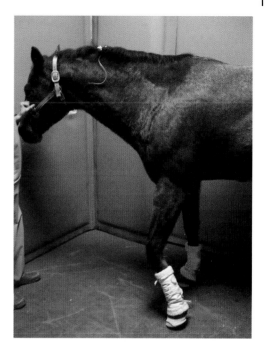

Figure 8.1 A horse after recovering from anesthesia with inability to put weight on the left forelimb demonstrating a "dropped elbow."

the degree to which dysfunction relates to each tissue may not be clear, particularly in the early stages of disease (Young 2005).

Initial clinical signs of EAAM may be subtle and not recognized until hours later when affected horses might display lameness, visible muscle swelling, or biochemical indicators of muscle injury. In rare cases, biochemical and clinical evidence of muscle damage has appeared several days after anesthesia, though the reasons for such apparently delayed onset are unknown (Grint et al. 2007). Serum CK activity in horses with EAAM is often only mildly elevated immediately after anesthesia (~1000–5000 U/l), but frequently increases over the next 24–48 hours, and elevations can be profound (Waldron-Mease and Rosenberg 1979; Duke et al. 2006; Ayala et al. 2009, McKenzie et al. 2015). Therefore, serial monitoring of clinicopathologic variables, particularly muscle enzyme activities and serum electrolyte concentrations is recommended in any horse considered at risk of or potentially affected with EAAM. Some horses can have significant elevations in serum CK with relatively limited clinical signs if there is diffuse damage to a large amount of muscle mass. Conversely, significant clinical signs can occur with relatively limited increases in serum CK if a small area or single muscle group is severely damaged, such as the triceps (Ayala et al. 2009; McKenzie et al. 2015). As a result, serum CK should always be interpreted in conjunction with thorough physical examination, and should be serially monitored to determine need for systemic interventions including intravenous fluids, and to monitor progression and resolution of rhabdomyolysis. Given the dynamics of this enzyme, evaluation at 12-hour intervals is ideal in the early stages of disease. Serum CK is often reported as a cut-off value, typically between 2000 and 20 000 U/l, which can obscure the true magnitude of increase (Friend 1981; Overmann et al. 2010). If cut-off values are exceeded and the potential for significant rhabdomyolysis exists, manual dilution of samples should be performed to achieve an approximate maximum value (Overmann et al. 2010). Serum CK activity can exceed 1 million U/l in very severe rhabdomyolysis; remarkably, this is not always correlated with a fatal outcome (Collins et al. 1998). Furthermore, horses with massively elevated serum CK can also display spuriously high serum total CO_2 concentrations and negative anion gap if these values are determined on a chemistry analyzer versus a blood gas analyzer. This results from interference of enzymatic reactions in the analyzer generated by release of pyruvate and lactate dehydrogenase from injured muscle cells (Overmann et al. 2010). Serum aspartate aminotransferase (AST) is less labile than CK and is also useful in determining immensity of damage and progress over time, particularly if CK has normalized. Horses with severe muscle damage will have AST values exceeding several thousand U/l,

with a maximum ceiling of approximately 45 000 U/l; values above 20 000 U/l are uncommon and indicate profound generalized rhabdomyolysis (Friend 1981; Collins et al. 1998). Diagnostic ultrasound can be performed on visibly affected muscle groups to evaluate local swelling and edema, and to differentiate probable EAAM from a traumatic muscle tear sustained during anesthetic recovery. Ultrasound is particularly useful if the contralateral muscle appears normal and can provide an appropriate comparison (Walmsley et al. 2010).

Horses with suspected or confirmed EAAM should be treated promptly and aggressively, to limit pain and muscle swelling, to correct acid–base and electrolyte abnormalities, and to reduce the deleterious effects of myoglobinuria. The disorder is often progressive, and horses that are initially weight bearing and standing can become non-weight bearing or even recumbent as muscle swelling and damage progresses over the next 24–28 hours, hence early treatment and close observation over time is warranted. Serial monitoring of biochemical variables including blood urea nitrogen (BUN) and creatinine, CK and AST, serum electrolytes and acid–base status is indicated. Horses with visible myoglobinuria should receive intravenous or nasogastric fluids at least until urine color returns to normal and any perfusion and electrolyte anomalies are resolved. Blood and urine pH should be assessed, since the production of acid urine can greatly enhance the nephrotoxicity of myoglobin. Horses with disturbed acid–base status (blood pH < 7.2, urine pH < 7.0) and myoglobinuria might benefit from inclusion of sodium bicarbonate in intravenous fluids until normal values are achieved (Waldron-Mease 1978). Myoglobinuria is usually a transient phenomenon since this product is cleared rapidly from the serum, so careful attention should be paid to urinations for resolution over time. Profound muscle swelling can damage peripheral nerves and exacerbate discomfort and muscle necrosis, and surgical fasciotomy

Figure 8.2 A horse with equine anesthesia associated myopathy with severe swelling of the epaxial and gluteal musculature. Surgical fasciotomy was performed to relieve elevated intra- and inter-fascial compartment pressure.

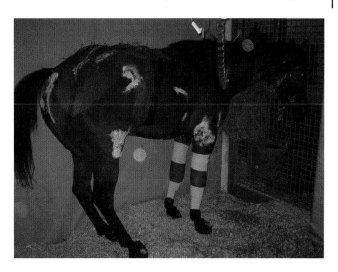

might be required in severe cases to relieve elevated pressure in intra- and inter-fascial compartments (Figure 8.2).

Pain management can be very challenging in horses with severe focal myopathy causing non-weight-bearing lameness, and multi-modal analgesia is indicated. Non-steroidal anti-inflammatory agents are valuable, but should be applied with caution if patients are azotemic, visibly myoglobinuric, receiving concurrent nephrotoxic drugs, or have other contraindications to their use (Cook and Blikslager 2015). Acepromazine has also been utilized empirically in EAAM for its sedative, relaxant, and vasodilatory effects and can be given by intermittent administration orally or parenterally. Opioid medications including morphine and butorphanol can be useful adjunct analgesics in horses with significant discomfort. Intermittent administration may be adequate; however, more severe pain may respond more favorably to constant rate infusions of these drugs. Horses should be monitored for potential adverse effects including excitement, compulsive walking, indicators of reduced gastrointestinal motility, and urinary retention, particularly if receiving high intermittent doses or constant rate infusions of opioids (Clutton 2010; Gozalo-Marcilla et al. 2014; Sanchez and Robertson 2014).

Constant rate infusions of other analgesic drugs including lidocaine and ketamine can be beneficial in horses with severe discomfort. Horses with severe pain creating danger to themselves and their handlers may require administration of a combination of drugs by bolus and constant rate infusion, including alpha-2 agonists, to permit additional measures such as placement of epidural medication to reduce acute or ongoing distress. Epidural injection or epidural catheter placement with intermittent or constant infusions of analgesic drugs should be strongly considered in horses with profound pain inhibiting weight bearing. This is particularly important if initial pain control measures fail to achieve reasonable comfort within 12 hours, to reduce the risk of supporting limb laminitis. The combination of morphine with xylazine or detomidine can provide potent relief when one or more limbs are partially or totally non-weight bearing (Natalini 2010). The volume of injection can be increased in horses with forelimb involvement to promote cranial analgesia. As pain improves, analgesic drugs can be reduced or removed in a serial fashion over time while monitoring the patient's progress. The process should commence by removing agents most likely to produce side effects and/or that are the most expensive or inconvenient to administer. Ideally, only a single

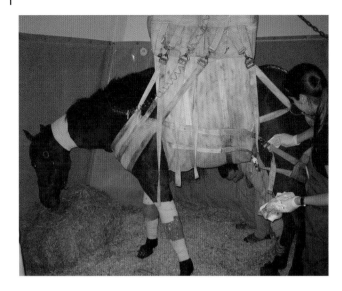

Figure 8.3 A horse with equine anesthesia associated myopathy in a sling to assist the horse with remaining in a standing position.

medication is manipulated at any time to reduce risk of compromising clinical stability and to accurately assess the effect of specific changes.

Horses should be encouraged to remain standing if possible, and may require a lift or sling to assist them to rise (Figure 8.3). If they are recumbent and slinging is not tolerated or feasible, then attempts should be made to rotate lateral recumbency frequently or to maintain them in sternal position in a deeply bedded stall. Manual assistance to stand several times a day can help relieve compression of musculature, but must be performed with attention to the risk of additional injury. Limbs should be wrapped and shoes removed or wrapped to help prevent additional trauma. Cryotherapy consisting of ice packs or cold-water hydrotherapy over localized areas of muscle damage may assist with pain management and recovery (Figure 8.4). Horses with severe focal or diffuse rhabdomyolysis may benefit from the administration of dantrolene sodium (4–6 mg/kg, every 12 hours per os to a recently fed horse) (McKenzie et al. 2010). This drug prevents additional muscle necrosis and potentially speeds recovery and reduces muscular pain. Dosing should begin as soon as recognition of a muscular complication is made. Administration of dantrolene via nasogastric tube can be performed as soon as a swallowing reflex is present in the recovering patient if feasible in a manner that prevents risk to the operator (Waldron-Mease and Rosenberg 1979).

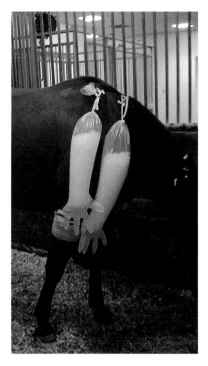

Figure 8.4 Treatment of a horse with equine anesthesia associated myopathy with cryotherapy using ice packs placed over the affected muscles.

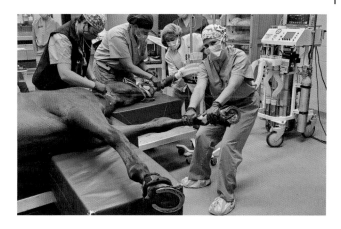

Figure 8.5 A horse in lateral recumbency during anesthesia. The down forelimb is manually pulled forward to minimize pressure on the dependent muscles and nerves.

Prevention of EAAM should be approached in a multi-faceted manner due to the range of contributing factors. Tactics include careful limb positioning to protect dependent musculature, minimizing duration of anesthesia, and maintaining mean arterial pressure at values above 70 mmHg, which may not prevent but can potentially reduce severity (Duke et al. 2006). In laterally recumbent horses, the dependent front limbs should be pulled forward to minimize pressure from bones on large nerve bundles and non-dependent limbs should be placed in a neutral position and supported with padding or stirrups (Figures 8.5 and 8.6). Placing horses on an adequately padded surface is critical, and since the duration of procedures can be variable and challenging to predict, padding should be considered even for procedures expected to be transient in nature. Padding should be thick and soft enough to allow for a diffuse area of contact with the horse's body to minimize pressure localization on small areas. If procedures are to extend significantly beyond their expected duration, then re-assessment of patient positioning and padding should be made to determine if there are beneficial alterations that could be feasibly achieved to avoid complications. Specialized recovery systems including air mattresses, pools, and rope systems may reduce the risk of additional muscular trauma related to prolonged or violent recovery.

Prevention of EAAM can potentially also be achieved by premedication with dantrolene sodium in horses considered at high risk. Studies demonstrate substantially lower serum CK activities in horses anesthetized after dantrolene administration than after sham treatment, even under hypotensive conditions (McKenzie and Mosley 2010; McKenzie et al. 2015). A dose of 4–6 mg/kg

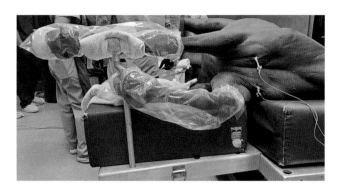

Figure 8.6 A horse in lateral recumbency during anesthesia. Padded stirrups are used to maintain the limbs in a neutral position to the trunk to minimize strain and pressure on the musculature.

can be provided orally or by nasogastric tube one to two hours prior to anesthesia (McKenzie et al. 2015). It should be noted that dantrolene absorption is minimal in horses fasted for 12 hours, and optimal in horses fed in the 4 hours preceding administration, which can interfere with standard pre-anesthesia fasting protocols (McKenzie et al. 2010). Other potential disadvantages of dantrolene administration include a negative effect on cardiac output, and potential development of hyperkalemia in anesthetized horses approximately two hours after administration of the drug, and one hour after commencement of anesthesia (McKenzie et al. 2015). These findings might relate to the dose used in the reporting study (6 mg/kg) and protective effects are possibly achieved at lower doses. However, substantial inter-individual variability in plasma concentrations after treatment makes determination of an appropriate and reliable oral dose challenging. Currently, premedication with dantrolene should be considered only for horses considered at high risk of EAAM and avoided in horses susceptible to hyperkalemic periodic paralysis (HYPP). Horses that receive dantrolene prior to anesthesia should have serial monitoring of blood potassium concentrations and cardiac rhythm performed throughout anesthesia (McKenzie et al. 2015).

Hyperkalemic Periodic Paralysis (HYPP)

HYPP is a well-described hereditary muscular disorder that predominantly affects Quarter horses and related breeds including Paints, Palominos, Appaloosas, and the Pony of the Americas breed (Naylor 1997). The disease is associated with a point mutation in the SCN4A gene encoding the alpha subunit of the skeletal muscle sodium channel, and is heritable in a codominant autosomal fashion (Naylor et al. 1999; Mickelson and Valberg 2015). This results in a higher resting membrane potential in muscle fibers containing mutant sodium

channels, increasing their susceptibility to depolarization, particularly in the presence of high potassium concentrations (Pickar et al. 1991). Clinically, this is most often reflected by muscle fasciculations with subsequent weakness as a result of depolarization block. Abnormal muscular activity during clinical episodes of disease promotes efflux of potassium into the extracellular environment in many, but not all affected horses, evidenced by an increase in serum potassium concentration.

The genetic mutation associated with HYPP has been previously estimated to occur with a prevalence of 4.4% in the general Quarter horse population, and remarkably, exceeded 55% in a genetic survey of elite Halter horses (Tryon et al. 2009). This is likely the result of positive selection pressure related to enhanced muscle mass in affected animals (Naylor 1994; Bowling et al. 1996; Tryon et al. 2009; Mickelson and Valberg 2015). Since 2007, foals that test homozygous for the relevant mutation cannot be registered with the American Quarter Horse Association; however, there is no evidence that this has reduced the prevalence of the disorder, perhaps unsurprising since most horses that carry the defect are heterozygotes (Mickelson and Valberg 2015). Horses that carry the mutation can be asymptomatic, or may display episodic weakness, third eyelid protrusion, facial myotonia, sweating and muscle fasciculations. Homozygous animals may also display dysphagia as foals, or respiratory compromise with stridor, respiratory distress, and hypercapnia due to laryngeal and pharyngeal dysfunction (Meyer et al. 1999). Hyperkalemia is a common corollary of abnormal muscle activity and can result in cardiac arrhythmias. Horses often display clinical episodes of HYPP from two to three years of age onward, and horses under or recovering from anesthesia are at particular risk, even in their first year of life (Cornick et al. 1994; Bailey et al. 1996; Baetge 2007). It is unclear why anesthesia might enhance susceptibility to clinical episodes of HYPP.

A clinical HYPP event during anesthesia is possible even in horses that have previously been anesthetized without complication (Cornick et al. 1994; Pang et al. 2011). Clinical signs may be mild and nonspecific, reflected simply by prolonged recovery and ineffective attempts to stand. Severe signs include fasciculations, tachycardia, rigidity, sweating, hypercapnia, hypertension, and cardiac arrhythmias (Baetge 2007). Hyperkalemia can develop as a progressive phenomenon over time, hence serial sampling during anesthesia is recommended in any patient with known or possible HYPP (Baetge 2007). Electrocardiogram analysis can reveal development of abnormalities consistent with hyperkalemia, indicating the need for rapid pharmacologic intervention. Changes to the electrocardiogram (ECG) observed in hyperkalemic horses include widening of the P wave with decreased amplitude, and eventual obliteration of P wave activity. The P-R interval and T wave amplitude might both increase (Carpenter and Evans 2005). The QRS interval may become prolonged and begin merging with the T wave, with irregular ventricular rate preceding ventricular fibrillation. It should be noted that there is poor correlation between heart rate and plasma potassium concentration, and absence of ECG changes does not rule out the potential for severe hyperkalemia to be present. Horses can display severe cardiac rhythm anomalies once plasma potassium reaches or exceeds 5.5 mEq/l. Treatment to address hyperkalemia is prudent if plasma potassium reaches or exceeds this level or displays a progressive increase, regardless of the underlying provoking condition (Glazier et al. 1982; Meyer et al. 1999; McKenzie et al. 2015; Langdon Fielding 2015).

Recognition of an HYPP episode during anesthesia should prompt emergency measures to address hypercapnia and hyperkalemia (Table 8.1). Affected horses should be ventilated appropriately to maintain acceptable arterial partial pressure of CO_2 as an aid to increase blood pH. Infusion of crystalloid solutions with added potassium, or whole blood should be ceased and replaced with crystalloid fluids (lactated Ringer's solution [LRS], Plasmalyte) with no external additives. These formulations contain minimal potassium, exerting a dilutional effect on plasma potassium concentrations, and also provide a pH buffering effect which may help further reduce plasma potassium through cellular ion exchange (Dépret et al. 2019). The use of normal saline has recently been questioned as this solution is acidifying and can increase plasma potassium concentration and exacerbate acid–base aberrations (Khajavi et al. 2008; Cunha et al. 2010; Li et al. 2016; González-Castro et al. 2018; Dépret et al. 2019). Hyperkalemia can also be addressed via the administration of dextrose and insulin, and calcium gluconate to enhance intracellular movement of potassium and reduce the risk of cardiac arrhythmias (Langdon Fielding 2015; Dépret et al. 2019). Sodium bicarbonate also represents a traditional treatment for hyperkalemia; however, hypertonic saline is similarly effective in decreasing plasma potassium concentration and preventing cardiac arrhythmia (Trefz et al. 2017). This likely reflects vascular expansion, diuresis, and hypernatremia-mediated intracellular movement of potassium. Additionally, hypertonic saline increases the velocity of the rising action potential, which is depressed during hyperkalemia, and therefore may act as a membrane stabilizer similarly to calcium (Dépret et al. 2019). Administration of crystalloid fluids after administration of hypertonic saline is indicated to prevent detrimental cellular dehydration and chloride-induced acidemia.

Treatment of HYPP usually results in prompt improvement in serum potassium concentration, which should continue to be serially monitored as the horse recovers. Serial measurement of serum muscle enzyme activity can also be performed every 2–12 hours after anesthesia ends. Typically, HYPP causes only mild elevations in serum CK; however, measurement can help to distinguish HYPP from other disorders such as malignant hyperthermia,

Table 8.1 Options for emergency treatment of hyperkalemia in horses (Mushiyakh et al. 2012; Langdon Fielding 2015).

Drug	Dose	Mode of action	Comments
Calcium gluconate	• 0.2–0.5 ml/kg of 20–23% solution in 1–2 l of IV fluid over 20 min	• Cardioprotective • Enhances cardiac output • Rapid onset of action	• Administer slowly • Caution regarding precipitation with other products
Dextrose	• 5–6 ml/kg of 5% solution IV • 1 ml/kg of 50% solution in 1 l of crystalloid fluids	• Prompts intracellular movement of potassium • May take 10–20 minutes for effect	• Avoid extravasation of concentrated solutions • Hyperglycemia and diuresis at high rates of administration
Insulin	• 0.1–0.2 U/kg IV • Ideally administer with dextrose	• Prompts intracellular movement of potassium • May take 10–20 minutes for effect	• Monitor for hypoglycemia after administration
Sodium bicarbonate	• 1–2 mEq/kg of 1.3% sodium bicarbonate solution • Or dilute hypertonic solutions in non-calcium containing fluids and give IV over 20 min	Hypernatremia likely prompts vascular expansion, diuresis, and intracellular movement of potassium	• Watch for respiratory acidosis • Precipitation with calcium containing fluids • Appropriate choice if concurrent significant metabolic acidosis
Isotonic crystalloid fluid bolus	2–5 ml/kg/h IV	Increase urinary potassium excretion	• Ensure no additive to fluids
Furosemide	1–2 mg/kg IV	• Enhanced excretion of potassium in urine	• May be contraindicated in patients receiving gentamicin

and can also document muscle injury if prolonged or violent anesthetic recovery is encountered in horses with HYPP.

For horses with suspected HYPP and without an established genetic profile, owners should be encouraged to permit polymerase chain reaction (PCR) testing for the causative mutation on whole blood or plucked hair samples. Testing for other genetic disorders can be accomplished at the same time and should be encouraged for breeding stock (Tryon et al. 2009; Mickelson and Valberg 2015). Samples should be submitted to laboratories offering scientifically validated genetic testing procedures.

Preparing for future episodes of anesthesia in horses with suspected or confirmed HYPP is important and may help to prevent clinical disease arising during the anesthesia process. For elective procedures, the risk of clinical episodes may be reduced if horses are prepared in advance by feeding a low potassium ration and treated with the potassium wasting diuretic, acetazolamide administered at 2–4 mg/kg per os at 8–12-hour intervals for several days or weeks before planned anesthesia (Langdon Fielding 2015). Additionally, minimizing stressful events that may precipitate an episode, in the days prior to an anesthetic event, may be helpful. Transporting a suspected or confirmed HYPP horse several days prior instead of the day of anesthesia is recommended to allow for acclimation, monitoring of clinical signs, and verification of diet and acetazolamide administration.

Pre-existing ER Disorders

Exertional rhabdomyolysis (ER), the development of abnormal muscle necrosis with exercise, is usually recognized by signs of stiffness, reluctance to move, inappropriate sweating, and other indications of exercise-induced muscular damage. It is a common phenomenon in several equine breeds, including Thoroughbreds, Quarter horses, Standardbreds, Arabians, and polo ponies (Valberg 2018). Multiple reports, some anecdotal, suggest that horses with previously known ER, and fit athletic horses, are more prone to adverse muscular events under anesthesia. This can contribute to concern when these horses require anesthesia (Klein 1978; Hildebrand et al. 1990; Aleman et al. 2009; Auckburally and Flaherty 2009a).

Polysaccharide storage myopathy (PSSM) in Quarter horses and related breeds is an autosomal dominant glycogen storage disorder linked to a gain of function mutation in the glycogen synthase 1 gene (*GYS1*), resulting in abnormal muscle glycogen metabolism. This mutation has an estimated prevalence of approximately 6–10% in the general American Quarter horse population, and up to 28% in elite Halter Quarter horses (Tryon et al. 2009; Valberg 2018). PSSM is a very prevalent disorder in specific draft breeds, particularly Belgians and Percherons in North America, with reported prevalences in one study of 38.9% and 62.4% in each breed, respectively (McCue et al. 2010). Horses with the *GYS1* mutation are often asymptomatic, and the most common clinical presentation in light breed horses is ER, and in draft horses, muscular weakness and atrophy. There is no definitive evidence that possession of the *GYS1* mutation alone increases the risk of complications with general anesthesia. However, one case report attributed prolonged recumbency in anesthetic recovery to PSSM in a Belgian draft filly, and PSSM was linked to generalized post-operative rhabdomyolysis in a draft horse in another report (Bloom et al. 1999; Kraus et al. 2003). It seems possible this is coincidental given the high prevalence of PSSM in some draft breeds, and the recognized challenges of anesthetizing these horses even when they are completely healthy (Kraus et al. 2003; Rothenbuhler et al. 2006; McCue et al. 2010). However, muscle damage in horses with PSSM can be evoked by stimuli other than exercise, including respiratory infections. The previously described Belgian filly also developed bilateral triceps myopathy several days after anesthesia, and the role of PSSM and its association to the preceding anesthesia event in this complication is not clear (Bloom et al. 1999). Furthermore, a fraction of Quarter horses with PSSM1 also carry the *RYR1* mutation linked to malignant hyperthermia (MH), which can promote disease associated with anesthesia (McCue et al. 2009; Aleman et al. 2009).

Individuals with PSSM might be detected ahead of anesthesia based on historical reports of ER, pre-existing genetic testing results, or detection of elevated serum CK and/or AST values on pre-anesthesia blood work or after an exercise test. Halter Quarter horses and draft horses have a high prevalence of PSSM, but also tend to be heavily muscled, such that risk of muscle injury might relate to body mass rather than to PSSM. Nonetheless, recognition and directed monitoring of individuals with PSSM undergoing anesthesia is prudent.

Thoroughbred and Standardbred racehorses appear to share an analogous ER disorder with each other, which has also been suggested to increase their vulnerability to adverse muscular events under anesthesia (Klein 1978; Hildebrand et al. 1990). This disorder is commonly attributed to a heritable abnormality of skeletal muscle cell calcium metabolism; however, it has proven remarkably challenging to identify the genetic signature, suggesting the disorder might have complex inheritance (Mickelson and Valberg 2015; Norton et al. 2016). Currently referred to as *recurrent exertional rhabdomyolysis* (RER), this disorder is reported to have a 5–9% prevalence in Thoroughbred and Standardbred horses. For both breeds, young females, and fit individuals, appear most predisposed to clinical disease, though this sex difference resolves with age (MacLeay et al. 1999; Isgren et al. 2010). Thoroughbred horses with this disorder have a lower contracture threshold of intercostal muscle tissue in response to halothane and caffeine, which emulates a feature of MH. Application of dantrolene in an *in vitro* model normalized muscle contracture responses in these horses, and ER can be prevented in affected horses by oral administration of dantrolene prior to exercise, potentially also supporting the theory of a calcium regulation anomaly (McKenzie et al. 2004). It is not known if RER links with reports of a higher incidence of adverse muscular events under general anesthesia in Standardbreds and Thoroughbreds. The *RYR1* mutation linked to MH in Quarter horses has not been demonstrated in Thoroughbreds or Standardbreds at this time. Horses with RER are unlikely to be recognized in advance of anesthesia unless clients provide a history of previous episodes of clinical disease. Muscle enzyme activity is usually unremarkable if there has been no recent clinical episode and submaximal exercise testing is unlikely to be rewarding in these breeds. Management of horses with suspected RER undergoing anesthesia should therefore focus on monitoring of blood pressure, arterial gas characteristics, and periodic assessment of serum CK commencing two to four hours after anesthesia ceases to evaluate any concerning or inappropriate increases. If evidence of local or generalized muscle reactions occur, horses can be managed according to severity as described for EAAM.

Malignant Hyperthermia (MH)

MH is a rare genetic disorder that can cause severe diffuse rhabdomyolysis and death associated with exposure to anesthetic and other agents. Clinical signs reflect uncontrolled calcium release from the sarcoplasmic reticulum of skeletal muscle cells via the calcium release channel (the *RYR1* receptor), resulting in sustained muscle contraction, profound muscle hypermetabolism, and heat production. Affected horses display a progressive increase in body temperature, hyperventilation, tachycardia, excessive sweating, extrusion of the third eyelid, rigidity, and fasciculations. Myoglobinuria and violent anesthetic recovery may also be observed. Rapid onset of profound rigor mortis is observed in horses that do not survive (Aleman et al. 2005). Clinicopathologic findings in MH include hemoconcentration, hyperkalemia, hyper- or hypocalcemia, hyper- or hypophosphatemia, metabolic and respiratory acidosis, relative hypoxemia, hyperlactatemia, and elevations in serum CK and AST (Friend 1981; Aleman et al. 2009). Rapid rise in end-tidal partial pressure of CO_2 despite adjustment to mechanical ventilation parameters is frequently the first clinical indication of MH, occurring in conjunction with rising body temperature (Aleman et al. 2005). Hypoxemia and acidosis are profound in advanced disease, and the anesthesia circuit may become very hot to touch and carbon dioxide absorbent may become quickly exhausted (Aleman et al. 2005). Peracute death may be associated with minimal derangement of serum muscle enzyme activities in conjunction with severe derangements in blood gas variables.

A point mutation in exon 46 of the *RYR1* gene resulting in a substitution error has been documented in Quarter horses with clinical disease represented by anesthesia-induced MH and also ER (Aleman et al. 2009). The mutation is heritable in an autosomal dominant fashion, but appears only to occur as a heterozygous trait, suggesting early or in utero mortality might occur with homozygous status (Aleman et al. 2004, 2009). The mutation is uncommon, with one study reporting a prevalence of 1.3% in a random selection of 225 Quarter horses (Nieto and Aleman 2009). The propensity for horses carrying the mutation to display signs of MH when exposed to anesthetic agents is not clear. A recent study of horses carrying the genetic mutation associated with equine MH reported a mortality of 100% in all anesthetized horses (Johnston et al. 2004; Aleman et al. 2009). Three of these horses were anesthetized with halothane and two with isoflurane (Aleman et al. 2009). This would suggest that although the prevalence of the mutation is low, the probability of severe adverse reactions to inhalant anesthesia and subsequent mortality is high.

Clinical signs mimicking MH have also been reported in Thoroughbred horses, particularly those in training, despite lack of documentation of the known equine MH mutation in this breed (Klein 1978; Waldron-Mease 1978; Mickelson and Valberg 2015). Additionally, MH-like reactions have also been reported in horses receiving relatively short duration injectable anesthesia with xylazine and ketamine (anecdotal report) and hyperthermia with delayed onset diffuse myopathy was reported in a horse receiving a combination infusion of guaifenesin, detomidine, and ketamine (Grint et al. 2007). In horses receiving injectable drugs, the possibility of contamination of injected products with endotoxin or other impurities must also be considered. Although muscle contracture testing and other *in vitro* techniques have been applied in several studies to try to detect underlying propensity for MH in a variety of equine breeds, these are technically challenging procedures typically limited to research investigations (Hildebrand et al. 1990; Lentz et al. 1999a, 1999b; Ward et al. 2000).

Severe diffuse rhabdomyolysis without typical accompanying signs of MH has also been reported in horses during or soon after anesthesia, and can affect non-dependent musculature and internal musculature such as the diaphragm, tongue, and myocardium (Klein 1978; Friend 1981; Manley et al. 1983; Aleman et al. 2005). Disease has typically been reported in adults, but also in foals (Short and White 1978; Manley et al. 1983), with Thoroughbreds, Quarter Horses, Appaloosas, Arabians, and pony breeds affected. Occasionally, evidence of muscle damage may be delayed for several days (Grint et al. 2007). It is possible that this syndrome represents a form of MH or EAAM.

Treatment of MH must commence as soon as complications are recognized, and early recognition is critical to improving survival (Table 8.2). Unfortunately, some early clinical signs, such as tachycardia and muscle activity may be confused with a light plane of anesthesia (Waldron-Mease 1978). However, progression of signs commonly occurs, resulting in eventual recognition of the disorder. Administration of anesthetic agents should be ceased immediately, and the patient ventilated

Table 8.2 Emergency management of suspected malignant hyperthermia in anesthetized horses.

- Discontinue inhalant anesthetic exposure and transition to an intravenous protocol
- Increase ventilation rate and tidal volume with 100% oxygen
- Administer dantrolene (1 mg/kg IV or 4 mg/kg via nasogastric tube) if available
- Monitor core temperature
- Apply active cooling
  - Ice packs
  - Alcohol bath
  - Fans
  - Cool water skin bath, gastric lavage, and enema
  - Cool intravenous crystalloid fluids
- Serial blood gas and electrolyte analysis to address metabolic and respiratory abnormalities.

with 100% oxygen. Horses should be removed from the original anesthetic circuit and placed on another if possible to decrease exposure to residual inhalant anesthetic. Replacement of inhalant agents with intravenous agents to maintain anesthesia can be used if needed to bring active procedures to a point where they can be safely truncated (Waldron-Mease 1978). Although not reviewed in horses with MH, a combination of propofol and an alpha-2 agonist for total intravenous anesthesia has been used successfully in humans with MH and might represent an option for some equine cases (Naquib et al. 2011; Schieren et al. 2017). Minute ventilation should be increased as appropriate to address hypercapnia, though a ventilation ceiling may be reached due to the abnormal unregulated metabolic processes that are occurring. Emergency measures should also focus on documenting and controlling body temperature, acid–base anomalies, and hyperkalemia.

Active cooling should be performed incorporating combinations of wet towels, cold-water gastric lavage and enemas, fans, application of alcohol to the skin, and administration of cool crystalloid intravenous fluids with serial temperature monitoring. Serial arterial blood gas analysis is valuable to document critical acid–base and electrolyte abnormalities that require treatment, including acidosis and hyperkalemia. If hyperkalemia is progressive, profound, or associated with cardiac rhythm abnormalities, emergency drug administration can include dextrose, insulin, and/or calcium gluconate. Administration of bicarbonate should be performed with caution to avoid exacerbation of respiratory acidosis. If a nasogastric tube is in place, or as soon as one can be feasibly placed, horses can be administered dantrolene sodium at 4–6 mg/kg, which can be repeated at 8–12-hour intervals. Intravenous formulations of this drug are not usually available for veterinary use due to the large volumes required and associated expense, however, if available, a dose of 1 mg/kg IV is likely appropriate (Court et al. 1987). Even with aggressive treatment, mortality rates in horses with clinical MH is likely to be high.

If stabilized, horses should be moved into a safe environment for recovery. Recovery quite often will be violent and additional steps to improve safety and reduce trauma should be considered including head protection and rope or sling assistance. Once standing, treatment of affected horses is very similar to that described for EAAM. Therapeutic measures should focus on restoration of circulating volume and prevention of renal damage, control of pain and inflammation, correction of fluid and electrolyte anomalies, prevention of ongoing muscle necrosis, and high-quality nursing care.

Recovered animals requiring future anesthetic events may benefit from premedication with dantrolene sodium, though there is currently no confirmed evidence that dantrolene has efficacy for specifically preventing MH in horses. However, dantrolene apparently reduces muscle damage in horses with ER and in healthy horses undergoing deliberately hypotensive general anesthesia (McKenzie et al. 2004; McKenzie et al. 2015). If possible, anesthesia should be achieved in susceptible horses via total intravenous anes-thesia as previously mentioned, with total avoidance of inhalant anesthetics. (Aleman et al. 2009; Schieren et al. 2017). Horses should be tested for the known equine MH mutation, though it is unlikely to be identi-fied outside of Quarter horses or related breeds (Paints, Appaloosas). Suspect horses should also be tested for HYPP, due to clini-cal similarities between these syndromes (Cornick et al. 1994; Pang et al. 2011).

Myofibrillar Myopathy

Myofibrillar myopathy is a newly recognized disorder that contributes to ER in Arabian and Warmblood horses (Valberg et al. 2016, 2017). The etiology and pathophysiology of this con-dition is currently poorly understood, and the implications for anesthesia unknown.

Glycogen Branching Enzyme Deficiency

Glycogen branching enzyme deficiency (GBED) is a fatal glycogen storage disorder of Quarter Horse and Paint foals, heritable in an autosomal recessive fashion. Disease arises from a missense mutation in the glyco-gen branching enzyme 1 gene (*GBE1*). This results in negligible production of this essen-tial enzyme, which is responsible for produc-ing normally configured glycogen molecules in numerous tissues (Valberg et al. 2001; Ward et al. 2004). Clinical signs only occur in homozygous animals and likely relate to ina-bility to store glycogen and mobilize glucose for normal tissue metabolism resulting in sudden cardiac death or respiratory failure (Valberg et al. 2001; Ward et al. 2004). The vast majority of affected individuals are believed to be aborted; however, some foals are born live, and typically die in the first days to weeks of life. Anecdotally, however, at least one case has been described to sur-vive to nearly 18 weeks of life before suc-cumbing to this invariably fatal disease. The prevalence of heterozygous carriers in the general population is reported to be approxi-mately 8–9% in Quarter Horses and 7% in Paint horses (Wagner et al. 2002).

The potential for anesthesiologists to encounter a foal with GBED is low; however, foals are prone to several disorders in early life including uroabdomen, umbilical disorders, traumatic injuries, and colic that can require anesthesia. Complicating this picture is the fact that GBED is commonly overlooked, and clinical signs are often attributed to other dis-orders including sepsis, hypothyroidism, or neonatal maladjustment syndrome. Ideally, GBED-affected foals are recognized before extended medical or surgical care occur to avoid futile expenditure. Clinically, foals may appear relatively normal, or may be persis-tently or episodically weak and may have hypothermia and flexural deformities of all limbs. Serial hematologic and clinical pathol-ogy monitoring may identify persistent leuko-penia, intermittent hypoglycemia, and moderately high serum CK (1000–15 000 U/l), AST, and GGT activities (Valberg et al. 2001). Some foals will display episodic seizure activ-ity related to recurrent hypoglycemia, and some will display respiratory failure with hypercapnia and respiratory acidosis; foals can also display sudden death related to probable cardiac arrhythmia (Valberg et al. 2001).

Definitive diagnosis of GBED can be achieved via histopathologic examination of tissues, particularly skeletal muscle, cardiac muscle, and liver. Findings include reduced or absent normal background staining with Periodic Acid Schiff (PAS) reflecting absence of normal glycogen in tissues, and variable globular or crystalline PAS positive intracellu-lar inclusions in skeletal muscle and cardiac Purkinje fibers (Valberg et al. 2001). Genetic testing can also be performed at laboratories offering scientifically validated testing proce-dures on hair or whole blood samples to iden-tify the causative mutation. Since the dam and sire must both carry the trait, one or both can be tested for heterozygote status if samples from the foal are not available.

General Considerations for Anesthetizing Horses with Emphasis on Muscular Preservation

Factors Associated with Muscular or Peripheral Nerve Injury in Anesthetized Horses

Factors that might exacerbate or create neuromuscular injury in horses during anesthesia were previously described, and include ischemia related to positioning, prolonged compression or tourniquet application, hypotension, blunt trauma, surgical injury, administration of pharmacologic agents, and contributions from underlying muscle disorders (Dodman et al. 1988; Lindsay et al. 1989; Bailey et al. 1996; Bloom et al. 1999; Wong and Chung 2000; Johnston et al. 2004; Franci et al. 2006). Animals encountering prolonged or violent anesthetic recovery for any reason are at risk of additional muscular trauma. Since muscle damage often represents a compound event, it can be challenging to definitively identify the most significant contributing factors in specific individuals. Nonetheless, recognizing as many of these factors as possible in advance can help to prevent problems, or might mitigate serious damage. Thus, consideration of the muscular system should be included in any anesthetic plan, particularly in horses with known or suspected diseases or abnormalities.

Pre-emptive Evaluation

Evaluation of horses prior to anesthesia should begin with a complete history and physical examination. This presents the ideal opportunity to establish the possibility of pre-existing muscular disease and to assess the risk for muscle-related complications during or after anesthesia. Patient signalment can indicate potential risk for specific muscular disorders or muscle damage under anesthesia (Table 8.3). This is particularly the case for draft breeds with high body mass, and for breeds with a high prevalence of HYPP, which greatly complicates anesthesia when clinical episodes occur (Bailey et al. 1996; Carpenter and Evans 2005; Rothenbuhler et al. 2006; Baetge 2007). Breeds with known predispositions to muscular disorders should be noted and carefully evaluated prior to anesthesia, and establishing any known information about genetic status prior to anesthetizing members of these breeds is strongly recommended. Some of these disorders create aberrations of muscle enzymes on screening blood work, and awareness of their presence can aid more directed monitoring during anesthesia and in the post-anesthesia period. Ideally, horses with a known muscular disorder are identified in advance of anesthesia to permit tailored management. Careful historical evaluation may in some cases reveal prior indications of muscle disease, problematic prior anesthesia events, or genetic testing results for HYPP, PSSM, or MH. However, such information often passes undisclosed unless specific questioning is employed. Physical examination should be thorough and should include assessment of muscle mass and symmetry, palpation of musculature for abnormalities including pain, swelling, tissue defects, and percussion dimpling.

Pre-anesthesia clinical pathology assessment is strongly encouraged regardless of the age or apparent health status of the horse. Values of particular importance for assessing the muscular system include the muscle-derived enzymes CK and AST, and the muscle product creatinine which is an indicator of muscle mass and renal function (Stockham and Scott 2008). Ideally, the liver-derived enzyme gammaglutamyl transferase (GGT) should also be evaluated to distinguish muscle pathology from liver pathology in horses with elevations of AST due to the latter enzyme's shared origin from muscle and liver tissue. BUN and creatinine should be assessed because azotemia may be documented post-anesthesia in horses with significant rhabdomyolysis, and an absence of pre-existing

Table 8.3 Currently recognized muscular disorders of horses with potential implications for anesthesia.

Muscular disorder	Affected breeds	Gene and product affected	Implications for anesthesia	Signs relevant to anesthesia	Validated genetic testing available?
Hyperkalemic periodic paralysis (HYPP)	Quarter Horse Paint Appaloosa Pony of the Americas	*SCN4A* Alpha subunit of the skeletal muscle sodium channel	Severe. Anesthesia appears to stimulate clinical disease	Fasciculations Weakness Prolonged recovery Hyperkalemia Variable CK	Yes
Type 1 polysaccharide storage myopathy (PSSM1)	Quarter, Horse, Paint, Appaloosa Belgian, Percheron	*GYS1* Muscle glycogen synthase	Unclear. Anesthetic myopathy and prolonged recovery suggested in individual case reports	Potentially signs of anesthetic myopathy or prolonged recovery	Yes
Type 2 polysaccharide storage myopathy (PSSM2)	Warmblood Quarter Horse	Unknown	Unknown	Unknown	Not currently
Recurrent exertional rhabdomyolysis (RER)	Thoroughbred Standardbred	Unknown, possibly linked to altered intramuscular calcium regulation	Anecdotal association with mild-to-severe myopathy	Potentially signs of anesthetic myopathy or MH Increased serum CK	Not currently
Glycogen branching enzyme deficiency (GBED)	Quarter Horse Paint	*GBE1* Glycogen branching enzyme	Invariably fatal in early life, though cases have survived through general anesthesia	Weakness Prolonged recovery Hypoglycemia Hypercapnia	Yes
Malignant hyperthermia (MH)	Quarter Horse Thoroughbred	*RYR1* Skeletal muscle ryanodine receptor (Quarter Horses, mutation not reported in Thoroughbred)	Severe. Profound. Severe generalized hypermetabolism and rhabdomyolysis Very high fatality rate with general anesthesia	Tachycardia Rigidity Sweating Third eyelid extrusion Violent recovery Metabolic and respiratory acidosis Hyperkalemia Rising CK	Yes
Myofibrillar myopathy (MFM)	Arabian Warmblood	Unknown	Unknown	Unknown	Not currently

information on serum BUN and creatinine complicates accurate diagnosis, assessment, and treatment of azotemic disorders. Ideally, a minimum biochemistry panel for assessment of the muscular system should therefore include CK, AST, GGT, BUN, creatinine, and potassium. Assessment of additional variables including other serum electrolyte concentrations, blood gas, and hemogram variables is also often relevant prior to anesthesia of patients with known or suspected muscular disorders.

Elevations in serum CK activity are typically indicative of muscle disorders associated with muscle necrosis. This enzyme is contained within the myofiber cytosol and reaches substantial serum or plasma activity rapidly within four to six hours after release from damaged muscle tissue (Stockham and Scott 2008). Due to its brief half-life, serum CK activity declines rapidly over 24–72 hours unless ongoing muscle injury occurs. AST activity increases in response to muscle or liver injury, peaking between 12 and 48 hours after injury and remaining elevated for 10–14 days. Hence, concurrent measurement of AST and GGT with CK are encouraged to accurately determine the timeline of muscle injury, as well as to distinguish liver from muscle pathology (Stockham and Scott 2008). Elevation of AST without concurrent increases in CK or GGT is most consistent with muscular injury three to ten days previously. Assessment of serum electrolyte concentrations in clinically sick horses and whenever significant muscle disease is suspected is also encouraged. Serum potassium concentrations are of particular interest because they can increase in response to severe muscle damage and with episodes of HYPP or MH in horses, promoting risk of complicated cardiac arrhythmias under anesthesia (Aleman et al. 2009; Pang et al. 2011; McKenzie et al. 2015). Furthermore, horses with HYPP are at risk of episodes of clinical disease as a result of concurrent disorders that elevate serum potassium, which include urinary tract rupture or obstruction, and potentially premedication with dantrolene sodium prior to anesthesia (McKenzie et al. 2015).

Elevation of serum CK activity is a common finding in many equine patients destined for anesthesia. The majority of the time, increases are mild, and relate to muscular trauma including thrashing and recumbency in response to abdominal pain, accidental injuries, and the intramuscular administration of sedatives or other drugs. Recent prolonged exercise, such as endurance racing, also provokes increases in serum CK activity (Schott et al. 2006). Elevations of 1000–2000 IU/l is common in these circumstances, particularly in horses with the complaint of colic, and are typically of minimal concern. However, occasionally muscle enzyme aberrations, even seemingly minor, are indicators of muscular disorders that can potentially complicate anesthesia (Bloom et al. 1999). Horses that have increases in serum CK prior to anesthesia that are unable to be explained or that reach or exceed several thousand units/liter should be carefully examined for any other evidence of muscle disease, and historical questioning revisited to determine additional relevant information including recent exercise activities. It should be borne in mind that degree of perturbation in CK often correlates poorly with clinical severity or significance. For example, severe, focal muscle trauma can create relatively mild elevations of CK and AST, despite considerable consequences for the function of the affected muscle. Examples include damage to the gracilis, gluteal, or semimembranosus or semitendinosus muscles, which could impede affected horses from rising after anesthesia (Dabareiner et al. 2004; Walmsley et al. 2010). Similarly, some disorders, such as PSSM, can occasionally generate massive increases in muscle enzyme activity with limited clinical signs. Generally, if no preceding physical or historical reason for increased muscle enzyme activity can be identified, and if concurrent increases in serum CK and AST activity are apparent, suggesting chronicity of muscular disease, a pre-existing disorder is likely present. Low-grade persistent elevations of CK and/or AST (of up to several hundred IU/l) are common in horses with PSSM (Valberg et al. 1997). Thoroughbred horses with elevated muscle enzyme activity may have underlying RER, potentially increasing the risk of muscular damage with anesthesia (Klein 1978; Waldron-Mease 1978; Lentz et al. 1999a). HYPP does not typically cause substantial muscle necrosis, and horses with this trait therefore often have unremarkable or mildly abnormal serum muscle enzyme activities in spite of the potential for severe clinical disease (Naylor et al. 1999).

Healthy foals typically have normal or low serum CK activity after birth, reflecting their low muscle mass, but can have substantial elevations in serum creatinine in the first few days of life despite normal renal function (Axon and Palmer 2008). Elevations in serum CK in foals most often reflects birth trauma, asphyxia, recumbency or rolling in sick or painful foals, and intramuscular injection (Axon and Palmer 2008). The potential for anesthesia of foals with serious underlying muscle disorders exists due to the inherent challenges associated with prompt identification of some of these diseases and the necessity of anesthesia to address severe disorders in early life, including complicated colic, uroabdomen, regional infections of joints, bones or the umbilicus, fractures, and wounds. Certainly, there are multiple reported instances of foals or yearlings with severe underlying muscular disorders being unwittingly anesthetized, which promotes recognition of the disorder when unexpected complications related to these conditions are encountered (Manley et al. 1983; Cornick et al. 1994; Bloom et al. 1999; Valberg et al. 2001).

Where horses or foals are suspected or known to have a pre-existing muscular disorder, or when they are considered at higher risk of developing complications associated with anesthesia, preceding conversation with the client should thoroughly encompass risk and expectations.

Induction

Preservation of the muscular system during induction is largely restricted to preventing injury. Close attention must be paid to preventing injury during descent to recumbency through adequate sedation, adequate control of the horse through physical means including appropriate numbers of personnel, ropes, restrictive movement induction gates, or other measures, and providing a safe surface for the horse to collapse onto (Coumbe 2005). Removal of shoes or wrapping of the feet and wrapping limbs prior to anesthesia can reduce the risk of blunt injury to musculature by inadvertent contact with shoes or hooves (Clark-Price 2013). As previously described, minimal information is available on how commonly used anesthetic and analgesic agents interact with equine skeletal muscle; therefore, the selection of premedicants, induction and maintenance agents, and analgesic drugs should be based on the individual horse and the reason for which it is being anesthetized (Raisis 2005).

Maintenance (Monitoring)

Decreases in cardiac output and systemic blood pressure are well-defined consequences of general anesthesia in horses and can result in impaired perfusion of their large skeletal muscle mass. Consequently, oxygen delivery and removal of metabolic waste also diminishes, leading to tissue hypoxia and decreased tissue pH. Cardiac output measurement in adult horses requires specialized equipment and expertise and is therefore not currently routinely performed (Shih 2013). Blood pressure measurement is frequently utilized as a surrogate measure even though it may be a poor indicator of forward blood flow and tissue perfusion (Edner et al. 2002). However, combined with information from other modalities, including pulse oximetry, arterial blood gas analysis, blood lactate measurement, mucous membrane color, and capillary refill time, arterial blood pressure measurement can give indications regarding cardiac function and the potential effect of blood pressure changes (Trim 2005). Direct measurement of arterial blood pressure via intra-arterial cannula placement is recommended since indirect measurement in horses has been shown to have variable correlation with direct measurement, and poor correlation with cardiac output (Bailey et al. 1994; Giguère et al. 2005; Tearney et al. 2016). MAP represents the average blood pressure during a single cardiac cycle and is determined by cardiac output, systemic vascular resistance, and central venous pressure. It is also a key contributor to perfusion pressure of organs in the body, and therefore accurate measurement is critical in horses where concern for perfusion of skeletal muscle is important. It has been recommended that MAP be maintained above 70 mmHg in anesthetized adult horses, which may reduce the severity of muscle injury incurred during anesthesia (Grandy et al. 1987; Duke et al. 2006). However, it must be recognized that this recommendation was based on small numbers of horses anesthetized with halothane; it is unclear if similar recommendations apply to the more modern inhalants such as isoflurane and sevoflurane (Duke et al. 2006). Also, as previously described, a clear link between myopathy and blood pressure was not identified in a large-scale study (Johnston et al. 2004; Young 2005). Furthermore, pressure external to the capillaries, referred to by some sources as intracompartmental pressure, acts counter to MAP and can compromise muscular perfusion contributing to injury (Lindsay et al. 1980; Young 2005). The difference between these two variables describes the "perfusion pressure," which is not typically measured except in experimental situations. A perfusion pressure greater than 30 mmHg has been recommended to maintain adequate microcirculation in tissues, and can be compromised by high intracompartmental pressure, which is commonly encountered in the dependent musculature during routine anesthesia (Lindsay et al. 1980; Young 2005). Differences in local tissue metabolism, such as those demonstrated between healthy horses and horses with colic in a muscle microdialysis study are likely also relevant to the development of muscular injury (Edner et al. 2009). Clearly, relying on MAP alone to maintain a healthy muscular microenvironment is a simplistic approach that cannot reliably prevent muscular damage, though it may reduce severity, and does not effectively explain the development of damage in nondependent musculature of anesthetized horses (Short and White 1978; Young 2005). In addition, horses demonstrating MH or MH-like reactions under anesthesia may be hypertensive rather than hypotensive (Waldron-Mease 1978). More accessible and convenient methods of measuring cardiac output and the muscular microenvironment in anesthetized horses may clarify factors contributing to muscular injury during anesthesia.

Other aspects of monitoring that are important for early identification of muscular complications include heart rate, respiratory rate, skin and body temperature, and muscle tone and activity. Alterations can be early indicators of MH and HYPP (Manley et al. 1983; Cornick et al. 1994; Aleman et al. 2009; Pang et al. 2011). Serial arterial blood gas analysis monitoring is valuable particularly to track blood potassium concentration, pH, and contributing variables, which can become progressively deranged over time with these disorders. Monitoring of end-tidal partial pressure of CO_2 is also important since inappropriate increases can also be an early indicator of MH or MH-like reactions in anesthetized horses (Aleman et al. 2009).

Positioning and Padding the Recumbent Horse

As previously mentioned, appropriate positioning and padding of the recumbent equine patient is a critical feature in the prevention of myopathy (Johnson 2005). Placement of an anesthetized horse on thin, noncompliant padding or hard surfaces can result in compression of vascular beds, ischemia, and reperfusion injury of skeletal muscles (Clark-Price et al. 2012). Occlusion of venous drainage from compressed musculature can result in reduced perfusion pressure in the tissue, in spite of adequate arterial blood pressure (Johnson 2005; Young 2005). The combination of optimal positioning and padding with maintenance of adequate arterial pressure therefore promotes the likelihood of adequate muscle tissue perfusion during procedures, though should never be regarded as fail-safe. Horses in lateral recumbency are reportedly much more likely to encounter clinical signs of myopathy, particularly in large muscle groups of the dependent limbs including the triceps of the non-dependent forelimb (Johnston et al. 2004; Coumbe 2005). Positioning of the limbs to reduce the likelihood of complications can be achieved with stirrups or padding placed between the limbs, to relieve weight on the dependent limb musculature by providing support in a manner that emulates a standing position with the limbs parallel to each other and the ground surface. The lower forelimb should be pulled forward to reduce pressure on the dependent triceps mass and radial nerve, while keeping the heavily muscled portion of the limb well back from the table or pad edge

(Coumbe 2005; Johnson 2005). Horses in lateral recumbency on firm or non-padded surfaces can have a semi-inflated rubber tube placed under the dependent shoulder to help reduce trauma and compression of the radial nerve and triceps musculature (Figure 8.7). Periodic repositioning of the limbs has also been previously recommended for horses undergoing prolonged anesthesia events (Gleed and Short 1980). Horses in lateral recumbency are also at risk of developing myopathy of the dependent masseter muscle, so attention to padding and position should extend to the head, and halters should be removed to prevent damage resulting from contact with the buccal branch of the facial nerve (Clark-Price et al. 2012).

Horses in dorsal recumbency can also develop significant muscular damage involving the epaxial and gluteal musculature, bilaterally or unilaterally if asymmetric positioning occurs (Coumbe 2005) (Figure 8.8). Severe damage to the pectineus, gracilis, and adductor muscles with fatal consequences has also been reported in five horses undergoing prolonged anesthesia while positioned in dorsal recumbency, potentially related to occlusion of the medial circumflex femoral artery (Dodman et al. 1988). In conjunction with careful positioning, horses should be placed on thick padding of at least 30 cm depth to distribute pressure associated with body mass, and

Figure 8.7 A horse in lateral recumbency on a hard surface during anesthesia. A small head pad and a semi-inflated rubber tube has been placed under the horse to minimize trauma and compression of dependent muscle groups.

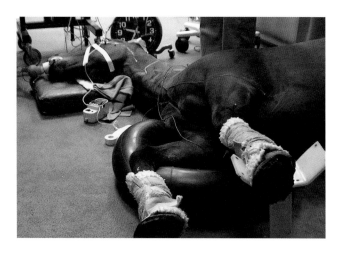

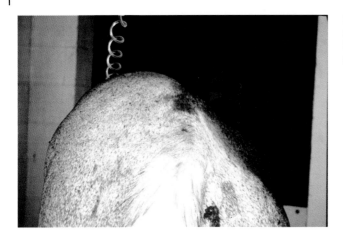

Figure 8.8 Severe unilateral gluteal swelling in a horse as a result of improper padding/position during anesthesia in dorsal recumbency.

padding should extend appropriately beyond the croup as well as distally below the shoulders and up the neck of the recumbent horse (Johnson 2005).

Recovery

There are minimal reports available for recovery recommendations for horses with muscular injury or disease. However, following general "good practice" steps to promote quiet recoveries of appropriate duration are important to prevent trauma from occurring in the recovery period and are described (Auckburally and Flaherty 2009b, Clark-Price 2013). Providing a safe environment (recovery stall) and the use of analgesic and sedative medications to promote a smooth transition to standing are useful in improving recovery quality. The recovery stall should be padded and free of dangerous objects. Movement to standing position in horses with muscular injury may require assistance with head and tail ropes and in severe cases may require the use of a sling (Coumbe 2005; Clark-Price 2013). Recovery time should be recorded and monitored carefully, and based on clinician experience, procedure performed, length of anesthesia, and administered sedatives, recoveries that are particularly prolonged should encourage investigation to determine if injury has occurred. When no obvious injury or condition can be identified, then additional steps to encourage movement and attempts to rise should be considered (Clark-Price 2013). This can include reversal of alpha-2 agents, manual encouragement methods, and application of lifts or slings (Auckburally and Flaherty 2009b).

Horses with a muscular disorder exacerbated by or acquired during anesthesia, such as EAAM, HYPP, PSSM, and MH, often display clinical signs during recovery that may not initially reflect obvious muscle pain or dysfunction, delaying recognition of their origin. These can include delayed recovery with slow return to movement, or repeated futile attempts to achieve sternal recumbency or to stand (Bloom et al. 1999; Young 2005; Auckburally and Flaherty 2009b). Horses with EAAM can occasionally display aberrant and almost manic behavior, with vocalization, thrashing, repeated violent attempts to rise, and even rearing and bucking, likely as a reaction to severe persistent pain. Some horses will be obviously lame on a specific limb once standing, with knuckling, buckling, and refusal to weight bear, pronounced fasciculations, excessive sweating, and collapse. Pain may be extreme with non-weight-bearing lameness, requiring immediate intervention to reduce pain and to prevent the horse from returning to a recumbent position. Horses with MH may display rigidity, fasciculations, excessive sweating, tachypnea, exposure of the third eyelid, and semi-consciousness (Aleman et al. 2009). Spontaneous death during the recovery period can be a substantial risk associated with MH and HYPP.

Post-anesthetic Monitoring

Monitoring of horses that have encountered a neuromuscular complication will depend upon the individual and the specific problem; however, basic tenets are usually applicable in most cases. Horses should be observed at appropriate intervals, which may be as frequent as 30 minutes or as little as twice a day depending on the degree of dysfunction. Physical assessment should include evaluation of demeanor and appetite, limb position, and degree of lameness. Pain scoring systems can be utilized to assess recovery, comfort, and efficacy of therapy (de Grauw and van Loon 2016). Affected muscle groups can be visually assessed for progression or resolution of swelling, and muscles can be palpated for firmness and reactivity. Clinical pathology monitoring can aid tracking of progression of disease and recovery. Horses with EAAM may have minimal swelling and relatively mild elevations in serum CK in the first hours after recovery, but these can progressively increase over the next 24–48 hours and should be serially assessed at 12-hour intervals (Figure 8.9) (Waldron-Mease and Rosenberg 1979; McKenzie et al. 2015).

Severe muscle damage can also result in biochemical aberrations including azotemia, hyperkalemia, hypophosphatemia, and hypocalcemia; therefore, monitoring of serum variables over time is often relevant. Urinations should be monitored for the presence of discoloration suggesting myoglobin, and periodic urine dipstick testing can also be utilized to detect occult myoglobinuria, since a high level of pigmenturia is required to create gross urine discoloration.

Conclusion

In summary, muscular disorders are common in horses, but uncommonly recognized, and some carry serious implications for general anesthesia. General anesthesia also poses some risk to muscular health in horses of all ages and breeds, though specific factors such as body mass, underlying disorders, and management of the patient influence individual vulnerability to neuromuscular complications. Clinicians should be informed and aware of potential risks for each patient, ensure appropriate monitoring before, during, and after anesthesia, and strive to recognize and respond to factors that affect muscular health in a timely manner.

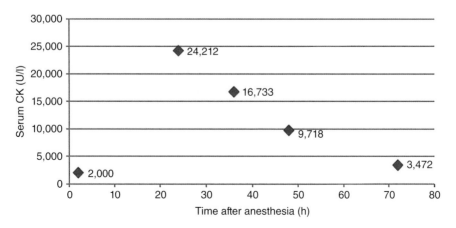

Figure 8.9 Graphical display of serum creatine kinase (CK) activity over time in a horse with severe muscle damage after anesthesia. Initial elevation of CK may be minimal but progressively increase over time necessitating serial monitoring.

References

Aleman, M., Riehl, J., Aldridge, B.M. et al. (2004). Association of a mutation in the ryanodine receptor 1 gene with equine malignant hyperthermia. *Muscle & Nerve* 30: 356–365.

Aleman, M., Brosnan, R.J., Williams, D.C. et al. (2005). Malignant hyperthermia in a horse anesthetized with halothane. *Journal of Veterinary Internal Medicine* 19 (3): 363–366.

Aleman, M., Nieto, J.E., and Magdesian, K.G. (2009). Malignant hyperthermia associated with ryanodine receptor 1 (C7360G) mutation in Quarter Horses. *Journal of Veterinary Internal Medicine* 23 (2): 329–334.

Aoki, M., Wakuno, A., Kushiro, A. et al. (2017). Evaluation of total intravenous anesthesia with propofol-guaifenesin-medetomidine and alfaxalone-guaifenesin-medetomidine in Thoroughbred horses undergoing castration. *Journal of Veterinary Medical Science* 79 (12): 2011–2018.

Auckburally, A. and Flaherty, D. (2009a). Recovery from anaesthesia in horses. 1. What can go wrong? *In Practice* 31: 340–347.

Auckburally, A. and Flaherty, D. (2009b). Recovery from anesthesia in horses. 2. Avoiding complications. *In Practice* 31: 362–369.

Axon, J.E. and Palmer, J.E. (2008). Clinical pathology of the foal. *The Veterinary Clinics of North America. Equine Practice* 24 (2): 357–385.

Ayala, I., Rodríguez, M.J., Aguirre, C. et al. (2009). Postanesthetic brachial triceps myonecrosis in a Spanish-bred horse. *Canadian Veterinary Journal* 50 (2): 189–193.

Baetge, C.L. (2007). Anesthesia case of the month. Hyperkalemic periodic paralysis. *Journal of the American Veterinary Medical Association* 230 (1): 33–36.

Bailey, J.E., Dunlop, C.I., Chapman, P.L. et al. (1994). Indirect Doppler ultrasonic measurement of arterial blood pressure results in a large measurement error in dorsally recumbent anaesthetized horses. *Equine Veterinary Journal* 16 (1): 70–73.

Bailey, J.E., Pablo, L., and Hubbell, J.A. (1996). Hyperkalemic periodic paralysis episode during halothane anesthesia in a horse. *Journal of the American Veterinary Medical Association* 208 (11): 1859–1865.

Beech, J., Lindborg, S., Fletcher, J.E. et al. (1993). Caffeine contractures, twitch characteristics and the threshold for Ca(2+)-induced Ca2+ release in skeletal muscle from horses with chronic intermittent rhabdomyolysis. *Research in Veterinary Science* 54 (1): 110–117.

Bellei, M.H., Kerr, C., McGurrin, M.K. et al. (2007). Management and complications of anesthesia for transvenous electrical cardioversion of atrial fibrillation in horses: 62 cases (2002–2006). *Journal of the American Veterinary Medical Association* 231 (8): 1225–1230.

Berry, S.H. (2015). Injectable anesthetics. In: *Veterinary Anesthesia and Analgesia the Fifth Edition of Lumb and Jones* (eds. K.A. Grimm, L.A. Lamont, W.J. Tranquilli, et al.), 277–296. Ames, IA: Wiley.

Bettschart-Wolfensberger, R. (2015). Horses. In: *Veterinary Anesthesia and Analgesia the Fifth Edition of Lumb and Jones* (eds. K.A. Grimm, L.A. Lamont, W.J. Tranquilli, et al.), 857–866. Ames, IA: Wiley.

Bidwell, L.A., Bramlage, L.R., and Rood, W.A. (2004). Fatality rates associated with equine general anesthesia. *Proceedings of the 50th annual convention of the American Association of Equine Practitioners* 50: 492–493.

Bidwell, L.A., Bramlage, L.R., and Rood, W.A. (2007). Equine perioperative fatalities associated with general anaesthesia at a private practice-a retrospective case series. *Veterinary Anesthesia and Analgesia* 34 (1): 23–30.

Bloom, B.A., Valentine, B.A., Gleed, R.D. et al. (1999). Postanaesthetic recumbency in a Belgian filly with polysaccharide storage myopathy. *Veterinary Record* 144 (3): 73–75.

Bowling, A.T., Byrns, G., and Spier, S. (1996). Evidence for a single pedigree source of the hyperkalemic periodic paralysis susceptibility gene in quarter horses. *Animal Genetics* 2 (4): 279–281.

Carpenter, R.E. and Evans, A.T. (2005). Anesthesia case of the month. Hyperkalemia. *Journal of the American Veterinary Medical Association* 226 (6): 874–876.

Clark-Price, S.C. (2013). Recovery of horses from anesthesia. *The Veterinary Clinics of North America. Equine Practice* 29 (1): 223–242.

Clark-Price, S.C., Gutierrez-Nibeyro, S.D., and Santos, M.P. (2012). Anesthesia case of the month. *EPAM. Journal of the American Veterinary Medical Association* 240 (1): 40–44.

Clutton, R.E. (2010). Opioid analgesia in horses. *Veterinary Clinics of North America. Equine Practice* 26 (3): 493–514.

Collins, N.D., LeRoy, B.E., and Vap, L. (1998). Artifactually increased serum bicarbonate values in two horses and a calf with severe rhabdomyolysis. *Veterinary Clinical Pathology* 27 (3): 85–90.

Cook, V.L. and Blikslager, A.T. (2015). The use of nonsteroidal anti-inflammatory drugs in critically ill horses. *Journal of Veterinary Emergency and Critical Care* 51 (1): 76–88.

Cooper, G.M. (2000). Actin, myosin, and cell movement. In: *The Cell: A Molecular Approach*, 2e (ed. G.M. Cooper). Sunderland, MA: Sinauer Associates https://www.ncbi. nlm.nih.gov/books/NBK9961.

Cornick, J.L., Seahorn, T.L., and Hartsfield, S.M. (1994). Hyperthermia during isoflurane anaesthesia in a horse with suspected hyperkalaemic periodic paralysis. *Equine Veterinary Journal* 26 (6): 511–514.

Coumbe, K. (2005). Anesthetic complications and emergencies: part 2. *Equine Veterinary Education* 7: 81–88.

Court, M.H., Engelking, L.R., Dodman, N.H. et al. (1987). Pharmacokinetics of dantrolene sodium in horses. *Journal of Veterinary Pharmacology and Therapeutics* 10: 218–226.

Crook, T.C., Cruickshank, S.E., McGowan, C.M. et al. (2008). Comparative anatomy and muscle architecture of selected hind limb muscles in the Quarter Horse and Arab. *Journal of Anatomy* 212 (2): 144–152.

Crook, T.C., Cruickshank, S.E., McGowan, C.M. et al. (2010). A comparison of the moment arms of pelvic limb muscles in horses bred for acceleration (Quarter Horse) and endurance (Arab). *Journal of Anatomy* 217 (1): 26–37.

Cunha, M.G., Freitas, G.C., Carregaro, A.B. et al. (2010). Renal and cardiorespiratory effects of treatment with lactated Ringer's solution or physiologic saline (0.9% NaCl) solution in cats with experimentally induced urethral obstruction. *American Journal of Veterinary Research* 71 (7): 840–846.

Dabareiner, R.M., Schmitz, D.G., Honnas, C.M. et al. (2004). Gracilis muscle injury as a cause of lameness in two horses. *Journal of the American Veterinary Medical Association* 224 (10): 1630–1633. 1605–1606.

Dancker, C., Hopster, K., Rohn, K. et al. (2018). Effects of dobutamine, dopamine, phenylephrine and noradrenaline on systemic haemodynamics and intestinal perfusion in isoflurane anaesthetized horses. *Equine Veterinary Journal* 50 (1): 104–110.

Dépret, F., Peacock, W.F., Liu, K.D. et al. (2019). Management of hyperkalemia in the acutely ill patient. *Annals of Intensive Care* 9 (1): 32.

Dodman, N.H., Williams, R., Court, M.H. et al. (1988). Postanesthetic hind limb adductor myopathy in five horses. *Journal of the American Veterinary Medical Association* 193 (1): 83–86.

Dugdale, A.H. and Taylor, P.M. (2016). Equine anaesthesia-associated mortality: where are we now? *Veterinary Anaesthesia and Analgesia* 43 (3): 242–255.

Duke, T., Filzek, U., Read, M.R. et al. (2006). Clinical observations surrounding an increased incidence of postanesthetic myopathy in halothane-anesthetized horses. *Veterinary Anaesthesia and Analgesia* 33: 122–127.

Durongphongtorn, S., McDonell, W.N., Kerr, C.L. et al. (2006). Comparison of hemodynamic, clinicopathologic, and gastrointestinal motility effects and recovery characteristics of anesthesia with isoflurane and halothane in horses undergoing arthroscopic surgery. *American Journal of Veterinary Research* 67 (1): 32–42.

Edner, A., Nyman, G., and Essén-Gustavsson, B. (2002). The relationship of muscle perfusion and metabolism with cardiovascular variables before and after detomidine injection during propofol-ketamine anaesthesia in horses. *Veterinary Anesthesia and Analgesia* 29 (4): 182–199.

Edner, A., Essén-Gustavsson, B., and Nyman, G. (2005). Muscle metabolic changes associated with long-term inhalation anaesthesia in the horse analysed by muscle biopsy and microdialysis techniques. *Journal of Veterinary Medicine. A, Physiology, Pathology, Clinical Medicine* 52 (2): 99–107.

Edner, A.H., Essén-Gustavsson, B., and Nyman, G.C. (2009). Metabolism during anaesthesia and recovery in colic and healthy horses: a microdialysis study. *Acta Veternaria Scandinavica* 10: 51.

Fisher, R.J. (1984). A field trial of ketamine anaesthesia in the horse. *Equine Veterinary Journal* 16 (3): 176–179.

Franci, P., Leece, E.A., and Brearley, J.C. (2006). Post anaesthetic myopathy/neuropathy in horses undergoing magnetic resonance imaging compared to horses undergoing surgery. *Equine Veterinary Journal* 38 (6): 497–501.

Friend, S.C. (1981). Postanesthetic myonecrosis in horses. *Canadian Veterinary Journal* 22 (12): 367–371.

Funk, K.A. (1973). Glyceryl guaiacolate: some effects and indications in horses. *Equine Veterinary Journal* 5 (1): 15–19.

Giguère, S., Knowles, H.A. Jr., Valverde, A. et al. (2005). Accuracy of indirect measurement of blood pressure in neonatal foals. *Journal of Veterinary Internal Medicine* 19 (4): 571–576.

Glazier, D.B., Littledike, E.T., and Evans, R.D. (1982). Electrocardiographic changes in induced hyperkalemia in ponies. *American Journal of Veterinary Research* 43 (11): 1934–1937.

Gleed, R. and Short, C.E. (1980). A retrospective study of the anesthetic management of adult draft horses. *Veterinary Medicine, Small Animal Clinician* 75 (9): 1409–1416.

Goetz, T.E., Manohar, M., Nganwa, D. et al. (1989). A study of the effect of isoflurane anaesthesia on equine skeletal muscle perfusion. *Equine Veterinary Journal. Supplement* 7: 133–137.

González-Castro, A., Ortiz-Lasa, M., Rodriguez-Borregan, J.C. et al. (2018). Influence of proportion of normal saline administration in the perioperative period of renal transplantation on kalemia levels. *Transplantation Proceedings* 50 (2): 569–571.

Goodwin, W.A., Keates, H.L., Pasloske, K. et al. (2011). The pharmacokinetics and pharmacodynamics of the injectable anaesthetic alfaxalone in the horse. *Veterinary Anaesthesia and Analgesia* 38 (5): 431–438.

Goodwin, W.A., Keates, H.L., Pearson, M. et al. (2013). Alfaxalone and medetomidine intravenous infusion to maintain anaesthesia in colts undergoing field castration. *Equine Veterinary Journal* 45 (3): 315–319.

Gozalo-Marcilla, M., Gasthuys, F., and Schauvliege, S. (2014). Partial intravenous anaesthesia in the horse: a review of intravenous agents used to supplement equine inhalation anaesthesia. Part 1: lidocaine and ketamine. *Veterinary Anesthesia and Analgesia* 41 (4): 335–345.

Grandy, J.L., Steffey, E.P., Hodgson, D.S. et al. (1987). Arterial hypotension and the development of postanesthetic myopathy in halothane-anesthetized horses. *American Journal of Veterinary Research* 48 (2): 192–197.

de Grauw, J.C. and van Loon, J.P. (2016). Systematic pain assessment in horses. *Veterinary Journal* 209: 14–22.

Grint, N., Gorvy, D., and Dugdale, A. (2007). Hyperthermia and delayed-onset myopathy after recovery from anesthesia in a horse. *Journal of Equine Veterinary Science* 27 (5): 221–227.

Gustafsson, U., Sjöberg, F., Lewis, D.H. et al. (1995). Influence of pentobarbital, propofol and ketamine on skeletal muscle capillary perfusion during hemorrhage: a comparative study in the rabbit. *International Journal of Microcirculation, Clinical and Experimental* 15 (4): 163–169.

Hennig, G.E., Court, M.H., and King, V.L. (1995). The effect of xylazine on equine muscle surface capillary blood flow. *Journal of Veterinary Pharmacology and Therapeutics* 18: 388–390.

Hildebrand, S.V., Arpin, D., and Cardinet, G. (1990). Contracture test and histologic and histochemical analyses of muscle biopsy specimens from horses with exertional rhabdomyolysis. *Journal of the American Veterinary Medical Association* 196 (7): 1077–1083.

Hubbell, J.A., Kelly, E.M., Aarnes, T.K. et al. (2013). Pharmacokinetics of midazolam after intravenous administration to horses. *Equine Veterinary Journal* 45 (6): 721–725.

Isgren, C.M., Upjohn, M.M., Fernandez-Fuente, M. et al. (2010). Epidemiology of exertional rhabdomyolysis susceptibility in Standardbred horses reveals associated risk factors and underlying enhanced performance. *PLoS One* 5 (7): e11594.

Johnson, C.B. (2005). Positioning the anaesthetized horse. *Equine Veterinary Education* 7: 30–40.

Johnston, G.M., Eastment, J.K., Wood, J. et al. (2002). The confidential enquiry into perioperative equine fatalities (CEPEF): mortality results of phases 1 and 2. *Veterinary Anesthesia and Analgesia* 29 (4): 159–170.

Johnston, G.M., Eastment, J.K., Taylor, P.M. et al. (2004). Is isoflurane safer than halothane in equine anaesthesia? Results from a prospective multicentre randomised controlled trial. *Equine Veterinary Journal* 36 (1): 64–71.

Kearns, C.F., McKeever, K.H., and Abe, T. (2002). Overview of horse body composition and muscle architecture: implications for performance. *Veterinary Journal* 164 (3): 224–234.

Keates, H.L., van Eps, A.W., and Pearson, M.R. (2012). Alfaxalone compared with ketamine for induction of anaesthesia in horses following xylazine and guaifenesin. *Veterinary Anaesthesia and Analgesia* 39 (6): 591–598.

Keshavarz, M., Showraki, A., and Emamghoreishi, M. (2013). Anticonvulsant effect of guaifenesin against pentylenetetrazol-induced seizure in mice. *Iranian Journal of Medical Sciences* 38 (2): 116–121.

Khajavi, M.R., Etezadi, F., Moharari, R.S. et al. (2008). Effects of normal saline vs. lactate Ringer's during renal transplantation. *Renal Failure* 30: 535–539.

Klein, L. (1978). A review of 50 cases of post-operative myopathy in the horse – intrinsic and management factors affecting risk. *Proceedings of the 24th annual convention of the American Association of Equine Practitioners* 24: 89–94.

Krajčová, A., Løvsletten, N.G., Waldauf, P. et al. (2018). Effects of propofol on cellular bioenergetics in human skeletal muscle cells. *Critical Care Medicine* 46 (3): e206–e212.

Kraus, B.M., Parente, E.J., and Tulleners, E.P. (2003). Laryngoplasty with ventriculectomy or ventriculocordectomy in 104 draft horses (1992–2000). *Veterinary Surgery* 32 (6): 530–538.

Langdon Fielding, C. (2015). Potassium homeostasis and derangements. In: *Equine Fluid Therapy*, 1e (eds. C. Langdon Fielding and K.G. Magdesian), 27–44. Ames, IA: Wiley.

Lee, Y.-H., Clarke, K.W., and Alibhai, H.I.K. (1998). Effects on the intramuscular blood flow and cardiopulmonary function of anaesthetized ponies of changing from halothane to isoflurane maintenance and vice versa. *Veterinary Record* 143: 629–633.

Lentz, L.R., Valberg, S.J., Balog, E.M. et al. (1999a). Abnormal regulation of muscle contraction in horses with recurrent exertional rhabdomyolysis. *American Journal of Veterinary Research* 60 (8): 992–999.

Lentz, L.R., Valberg, S.J., Mickelson, J.R. et al. (1999b). *in vitro* contractile responses and contracture testing of skeletal muscle from Quarter Horses with exertional rhabdomyolysis. *American Journal of Veterinary Research* 60 (6): 684–688.

Li, H., Sun, S.R., Yap, J.Q. et al. (2016). 0.9% saline is neither normal nor physiological. *Journal of Zhejiang University* 17 (3): 181–187.

Lindsay, W.A., McDonell, W., and Bignell, W. (1980). Equine postanesthetic forelimb lameness: intracompartmental muscle pressure changes and biochemical patterns. *American Journal of Veterinary Research* 41 (12): 1919–1924.

Lindsay, W.A., Robinson, G.M., Brunson, D.B. et al. (1989). Induction of equine postanesthetic myositis after halothane-induced hypotension. *American Journal of Veterinary Research* 50 (3): 404–410.

Lodish, H., Berk, A., Zipursky, S.L. et al. (2000). Muscle: a specialized contractile machine. In: *Molecular Cell Biology*, 4e (eds. H. Lodish, A. Berk, S.L. Zipursky, et al.). New York, NY: W. H. Freeman https://www.ncbi.nlm.nih.gov/books/NBK21670.

Luther, P.K. (2009). The vertebrate muscle Z-disc: sarcomere anchor for structure and signaling. *Journal of Muscle Research and Cell Motility* 30 (5–6): 171–185.

MacLeay, J.M., Sorum, S.A., Valberg, S.J. et al. (1999). Epidemiologic analysis of factors influencing exertional rhabdomyolysis in Thoroughbreds. *American Journal of Veterinary Research* 60 (12): 1562–1566.

Mama, K.R., Steffey, E.P., and Pascoe, P.J. (1996). Evaluation of propofol for general anesthesia in premedicated horses. *American Journal of Veterinary Research* 57 (4): 512–516.

Manley, S.V., Kelly, A.B., and Hodgson, D. (1983). Malignant hyperthermia-like reactions in three anesthetized horses. *Journal of the American Veterinary Medical Association* 183 (1): 85–89.

Marntell, S., Nyman, G., Funkquist, P. et al. (2005). Effects of acepromazine on pulmonary gas exchange and circulation during sedation and dissociative anaesthesia in horses. *Veterinary Anaesthesia and Analgesia* 32 (2): 83–93.

Matthews, N.S., Hartsfield, S.M., Cornick, J.L. et al. (1991). A comparison of injectable anesthetic combinations in horses. *Veterinary Surgery* 20 (4): 268–273.

McCue, M.E., Valberg, S.J., Jackson, M. et al. (2009). Polysaccharide storage myopathy phenotype in quarter horse-related breeds is modified by the presence of an RYR1 mutation. *Neuromuscular Disorders* 19 (1): 37–43.

McCue, M.E., Anderson, S.M., Valberg, S.J. et al. (2010). Estimated prevalence of the type 1 polysaccharide storage myopathy mutation in selected north American and European breeds. *Animal Genetics* 41 (Supplement 2): 145–149.

McKenzie, E.C. and Mosley, C. (2010). Dantrolene sodium prevents myopathy in horses undergoing hypotensive anesthesia. In: abstracts presented at the 34th American College of Veterinary Anesthesiologists Annual Meeting, 9th–12th September 2009, Chicago, IL, USA. *Veterinary Anaesthesia and Analgesia* 37: 1–16.

McKenzie, E.C., Valberg, S.J., Godden, S.M. et al. (2004). Effect of oral administration of dantrolene sodium on serum creatine kinase activity after exercise in horses with recurrent exertional rhabdomyolysis. *American Journal of Veterinary Research* 65 (1): 74–79.

McKenzie, E.C., Garrett, R.L., Payton, M.E. et al. (2010). Effect of feed restriction on plasma dantrolene concentrations in horses. *Equine Veterinary Journal. Supplement* 38: 613–617.

McKenzie, E.C., Di Concetto, S., Payton, M.E. et al. (2015). Effect of dantrolene premedication on various cardiac and biochemical variables and the recovery of healthy isoflurane-anesthetized horses. *American Journal of Veterinary Research* 76 (4): 293–301.

Meyer, T.S., Fedde, M.R., Cox, J.H. et al. (1999). Hyperkalaemic periodic paralysis in horses: a review. *Equine Veterinary Journal* 31 (5): 362–367.

Mickelson, J.R. and Valberg, S.J. (2015). The genetics of skeletal muscle disorders in horses. *Annual Review of Animal Biosciences* 3: 197–217.

Muir, W.W., Sams, R.A., Huffman, R.H. et al. (1982). Pharmacodynamic and pharmacokinetic properties of diazepam in horses. *American Journal of Veterinary Research* 43 (10): 1756–1762.

Mushiyakh, Y., Dangaria, H., Qavi, S. et al. (2012). Treatment and pathogenesis of acute hyperkalemia. *Journal of Community Hospital Internal Medicine Perspectives* 1 (4): 1–6.

Naquib, A., McKee, C., Phillips, A. et al. (2011). Dexmedetomidine as the primary anesthetic agent during cardiac surgery in an infant with a family history of malignant hyperthermia. *Saudi Journal of Anaesthesia* 5 (4): 426–429.

Natalini, C.C. (2010). Spinal anesthetics and analgesics in the horse. *The Veterinary Clinics of North America. Equine Practice* 26 (3): 551–564.

Naylor, J.M. (1994). Selection of quarter horses affected with hyperkalemic periodic paralysis by show judges. *Journal of the American Veterinary Medical Association* 204 (6): 926–928.

Naylor, J.M. (1997). Hyperkalemic periodic paralysis. *The Veterinary Clinics of North America. Equine Practice* 13 (1): 129–144.

Naylor, J.M., Nickel, D.D., Trimino, G. et al. (1999). Hyperkalaemic periodic paralysis in homozygous and heterozygous horses: a co-dominant genetic condition. *Equine Veterinary Journal* 31 (2): 153–159.

Nieto, J.E. and Aleman, M. (2009). A rapid detection method for the ryanodine receptor 1 (C7360G) mutation in Quarter Horses. *Journal of Veterinary Internal Medicine* 23 (3): 619–622.

Nolan, A.M. and Hall, L.W. (1985). Total intravenous anaesthesia in the horse with propofol. *Equine Veterinary Journal* 17 (5): 394–398.

Norton, E.M., Mickelson, J.R., Binns, M.M. et al. (2016). Heritability of recurrent exertional rhabdomyolysis in standardbred and thoroughbred racehorses derived from SNP genotyping data. *Journal of Heredity* 107 (6): 537–543.

Nowrouzian, I., Scheles, H.F., Ghodsian, I. et al. (1981). Evaluation of the anaesthetic properties of ketamine and ketamine/ xylazine/atropine combination in sheep. *Veterinary Record* 108 (16): 354–356.

Oku, K., Ohta, M., Katoh, T. et al. (2006). Cardiovascular effects of continuous propofol infusion in horses. *Journal of Veterinary Medical Science* 68 (8): 773–778.

Olkkola, K.T. and Ahonen, J. (2008). Midazolam and other benzodiazepines. *Handbook of Experimental Pharmacology* 182: 335–360.

Overmann, J.A., Finno, C., and Sharkey, L.C. (2010). What is your diagnosis? Increased total CO_2 concentration and negative anion gap in a foal. *Veterinary Clinical Pathology* 39 (4): 515–516.

Palmeri, A. and Wiesendanger, M. (1990). Concomitant depression of locus coeruleus neurons and of flexor reflexes by an alpha 2-adrenergic agonist in rats: a possible mechanism for an alpha-2 mediated muscle relaxation. *Neuroscience* 34 (1): 177–187.

Pang, D.S., Panizzi, L., and Paterson, J.M. (2011). Successful treatment of hyperkalaemic periodic paralysis in a horse during isoflurane anaesthesia. *Veterinary Anaesthesia and Analgesia* 38 (2): 113–120.

Pickar, J.G., Spier, S.J., Snyder, J.R. et al. (1991). Altered ionic permeability in skeletal muscle from horses with hyperkalemic periodic paralysis. *The American Journal of Physiology* 260: C926–C933.

Piercy, R.J. and Rivero, J. (2012). Muscle disorders of equine athletes. In: *Equine Sports Medicine and Surgery*, 2e (eds. K.W. Hinchcliff, A.J. Kaneps and R.J. Geor), 109–143. New York, NY: Saunders Elsevier.

Poole, D.C. and Erickson, H.H. (2011). Highly athletic terrestrial mammals: horses and dogs. *Comprehensive Physiology* 1 (1): 1–37.

Portier, K., Crouzier, D., Guichardant, M. et al. (2009). Effects of high and low inspired fractions of oxygen on horse erythrocyte membrane properties, blood viscosity and muscle oxygenation during anaesthesia. *Veterinary Anaesthesia and Analgesia* 36: 287–298.

Posner, L.P., Kasten, J.I., and Kata, C. (2013). Propofol with ketamine following sedation with xylazine for routine induction of general anaesthesia in horses. *Veterinary Record* 173 (22): 550.

Raisis, A.L. (2005). Skeletal muscle blood flow in anaesthetized horses. Part II: effects of anaesthetics and vasoactive agents. *Veterinary Anaesthesia and Analgesia* 32 (6): 331–337.

Raisis, A.L., Young, L.E., Blissitt, K.J. et al. (2000). Effect of a 30-minute infusion of dobutamine hydrochloride on hind limb blood flow and hemodynamics in halothane-anesthetized horses. *American Journal of Veterinary Research* 61 (10): 1282–1288.

Reich, D.L. and Silvay, G. (1989). Ketamine: an update on the first twenty-five years of clinical experience. *Canadian Journal of Anesthesia* 36 (2): 186–197.

Rothenbuhler, R., Hawkins, J.F., Adams, S.B. et al. (2006). Evaluation of surgical treatment for signs of acute abdominal pain in draft horses: 72 cases (1983–2002). *Journal of the American Veterinary Medical Association* 228 (10): 1546–1550.

Sanchez, L.C. and Robertson, S.A. (2014). Pain control in horses: what do we really know? *Equine Veterinary Journal* 46 (4): 517–523.

Schier, M.F., Raisis, A.L., Secombe, C.J. et al. (2016). Effects of dobutamine hydrochloride on cardiovascular function in horses anesthetized with isoflurane with or without acepromazine maleate premedication. *American Journal of Veterinary Research* 77 (12): 1318–1324.

Schieren, M., Defosse, J., Böhmer, A. et al. (2017). Anaesthetic management of patient with myopathies. *European Journal of Anaesthesiology* 34 (10): 641–649.

Schott, H.C., Marlin, D.J., Geor, R.J. et al. (2006). Changes in selected physiological and laboratory measurements in elite horses competing in a 160 km endurance ride. *Equine Veterinary Journal. Supplement* 36: 37–42.

Senior, J.M., Pinchbeck, G.L., Allister, R. et al. (2007). Reported morbidities following 861 anaesthetics given at four equine hospitals. *Veterinary Record* 160: 407–408.

Serteyn, D., Lavergne, L., Coppens, P. et al. (1988). Equine post anaesthetic myositis: muscular post ischaemic hyperaemia measured by laser Doppler flowmetry. *Veterinary Record* 123 (5): 126–128.

Shih, A. (2013). Cardiac output monitoring in horses. *The Veterinary Clinics of North America. Equine Practice* 29 (1): 155–167.

Short, C.E. and White, K.K. (1978). Anesthetic/surgical stress-induced myopathy (myositis) Part I: Clinical occurrences. *Proceedings of the 24th Annual Meeting of the American Association of Equine Practitioners*, 101–106.

Stäuble, C.G., Stäuble, R.B., Schaller, S.J. et al. (2015). Effects of single-shot and steady-state propofol anaesthesia on rocuronium dose–response relationship: a randomised trial. *Acta Anaesthesiologica Scandinavica* 59 (7): 902–911.

Steffey, E.P. and Howland, D. Jr. (1980). Comparison of circulatory and respiratory effects of isoflurane and halothane anesthesia in horses. *American Journal of Veterinary Research* 41 (5): 821–825.

Steffey, E.P., Mama, K.R., Galey, F.D. et al. (2005). Effects of sevoflurane dose and mode of ventilation on cardiopulmonary function and blood biochemical variables in horses. *American Journal of Veterinary Research* 66 (4): 606–614.

Stockham, S.L. and Scott, M.A. (2008). Enzymes. In: *Fundamentals of Veterinary Clinical Pathology*, 2e (eds. S.L. Stockham and M.A. Scott), 639–674. Ames, IA: Blackwell Publishing.

Tearney, C.C., Guedes, A.G., and Brosnan, R.J. (2016). Equivalence between invasive and oscillometric blood pressures at different anatomic locations in healthy normotensive anaesthetized horses. *Equine Veterinary Journal* 48 (3): 357–361.

Teixeira Neto, F.J., McDonell, W.N., Black, W.D. et al. (2004). Effects of glycopyrrolate on cardiorespiratory function in horses anesthetized with halothane and xylazine.

American Journal of Veterinary Research 65 (4): 456–463.

Trefz, F.M., Constable, P.D., and Lorenz, I. (2017). Effect of intravenous small-volume hypertonic sodium bicarbonate, sodium chloride, and glucose solutions in decreasing plasma potassium concentration in hyperkalemic neonatal calves with diarrhea. *Journal of Veterinary Internal Medicine* 31 (3): 907–921.

Trim, C.M. (2005). Monitoring during anesthesia: techniques and interpretation. *Equine Veterinary Education* 7: 30–40.

Trim, C.M. and Mason, J. (1973). Post-anaesthetic forelimb lameness in horses. *Equine Veterinary Journal* 5 (2): 71–76.

Tryon, R.C., Penedo, M.C., McCue, M.E. et al. (2009). Evaluation of allele frequencies of inherited disease genes in subgroups of American Quarter Horses. *Journal of the American Veterinary Medical Association* 234 (1): 120–125.

Umar, M.A., Fukui, S., Kawase, K. et al. (2015). Cardiovascular effects of total intravenous anesthesia using ketamine-medetomidine-propofol (KMP-TIVA) in horses undergoing surgery. *Journal of Veterinary Medical Science* 77 (3): 281–288.

Valberg, S.J. (2014). Muscle anatomy, physiology and adaptations to exercise and training. In: *Equine Sports Medicine and Surgery*, 2e (eds. K.W. Hinchcliff, A.J. Kaneps and R.J. Geor), 174–201. New York, NY: Saunders Elsevier.

Valberg, S.J. (2018). Muscle conditions affecting sport horses. *The Veterinary Clinics of North America. Equine Practice* 34 (2): 253–276.

Valberg, S.J., MacLeay, J.M., and Mickelson, J.R. (1997). Exertional rhabdomyolysis and polysaccharide storage myopathy in horses. *Compendium on Continuing Education for the Practicing Veterinarian* 19 (9): 1077–1085.

Valberg, S.J., Ward, T.L., Rush, B. et al. (2001). Glycogen branching enzyme deficiency in quarter horse foals. *Journal of Veterinary Internal Medicine* 15 (6): 572–580.

Valberg, S.J., McKenzie, E.C., Eyrich, L.V. et al. (2016). Suspected myofibrillar myopathy in Arabian horses with a history of exertional rhabdomyolysis. *Equine Veterinary Journal* 48 (5): 548–556.

Valberg, S.J., Nicholson, A.M., Lewis, S.S. et al. (2017). Clinical and histopathological features of myofibrillar myopathy in Warmblood horses. *Equine Veterinary Journal* 49 (6): 739–745.

Vien, A. and Chhabra, N. (2017). Ketamine-induced muscle rigidity during procedural sedation mitigated by intravenous midazolam. *The American Journal of Emergency Medicine* 35 (1): 200.

Wagner, A.E., Mama, K.R., Steffey, E.P. et al. (2002). Behavioral responses following eight anesthetic induction protocols in horses. *Veterinary Anesthesia and Analgesia* 29 (4): 207–211.

Wakuno, A., Aoki, M., Kushiro, A. et al. (2017). Comparison of alfaxalone, ketamine and thiopental for anaesthetic induction and recovery in Thoroughbred horses premedicated with medetomidine and midazolam. *Equine Veterinary Journal* 49 (1): 94–98.

Waldron-Mease, E. (1978). Correlation of post-operative and exercise-induced equine myopathy with the defect malignant hyperthermia. *Proceedings of the 24th annual convention of the American Association of Equine Practitioners* 24: 95–99.

Waldron-Mease, E. and Rosenberg, H. (1979). Post anesthetic myositis in the horse associated with *in vitro* malignant hyperthermia susceptibility. *Veterinary Science Communications* 3: 45–50.

Walmsley, E.A., Steel, C.M., Richardson, J.L. et al. (2010). Muscle strain injuries of the hindlimb in eight horses: diagnostic imaging, management and outcomes. *Australian Veterinary Journal* 88 (8): 313–321.

Ward, T.L., Valberg, S.J., Gallant, E.M. et al. (2000). Calcium regulation by skeletal muscle membranes of horses with recurrent exertional rhabdomyolysis. *American Journal of Veterinary Research* 61 (3): 242–247.

Ward, T.L., Valberg, S.J., Adelson, D.L. et al. (2004). Glycogen branching enzyme (GBE1) mutation causing equine glycogen storage disease IV. *Mammalian Genome* 15 (7): 570–577.

Wong, S.F. and Chung, F. (2000). Succinylcholine-associated postoperative myalgia. *Anaesthesia* 55 (2): 144–152.

Wooldridge, A.A., Eades, S.C., Hosgood, G.L. et al. (2002). *in vitro* effects of oxytocin, acepromazine, detomidine, xylazine, butorphanol, terbutaline, isoproterenol, and dantrolene on smooth and skeletal muscles of the equine esophagus. *American Journal of Veterinary Research* 63 (12): 1732–1737.

Young, S.S. (2005). Post anaesthetic myopathy. *Equine Veterinary Education, Manual* 7: 60–63.

9

Anesthetic Management for Laparoscopic and Thoracoscopic Procedures

Rachel Hector and Dean Hendrickson

Department of Clinical Sciences, College of Veterinary Medicine and Biomedical Science, Colorado State University, 300 West Drake Road, Fort Collins, CO, 80523, USA

Considerations for Laparoscopy and Thoracoscopy

Due to benefits such as decreased pain, reduced tissue damage, and quicker return to performance, laparoscopic and thoracoscopic procedures are increasing in popularity. In the horse, these may be done under standing sedation or general anesthesia. For standing procedures, stocks that allow access for surgeons while also providing restraint for the horse are highly recommended. For procedures performed in the recumbent horse, the ability of the surgical table to be tilted (e.g. to allow the surgeon access to the caudal abdominal organs) is a key feature. However, the anesthetist must also consider the impact to physiological parameters and accuracy of measurements as the horse is moved. These are in addition to the alterations resulting from insufflation of gas to facilitate surgical visualization. Effects on cardiovascular parameters, oxygenation, ventilation, and intracranial pressure (ICP) are summarized in the following text.

Cardiovascular Effects

In addition to the dose-dependent effects of inhaled anesthetics on cardiovascular function, changes in positioning (tilt) and abdominal gas insufflation can alter cardiac output and blood pressure in horses. For example, cardiac output and mean arterial blood pressure (typically measured in the facial artery) improve in Trendelenburg position as the tilting angle becomes steeper. This is thought to be related to gravitationally increased venous return from the caudal vena cava and resulting larger stroke volume. There is likely to be some additional effect via the sympathetic nervous system resulting from concurrent increases in arterial carbon dioxide (Hofmeister et al. 2008). Abdominal insufflation alone has also been reported to improve blood pressure in horses undergoing laparoscopy (Donaldson et al. 1998), though it should be noted that this may be a result of increased vasomotor tone rather than cardiac output (Grabowski and Talamini 2009). Pressures in the hind portion of the body have not been well quantitated, and concerns for myopathy and neuropathy with long periods of Trendelenburg remain unknown.

In reverse Trendelenburg, arterial blood pressure and cardiac output decrease, and patients may require additional inotropic support to maintain blood pressure. However, rarely are horses anesthetized with such a steep head up angle that this has a clinically significant effect on cardiac output and oxygen delivery to tissues (Binetti et al. 2018; Schauvliege et al. 2018).

Equine Anesthesia and Co-Existing Disease, First Edition. Stuart Clark-Price and Khursheed Mama.

Hemodynamic changes related to positioning and insufflation are generally transient, and blood pressure and cardiac output return to baseline when horses are returned to horizontal positioning and a normal intra-abdominal pressure (Binetti et al. 2018; Hofmeister et al. 2008).

If the thorax is insufflated during thoracoscopy, it has been shown that as pleural pressure increases cardiac output decreases in dorsally recumbent horses (likely because of compression of venous return to the heart). The decrease in cardiac output is similar across a range of pleural pressures, but the lowest possible pleural pressure is recommended to maintain both cardiovascular and pulmonary function (less than 2 mmHg). As with abdominal de-sufflation, cardiac output normalizes with pleural de-sufflation (Bohaychuk-Preuss et al. 2017). During thoracoscopy, additional considerations include the potential for ventricular arrhythmias (e.g. ventricular premature contractions, ventricular tachycardia) that may be elicited if the heart is directly manipulated (Hardy et al. 1992). These can also be seen in the absence of cardiac manipulation in systemically ill horses (Díaz et al. 2014).

Respiratory Effects

Insufflation of gas into the abdomen facilitates visualization of abdominal organs but negatively affects the ability of the lungs to expand. Additionally, during laparoscopy for caudal abdominal procedures as for example removal of a cryptorchid testicle, horses are often placed in Trendelenburg position causing cranial displacement of the viscera (Figure 9.1). This further decreases lung volumes and compliance and compounds the negative effects of abdominal insufflation on pulmonary function.

Abdominally insufflated horses in Trendelenburg have significantly lower arterial oxygen values compared to horizontal positioning. Though oxygenation improves, it does not return to baseline with return to horizontal positioning and subsequent abdominal de-sufflation (Hofmeister et al. 2008). In one study without abdominal insufflation, when head down horses were subsequently converted to a head up (reverse Trendelenburg) position, the arterial oxygenation remained low compared to horses that had been positioned in the opposite order due to early development of atelectasis. This

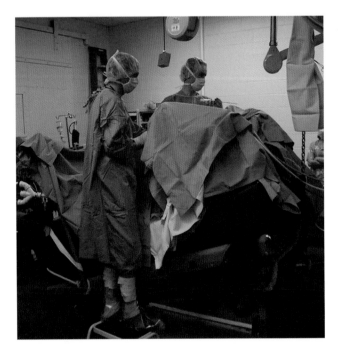

Figure 9.1 Horse placed in Trendelenburg to facilitate visualization of caudal abdominal organs during laparoscopy. *Source:* Courtesy of Dr. Dean Hendrickson.

information also suggests there may be some oxygenation benefit to providing a period of reverse Trendelenburg at the beginning of anesthesia when Trendelenburg position is required later in the procedure (Binetti et al. 2018).

Considering the effect on lung volumes and compliance, it is not surprising that Trendelenburg positioning and abdominal insufflation also lead to increases in arterial carbon dioxide concentration, especially if ventilation is pressure-limited. The use of carbon dioxide as a common surgical insufflation gas also causes hypercapnia because carbon dioxide diffuses readily into the bloodstream (Hofmeister et al. 2008; Binetti et al. 2018). Historically, many gases including air, helium, and nitrous oxide have been used for insufflation. Today, carbon dioxide is almost exclusively used because of reduced risk of fatal complications such as combustion or gas embolism. While gas embolism is still possible with carbon dioxide, its diffusibility in blood mitigates the risk (Neuhaus et al. 2001; Ikechebelu et al. 2005).

While not all thoracoscopic procedures require insufflation of gas, the lung does passively collapse and oxygenation is negatively affected. In horses that are insufflated with carbon dioxide, insufflation pressures of 2 mmHg or less appear to preserve acceptable pulmonary function. When higher thoracic insufflation pressures are used (over 5 mmHg), oxygenation is significantly affected and horses are likely to be hypoxemic. Interestingly, subsequent desufflation does not restore baseline pulmonary function (Bohaychuk-Preuss et al. 2017).

A unique consideration for horses undergoing thoracoscopy is the potential need for *one lung ventilation* (OLV). This is used to provide optimal visualization and surgical access. In human and small animal surgery, OLV is most commonly achieved using a commercially produced double-lumen endotracheal tube or endobronchial blocking device. Less commonly, a long endotracheal tube can be used to perform a purposeful endobronchial intubation (Mayhew et al. 2012). Commercial devices sized to facilitate OLV are not readily available for horses but techniques to isolate lung fields have been described, including the fabrication of a double-lumen endotracheal tube (Elliott et al. 1991) or endobronchial blocker. One endobronchial blocking technique slides a 10 mm cuffed endotracheal tube in the lumen of a 26 mm endotracheal tube through a hole placed at the distal end of the larger tube. The "tube in tube" is then guided such that the small tube sits in the desired bronchus, blocking it as the cuff is inflated. Guidance is provided by video endoscopy. This technique, however, requires a tracheostomy because the length of the commercially available tubes is not sufficient to reach the bronchus from the oral cavity (Bauquier et al. 2010). An alternate technique allowing for orotracheal intubation and bronchial blockade is described using a 26 mm endotracheal tube with a long broncho-alveolar-lavage catheter (with balloon) inserted in a similar fashion and used as an endobronchial blocker when inflated (Gozalo-Marcilla et al. 2012).

Because of the potential for displacement of the blocker and occlusion of the entire airway at the carina, blockers should be placed, and position confirmed when the horse is appropriately positioned on the surgical table and no longer needs to be moved. Capnography is a useful tool during OLV to ensure the bronchial blocker has not slipped out of place: occlusion of the entire trachea will cause the capnogram to acutely disappear. Should this occur, the bronchial blocker balloon should be deflated immediately, and re-positioned.

Management of OLV has been well described in human and small animal medicine (Mayhew and Friedberg 2008; Mayhew et al. 2012; Schisler and Lohser 2019) but there is limited experience with it in horses. OLV effectively creates a large physiologic shunt, as the collapsed lung is perfused, but not ventilated and extensive venous admixture occurs. Therefore, large alveolar to arterial oxygen tension gradients and hypoxemia are expected. In theory, hypoxic pulmonary vasoconstriction (HPV) occurs to direct more blood flow to the ventilated lung to maintain ventilation-perfusion matching. However, horses do not have as robust an HPV response compared to other species (MacEachern et al. 2004; Elliott et al. 1991) and inhalant anesthetics also dose dependently blunt this response. Though not studied in horses, total intravenous anesthesia is a beneficial management strategy in humans (Cho et al. 2017).

In human medicine, a major concern is balancing the potential for lung injury with strategies used to treat and prevent resultant hypoxemia. Ventilator-induced lung injury is a possibility in any mechanically ventilated human patient, and OLV predisposes patients to acute lung injury (ALI) (Lohser and Slinger 2015). Protective ventilation strategies using low tidal volumes, low-level positive end-expiratory pressure (PEEP), PEEP titration, and permissive hypercapnia are now routine practice, though the pathology of OLV associated ALI is multifactorial (Schisler and Lohser 2019). These strategies have not been investigated in horses.

Other Considerations

Though often overlooked in equine anesthesia, horses in a head down position in dorsal recumbency have dramatic increases in *ICP* leading to significant intracranial hypertension. Both inhalant anesthesia and hypercapnia cause cerebral vasodilation and altered autoregulation of cerebral blood flow. This is compounded by hydrostatic pressure changes associated with positioning (Brosnan et al. 2002) and likely abdominal insufflation. Whether this is of clinical importance in horses without risk factors for increased ICP is unknown. However, clinical signs of increased ICP in humans include headaches, nausea, blurred vision, and confusion (Dunn 2002; Leinonen et al. 2018), which have the potential to influence the recovery phase from anesthesia.

Additionally, *facial and nasal swelling* is more likely to develop in a head down position, particularly in horses that are hypoproteinemic or volume overloaded. Maintaining airway patency in recovery becomes an important consideration due to the resulting nasal edema. The patient management team should be prepared to manage this prior to extubation if it occurs.

Surgical complications can also occur, especially associated with cannula placement for laparoscopy. These include inadvertent vessel or organ puncture (Figure 9.2). Hemorrhage is rarely a significant problem in the horse, but bowel damage can be critical. Reducing the amount of feed in the colon is beneficial for mitigating this risk: pre-anesthetic fasting of at least 24 hours is recommended (Hendrickson 2008).

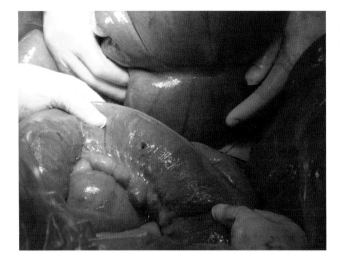

Figure 9.2 Inadvertent bowel puncture during placement of the cannula. *Source:* Courtesy of Dr. Dean Hendrickson.

Standing Sedation and Local Anesthesia

Many procedures can be performed successfully in horses using standing sedation, including ovariectomy and cryptorchidectomy, cystotomy, intestinal and pulmonary biopsies, nephrosplenic space ablation, and diaphragmatic hernia repair (Hendrickson and Wilson 1997; Hanson and Galuppo 1999; Epstein and Parente 2006; Schambourg and Marcoux 2006; Relave et al. 2008; Lund et al. 2013; Gialletti et al. 2018). This section will briefly review sedation and locoregional anesthetic techniques used for standing surgery. Considerations for general anesthesia are provided later in the chapter.

Sedative Drugs

Several drugs or drug combinations can be used for sedation, but α2-adrenoreceptor agonists (α2-agonists) form the foundation of many protocols. Acepromazine and opioids can be used in conjunction with α2-agonists to augment sedation or analgesia. Table 9.1 provides a summary of selected information relevant to dosing and attributes of these drugs. Additionally, sample sedation protocols are outlined in Table 9.2.

α2-Adrenoreceptor Agonists

Several excellent sources on the use of different α2-agonists in horses exist (England and Clarke 1996; Valverde 2010; Gozalo-Marcilla et al. 2015). The qualities of each α2-agonist can be used advantageously depending on the chosen sedative technique. For example, a short-acting drug such as xylazine or dex/medetomidine is ideal for titration by infusion or as a bolus when only a limited amount of additional sedation time is required. Long-acting drugs such as detomidine and romifidine are well suited for bolus dosing for longer procedures. There is no one protocol that will work for every horse, and combinations of the different α2-agonists can allow utilization of each drug's individual benefits.

Acepromazine

Acepromazine is a long-acting phenothiazine tranquilizer that typically results in dose-dependent, mild-to-moderate anxiolytic effect when given alone (Ballard et al. 1982; Knych et al. 2018). It has been used with opioids and α2-agonists as an adjunct to sedation for standing procedures and is thought to be particularly beneficial when given to an undisturbed horse before it is brought into the surgical area. Hypotension can be a significant side effect in a volume depleted animal. Avoiding the use of acepromazine in stallions is advocated by some, but evidence suggests that this complication is likely dose dependent (Ballard et al. 1982) and uncommon (Driessen et al. 2011).

Opioids

Opioids, such as butorphanol, morphine, hydromorphone, or methadone, typically improve the quality of sedation provided by α2-agonists; when given in the absence of sedatives or tranquilizers to healthy, non-painful horses, opioids tend to cause central excitement and increased locomotor activity (Clutton 2010). Experimental and clinical studies conflict with respect to the analgesic efficacy of opioids in horses, and controversy exists in part due to the risk of undesirable side effects (Clutton 2010; Figueiredo et al. 2012). These include reducing gastrointestinal motility and fecal retention (Boscan et al. 2006). However, appropriately used clinically relevant doses of opioids do not appear to predispose horses to post-operative colic (Andersen et al. 2006; Skrzypczak et al. 2020).

Intravenous and Adjunctive Administration Techniques

Sedation can be administered by varying routes but is most commonly given IV in bolus dosing or as an infusion, generally through an IV catheter. Alternate routes for drug administration are also included.

Table 9.1 Drugs used for standing sedation in horses and suggested dose ranges.

Drug	Suggested doses	Notes
Tranquilizer		
Acepromazine	IV: 0.005–0.03 mg/kg IM: 0.02–0.04 mg/kg	Several minutes time for onset even if given IV.
α2-agonists		
Dexmedetomidine	IV: 0.003–0.005 mg/kg IV CRI: 0.001–0.008 mg/kg/h Epidural: 0.005 mg/kg	Short duration of action (<20 minutes): CRI route ideal for longer procedures. Epidural dosing not extensively studied in equids.
Medetomidine	IV: 0.007–0.01 mg/kg IV CRI: 0.003–0.005 mg/kg	
Xylazine	IV: 0.5–1 mg/kg IV CRI: 0.3–1 mg/kg/h Epidural: 0.2 mg/kg	
Detomidine	IV: 0.005–0.02 mg/kg IV CRI: 0.005–0.02 mg/kg/h Epidural: 0.015–0.03 mg/kg	
Romifidine	IV: 0.02–0.08 mg/kg IV CRI: 0.03–0.05 mg/kg/h Epidural: 0.03–0.06 mg/kg	Less ataxia compared to other α2-agonists. Reported poor efficacy by epidural route.
Opioids		
Butorphanol	IV: 0.01–0.04 mg/kg IV CRI: 0.01–0.02 mg/kg/h	
Nalbuphine	IV: 0.03–0.06 mg/kg	
Buprenorphine	IV: 0.003–0.005 Epidural: 0.004	Several hour duration of effect when given systemically. Large doses can lead to opioid-induced excitement in the absence of long-lasting sedation. Acepromazine administration may help decrease associated locomotor activity.
Morphine	IV: 0.05–0.2 IV CRI: 0.03–0.1 mg/kg/h Epidural: 0.1–0.2 mg/kg	
Methadone	IV: 0.1–0.2 mg/kg IV CRI: 0.05 mg/kg/h (Gozalla-Marcillo et al. 2019) Epidural: 0.1 mg/kg	
Hydromorphone	IV: 0.01–0.04 mg/kg Epidural: 0.04 mg/kg	CRI dosing has not been established but could be extrapolated from bolus dose data.
Meperidine	IV: 1 mg/kg Epidural: 0.3–0.8 mg/kg	

IV = intravenous; IV CRI = intravenous constant rate infusion; IM = intramuscular. Doses should be adjusted to the patient and used in conjunction with appropriate local/regional anesthesia.

Table 9.2 Sample sedation protocols for a 500 kg horse undergoing standing surgery.

	Initial sedation	Infusion	Top-up sedation
Protocol 1	Acepromazine 5 mg IV in stall 15 minutes prior to additional sedation. Detomidine 8 mg IV in surgical area.	Detomidine 2–5 mg/h and dexmedetomidine 1 mg/h on infusion pumps.	If needed, detomidine 1–2 mg IV bolus or dexmedetomidine 0.25–0.5 mg IV bolus if briefer sedation required.
Protocol 2	Xylazine 300 mg and methadone 25 mg IV in surgical area.	800–1600 mg in 0.5–1 l IV fluid dripped to effect. Example: 0.75 mg/kg/h is 1 drop/second of 1.6 mg/ml xylazine using a 15 drop/ml drip set: rate can be adjusted up or down as needed.	If needed, xylazine 80–160 ml bolus from bag (50–100 mg IV). Methadone 25 mg IV every two hours.
Protocol 3	Romifidine 30 mg and morphine 25 mg IV in surgical area.	None.	Romifidine 20–30 mg IV and morphine 10–20 mg IV bolus every 45–90 minutes. Dexmedetomidine 0.25–0.5 mg IV bolus if briefer sedation required.
Protocol 4	Detomidine 5 mg and butorphanol 5 mg IV in surgical area.	10–20 mg in 0.5–1 l IV fluid dripped to effect. Example: 0.01 mg/kg/h is 1 drop/second of 0.02 mg/ml detomidine using a 15 drop/ml drip set: rate can be adjusted up or down as needed.	If needed, detomidine 50–150 ml bolus from bag (1–3 mg IV). Dexmedetomidine 0.25–0.5 mg IV bolus if briefer sedation required. Butorphanol 5 mg IV every 45 minutes.

Protocols are author-provided examples only. Actual sedation should be individualized to the patient and used in conjunction with appropriate local/regional anesthesia.

Intravenous Bolus

Administration of single boluses of sedative drugs throughout the procedure is a common technique. An IV catheter is not required but is strongly recommended. Most procedures will require some amount of redosing, and a short-term IV catheter minimizes the trauma and hassle associated with multiple off-the-needle injections. This improves both patient compliance and surgical working conditions, in addition to reducing the risk of inadvertent intracarotid injection. While IV bolus dosing is easy, it can create over-sedation during some parts of the procedure while providing insufficient sedation at other times.

Intravenous Infusion

A continuous infusion of sedative drugs in a bag of IV fluids provides an alternative and allows for adjustment of the drip rate in accordance with the horse's level of sedation. This technique is simple, and it does not require specialized equipment. However, if a combination of drugs is used in the bag, one drug cannot be delivered without also administering the other. Administration of individual drugs using syringe or fluid pumps allow for more precise control.

Epidurals

Epidural administration of α2-agonists and opioids can provide analgesia for standing laparoscopic procedures. Some also are readily absorbed from the epidural space (Skarda 1994). For example, detomidine administered epidurally to mares undergoing ovariectomy provided similar surgical conditions to an intravenous detomidine infusion (Virgin et al. 2010). Because of analgesia and/or enhanced systemic sedation, horses may require less total systemic drug when receiving an epidural (Van Hoogmoed and Galuppo 2005). Epidural injections are typically performed at the first inter-coccygeal joint (Co1-Co2) or the sacrococcygeal junction; compared to a lumbosacral epidural injection, it is technically easier to perform at this location and there is no risk of entering the subarachnoid space. For additional information on how to perform an epidural injection, please refer to Michou and Leece 2012.

Epidural drugs are diluted to a volume intended to reach the desired sensory innervation for the surgical site. The paralumbar fossa receives sensory innervation from branches of spinal nerves T18, L1 and L2; therefore, a volume of approximately 15–20 ml is required for cranial migration from the intercoccygeal injection site. Slow injection of this volume is advised as administration may be uncomfortable for the horse (Hendrickson et al. 1998; Natalini and Linardi 2006). Because this dermatome is cranial to both the sensory and motor innervation to the hind limbs (L4-S2) (Singh 2017), local anesthetics should not be used in this scenario. High doses of certain alpha-2 agonists can also cause hind limb weakness and occasionally recumbency (Wittern et al. 1998) (Figure 9.3). If long-term epidural analgesia is required, an indwelling epidural catheter (Figure 9.4) can be placed (Robinson and Natalini 2002).

Local Anesthetic Techniques

Desensitization of the surgical site with a local anesthetic is frequently needed for compliance and improved analgesia in standing surgery. Lidocaine, mepivacaine, bupivacaine, and ropivacaine are all local anesthetics that are used in used in horses. Additional information specific to their similarities and differences is available elsewhere. (Campoy and Read 2013)

An extended duration, liposomal encapsulated bupivacaine formulation (Nocita®) is now available in veterinary medicine. Though it is not

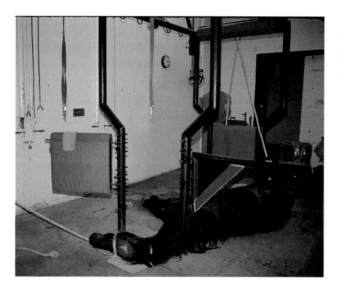

Figure 9.3 Recumbency observed following epidural drug administration prior to planned laparoscopic procedure. *Source:* Courtesy of Dr. Dean Hendrickson.

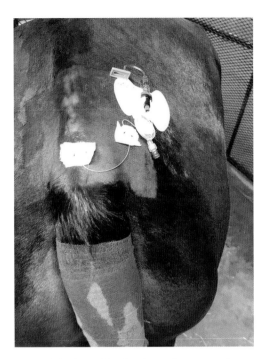

Figure 9.4 An epidural catheter for repeated delivery of epidural drugs. *Source:* Courtesy of Dr. Rachel Hector.

licensed for horses, it is becoming popular for a variety of purposes in equine surgery. It is meant to be used by infiltration in the surgical incision and provides local anesthesia of the surgical site for approximately 72 hours in dogs, which could significantly reduce the need for systemic analgesics (e.g. non-steroidal anti-inflammatory drugs) post-operatively. Recommendations for horses are primarily anecdotal but research is emerging (Knych et al. 2019; Griffenhagen et al. 2019; McCracken et al. 2020). Caution should be exercised when administered in the vicinity of motor nerves due to potential risk of prolonged motor paralysis.

Local Anesthesia for Laparoscopy

Skin and Body Wall
The skin and body wall can be desensitized using one or a combination of methods, but most commonly local anesthetic is administered at the portal incisions. The area of desensitization may be extended to facilitate removal of abdominal tissues during the procedure. Full thickness portal blocks are advantageous in that they take less local anesthetic, allow for flexibility in the placement of portal sites, and are technically easy to perform. Regional blocks as used for flank laparotomy including the inverted L block and paravertebral block are therefore almost never used for laparoscopic procedures.

Ovaries and Intra-abdominal Testes
When performing laparoscopic cryptorchidectomy, local anesthesia of the intra-abdominal testes is performed using a laparoscopic needle and approximately 10–15 ml of lidocaine injected into the testes or the mesorchium. Without a local block, stallions are more likely to be responsive to testicular manipulation and display behaviors such as stomping or kicking. Although a blinded clinical study detected no statistical difference in pain scores between the two injection sites, the authors subjectively assessed mesorchium injection to be more effective (Joyce and Hendrickson 2006).

Similarly, injection of lidocaine directly into the ovary while simpler to perform was found to be less effective than injection of local anesthetic into the mesovarium when handling the ovary or ovarian pedicle during laparoscopic ovariectomy (Palmer 1993; Farstvedt and Hendrickson 2005). Some mares, however, are reactive to needle insertion. Hence a recent study compared irrigation of the ovarian pedicle with mepivacaine to injection in the mesovarium and found both provided equal levels of analgesia. Irrigation also reduces risk of inadvertent damage to other structures (Koch et al. 2020).

Kidney and Bladder
For laparoscopic nephrectomy, local anesthesia is provided by infusing 15–20 ml of drug into the retroperitoneal space caudal to the kidney using a laparoscopic needle directed through the peritoneum axial and caudal to the nephrosplenic ligament (Keoughan et al. 2003). Local anesthesia of the bladder has

been used in conscious people undergoing surgery despite potential discomfort associated with administration. (Engberg et al. 1983). Intravesicular infusion of lidocaine is also reported to be effective for treatment of bladder pain associated with chronic interstitial cystitis in people (Nickel et al. 2012). Use of an intraluminal local anesthetic technique has been reported once in anesthetized horses and was deemed helpful in bladder exteriorization and removal of cystic calculi (Russell and Pollock 2012).

Local Anesthesia for Thoracoscopy

Skin and Body Wall

Portal blocks can be performed in the thoracic body wall using a similar technique as described for the abdomen. However, the thoracic body wall is not as thick as the abdominal wall, and therefore less depth and less volume of local anesthetic is required at each site. If local anesthetic is inadvertently injected into the pleural space, the primary issue will be lack of anesthetic effect at the incision. Interestingly, even when sites are blocked, horses are reported to be less reactive to thoracoscopy through the 12th versus 8th intercostal space (Klohnen and Peroni 2000).

Specific intercostal nerve blocks can also be performed to facilitate thoracoscopy in horses (Laverty et al. 1996; Hassel 2007; Hilton et al. 2010). Briefly, at the most proximal palpable point on the chosen rib, a 22 or 20 gauge 1 inch (2.5 cm) needle is inserted perpendicular to the caudal aspect of the rib. Once the needle hits bone, it is directed caudally off the edge of the rib into the intercostal muscle. After aspiration to confirm the needle is not located in a vessel or the pleural space, local anesthetic is administered. The intercostal block is associated with a higher degree of systemic local anesthetic uptake compared to other sites, so attention to local anesthetic dose is particularly important (Chan et al. 1991). In other species, it is recommended to block at least two rib spaces cranial and caudal to the incision site to be sure all sensory innervation is blocked.

Specific Considerations for Standing Thoracoscopy

Oxygen can be supplemented in standing surgery using nasal insufflation tubing and high flow oxygen (10–15 l/min), particularly in horses with extensive pre-existing thoracic disease (e.g. pleuropneumonia). Creation of a pneumothorax and pulmonary collapse is an unavoidable component of standing thoracoscopy. Although generally well tolerated because of normal ventilation of the contralateral lung when the mediastinum is intact, healthy horses with prolonged pneumothorax do have lower than normal oxygen tensions, especially during thoracoscopy of the left hemithorax (Klohnen and Peroni 2000). While carbon dioxide insufflation is not usually required, it is tolerated for short periods, but bilateral pneumothorax is more likely to occur (Penha et al. 2008). Although negative pressure is re-established in the thorax via post-procedure suction, horses should be monitored for signs of residual pneumothorax; a leak can be created if lung parenchyma is damaged during the procedure, and a pneumothorax can be re-created.

General Anesthesia

In some cases, the nature of the procedure or temperament of the horse preclude performing standing surgery. This section will briefly review anesthetic techniques as well as the unique challenges faced during laparoscopic and thoracoscopic procedures performed under general anesthesia. Standard equine anesthesia protocols typically consist of pre-anesthetic sedation, an intravenously administered anesthetic induction agent and adjunctive drug, inhaled or injectable anesthetic maintenance, and if appropriate post-anesthetic sedation. Table 9.3

Table 9.3   Selected sedation and induction drugs used in equine anesthesia and their suggested doses.

Sedatives and tranquilizers	Intravenous dose
Dexmedetomidine	Pre-anesthetic: to effect up to 0.007 mg/kg Recovery: 0.001–0.002 mg/kg
Medetomidine	Pre-anesthetic: to effect up to 0.01 mg/kg Recovery: 0.002–0.003 mg/kg
Xylazine	Pre-anesthetic: to effect up to 1 mg/kg Recovery: 0.1–0.2 mg/kg
Detomidine	Pre-anesthetic: to effect up to 0.02 mg/kg Recovery: 0.002–0.004 mg/kg
Romifidine	Pre-anesthetic: to effect up to 0.1 mg/kg Recovery: 0.01–0.02 mg/kg
Acepromazine	0.005–0.02 mg/kg
Butorphanol	0.01–0.05 mg/kg
Morphine	0.05–0.2 mg/kg
Methadone	0.1–0.2 mg/kg
Hydromorphone	0.01–0.04 mg/kg
Induction	
Ketamine	2–3 mg/kg combined with one or more adjunct drug below
Adjunct drugs	
Midazolam/diazepam	0.02–0.1 mg/kg following ketamine
Propofol	0.5–1 mg/kg following ketamine
Guaifenesin	50–100 mg/kg to effect prior to ketamine

lists examples of drugs and doses. The interested reader is referred to other sources specific to equine anesthesia for additional information or details not covered in the following section, such as techniques for partial or total intravenous anesthesia (Muir and Hubbell 2009; Clark-Price 2013).

Pre-anesthetic Sedation

Good sedation is a prerequisite to anesthetic induction in horses. Choice of a specific drugs will depend on the systemic health status of the horse, personal experience, desired drug volume, duration of drug effect, expected length of procedure, and drug availability and cost.

It is important to recognize that after a single IV dose, *α2-agonists* cause a marked increase in systemic vascular resistance, bradycardia, bradyarrhythmias, and a profound reduction in cardiac output. Over time, peripheral vascular tone decreases, but due to persistent decreases in sympathetic outflow, bradycardia and bradyarrhythmias can last for a period from 20 minutes to over 2 hours depending on the drug used (Rezende et al. 2015; Freeman et al. 2002; Wojtasiak-Wypart et al. 2012). In addition, one should also keep in mind that certain drugs will significantly reduce gastrointestinal motility.

Acepromazine can maintain anxiolysis preoperatively and dose dependently maintain this effect during anesthetic recovery. Cardiovascularly, acepromazine causes α1-adrenoreceptor antagonist mediated vasodilation and significant systemic arterial hypotension (Marroum et al. 1994; Pequito et al. 2013).

Opioids improve quality of sedation provided by aforementioned drugs prior to anesthetic induction and can be particularly helpful in horses that remain reactive following their administration. Though studies conflict, most of the published work shows that horses receiving opioids at common clinical doses have no increased risk of post-anesthesia gastrointestinal dysfunction (Mircica et al. 2003; Andersen et al. 2006; Love et al. 2006; Sano et al. 2011; Devine et al. 2013). The risk however increases when high doses are administered (Mama et al. 1993; Sellon et al. 2001; Knych et al. 2018).

Anesthesia Induction

This is typically achieved using a combination of an intravenous anesthetic agent and adjunct muscle relaxant as detailed in Table 9.3. Following appropriate sedation, most provide good anesthetic induction quality, and selection should again be based on what is likely to minimize side effects. For example, guaifenesin allows for a reduction in dose of the alpha-2 agonist (Hubbell et al. 1980; Matthews et al. 1997). This could be particularly beneficial in a cardiovascularly unstable horse that could be further compromised as a result of positioning and insufflation.

Maintenance

Isoflurane, sevoflurane, and less commonly desflurane are inhalant anesthetics currently used for maintenance of anesthesia in horses. While sevoflurane offers the ability to more rapidly change anesthetic depth and shorten recovery, this effect may be blunted by injectable sedative and anesthetic drugs. (Grosenbaugh and Muir 1998; Matthews et al. 1998; Hubbell 1999; Read et al. 2002; Valverde et al. 2005; Leece et al. 2008). Desflurane conversely is associated with smooth recoveries from general anesthesia irrespective of other drugs provided (Clarke et al. 1996; Steffey et al. 2009; Aarnes et al. 2014; Valente et al. 2015). Cardiorespiratory effects of

the drugs are largely similar although one study suggests that horses anesthetized with sevoflurane require less inotropic support to maintain blood pressure (Driessen et al. 2006). Nitrous oxide can be used to reduce the dose, and thus cardiorespiratory effects, of other inhaled agents (Testa et al. 1990). However, nitrous oxide, by virtue of its blood: gas partition coefficient, has a tendency to enter gas filled spaces in the body. This includes the bowel and abdomen insufflated with carbon dioxide. The concentration of nitrous oxide in these spaces increases over time, increasing the risk of potential gas embolism or possible combustion (Diemunsch et al. 2000; Becker and Rosenberg 2008).

To summarize, when choosing drugs for horses undergoing laparoscopy or thoracoscopy under general anesthesia, beneficial and side effects of these drugs or drug classes should be considered as they might compound side effects resulting from long periods of fasting (e.g. ileus, vascular volume changes) as often required prior to laparoscopic intervention, the cardiovascular, respiratory, and noxious effects of carbon dioxide insufflation into the abdomen, and postural changes (e.g. hypotension).

Anesthetic Monitoring and Support

Recommendations for monitoring and support and considerations of the same are similar to those for any horse undergoing procedures under general anesthesia and may include non-invasive and invasive measures. Two non-invasive and continuous tools namely pulse oximetry and capnography while easily applied may have limitations during laparoscopy and thoracoscopy as they do not accurately and consistently inform on oxygenation and ventilation in horses (Koenig et al. 2003). Arterial blood gas analysis is the gold standard for assessing oxygenation and ventilation and is especially important in horses undergoing laparoscopy and thoracoscopy. Capnography may however be especially useful in situations when OLV is used and has importance in diagnosing intravascular insufflation gas (carbon dioxide) embolization.

Oxygenation and Ventilation

Preoxygenation

Preoxygenation is recommended in horses with existing thoracic disease or those with abdominal distention (e.g. animal with nephrosplenic entrapment) that either are or are likely to become hypoxemic following sedation and during anesthesia induction. This is generally well tolerated when achieved by placing soft nasal insufflation tubing to the level of the medial canthus of the eye and delivering an oxygen flow rate of 15 l/min (in the adult horse) (Wilson et al. 2006; Van Oostrom et al. 2017). Upon recumbency and endotracheal intubation insufflation may be continued or breathing supplemented with a demand valve until the horse is transitioned to the anesthesia machine.

Management of Oxygenation During the Peri-anesthetic Period

In lateral recumbency, anesthetized horses usually oxygenate well even if spontaneously ventilating. (Steffey et al. 1977; Day et al. 1995), but they experience profound ventilation/perfusion (V/Q) mismatches in dorsal recumbency and have a tendency toward poor oxygenation despite mechanical ventilation and a high FiO_2. Shunt fraction increases over time and is more significant as body weight increases (Marntell et al. 2005; Auckburally and Nyman 2017).

When trying to improve arterial oxygenation, application of recruitment maneuvers and the addition of PEEP are often useful (Hopster et al. 2011). However, it is important to ensure that cardiac output is not detrimentally influenced as this has a large role in maintaining oxygen delivery (Hopster et al. 2011). Cardiac output is not directly measured in routine equine clinical cases, but a ventilation-related decrease may be presumed if a concurrent decrease in mean arterial pressure occurs even in the absence of signs of change on the anesthetic monitor (Ambrósio et al. 2013).

Given a period of hypoxemia occurs in even healthy, well-oxygenated horses upon placement in the recovery stall on room air (Mason et al. 1987), oxygen administration, which can temper the severity, should be continued into the recovery period. This is critical in the horse that demonstrated hypoxemia during the procedure. Further benefit can be achieved with positive pressure ventilation using a demand valve (Mason et al. 1987).

Management of Ventilation During the Anesthetic Period

As stated earlier, abdominal insufflation and Trendelenburg positioning during laparoscopic interventions lead to hypercapnia (Hofmeister et al. 2008; Binetti et al. 2018). Mild-to-moderate hypercapnia has a positive sympathetic effect and results in an increase in cardiac output (Wagner and Bednarski 1990; Khanna et al. 1995). While ventilation may be necessary to mitigate the negative influence of continued increases in carbon dioxide on pH and oxygenation, permissive hypercapnia may be adopted to take advantage of the cardiovascular benefits of elevations in carbon dioxide and avoid the negative cardiovascular effects of more aggressive positive pressure ventilation (Cardenas et al. 1996; Kelleher et al. 2013).

Cardiovascular Monitoring and Support

Inhaled anesthetics dose dependently depress cardiovascular function in horses, even those that are systemically healthy, with many horses requiring inotropic support. Prolonged hypotension (mean arterial blood pressure <60 mmHg) provides insufficient organ blood flow, particularly to dependent muscles, and predisposes horses to serious complications in recovery (e.g. myopathy) (Grandy et al. 1987). As such, a safe recommendation is to keep the average horse's mean arterial pressure over 70 mmHg and that of a very large or heavily muscled horse over 80 mmHg.

While newer non-invasive technology can provide relatively accurate blood pressure measurements (Tünsmeyer et al. 2015), the authors recommend direct blood pressure measurement be performed in horses undergoing laparoscopic and thoracoscopic procedures under anesthesia due to the potential complications highlighted previously. For accuracy to be maintained however, the transducer must be re-positioned and zero verified with postural changes. Presence of an arterial catheter also facilitates obtaining blood samples for blood gas analysis. Additionally, the use of an electrocardiogram to assess heart rate and rhythm is standard of care but has an additional role in thoracoscopy where rhythm changes may be evident with thoracic intervention.

Recovery

Management of recovery including post-operative analgesics does not differ significantly than for other procedures in horses undergoing laparoscopy or thoracoscopy. While overall post-operative pain is decreased compared to open laparotomy or thoracotomy (Holzer et al. 2006; Rodríguez-Torres et al. 2019), significant discomfort is reported in people following carbon dioxide administration and peritoneal distention: most commonly referred pain in the shoulder region, even up to 24 hours after the procedure. This is thought to be related to irritation of the phrenic nerve from the dry insufflation gas and attempts at reducing the same have focused on humidifying the gases, decreasing insufflation pressure, and lavaging the peritoneal cavity with warm fluids or local anesthetics (Kaloo et al. 2019). It is not known whether this referred pain occurs in horses. Local anesthetic techniques described earlier may also be applied to horses undergoing procedures using general anesthesia. Intraoperative local or regional anesthetic techniques reduce inhalant and injectable anesthetic requirements and have also been shown to reduce post-operative pain even beyond their duration of effect (Woolf and Chong 1993; Roberge and McEwen 1998; Ilkiw 1999; Hodgson and Liu 2001; Portier et al. 2009; Barreveld et al. 2013).

As previously mentioned, administration of oxygen is prudent and maintaining the airway as long as possible in recovery is beneficial, particularly in horses with pre-existing thoracic disease. Horses tolerate a nasotracheal or orotracheal tube well even while standing. If secured properly, this tube can be left in place for the entire recovery, facilitating delivery of oxygen via insufflation and demand valve breaths as necessary. Emergency airway access supplies should also always be readily available.

References

Aarnes, T.K., Bednarski, R.M., Bertone, A.L. et al. (2014). Recovery from desflurane anesthesia in horses with and without post-anesthetic xylazine. *Canadian Journal of Veterinary Research* 78(2): 103–109.

Ambrósio, A.M., Ida, K.K., Souto, M.T. et al. (2013). Effects of positive end-expiratory pressure titration on gas exchange, respiratory mechanics and hemodynamics in anesthetized horses. *Veterinary Anaesthesia and Analgesia* 40(6): 564–572.

Andersen, M.S., Clark, L., Dyson, S.J., and Newton, J.R. (2006). Risk factors for colic in horses after general anaesthesia for MRI or nonabdominal surgery: absence of evidence of effect from perianaesthetic morphine. *Equine Veterinary Journal* 38(4): 368–374.

Auckburally, A. and Nyman, G. (2017). Review of hypoxaemia in anaesthetized horses: predisposing factors, consequences and management. *Veterinary Anaesthesia and Analgesia* 44(3): 397–408.

Ballard, S., Shults, T., Kownacki, A.A. et al. (1982). The pharmacokinetics, pharmacological responses and behavioral effects of acepromazine in the horse. *Journal of Veterinary Pharmacology and Therapeutics* 5(1): 21–31.

Barreveld, A., Witte, J., Chahal, H. et al. (2013). Preventive analgesia by local anesthetics: the reduction of postoperative pain by peripheral nerve blocks and intravenous drugs. *Anesthesia and Analgesia* 116(5): 1141.

Bauquier, S.H., Dusavage, S., and Driessen, B. (2010). Anaesthesia and ventilation strategy in a horse undergoing pulmonectomy. *Equine Veterinary Education* 22(5): 231–236.

Becker, D.E. and Rosenberg, M. (2008). Nitrous oxide and the inhalation anesthetics. *Anesthesia Progress* 55(4): 124–131.

Binetti, A., Mosing, M., Sacks, M. et al. (2018). Impact of Trendelenburg (head down) and reverse Trendelenburg (head up) position on respiratory and cardiovascular function in anaesthetized horses. *Veterinary Anaesthesia and Analgesia* 45(6): 760–771.

Bohaychuk-Preuss, K.S., Carrozzo, M.V., and Duke-Novakovski, T. (2017). Cardiopulmonary effects of pleural insufflation with CO2 during two-lung ventilation in dorsally recumbent anesthetized horses. *Veterinary Anaesthesia and Analgesia* 44(3): 483–491.

Boscan, P., Van Hoogmoed, L.M., Farver, T.B., and Snyder, J.R. (2006). Evaluation of the effects of the opioid agonist morphine on gastrointestinal tract function in horses. *American Journal of Veterinary Research* 67(6): 992–997.

Brosnan, R.J., Steffey, E.P., LeCouteur, R.A. et al. (2002). Effects of body position on intracranial and cerebral perfusion pressures in isoflurane-anesthetized horses. *Journal of Applied Physiology* 92(6): 2542–2546.

Campoy, L. and Read, M.R. (2013). *Small Animal Regional Anesthesia and Analgesia*. Ames, IA: Wiley.

Cardenas, V.J., Zwischenberger, J.B., Tao, W. et al. (1996). Correction of blood pH attenuates changes in hemodynamics and organ blood flow during permissive hypercapnia. *Critical Care Medicine* 24(5): 827–834.

Chan, V.W., Chung, F., Cheng, D.C. et al. (1991). Analgesic and pulmonary effects of continuous intercostal nerve block following thoracotomy. *Canadian Journal of Anaesthesia* 38(6): 733–739.

Cho, Y.J., Kim, T.K., Hong, D.M. et al. (2017). Effect of desflurane-remifentanil vs. propofol-remifentanil anesthesia on arterial oxygenation during one-lung ventilation for thoracoscopic surgery: a prospective randomized trial. *BMC Anesthesiology* 17(1): 9.

Clarke, K.W., Song, D.Y., Lee, Y.H., and Alibhai, H.I. (1996). Desflurane anaesthesia in the horse: minimum alveolar concentration following induction of anaesthesia with xylazine and ketamine. *Journal of Veterinary Anaesthesia* 23(2): 56–59.

Clark-Price, S.C. (2013). Topics in equine anesthesia. *Veterinary Clinics: Equine Practice* 29(1): ix–x.

Clutton, R.E. (2010). Opioid analgesia in horses. *Veterinary Clinics: Equine Practice* 26 (3): 493–514.

Day, T.K., Gaynor, J.S., Muir, W.W. III et al. (1995). Blood gas values during intermittent positive pressure ventilation and spontaneous ventilation in 160 anesthetized horses positioned in lateral or dorsal recumbency. *Veterinary Surgery* 24(3): 266–276.

Devine, E.P., KuKanich, B., and Beard, W.L. (2013). Pharmacokinetics of intramuscularly administered morphine in horses. *Journal of the American Veterinary Medical Association* 243(1): 105–112.

Díaz, O.M., Durando, M.M., Birks, E.K., and Reef, V.B. (2014). Cardiac troponin I concentrations in horses with colic. *Journal of the American Veterinary Medical Association* 245(1): 118–125.

Diemunsch, P.A., Torp, K.D., Van Dorsselaer, T. et al. (2000). Nitrous oxide fraction in the carbon dioxide pneumoperitoneum during laparoscopy under general inhaled anesthesia in pigs. *Anesthesia & Analgesia* 90(4): 951–953.

Donaldson, L.L., Trostle, S.S., and White, N.A. (1998). Cardiopulmonary changes associated with abdominal insufflation of carbon dioxide in mechanically ventilated, dorsally recumbent, halothane anaesthetised horses. *Equine Veterinary Journal* 30 (2): 144–151.

Driessen, B., Nann, L., Benton, R., and Boston, R. (2006). Differences in need for hemodynamic support in horses anesthetized with sevoflurane as compared to isoflurane. *Veterinary Anaesthesia and Analgesia* 33 (6): 356–367.

Driessen, B., Zarucco, L., Kalir, B., and Bertolotti, L. (2011). Contemporary use of acepromazine in the anaesthetic management of male horses and ponies: a retrospective study and opinion poll. *Equine Veterinary Journal* 43 (1): 88–98.

Dunn, L.T. (2002). Raised intracranial pressure. *Journal of Neurology, Neurosurgery & Psychiatry* 73 (Suppl 1): i23–i27.

Elliott, A.R., Steffey, E.P., Jarvis, K.A., and Marshall, B.E. (1991). Unilateral hypoxic pulmonary vasoconstriction in the dog, pony and miniature swine. *Respiration Physiology* 85 (3): 355–369.

Engberg, A., Spångberg, A., and Urnes, T. (1983). Transurethral resection of bladder tumors under local anesthesia. *Urology* 22 (4): 385–387.

England, G.C. and Clarke, K.W. (1996). Alpha2 adrenoceptor agonists in the horse – a review. *British Veterinary Journal* 152 (6): 641–657.

Epstein, K.L. and Parente, E.J. (2006). Laparoscopic obliteration of the nephrosplenic space using polypropylene mesh in five horses. *Veterinary Surgery* 35 (5): 431–437.

Farstvedt, E.G. and Hendrickson, D.A. (2005). Intraoperative pain responses following intraovarian versus mesovarian injection of lidocaine in mares undergoing laparoscopic ovariectomy. *Journal of the American Veterinary Medical Association* 227 (4): 593–596.

Figueiredo, J.P., Muir, W.W., and Sams, R. (2012). Cardiorespiratory, gastrointestinal, and analgesic effects of morphine sulfate in conscious healthy horses. *American Journal of Veterinary Research* 73 (6): 799–808.

Freeman, S.L., Bowen, I.M., Bettschart-Wolfensberger, R. et al. (2002). Cardiovascular effects of romifidine in the standing horse. *Research in Veterinary Science* 72 (2): 123–129.

Gialletti, R., Corsalini, J., Lotto, E. et al. (2018). Standing thoracoscopic diaphragmatic hernia repair using a dual-facing mesh in a horse. *Journal of Equine Veterinary Science* 62: 13–17.

Gozalo-Marcilla, M., Schauvliege, S., Torfs, S. et al. (2012). An alternative for one lung ventilation in an adult horse requiring thoracotomy. *Vlaams Diergeneeskundig Tijdschrift* 81 (2): 98–101.

Gozalo-Marcilla, M., Gasthuys, F., and Schauvliege, S. (2015). Partial intravenous anaesthesia in the horse: a review of intravenous agents used to supplement equine inhalation anaesthesia. Part 2: opioids and alpha-2 adrenoceptor agonists. *Veterinary Anaesthesia and Analgesia* 42 (1): 1–6.

Gozalo-Marcilla, M., De Oliverira, A.R., Fonseca, M.W. et al. (2019). Sedative and antinociceptive effects of different detomidine constant rate infusions, with or without methadone in standing horses. *Equine Veterinary Journal* 51 (4): 530–536.

Grabowski, J.E. and Talamini, M.A. (2009). Physiological effects of pneumoperitoneum. *Journal of Gastrointestinal Surgery* 13 (5): 1009–1016.

Grandy, J.L., Steffey, E.P., Hodgson, D.S., and Woliner, M.J. (1987). Arterial hypotension and the development of postanesthetic myopathy in halothane-anesthetized horses. *American Journal of Veterinary Research* 48 (2): 192–197.

Griffenhagen, G., Pezzanite, L., Hendrickson, D., and Moorman, V. (2019). Liposomal encapsulated bupivacaine provides longer duration analgesia than bupivacaine HCl when administered as an abaxial sesamoid block in horses. *Veterinary Anaesthesia and Analgesia* 46 (6): 831–836.

Grosenbaugh, D.A. and Muir, W.W. (1998). Cardiorespiratory effects of sevoflurane, isoflurane, and halothane anesthesia in horses. *American Journal of Veterinary Research* 59 (1): 101–106.

Hanson, C.A. and Galuppo, L.D. (1999). Bilateral laparoscopic ovariectomy in standing mares: 22 cases. *Veterinary Surgery* 28 (2): 106–112.

Hardy, J., Robertson, J.T., and Reed, S.M. (1992). Constrictive pericarditis in a mare: attempted treatment by partial pericardiectomy. *Equine Veterinary Journal* 24 (2): 151–154.

Hassel, D.M. (2007). Thoracic trauma in horses. *Veterinary Clinics of North America. Equine Practice* 23 (1): 67–80.

Hendrickson, D.A. (2008). Complications of laparoscopic surgery. *Veterinary Clinics of North America. Equine Practice* 24 (3): 557–571.

Hendrickson, D.A. and Wilson, D.G. (1997). Laparoscopic cryptorchid castration in standing horses. *Veterinary Surgery* 26(4): 335–339.

Hendrickson, D.A., Southwood, L.L., Lopez, M.J. et al. (1998). Cranial migration of different volumes of new-methylene blue after caudal epidural injection in the horse. *Equine Practice (USA)* 20: 12–14.

Hilton, H., Aleman, M., Madigan, J., and Nieto, J. (2010). Standing lateral thoracotomy in horses: indications, complications, and outcomes. *Veterinary Surgery* 39(7): 847–855.

Hodgson, P.S. and Liu, S.S. (2001). Epidural lidocaine decreases sevoflurane requirement for adequate depth of anesthesia as measured by the Bispectral Index® monitor. *Anesthesiology* 94 (5): 799–803.

Hofmeister, E., Peroni, J.F., and Fisher, A.T. Jr. (2008). Effects of carbon dioxide insufflation and body position on blood gas values in horses anesthetized for laparoscopy. *Journal of Equine Veterinary Science* 28 (9): 549–553.

Holzer, A., Jirecek, S.T., Illievich, U.M. et al. (2006). Laparoscopic versus open myomectomy: a double-blind study to evaluate postoperative pain. *Anesthesia & Analgesia* 102 (5): 1480–1484.

Hopster, K., Kästner, S.B., Rohn, K., and Ohnesorge, B. (2011). Intermittent positive pressure ventilation with constant positive end-expiratory pressure and alveolar recruitment manoeuvre during inhalation anaesthesia in horses undergoing surgery for colic, and its influence on the early recovery period. *Veterinary Anaesthesia and Analgesia* 38 (3): 169–177.

Hubbell, J.A. (1999). Recovery from anaesthesia in horses. *Equine Veterinary Education* 11 (3): 160–167.

Hubbell, J.A., Muir, W.W., and Sams, R.A. (1980). Guaifenesin: cardiopulmonary effects and plasma concentrations in horses. *American Journal of Veterinary Research* 41 (11): 1751–1755.

Ikechebelu, J.I., Obi, R.A., Udigwe, G.O., and Joe-Ikechebelu, N.N. (2005). Comparison of carbon dioxide and room air pneumoperitoneum for day-case diagnostic laparoscopy. *Journal of Obstetrics and Gynaecology* 25 (2): 172–173.

Ilkiw, J.E. (1999). Balanced anesthetic techniques in dogs and cats. *Clinical Techniques in Small Animal Practice* 14 (1): 27–37.

Joyce, J. and Hendrickson, D.A. (2006). Comparison of intraoperative pain responses following intratesticular or mesorchial injection of lidocaine in standing horses undergoing laparoscopic cryptorchidectomy. *Journal of the American Veterinary Medical Association* 229 (11): 1779–1783.

Kaloo, P., Armstrong, S., Kaloo, C., and Jordan, V. (2019). Interventions to reduce shoulder pain following gynaecological laparoscopic procedures. *Cochrane Database of Systematic Reviews* 1 (1): 1–124.

Kelleher, M.E., Brosnan, R.J., Kass, P.H., and le Jeune, S.S. (2013). Use of physiologic and arterial blood gas variables to predict short-term survival in horses with large colon volvulus. *Veterinary Surgery* 42 (1): 107–113.

Keoughan, C.G., Rodgerson, D.H., and Brown, M.P. (2003). Hand-assisted laparoscopic left nephrectomy in standing horses. *Veterinary Surgery* 32 (3): 206–212.

Khanna, A.K., McDonell, W.N., Dyson, D.H., and Taylor, P.M. (1995). Cardiopulmonary effects of hypercapnia during controlled intermittent positive pressure ventilation in the horse. *Canadian Journal of Veterinary Research* 59 (3): 213.

Klohnen, A. and Peroni, J.F. (2000). Thoracoscopy in Horses. In: *Veterinary Clinics of North America: Equine Practice*, (eds. A.S. Turner and D.A. Hendrickson), 351–362. Philadelphia: WB Saunders.

Knych, H.K., Seminoff, K., McKemie, D.S., and Kass, P.H. (2018). Pharmacokinetics, pharmacodynamics, and metabolism of acepromazine following intravenous, oral, and sublingual administration to exercised thoroughbred horses. *Journal of Veterinary Pharmacology and Therapeutics* 41(4): 522–535.

Knych, H.K., Mama, K.R., Moore, C.E. et al. (2019). Plasma and synovial fluid concentrations and cartilage toxicity of bupivacaine following intra-articular administration of a liposomal formulation to horses. *Equine Veterinary Journal* 51(3): 408–414.

Koch, D.W., Easley, J.T., Hatzel, J.N. et al. (2020). Prospective randomized investigation of topical anesthesia during unilateral laparoscopic ovariectomy in horses. *Veterinary Surgery* 49: O54–O59.

Koenig, J., McDonell, W., and Valverde, A. (2003). Accuracy of pulse oximetry and capnography in healthy and compromised horses during spontaneous and controlled ventilation. *Canadian Journal of Veterinary Research* 67(3): 169.

Laverty, S., Lavoie, J.P., Pascoe, J.R., and Ducharme, N. (1996). Penetrating wounds of the thorax in 15 horses. *Equine Veterinary Journal* 28(3): 220–224.

Leece, E.A., Corletto, F., and Brearley, J.C. (2008). A comparison of recovery times and characteristics with sevoflurane and isoflurane anaesthesia in horses undergoing magnetic resonance imaging. *Veterinary Anaesthesia and Analgesia* 35(5): 383–391.

Leinonen, V., Vanninen, R., and Rauramaa, T. (2018). Raised intracranial pressure and brain edema. In: *Handbook of Clinical Neurology* (eds. G.G. Kovacs and I. Alafuzoff), vol. 145, 25–37. Elsevier.

Lohser, J. and Slinger, P. (2015). Lung injury after one-lung ventilation: a review of the pathophysiologic mechanisms affecting the ventilated and the collapsed lung. *Anesthesia & Analgesia* 121(2): 302–318.

Love, E.J., Geoffrey, L.J., and Murison, P.J. (2006). Morphine administration in horses anaesthetized for upper respiratory tract surgery. *Veterinary Anaesthesia and Analgesia* 33(3): 179–188.

Lund, C.M., Ragle, C.A., and Lutter, J.D. (2013). Laparoscopic removal of a bladder urolith in a standing horse. *Journal of the American Veterinary Medical Association* 243(9): 1323–1328.

MacEachern, K.E., Smith, G.L., and Nolan, A.M. (2004). Characteristics of the in vitro hypoxic pulmonary vasoconstrictor response in isolated equine and bovine pulmonary arterial rings. *Veterinary Anaesthesia and Analgesia* 31(4): 239–249.

Mama, K.R., Pascoe, P.J., Steffey, E.P. (1993). Evaluation of the interaction of mu and kappa opioid agonists on locomotor behavior in the horse. *Canadian Journal of Veterinary Research* 57(2): 106–109.

Marntell, S., Nyman, G., and Hedenstierna, G. (2005). High inspired oxygen concentrations increase intrapulmonary shunt in anaesthetized horses. *Veterinary Anaesthesia and Analgesia* 32(6): 338–347.

Marroum, P.J., Webb, A.I., Aeschbacher, G., and Curry, S.H. (1994). Pharmacokinetics and pharmacodynamics of acepromazine in horses. *American Journal of Veterinary Research* 55(10): 1428–1433.

Mason, D.E., Muir, W.W., and Wade, A. (1987). Arterial blood gas tensions in the horse during recovery from anesthesia. *Journal of the American Veterinary Medical Association* 190(8): 989–994.

Matthews, N.S., Peck, K.E., Mealey, K.L. et al. (1997). Pharmacokinetics and cardiopulmonary effects of guaifenesin in donkeys. *Journal of Veterinary Pharmacology and Therapeutics* 20(6): 442–446.

Matthews, N.S., Hartsfield, S.M., Mercer, D. et al. (1998). Recovery from sevoflurane anesthesia in horses: comparison to isoflurane and effect of postmedication with xylazine. *Veterinary Surgery* 27(5): 480–485.

Mayhew, P.D. and Friedberg, J.S. (2008). Video-assisted thoracoscopic resection of noninvasive thymomas using one-lung ventilation in two dogs. *Veterinary Surgery* 37(8): 756–762.

Mayhew, P.D., Culp, W.T., Pascoe, P.J. et al. (2012). Evaluation of blind thoracoscopic-assisted placement of three double-lumen endobronchial tube designs for one-lung ventilation in dogs. *Veterinary Surgery* 41(6): 664–670.

McCracken, M.J., Schumacher, J., Doherty, T.J. et al. (2020). Efficacy and duration of effect for liposomal bupivacaine when administered perineurally to the palmar digital nerves of horses. *American Journal of Veterinary Research* 81(5): 400–405.

Michou, J. and Leece, E. (2012). Sedation and analgesia in the standing horse 1. Drugs used for sedation and systemic analgesia. *In Practice* 34(9): 524–531.

Mircica, E., Clutton, R.E., Kyles, K.W., and Blissitt, K.J. (2003). Problems associated with perioperative morphine in horses: a retrospective case analysis. *Veterinary Anaesthesia and Analgesia* 30(3): 147–155.

Muir, W.W. and Hubbell, J.A.E. (2009). *Equine Anesthesia: Monitoring and Emergency Therapy*, 2e. Philadelphia, PA: Elsevier, Saunders.

Natalini, C.C. and Linardi, R.L. (2006). Analgesic effects of epidural administration of hydromorphone in horses. *American Journal of Veterinary Research* 67(1): 11–15.

Neuhaus, S.J., Gupta, A., and Watson, D.I. (2001). Helium and other alternative insufflation gases for laparoscopy. *Surgical Endoscopy* 15(6): 553–560.

Nickel, J.C., Jain, P., Shore, N. et al. (2012). Continuous intravesical lidocaine treatment for interstitial cystitis/bladder pain syndrome: safety and efficacy of a new drug delivery device. *Science Translational Medicine* 4(143): 143ra100.

Palmer, S.E. (1993). Standing laparoscopic laser technique for ovariectomy in five mares. *Journal of the American Veterinary Medical Association* 203(2): 279–283.

Penha, A., Machado, T., Silva, l., and Zoppa, A. (2008). Pneumothorax induced by controlled, continuous CO_2 infusion in horses: clinical evaluation. *Ars Veterinaria* 23(3): 120–124.

Pequito, M., Amory, H., de Moffarts, B. et al. (2013). Evaluation of acepromazine-induced hemodynamic alterations and reversal with norepinephrine infusion in standing horses. *The Canadian Veterinary Journal* 54 (2): 150.

Portier, K., Crouzier, D., Guichardant, M. et al. (2009). Effects of high and low inspired fractions of oxygen on horse erythrocyte membrane properties, blood viscosity and muscle oxygenation during anaesthesia. *Veterinary Anaesthesia and Analgesia* 36(4): 287–298.

Read, M.R., Read, E.K., Duke, T., and Wilson, D.G. (2002). Cardiopulmonary effects and induction and recovery characteristics of isoflurane and sevoflurane in foals. *Journal of the American Veterinary Medical Association* 221(3): 393–398.

Relave, F., David, F., Leclere, M. et al. (2008). Evaluation of a thoracoscopic technique using ligating loops to obtain large lung biopsies in standing healthy and heaves-affected horses. *Veterinary Surgery* 37(3): 232–240.

Rezende, M.L., Grimsrud, K.N., Stanley, S.D. et al. (2015). Pharmacokinetics and pharmacodynamics of intravenous dexmedetomidine in the horse. *Journal of Veterinary Pharmacology and Therapeutics* 38(1): 15–23.

Roberge, C.W. and McEwen, M. (1998). The effects of local anesthetics on postoperative pain. *AORN Journal* 68(6): 1003–1012.

Robinson, E.P. and Natalini, C.C. (2002). Epidural anesthesia and analgesia in horses. *The Veterinary Clinics of North America. Equine Practice* 18(1): 61–82.

Rodríguez-Torres, J., Lucena-Aguilera, M.D., Cabrera-Martos, I. et al. (2019). Musculoskeletal signs associated with shoulder pain in patients undergoing video-assisted thoracoscopic surgery. *Pain Medicine* 20(10): 1997–2003.

Russell, T. and Pollock, P.J. (2012). Local anesthesia and hydro-distension to facilitate cystic calculus removal in horses. *Veterinary Surgery* 41(5): 638–642.

Sano, H., Martin-Flores, M., Santos, L.C. et al. (2011). Effects of epidural morphine on gastrointestinal transit in unmedicated horses. *Veterinary Anaesthesia and Analgesia* 38(2): 121–126.

Schambourg, M.M. and Marcoux, M. (2006). Laparoscopic intestinal exploration and full-thickness intestinal biopsy in standing horses: a pilot study. *Veterinary Surgery* 35(7): 689 696.

Schauvliege, S., Binetti, A., Duchateau, L. et al. (2018). Cardiorespiratory effects of a 7° reverse Trendelenburg position in anaesthetized horses: a randomized clinical trial. *Veterinary Anaesthesia and Analgesia* 45(5): 648–657.

Schisler, T. and Lohser, J. (2019). Clinical management of one-lung ventilation. In: *Principles and Practice of Anesthesia for Thoracic Surgery*, (ed. P. Slinger) 107–129. New York: Springer.

Sellon, D.C, Monroe, V.L. Roberts, M.C. Papich, M.G. (2001) Pharmacokinetics and adverse effects of butorphanol administered by single intravenous injection or continuous intravenous infusion in horses. *American Journal of Veterinary Research* 62(2): 183–189.

Singh, B. (2017). *Dyce, Sack, and Wensing's Textbook of Veterinary Anatomy*, 5e. Philadelphia, PA: Elsevier, Saunders.

Skarda, R.T. (1994). Caudal analgesia induced by epidural or subarachnoid administration of detomidine hydrochloride solution in mares. *American Journal of Veterinary Research* 55(5): 670–680.

Skrzypczak, H., Reed, R., Barletta, M. et al. (2020). A retrospective evaluation of the effect of perianesthetic hydromorphone administration on the incidence of postanesthetic signs of colic in horses. *Veterinary Anaesthesia and Analgesia* 47(6): 757–762.

Steffey, E.P., Wheat, J.D., Meagher, D.M. et al. (1977). Body position and mode of ventilation influences arterial pH, oxygen, and carbon dioxide tensions in halothane-anesthetized horses. *American Journal of Veterinary Research* 38(3): 379–382.

Steffey, E.P., Mama, K.R., Brosnan, R.J. et al. (2009). Effect of administration of propofol and xylazine hydrochloride on recovery of horses after four hours of anesthesia with desflurane. *American Journal of Veterinary Research* 70(8): 956–963.

Testa, M., Raffe, M.R., and Robinson, E.P. (1990). Evaluation of 25%, 50%, and 67% nitrous oxide with halothane-oxygen for general anesthesia in horses. *Veterinary Surgery* 19(4): 308–312.

Tünsmeyer, J., Hopster, K., Feige, K., and Kästner, S.B. (2015). Agreement of high definition oscillometry with direct arterial blood pressure measurement at different blood pressure ranges in horses under general anaesthesia. *Veterinary Anaesthesia and Analgesia* 42(3): 286–291.

Valente, A.C., Brosnan, R.J., and Guedes, A.G. (2015). Desflurane and sevoflurane elimination kinetics and recovery quality in horses. *American Journal of Veterinary Research* 76(3): 201–207.

Valverde, A. (2010). Alpha-2 agonists as pain therapy in horses. *Veterinary Clinics: Equine Practice* 26(3): 515–532.

Valverde, A., Gunkel, C., Doherty, T.J. et al. (2005). Effect of a constant rate infusion of lidocaine on the quality of recovery from sevoflurane or isoflurane general anaesthesia in horses. *Equine Veterinary Journal* 37(6): 559–564.

Van Hoogmoed, L.M. and Galuppo, L.D. (2005). Laparoscopic ovariectomy using the endo-GIA stapling device and endo-catch pouches and evaluation of analgesic efficacy of epidural morphine sulfate in 10 mares. *Veterinary Surgery* 34(6): 646–650.

Van Oostrom, H., Schaap, M.W., and van Loon, J.P. (2017). Oxygen supplementation before induction of general anaesthesia in horses. *Equine Veterinary Journal* 49(1): 130–132.

Virgin, J., Hendrickson, D., Wallis, T., and Rao, S. (2010). Comparison of intraoperative behavioral and hormonal responses to noxious stimuli between mares sedated with caudal epidural detomidine hydrochloride or a continuous intravenous infusion of detomidine hydrochloride for standing laparoscopic ovariectomy. *Veterinary Surgery* 39(6): 754–760.

Wagner, A.E. and Bednarski, R.M. (1990). Hemodynamic effects of carbon dioxide during intermittent positive-pressure ventilation in horses. *American Journal of Veterinary Research* 51(12): 1922–1929.

Wilson, D.V., Schott, H.C. II, Robinson, N.E. et al. (2006). Response to nasopharyngeal oxygen administration in horses with lung disease. *Equine Veterinary Journal* 38(3): 219–223.

Wittern, C., Hendrickson, D.A., Trumble, T., and Wagner, A. (1998). Complications associated with administration of detomidine into the caudal epidural space in a horse. *Journal of the American Veterinary Medical Association* 213(4): 516–518.

Wojtasiak-Wypart, M., Soma, L.R., Rudy, J.A. et al. (2012). Pharmacokinetic profile and pharmacodynamic effects of romifidine hydrochloride in the horse. *Journal of Veterinary Pharmacology and Therapeutics* 35(5): 478–488.

Woolf, C.J. and Chong, M.S. (1993). Preemptive analgesia – treating postoperative pain by preventing the establishment of central sensitization. *Anesthesia & Analgesia* 77 (2): 362–379.

10

Anesthetic Management for Gastrointestinal Diseases
Diana Hassel and Khursheed Mama

Department of Clinical Sciences, College of Veterinary Medicine and Biomedical Sciences, Colorado State University, 300 West Drake Road, Fort Collins, CO, 80523, USA

Introduction

Gastrointestinal (GI) tract disease is among the most common reason to require general anesthesia on an urgent basis where time is of the essence for patient survival. The GI tract plays a vital role in fluid homeostasis, electrolyte balance, and nutrient acquisition both primarily and via fermentative processes. Most forms of injury to the equine GI tract will present hurdles for anesthetic management prior to induction, intraoperatively, and in the post-operative recovery period. This chapter will provide an overview of general considerations for the surgical GI equine patient as well as special considerations for specific GI diseases including esophageal obstruction, non-strangulating GI obstructions, strangulating obstructions, and conditions associated with septic processes.

General Considerations

In preparation for anesthesia of any horse or foal with surgical disease of the GI tract, there are several general considerations that apply that can impact the methods chosen for premedication, induction, anesthesia maintenance, and recovery. These include age, breed, gender, clinical examination findings, clinical pathological findings, presence of GI or stomach distension, level of pain, sedatives or analgesics available, exertion, fluid losses, electrolyte deficits, acid–base status, unique handling situations, and presence of pre-existing therapeutic agents administered both preoperatively and intraoperatively.

Signalment

The age of the foal or horse should be considered in the anesthetic planning process. Specific recommendations for anesthesia of the neonate can be found in Chapter 13 and those for the geriatric horse in Chapter 11. Breed considerations relative to temperament and body mass are important considerations with any anesthetic event, but even more so with horses with ischemic GI disease due to the prolonged nature of both the surgical procedure and recovery, as well as the accompanying systemic compromise. For example, utilizing alpha-2 agonists or other sedatives in the recovery period may be more likely in light breed horses prone to excitation such as some Arabian horses. Conversely, large draft breeds are more predisposed to difficulty standing during recovery from anesthesia due to development of myopathies or neuropathies (Rothenbuhler et al. 2006) and tools to assist them to stand such as a sling or the Large

Animal Lift (Large Animal Lift Enterprises LLC, Moses Lake, WA) may be necessary. Efforts toward reducing anesthesia duration in draft horses such as pre-surgical clipping of the abdomen are ideal to minimize time under general anesthesia. Gender considerations do not differ from elective anesthetic procedures, but in an emergency situation, these considerations may be overlooked such as potentially avoiding the use of acepromazine in breeding stallions (Wagner 2009); special considerations for anesthetic management of the pregnant mare may be found in Chapter 12.

Assessment of the Acute GI patient

A variety of procedures are commonly performed during assessment of the acute GI patient that can directly impact the anesthetic period. Physical examination parameters will include assessment of presence of dehydration through mucous membrane texture and skin turgor along with presence of hypovolemia by assessment of heart rate, mucous membrane color, capillary refill time, pulse quality from the facial artery, jugular refill time, temperature of extremities, mentation, and urine output. Stabilization of the pre-anesthetic patient with hypovolemia will be critical to success as most horses undergoing surgery for GI disease are positioned in dorsal recumbency, placing them at increased risk for hypotension and hypoxemia, even in the absence of pre-existing hypovolemia.

Other parameters including packed cell volume (PCV), total protein (TP), and lactate in peripheral blood, provide more critical quantitative estimates of anemia, dehydration, hypovolemia, and poor circulation. Elevations in PCV and lactate in the preoperative period are associated with reduced probability of survival, particularly in the presence of relatively low peripheral TP in horses with surgical disease of the small intestine (Proudman et al. 2005). Decreases in TP and colloid oncotic pressure associated with anesthesia (Boscan et al. 2007), and continued intravascular losses associated with increases in endothelial permeability

secondary to the systemic inflammatory response syndrome (SIRS) can further compromise the patient. Further, the use of synthetic colloids to promote intravascular volume support remains controversial due to increased risks relative to renal dysfunction and mortality in septic and critically ill human patients (Adamik et al. 2015). Convincing experimental studies and clinical investigations documenting this in equine and more broadly veterinary patients are however lacking.

Further initial assessment and therapeutic actions common in equine acute GI patients include abdominocentesis, passage of a nasogastric tube, and transcutaneous decompression of distended large intestine that may facilitate ventilation and improve oxygenation during the induction and early anesthetic period.

Gastric or Abdominal Distension

Gastric distention with fluid, gas, or feed material is a common finding in the adult acute surgical GI patient. Passage of a nasogastric tube (Figure 10.1) prior to induction of anesthesia is paramount to reducing the potential for aspiration pneumonia or the risk of gastric rupture upon induction. Presence of gastric distention may also exacerbate existing increases in intra-abdominal pressure (Barrett et al. 2013).

Generalized distention of the abdomen may result from a variety of sources, most commonly from gas accumulation within the ascending colon and cecum. However, fluid distention of small intestine, colon, or the peritoneal cavity may also contribute to generalized abdominal distention and increases in intra-abdominal pressure. Intra-abdominal hypertension and its sequelae have been documented in the horse (Brosnahan et al. 2009) and horses with GI obstruction are at particularly high risk. Abdominal distension presents not only challenges with ventilation and oxygenation, but the presence of intra-abdominal hypertension has the potential to contribute to hemodynamic derangements and multiple organ dysfunction (Roberts et al. 2016). Both transabdominal and transrectal trocarization

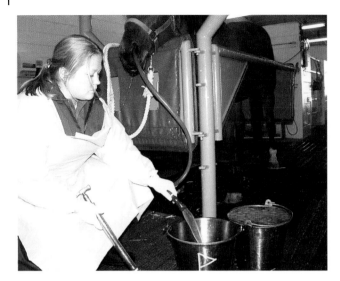

Figure 10.1 Placement of a nasogastric tube to reduce stomach contents and minimize gastric rupture or fluid aspiration during anesthesia induction.

in the preoperative period have been advocated as a method to decompress the abdomen in horses with severe large intestinal distension, as clinically relevant peritonitis is rare in those cases undergoing surgical exploration following trocarization (Schoster et al. 2020).

Pain

Many horses with surgical disease of the abdomen present in extreme pain making them fractious and sometimes difficult to stabilize in the preoperative period. Extreme pain may also make them refractory to sedation resulting in receipt of multiple doses of sedatives and analgesics such as xylazine, detomidine, and butorphanol. Compounding the situation is the need for rapid correction of the problem, as rapid correction of an ischemic process such as a colonic volvulus or a strangulating small intestinal lesion can markedly improve prognosis. General anesthesia must take place quickly to accomplish treatment of the underlying disease that may increase risk for anesthetic errors or result in insufficient volume resuscitation prior to induction. Interestingly, a large retrospective study correlated increased risk of intraoperative mortality with horses demonstrating less severe signs on pain on admission. This was attributed to either advanced devitalization of bowel since pain

can subside as ischemia advances, or delays in surgical intervention due to less obvious signs of pain (Proudman et al. 2006).

Exertion, Exhaustion, Trauma

Depending on the duration and severity of disease, horses with surgical abdominal lesions may present in a state of exhaustion with self-inflicted trauma from rolling and other colic-associated behaviors. This may manifest in the recovery period as a prolonged anesthetic recovery and reluctance or inability to stand in the postoperative period. This may be further influenced by high doses of drug received peri-operatively.

Anticipated Electrolyte and Acid/Base Imbalances

In addition to fluid losses from dehydration and hypovolemia for the more severe forms of surgical colic, there are anticipated changes in electrolyte concentrations in horses and foals with various forms of GI disease. The most common electrolyte disturbances identified in adult horses with surgical GI obstruction are hypomagnesemia, hypocalcemia, and hypokalemia.

The prevalence of total or ionized hypomagnesemia is reported to be 17–54% in horses with GI disease (Garcia-Lopez et al. 2001; Johansson et al. 2003). Magnesium is the second most abundant intracellular cation behind potassium and plays a critical role in over 300 enzymatic reactions involving ATP (Elin 1988). Hypomagnesemia is associated with increased cytokine production and systemic inflammation (Weglicki et al. 1992), and experimental endotoxin administration in horses results in acute decreases in both ionized and total magnesium concentrations (Toribio et al. 2005). Hypomagnesemia is concurrently observed with hypocalcemia in several GI diseases in horses (Garcia-Lopez et al. 2001; Toribio et al. 2001, 2005), and it is also frequently observed with hypokalemia in other species (Martin et al. 1994). The presence of hypomagnesemia may make patients refractory to treatment of both hypocalcemia and hypokalemia until serum magnesium concentrations are corrected (al-Ghamdi et al. 1994). This may place the patient at higher risk of post-operative ileus (Garcia-Lopez et al. 2001). Clinical signs of hypomagnesemia in horses that could have direct impact on anesthesia may include weakness, ataxia, ventricular arrhythmias, supraventricular tachycardia, atrial fibrillation, and seizures (Green et al. 1935; Marr 2004).

Hypokalemia in horses with GI disease is prevalent and believed to be associated with reduced intake, altered absorption, or excessive losses from secretory processes such as enteritis or colitis (Nappert and Johnson 2001). A whole-body deficit of potassium is expected in anorectic horses with surgical GI disease and consequences may include skeletal muscle weakness, paralysis, irregularities of cardiac rhythm, perturbed intestinal motility, and abnormal acid–base status (Johnson 1995). Restoration of potassium levels intraoperatively at a rate not to exceed 0.5 mEq/kg/h is appropriate. Rarely, hyperkalemia may be observed in the peri-operative equine GI patient and could be associated with intravascular hemolysis, severe metabolic acidosis, hyperkalemic periodic paralysis, severe myopathies, or malignant hyperthermia. Presence of serum hyperkalemia should be rapidly addressed with intravenous calcium, bicarbonate, or glucose and insulin to avoid fatal cardiac arrhythmias.

Hypocalcemia is associated with conditions commonly present in horses with surgical GI disease including colic, sepsis, endotoxemia, and acute renal failure. Signs of acute hypocalcemia may include muscle fasciculations, tremors, tetany, seizures, tachycardia, and cardiac arrhythmias. Hypocalcemia may also compound the development of ileus and can be addressed via supplementation intraoperatively at a dose of 50–100 ml of 23% calcium gluconate per 5 l volume of isotonic crystalloid (Johnson 1995). Fluid rates must be adjusted for the patient's body weight to deliver 10–30 mg/kg over 30–60 minutes.

The presence of both metabolic and respiratory acidosis during anesthesia is higher in colicky horses compared with controls (Edner et al. 2007), although significant reductions in serum bicarbonate at the time of presentation were not evident in horses that recovered from their colic episode (Nappert and Johnson 2001). Volume repletion should precede any attempts to correct a metabolic acidosis with bicarbonate therapy as the majority of surgical GI cases with metabolic acidosis suffer from impaired perfusion and accumulation of lactate. Intra-abdominal hypertension secondary to presence of gas or fluid accumulation in the GI tract, thoracic cavity (from diaphragmatic hernia), or peritoneal cavity can result in impaired ventilation and subsequent respiratory acidosis, resulting in increased requirements for ventilatory support.

Peri-procedural Handling

Horses with acute GI disease can present unique challenges in the peri-operative period. Preoperatively, they may present recumbent in a trailer and unable to stand or in a violently painful state where they continually collapse due to unrelenting pain. Some may require induction at a site distant from the surgical suite followed by transport during which there is a limited ability to monitor and support the patient. The Large Animal Rescue Glide (L.A.R.G.E., Inman, SC) can facilitate rapid transport of a recumbent horse from a trailer to the surgical suite when adequate numbers of people are available to facilitate movement of the horse. Special considerations for these critical patients may entail safety concerns for clinicians during IV catheter placement, anesthetic death from inability to properly stabilize the patient prior to induction, and impaired ventilation and oxygenation during the transport period. Endotracheal intubation and support of oxygenation and ventilation should be considered in these circumstances, with recognition that in the absence of rinsing out the oral cavity, contaminants may enter the airway. Solutions (e.g. hypertonic saline) with potential for improving circulation after small volume administration should be considered once the catheter is in place.

For mares presenting with colonic volvulus or other surgical GI conditions that are accompanied by their foal, attention must be paid to the foal to prevent injury from the mare and to provide a safe environment while the mare is in surgery. Alternatively, mares must be handled appropriately when the foal needs to undergo emergency surgery. To optimize the effectiveness of induction drugs along with sedatives for the mare, the mare and foal ideally should not be separated until the time of induction. Heavy sedation may still be required. Intravenous or intramuscular alpha-2 agonists alone or in combination with acepromazine or an opioid may be used.

Another complication following surgery for acute, GI disease includes a prolonged anesthetic recovery period with weakness and the inability of the horse to stand. During the transition from anesthesia and through the early recovery period, insufflation of oxygen via the endotracheal tube or nasal passage is routine, however, assistance of ventilation with a demand valve may be necessary in some horses. Maintenance of airway patency in horses with nasopharyngeal edema resulting from recumbency, and occasional treatment of pulmonary edema as a consequence of hypoproteinemia and other causes may be necessary. Additional support including IV fluids and electrolytes may also be continued during

recovery. Finally, recovery assistance, whether with ropes or mechanical lift/sling, should be considered in a horse that is weak and where the risk of injury is perceived to be increased. For example, an older mare following a postpartum colonic volvulus may benefit from recovery assistance.

Pharmacologic Agents for Peri-operative Treatment

Several pharmacologic agents are commonly used in the peri-operative period for the management of GI disease that may have a direct impact on anesthesia. These are not limited to, but may include alpha-2 agonists, opioids (systemic and epidural), local anesthetics (applied topically, via regional blocks or systemically as a constant rate infusion), n-acetyl butylscopolamine (Buscopan), non-steroidal anti-inflammatory drugs (NSAIDs), antibiotics, polymyxin B (for anti-endotoxic effects) and phenylephrine. A list of these agents and their potential impact on anesthetic and physiologic parameters is provided in Table 10.1.

Intraoperative Pharmacologic Management of Hypotension

Hypotension is commonly encountered in the anesthetic management of horses with acute GI disease, as a combination of dehydration and hypovolemia is expected, especially in horses with strangulating obstructions. These patients are also at high risk for SIRS commonly accompanied by increased vascular permeability and reduced oncotic pressure due to loss of albumin with subsequent intravascular fluid losses. In addition to fluid and electrolyte therapy as mentioned previously, inotropes and vasopressors are often required to maintain normotension and organ perfusion. Dobutamine (0.5–2 (3) µg/kg/min) is the most commonly selected inotrope as it works to combat decreases in myocardial contractility and resulting hypotension caused by inhaled anesthetics with minimal side effects when appropriately dosed (Ohta et al. 2013). While dobutamine may be diluted and gravity dripped, precise delivery using a syringe or fluid pump to ensure accurate dosing

Table 10.1 Pharmacologic agents commonly administered in the peri-operative period to horses undergoing surgical treatment of gastrointestinal disease and their potential physiologic impact.

Pharmacologic agent	Physiologic impact
Alpha-2 Adrenergic Agonists (e.g. xylazine, detomidine, romifidine)	Xylazine results in a transient increase in blood pressure followed by a decrease. It results in a decrease in heart rate and may potentiate first- and second-degree AV block (Morton et al. 2011). Other drugs in this class have similar actions but duration of these will vary. Alpha-2 adrenergic agonists produce sedation, analgesia, and muscle relaxation and decrease the requirement for anesthetic drugs.
Opioids – systemic or epidural (e.g. butorphanol, morphine)	Systemic morphine contributes to depression of gastrointestinal motility and gastric distension (Tessier et al. 2019) with prolonged gastrointestinal transit times even when administered epidurally (Sano et al. 2011). Opioids provide good analgesia but may produce excitement, agitation, and increased locomotor activity at higher dosages (Mama et al. 1993). They facilitate sedation in horses refractory to the alpha-2 agonists and are increasingly used for management of pain during recovery.
Local anesthetics – systemic or topical (e.g. lidocaine)	Lidocaine is frequently administered intraoperatively to reduce anesthetic inhalant requirements and in the post-operative period as a CRI (50 µg /kg/min) for its purported analgesic, anti-inflammatory and prokinetic effects (Cook et al. 2009a; Doherty and Frazier 1998). While other local anesthetics (e.g. bupivacaine) may be used regionally, their intravenous use is not advised due to significant cardiovascular side effects.
N-acetyl-butylscopolamine	Buscopan is an antispasmodic with anticholinergic effects used to treat spasmodic colic with a duration of action of 20–30 minutes. It results in an elevation in blood pressure and heart rate that can complicate physiologic assessment of pain (Hector and Mama 2018; Morton et al. 2011).
NSAIDs (e.g. flunixin meglumine, firocoxib)	NSAIDs are a prominent component of therapy in the peri-operative GI patient but have nephrotoxic effects that are exacerbated by pre-existing dehydration and hypovolemia. Nonspecific COX inhibition (e.g. flunixin) may impair mucosal recovery in ischemic-injured jejunum (Cook et al. 2009b).
Antibiotics (e.g. penicillin, aminoglycosides, fluroquinolones, cephalosporins)	Broad spectrum antibiotics are indicated prior to anesthesia for gastrointestinal disease, with penicillin and gentamicin used most commonly. Gentamicin has the potential to enhance neuromuscular blockade and cardiovascular depression under anesthesia and has nephrotoxic effects that should be considered in hypovolemic or dehydrated patients (Robertson and Scicluna 2009). Ataxia has been reported with rapid IV bolus administration of fluroquinolones (Bertone et al. 1998)
Polymyxin B	Polymyxin B has known nephrotoxic and neurotoxic effects including neuromuscular blockade, but these effects have not been reported in horses perhaps because doses used for endotoxemia are lower than antimicrobial uses. Primary concern is potential nephrotoxicity in uremic GI patients.

(Continued)

Table 10.1 (Continued)

Pharmacologic agent	Physiologic impact
Phenylephrine	A dose of 3 µg/kg/min for 15 minutes has been used to shrink splenic size in horses presenting with nephrosplenic entrapment. While splenic size is reported to shrink, success of non-surgical treatment (which can include jogging or rolling under anesthesia) is not uniform (Fultz et al. 2013; Pye and Nieto 2020). Bradycardia and hypertension are expected sequelae. Hypertension associated fatal bleeding has been reported in older horses (Frederick et al. 2010).

and minimize side effects is preferred. If tachycardia or tachydysrhythmias are observed following administration, a decrease in the dose is recommended. This response may indicate the horse is hypovolemic. In horses with severe hypovolemia or vasodilation resulting from sepsis or endotoxemia, drugs with predominantly alpha effects such as phenylephrine (0.25–1.0 µg/kg/min) may be utilized transiently in addition to fluid therapy (Ohta et al. 2013). Heart rate should be monitored as this may slow as blood pressure increases; this is commonly observed and may result in fatal hemorrhage (in older horses) when phenylephrine is administered (at higher doses) to the awake horse in an effort to reduce splenic size as noted previously (Frederick et al. 2010). While the increase in blood pressure is desirable, it is possible to compromise perfusion (due to vasoconstriction) with increasing doses. Considered use of dobutamine and phenylephrine together can be beneficial in this circumstance. Other vasoactive medications (e.g. dopamine, norepinephrine) have specific indications and the interested reader is referred to additional references (Craig et al. 2007; Lee et al. 1998; Swanson et al. 1985).

Case Management Example

Sixteen-year-old Thoroughbred mare weighing approximately 550 kg presents six weeks post partem with a foal at her side. She was found rolling two hours prior. Following initial evaluation on the farm and administration of 7 mg

detomidine and 500 mg flunixin intravenously, the mare and foal were loaded onto the trailer and presented to your surgical referral facility.

Upon presentation, the mare is difficult to keep standing, her heart rate is 88 beats per minute, respiratory rate is 46 breaths per minute, and you note marked abdominal distention. Gas distended bowel is palpated on brief rectal examination. Limited fluid is obtained from the nasogastric tube. An intravenous catheter is placed, and blood is collected for PCV, TP, venous pH, blood gases, electrolytes, lactate, and acid–base assessment. The PCV is 53%, TP 7.6 g/dl, pH 7.19, PvCO$_2$ 54 mmHg, PvO$_2$ 28 mmHg, K$^+$ 3.1 mEq/l, Ca^{2+} 1.24 mmol/l, Lactate 7.9 mmol/l, HCO$_3^-$ 20 mmol/l, BE – 4 mmol/l.

The mare is given 5 mg detomidine and 5 mg butorphanol IV to facilitate administration of 1 l of 7% hypertonic saline and 5 l of balanced crystalloid solution via a fluid pump as her abdomen is clipped in preparation for surgery. A colon volvulus is suspected. Antibiotics are also administered, and the mouth is rinsed. The foal is removed and sedated with 50 mg (approximately 1 mg/kg) IM xylazine. A decision on whether to leave the foal at the hospital or return to the farm is pending the outcome of the mare; food and water to be provided to the foal once sedation wears off.

Anesthesia is induced IV with guaifenesin (~25 mg/kg), midazolam (0.05 mg/kg), and ketamine (1 mg/kg) after the nasogastric tube is "uncorked." The mare is intubated in sternal recumbency and the demand valve used to administer intermittent breaths. The pulse is palpated prior to moving the horse and anesthetic depth assessed using ocular signs. The mare is transported to the operating room and hoisted onto the table in dorsal recumbency. She is immediately connected to an oxygen primed anesthesia machine and following assessment of her depth and with accounting for her disease, the sevoflurane is set at 2.5%. Intermittent breaths are provided (approximately 2 per minute) while support and monitoring equipment are connected.

These initially include an electrocardiogram, arterial catheter for direct blood pressure assessment, pulse oximeter, capnograph, IV fluids administered via a fluid pump, and a thermistor. An additional catheter is placed to allow for additional administration of gravity dripped fluids and additives. Based on preoperative values, 50 ml of 23% calcium gluconate and 80 mEq of potassium chloride (20 mEq already present in the bag) were added to the 5 l gravity drip bag. The surgeons are encouraged to scrub and prepare the surgical table to facilitate rapid intervention to relieve the abdominal distention.

Blood pressure readings were initially acceptable with a mean of 88 mmHg, but, following ventilation at 4 breaths per minute to an inspiratory pressure of 28 cm H_2O, this decreased to a mean of 62 mmHg, so dobutamine was initiated at 1 µg/kg/min via a syringe pump. A lidocaine infusion was also initiated at 50 µg/kg/min.

With dobutamine and surgical stimulation the mean arterial pressure rose to 68–72 mmHg. Following relieving of the gas in the cecum and exteriorization of the colon blood was again collected for assessment of previously described values. Adjustments to supportive medications, ventilation, and fluids are made based on these values which are periodically checked through the anesthesia period. Surgeons proceed to perform a pelvic flexure enterotomy and determine a resection is not needed. After complete exploration they begin closing the abdomen. The lidocaine is discontinued, and recovery stall is prepared. Oxygen for insufflation via the endotracheal tube is set up as well as towels to help dry the mare. The demand valve is also available if needed. In this case, it is decided to use ropes to assist the mare so 1 µg/kg dexmedetomidine is available in case of a need to sedate the mare while this is being set up

A final blood sample is obtained prior to disconnection of the anesthesia machine. The mare is administered 50 mg morphine intramuscularly at the conclusion of surgery. The nasogastric tube is removed once the mare is in lateral recumbency, and diluted phenylephrine is administered into each nasal passage. The tube is secured for recovery, and the decision is made to leave it in place until the mare is standing. The foal is kept on site and resedated during the mare's recovery in case its whinny triggers the mare to try stand to prior to her being ready.

Esophageal Obstruction

Diseases of the esophagus include esophageal obstruction, laceration, stricture, diverticula formation, megaesophagus, muscular hypertrophy, and a variety of congenital conditions. The most common disorder is esophageal obstruction or "choke" and will be the focus of this section. Choke is most frequently caused by feed impaction and may be complicated by functional neuromuscular disorders or anatomic abnormalities such as stenosis, stricture, diverticula, neoplasia, abscess formation, or cysts (Chiavaccini and Hassel 2010). Early clinical features of esophageal obstruction include distress, coughing, and nasal discharge containing feed material or saliva. Initial attempts to relieve the obstruction may be performed in the sedated horse. Consideration must be given to the potential for worsening respiratory difficulty with drugs used for sedation and obstruction of the nostril with passage of the naso-esophageal tube or endoscope. Nasal oxygen supplementation may be warranted in some circumstances. A balance between sufficient sedation to complete the procedure and minimizing side effects is key. Maintaining pharyngeal function such that the horse is able to protect its airway is also paramount. Drugs such as acepromazine which serve as tranquilizers often allow for a reduction in the alpha-2 dose needed and may have benefit. The influence of sedative and anesthetic medications on esophageal tone and motility is not well studied.

As duration of obstruction extends, the horse will become compromised due to dehydration, acid–base and electrolyte imbalances, and potential aspiration pneumonia. Risk for development of aspiration pneumonia is increased in horses younger than 1 year of age, older than 15 years of age, in horses with tachypnea, in those with moderate or severe tracheal contamination identified via endoscopy, and in horses undergoing general anesthesia for treatment of the obstruction (Chiavaccini and Hassel 2010). As with the scenario of the horse requiring anesthesia for colic surgery, managing dehydration, acid–base, and electrolytes is important. An animal with aspiration may face challenges with hypoxemia during recumbency. The anesthetist

should be prepared to intervene whether through supplementation of oxygen, intubation, ventilation, and adjunctive modalities (recruitment maneuvers, positive end-expiratory pressure, use of bronchodilators, etc.). The use of an endotracheal tube to protect the airway and the ability to suction the airway can be helpful.

Non-strangulating Obstructions of the Gastrointestinal Tract

Non-strangulating obstructions of the GI tract may be mechanical or functional in nature and most commonly involve the small or large intestine. Examples of conditions leading to non-strangulating GI obstructions are listed in Table 10.2, including specific conditions more commonly seen in the neonatal foal. Gastric or abdominal distension is a common characteristic of most

Table 10.2 Common non-strangulating or inflammatory disorders of the small and large intestine in horses and foals.

Location	Age	Disorder
Small intestine	Neonate	Duodenal ulceration/gastric outflow disorders
	Juvenile	Ascarid impaction (Figure 10.2)
	Adult	Duodenitis/proximal jejunitis
		Eosinophilic enteritis or other infiltrative enteritis
		Neoplasia – adenocarcinoma, lymphoma
		Ileal impaction
Large intestine	Neonate	Meconium impaction
		Atresia coli/recti/ani
	Adult	Left dorsal colonic displacement
		Right dorsal colonic displacement
		Other large colon displacements
		Cecal or colonic feed impaction
		Foreign body obstruction
		Enterolithiasis
		Sand impaction
		Fecalith obstruction
		Spasmodic (gas) colic

Figure 10.2   Image showing ascarid impaction.

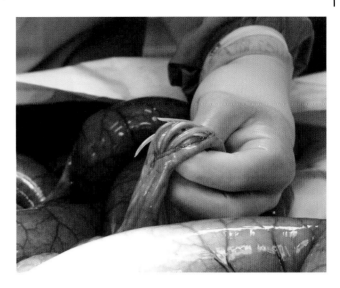

non-strangulating GI obstructions that can impact anesthetic management.

Strangulating Obstructions of the Gastrointestinal Tract and Conditions Causing Endotoxemia/SIRS/Sepsis

Strangulating obstructions most commonly involve either the small intestine or ascending colon, but the cecum and descending colon are also at risk. Ischemic injury (Figure 10.3) to the equine GI tract is particularly troubling as horses are exquisitely sensitive to endotoxin that is present in abundance in the intestinal lumen, so surgical cases are often accompanied by clinical evidence of SIRS. SIRS is a hallmark of sepsis and is characterized by systemic inflammation manifest by the presence of two or more of the following: (i) hyperthermia or hypothermia, (ii) tachycardia, (iii) tachypnea or hyperventilation, and (iv) leukopenia, leukocytosis, or >10% band neutrophils (Taylor 2015). A "toxic line" (Figure 10.4) may be observed when evaluating oral mucous

Figure 10.3   Devitalized bowel. Note the wire being grasped with the surgical instrument.

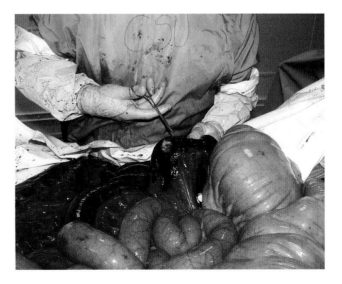

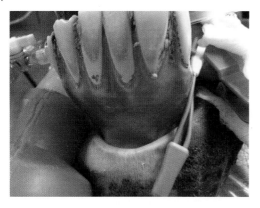

Figure 10.4 Image of oral mucus membranes with a "toxic line" in an anesthetized horse.

membranes. In addition, these patients are typically demonstrating extreme pain in combination with severe abdominal distension. Examples of conditions leading to SIRS in association with either strangulating GI obstruction or infectious disease processes are provided in Table 10.3.

Table 10.3 Common strangulating or infectious conditions affecting the gastrointestinal tract in adult horses that may be associated with SIRS.

Location	Disorder
Small intestine	Duodenitis/proximal jejunitis
	Strangulating lipoma
	Epiploic foramen entrapment
	Small intestinal volvulus
	Intussusception
	Mesenteric rent incarcerating small intestine
	Diaphragmatic hernia
Large intestine	Large colon volvulus
	Cecocecal or cecocolic intussusception
	Typhlocolitis, colitis, or typhlitis
	Infarction

Summary

Since GI disease presentations requiring anesthesia can be broad in their reach, beyond basic principles, the anesthetic plan should be directed at addressing the specific needs of the individual to maximize the chances for a favorable outcome.

References

Adamik, K.N., Yozova, I.D., and Regenscheit, N. (2015). Controversies in the use of hydroxyethyl starch solutions in small animal emergency and critical care. *Journal of Veterinary Emergency and Critical Care (San Antonio, Tex.)* 25: 20–47.

Barrett, E.J., Munsterman, A.S., and Hanson, R.R. (2013). Effects of gastric distension on intraabdominal pressures in horses. *Journal of Veterinary Emergency and Critical Care (San Antonio, Tex.)* 23: 423–428.

Bertone, A.L., Tremaine, W.H., Maccoris, D.G. et al. (1998). Effect of the chronic systemic administration of an injectable enrofloxacin solution on physical, musculoskeletal, and histologic parameters in adult horses.

Proceeding of the American Association of Equine Practitioners, pp. 252–253.

Boscan, P., Watson, Z., and Steffey, E.P. (2007). Plasma colloid osmotic pressure and total protein trends in horses during anesthesia. *Veterinary Anaesthesia and Analgesia* 34: 275–283.

Brosnahan, M.M., Holbrook, T.C., Gilliam, L.L. et al. (2009). Intra-abdominal hypertension in two adult horses. *Journal of Veterinary Emergency and Critical Care (San Antonio, Tex.)* 19: 174–180.

Chiavaccini, L. and Hassel, D.M. (2010). Clinical features and prognostic variables in 109 horses with esophageal obstruction (1992–2009).

Journal of Veterinary Internal Medicine 24: 1147–1152.

Cook, V.L., Jones Shults, J., McDowell, M.R. et al. (2009a). Anti-inflammatory effects of intravenously administered lidocaine hydrochloride on ischemia-injured jejunum in horses. *American Journal of Veterinary Research* 70: 1259–1268.

Cook, V.L., Meyer, C.T., Campbell, N.B., and Blikslager, A.T. (2009b). Effect of firocoxib or flunixin meglumine on recovery of ischemic-injured equine jejunum. *American Journal of Veterinary Research* 70: 992–1000.

Craig, C.A., Haskins, S.C., and Hildebrand, S.V. (2007). The cardiopulmonary effects of dobutamine and norepinephrine in isoflurane- anesthetized foals. *Veterinary Anaesthesia and Analgesia* 34: 377–387.

Doherty, T.J. and Frazier, D.L. (1998). Effect of intravenous lidocaine on halothane minimum alveolar concentration in ponies. *Equine Veterinary Journal* 30: 300–303.

Edner, A.H., Nyman, G.C., and Essen-Gustavsson, B. (2007). Metabolism before, during and after anesthesia in colic and healthy horses. *Acta Veterinaria Scandinavica* 49: 34.

Elin, R.J. (1988). Magnesium metabolism in health and disease. *Disease-a-Month* 34: 161–218.

Frederick, J., Guiguere, S., Butterworth, K. et al. (2010). Severe phenylephrine-associated hemorrhage in five aged horses. *Journal of the American Veterinary Medical Association* 237(7): 830–834.

Fultz, L.E., Peloso, J.G., Giguere, S., and Adams, A.R. (2013). Comparison of phenylephrine administration and exercise versus phenylephrine administration and a rolling procedure for the correction of nephrosplenic entrapment of the large colon in horses: 88 cases (2004–2010). *Journal of the American Veterinary Medical Association* 242(8): 1146–1151.

Garcia-Lopez, J.M., Provost, P.J., Rush, J.E. et al. (2001). Prevalence and prognostic importance of hypomagnesemia and hypocalcemia in horses that have colic surgery. *American Journal of Veterinary Research* 62: 7–12.

al-Ghamdi, S.M., Cameron, E.C., and Sutton, R.A. (1994). Magnesium deficiency: pathophysiologic and clinical overview. *American Journal of Kidney Diseases* 24: 737–752.

Green, H.H., Allcroft, W.M., and Montgomerie, R.F. (1935). Hypomagnesemia in equine transit tetany. *The Journal of Comparative Pathology and Therapeutics* 48: 74.

Hector, R.C. and Mama, K.R. (2018). Recognizing and treating pain in horses. In: *Equine Internal Medicine*, 138–157. St. Louis, Missouri: Elsevier.

Johansson, A.M., Gardner, S.Y., Jones, S.L. et al. (2003). Hypomagnesemia in hospitalized horses. *Journal of Veterinary Internal Medicine* 17: 860–867.

Johnson, P.J. (1995). Electrolyte and acid–base disturbances in the horse. *The Veterinary Clinics of North America. Equine Practice* 11: 491–514.

Lee, Y.H., Clarke, K.W., Alibhai, H.K., and Song, D. (1998). Effects of dopamine, dobutamine, dopexamine, phenylephrine and saline solution on intramuscular blood flow and other cardiopulmonary variables in halothane-anesthetized ponies. *American Journal of Veterinary Research* 59: 1463–1472.

Mama, K.R., Pascoe, P.J., and Steffey, E.P. (1993). Evaluation of the interaction of mu and kappa opioid agonists on locomotor behavior in the horse. *Canadian Journal of Veterinary Research* 57: 106–109.

Marr, C.M. (2004). Cardiac emergencies and problems of the critical care patient. *The Veterinary Clinics of North America. Equine Practice* 20: 217–230.

Martin, L.G., Matteson, V.L., Wingfield, W.E. et al. (1994). Abnormalities of Serum Magnesium in Critically Ill Dogs: Incidence and Implications. *Journal of Veterinary Emergency and Critical Care* 4: 15–20.

Morton, A.J., Varney, C.R., Ekiri, A.B., and Grosche, A. (2011). Cardiovascular effects of N-butylscopolammonium bromide and xylazine in horses. *Equine Veterinary Journal.* Supplement: 117–122.

Nappert, G. and Johnson, P.J. (2001). Determination of the acid–base status in 50 horses admitted with colic between December 1998 and May 1999. *The Canadian veterinary journal. La revue veterinaire canadienne* 42: 703–707.

Ohta, M., Kurimoto, S., Ishikawa, Y. et al. (2013). Cardiovascular effects of dobutamine and phenylephrine infusion in sevoflurane-anesthetized thoroughbred horses. *Journal of Veterinary Medical Science* 75(11): 1443–1448.

Proudman, C.J., Edwards, G.B., Barnes, J., and French, N.R. (2005). Factors affecting long-term survival of horses recovering from surgery of the small intestine. *Equine Veterinary Journal* 37: 360–365.

Proudman, C.J., Dugdale, A.H., Senior, J.M. et al. (2006). Pre-operative and anesthesia-related risk factors for mortality in equine colic cases. *Veterinary Journal* 171: 89–97.

Pye, J. and Nieto, J. (2020). The use of phenylephrine in the treatment of nephrosplenic entrapment of the large colon in horses. *Equine Veterinary Education* 32: 568–570.

Roberts, D.J., Ball, C.G., and Kirkpatrick, A.W. (2016). Increased pressure within the abdominal compartment: intra-abdominal hypertension and the abdominal compartment syndrome. *Current Opinion in Critical Care* 22: 174–185.

Robertson, J.T. and Scicluna, C. (2009). Preoperative evaluation: general considerations. In: *Equine Anesthesia – Monitoring and Emergency Therapy*, 2e, 121–130. St. Louis, MO: Saunders Elsevier.

Rothenbuhler, R., Hawkins, J.F., Adams, S.B. et al. (2006). Evaluation of surgical treatment for signs of acute abdominal pain in draft horses: 72 cases (1983–2002). *Journal of the American Veterinary Medical Association* 228: 1546–1550.

Sano, H., Martin-Flores, M., Santos, L.C. et al. (2011). Effects of epidural morphine on gastrointestinal transit in unmedicated horses. *Veterinary Anaesthesia and Analgesia* 38: 121–126.

Schoster, A., Altermatt, N., Torgerson, P.R., and Bischofberger, A.S. (2020). Outcome and complications following transrectal and transabdominal large intestinal trocarization in equids with colic: 228 cases (2004–2015). *Journal of the American Veterinary Medical Association* 257: 189–195.

Swanson, C.R., Mur, W.W., Bednarski, R.M. et al. (1985). Hemodynamic responses in halothane-anesthetized horses given infusions of dopamine or dobutamine. *American Journal of Veterinary Research* 46: 365–370.

Taylor, S. (2015). A review of equine sepsis. *Equine Veterinary Education* 27: 99–109.

Tessier, C., Pitaud, J.P., Thorin, C., and Touzot-Jourde, G. (2019). Systemic morphine administration causes gastric distention and hyperphagia in healthy horses. *Equine Veterinary Journal* 51: 653–657.

Toribio, R.E., Kohn, C.W., Chew, D.J. et al. (2001). Comparison of serum parathyroid hormone and ionized calcium and magnesium concentrations and fractional urinary clearance of calcium and phosphorus in healthy horses and horses with enterocolitis. *American Journal of Veterinary Research* 62: 938–947.

Toribio, R.E., Kohn, C.W., Hardy, J., and Rosol, T.J. (2005). Alterations in serum parathyroid hormone and electrolyte concentrations and urinary excretion of electrolytes in horses with induced endotoxemia. *Journal of Veterinary Internal Medicine* 19: 223–231.

Wagner, A.E. (2009). *The Case Against the Use of Acepromazine in Male Horses*, 20–21. Las Vegas, NV: American Association of Equine Practitioners Annual Convention.

Weglicki, W.B., Phillips, T.M., Freedman, A.M. et al. (1992). Magnesium-deficiency elevates circulating levels of inflammatory cytokines and endothelin. *Molecular and Cellular Biochemistry* 110: 169–173.

11

Anesthetic Management for Endocrine Diseases and Geriatric Horses

Bonnie Hay Kraus[1] and Philip Johnson[2]

[1] Department of Veterinary Clinical Sciences, College of Veterinary Medicine, Iowa State University, 1809 South Riverside Drive, Ames, IA, 50011, USA
[2] Department of Veterinary Medicine and Surgery, College of Veterinary Medicine, University of Missouri, 900 East Campus Drive, Columbia, MO, 65211, USA

Introduction

The understanding and recognition of equine endocrine disease has expanded significantly over the past decade. Endocrine disorders may have a primary cause or may be secondary to other systemic disease. Many of these disorders can be interlinked and affect multiple body systems. Aging horses are at increased risk for endocrine disease. The two most common endocrine diseases are pituitary *pars intermedia* dysfunction (PPID) and insulin dysregulation/equine metabolic syndrome (EMS/ID). Other endocrine diseases in aged horses may be associated with neoplasia (diabetes mellitus [DM], thyroid, parathyroid, and adrenal disease).

Pituitary *Pars Intermedia* Dysfunction (PPID, Equine Cushing Disease)

PPID is the most common endocrine disorder in geriatric horses, with a reported prevalence of ~21% in horses aged 15 years or older (McGowan et al. 2013; Miller et al. 2016). It is a clinical syndrome associated with hypertrichosis (hirsutism), chronic laminitis, epaxial muscle atrophy, weight loss, polyuria/polydipsia, and lethargy (Figure 11.1). PPID was originally and erroneously referred to as an equine manifestation of Cushing Disease due to similarities with humans and canine conditions. In those species, pituitary adenomas of the *pars distalis* (adenohypophysis) secrete excessive proopiomelano(lipo)cortin (POMC)-derived peptides, primarily ACTH (adrenocorticotropic hormone or corticotropin) and lead to secondary hyperadrenocorticism. In horses, increased secretion of POMC-peptides arises from melanotropes in the *pars intermedia* (PI) and results in increased secretion of numerous melanocortins with ACTH being a relatively minor product. Normally, melanocortin secretion by the PI is inhibited by dopamine from the hypothalamus. PPID is a neurodegenerative disease in which there is loss of the normal dopaminergic inhibition, leading to secondary endocrinopathy (McFarlane 2011; McFarlane and Toribio 2010).

Normal Anatomy/Physiology/Pathophysiology

The pituitary gland (hypophysis) lies within a bony cavity (the *sella turcica*) of the sphenoid

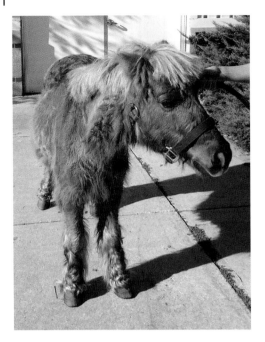

Figure 11.1 A 22-year-old pony with hypertrichosis as a result of pituitary *pars intermedia* dysfunction (PPID).

bone in the base of the skull (McFarlane 2011). The gland is divided into anterior and posterior lobes which have different embryological origins and functions. The posterior pituitary lobe (neurohypophysis or *pars nervosa*) consists of a collection of axons and nerve terminals originating in the hypothalamus (McFarlane 2011). The *pars nervosa* stores and secretes oxytocin and vasopressin (also known as antidiuretic hormone or ADH) (McFarlane 2011). The anterior pituitary (adenohypophysis) includes the *pars tuberalis* and the *pars distalis* (also called the *pars ventralis*). The *pars distalis* contains endocrine cells that synthesize, store, and release six different hormones in response to stimulating or inhibiting factors from the hypothalamus: growth hormone (GH, somatotropin), follicle stimulating hormone (FSH), luteinizing hormone (LH), prolactin (PRL), thyroid stimulating hormone (TSH, thyrotropin), and adrenocorticotrophic hormone (ACTH, corticotropin). The corticotropes of the *pars*

distalis produce the pre-pro-hormone POMC which is converted into beta-lipotropin and ACTH, which are subsequently released into the circulation.

The PI lies between the anterior and posterior pituitary lobes. The primary endocrine cells are melanotropes, which also produce POMC. PI-derived POMC undergoes further peptide cleavage and modification resulting in the secretory products (melanocortins): alpha melanocyte-stimulating hormone (α-MSH), beta-endorphin (β-END), corticotropin-like intermediate lobe peptide (CLIP), and ACTH (McFarlane 2011). Alpha-MSH exerts potent anti-inflammatory activity through inhibition of cytokine production and plays a role in metabolism and obesity (McFarlane 2011). The function of CLIP is not completely understood but it may enhance pancreatic insulin release, thus promoting hyperinsulinemia, a risk factor for endocrinopathic laminitis. β-END is a potent endogenous opioid agonist. Melanotrope-derived ACTH represents a significant minority (~2%) of the secreted output from the normal pituitary gland. For further detailed information on normal and pathologic equine pituitary function, the reader is referred to the referenced textbooks.

Overproduction of melanocortins is the endocrinological basis of PPID. In health, melanocortin secretion is tonically inhibited by dopamine released from the periventricular nuclei of the hypothalamus. PPID results from loss of this normal dopaminergic inhibition. Therefore, PPID is a primary neurodegenerative disease with secondary endocrinopathic consequences. Macroscopic enlargement of the pituitary gland is evident in some but not all cases of PPID, and histological examination is needed to identify small (micro) adenoma formation in the PI of affected pituitary glands. The overall clinical picture for PPID varies quite significantly between affected individuals due to heterogeneity in the PI-derived melanocortins produced by a given patient. For example, elevated levels of secreted β-END with enhanced opioid effectiveness in PPID cases may contribute to the lethargy and somnolence seen in some individuals.

Horses affected with PPID develop diminished systemic inflammatory responsiveness, possibly explained by the anti-inflammatory actions of elevated circulating melanocortin concentrations. Inhibited pain expression in the face of laminitis may lead to detrimental disruption of the digital lamellae in physically active PPID-affected individuals due to repeated uninhibited mechanical loading. Immunosenescence and inhibited inflammatory responsiveness also contribute to an increased risk of infection in PPID-affected horses.

Clinical Signs

A recent study suggested that age is the only risk factor for PPID (Ireland and McGowan 2018). Clinical manifestations, including laminitis, are reported to be more severe in the fall (autumn) season. Diagnosis of PPID in older horses that have developed inappropriate hirsutism (hypertrichosis, retention of the haircoat) is often presumptively made without corroborative endocrinological testing. PPID also occurs to an extent greater than previously recognized in younger horses (especially, ponies), and the clinical expression of PPID in these younger horses may not be so pathognomonic.

Although it is most commonly diagnosed in horses and ponies aged over 18 years, PPID has been diagnosed in ponies less than seven years of age. A diagnosis of PPID in the absence of inappropriate hirsutism can be challenging because several aspects of the clinical appearance of PPID could be attributed to other primary diseases (e.g. laminitis resulting from any cause) or the effects of advancing age. However, with time, horses affected with PPID eventually develop a characteristic physical appearance. Clinical abnormalities observed in younger horses include endocrinopathic laminitis, reduced athletic performance, lethargy, changed personality, and reduced shedding of haircoat and regional hypertrichosis, and changes in body morphology, including regional adiposity.

PPID should be suspected in mature and geriatric horses and ponies that are presented for diminishing athletic performance, ill-thrift, changing body condition (skeletal muscle atrophy, abdominal rotundity, regional adiposity), chronic laminitis, polyuria/polydipsia (PU/PD), and haircoat abnormalities. PPID-affected equids tend to lose skeletal muscle mass (especially from the gluteal and epaxial musculature), and to acquire a characteristic "regional" distribution of body fat. Paradoxically, some younger PPID-affected horses may be in normal or generally obese bodily condition. Endocrinopathic laminitis is usually recognized in horses and ponies with concomitant EMS/ID and presents as abnormalities of hoof structure and growth rather than lameness. Signs of laminitic pain (stiffness, lameness, etc.) may be diminished as a result of the combined anti-inflammatory (α-MSH) and analgesic (β-endorphin) actions of elevated circulating melanocortins in PPID. However, PPID-associated endocrinopathic laminitis can certainly cause very severe pain and lameness in some cases.

Other clinical problems that develop as a result of PPID include abnormalities of thermoregulation (inappropriate sweating or "hyperhidrosis," hypohidrosis, or anhidrosis), lethargy, infertility or inappropriate lactation (galactorrhea) in mares, suspensory ligament degeneration, blindness, and seizures. Ophthalmic (corneal) health is often compromised because the combination of increasing age and PPID elevates the risk of nonhealing or recurrent corneal ulcers in horses and lead to the development of corneal degeneration and calcific band keratopathy (Miller et al. 2013; Berryhill et al. 2017).

Reduced immune function due to elevated circulating levels of immunosuppressive factors (α-MSH, β-endorphin, and cortisol) can result in affected horses that are presented with opportunistic infections including equine protozoal myeloencephalitis, chronic dermatitis, tooth root infection, bronchopneumonia, and infection of the urinary tract.

Diagnosis

Although the diagnosis of PPID is commonly made based on the development of a characteristic clinical appearance, endocrine testing is important to establish the diagnosis in less advanced, less certain cases. Moreover, it is necessary to discriminate the clinical effects of PPID from those associated with advancing age in general. Many horses with PPID are often concomitantly affected with EMS/ID. EMS/ID requires its own specific testing and has its own line of specific treatment (see section on EMS/ID).

Endocrinological tests are utilized for establishing a diagnosis of PPID. The most straightforward test for PPID is to determine the plasma ACTH concentration and evaluate the result in light of seasonally appropriate reference intervals. An elevated plasma ACTH concentration is diagnostic for PPID in resting horses that are not concomitantly affected with either severe pain or systemic disease. Specific information on currently recommended testing methodologies can be found in the findings from the Equine Endocrinology Working Group (https://sites.tufts.edu/equineendogroup).

Endocrinopathic Laminitis

Previously, endocrinopathic laminitis was thought to be a clinical abnormality in early cases of PPID. However, recent recognition that insulin causes endocrinopathic laminitis has led to a revision of our understanding regarding the relationship between PPID and laminitis. Endocrinopathic laminitis is now attributed to a manifestation of hyperinsulinemia/ID and not directly to PPID. Thus, the endocrinopathic condition associated with insulin-mediated laminitis is equine metabolic syndrome or insulin dysregulation. These two conditions (PPID and EMS/ID) are regarded as independent diseases though some horses and ponies may develop both conditions. The development of PPID in EMS/ID-affected individuals is associated with more severe manifestations of endocrinopathic laminitis that may severely cripple horses.

PPID – Specific Implications for Anesthesia

A complete blood count (CBC) and serum/plasma biochemical analysis should be included in the pre-anesthetic work-up of all PPID-affected horses and ponies to provide information regarding overall health and evidence of significant co-morbidities that may or may not be evident upon review of the patient's medical history or following physical examination. There are usually no specific hematologic or serum/plasma biochemical abnormalities associated with the diagnosis of PPID, and abnormalities identified in geriatric horses may be interpreted as indicators of inflammation or disease due to age or co-morbidities, rather than PPID. Commonly identified but nonspecific abnormalities include leukocytosis (neutrophilia, lymphopenia), hyperfibrinogenemia, anemia, hypertriglyceridemia (more common in ponies), hyperglycemia, and increased liver enzymes. Hyperglycemia is the most commonly identified abnormality on serum/plasma biochemical analysis in these cases (McFarlane 2011). Elevated liver enzyme activities may be consistent with histopathologic hepatopathy in >70% of horses with PPID (Glover et al. 2009). Glycosuria is a common finding on urinalysis in horses with both PPID and hyperglycemia (Toribio 2010). Hyperglycemia in an aged horse, although nonspecific, should trigger consideration of PPID as it is present in 45–95% of horses with PPID (Toribio 2010). Horses and ponies with both PPID and hyperglycemia are also commonly affected with EMS/ID; hyperinsulinemia has been documented in ~32% of horses with PPID (McGowan et al. 2013). Clinically, hyperinsulinemia associated with normoglycemia is referred to as "compensated" insulin resistance (IR), and hyperinsulinemia with hyperglycemia is "decompensated" IR (or type-2 DM). Insulin resistance, EMS/ID, and diabetes are discussed in a separate section (see the following text).

Hyperglycemia

Human beings and dogs with endocrine abnormalities associated with glucose dysregulation (usually DM and/or IR) have higher complication and mortality rates attributed to the effects of altered glucose homeostasis on the cardiovascular, renal and central, peripheral, and autonomic nervous systems. The pathophysiology of many of these effects involves damage to the vascular endothelium throughout the body. Persistent hyperglycemia results in glycosylation of amino acids and stimulation of diacylglycerol synthesis and activation of protein kinase C causing blood vessel dysfunction (Frank and Tadros 2014). To date, there is little information regarding these effects in horses. It is unknown/undocumented whether horses develop hypertension and associated nephropathy, retinopathy, or peripheral or autonomic neuropathy. Systemic hypertension and left ventricular hypertrophy have been identified in ponies affected with chronic endocrinopathic laminitis (Rugh et al. 1987). Autonomic neuropathy has been documented in humans and dogs and results in altered parasympathetic and vasomotor tone, hypotension, decreased respiratory response to hypoxemia, and impaired thermoregulation, all of which provide concern during general anesthesia (Kadoi 2010a, b).

When identified in PPID-affected horses, hyperglycemia is usually mild and not sufficiently elevated to result in osmotic diuresis. With more severe degrees of hyperglycemia, osmotic diuresis and concomitant urinary loss of sodium and potassium may lead to hypovolemia. Some reports have suggested that polyuria/polydipsia occurs in ~30% of horses with PPID, perhaps a result of reduced antidiuretic hormone secretion, increased thirst due to hypercortisolism, or osmotic diuresis due to hyperglycemia/glycosuria. Moreover, inappropriate hyperhidrosis is commonly identified in PPID-affected individuals and is believed to result from melanocortin-induced abnormalities of thermoregulation.

These abnormalities may contribute to alterations in body fluid and electrolyte abnormalities or imbalances. Therefore, it is important to assess the patient's hydration and electrolyte status and correct any abnormalities prior to anesthesia whenever possible.

Musculoskeletal Considerations

Muscle wasting (sarcopenia) and weakness are common features of PPID and are most evident in the gluteal and epaxial musculature. Recently, a *postmortem* study comparing histopathologic changes in the suspensory ligaments of horses with PPID to old horses without PPID, and young horses revealed a possible association between PPID and degeneration of the suspensory ligament (Hofberger et al. 2015).

Approximately 30% of horses with PPID develop chronic hypercortisolism. Chronic hypercortisolism leads to osteoporosis in humans and therefore the risk of complicating pathological fractures should be considered when PPID-affected patients are being recovered from general anesthesia.

Weight loss, ligament degeneration, sarcopenia, myasthenia, and neurologic impairment represent significant risk factors for injury during anesthetic recovery for PPID patients. Careful attention should be paid to proper positioning and padding of these horses in an effort to prevent post-anesthetic myopathy/neuropathy. Anesthesia durations exceeding two hours, and especially greater than three hours, are associated with significantly higher mortality and so it is imperative to limit anesthesia duration to obviate these risks (Johnston et al. 1995). Rope assistance (tail or head and tail) during recovery may reduce mortality associated with musculoskeletal injuries (Bidwell et al. 2007; Niimura Del Barrio et al. 2018). When painful, laminitis may also contribute to difficulty achieving and maintaining a standing position following anesthesia. Providing appropriate analgesia and support during the recovery period may be helpful in reducing injury.

Drug Interactions in PPID Horses

Pergolide is the only drug presently approved for the treatment of PPID. It is used to support or re-establish dopaminergic control of melanotropes in the PI. Pergolide is a potent dopamine (D2) agonist that also may exert some adrenergic and 5-hydroxytryptamine effects. The administration of drugs that are antagonistic to the action of dopamine, such as phenothiazine tranquilizers (acepromazine), in horses being treated with pergolide may alter drug effectiveness.

Two of the melanocortins, α-MSH and β-END, may diminish PPID patients' responses to painful stimuli. Alpha-MSH decreases cytokine production and therefore exerts a potent anti-inflammatory effect, and β-END is a potent endogenous opioid receptor agonist. Butorphanol is a mu-antagonist, kappa agonist opioid commonly used in equine anesthetic patients as a premedication and as part of a multi-modal analgesia protocol. However, since it is a mu-antagonist, it may interact with endogenous β-endorphins to partially reverse analgesic effects. Morphine (0.05–0.15 mg/kg intravenous [IV]) loading doses followed by a constant rate infusion (CRI) (0.03–0.1 mg/kg/h [0.5–1.7 µg/kg/min]) have been safely used for analgesia in horses without adverse behavioral or disrupted locomotor functions that could adversely affect recovery (Valverde 2013). Use of mu-agonists at the lower end of the dose range, along with reliance on alternative classes of analgesic drugs for balanced anesthesia/analgesia techniques, may be warranted in these cases. Lidocaine, alpha-2 agonists (xylazine, detomidine, romifidine, dexmedetomidine), and ketamine have all been used alone or in combination to provide balanced anesthesia and have been reviewed elsewhere (Valverde 2013).

Geriatric Co-morbidities That May Affect Anesthetic Management

As noted above, PPID is most commonly diagnosed in geriatric horses (≥15 years of age) which now make up ~1/3 of the equine population (Ireland 2016). Along with the clinical and metabolic disturbances due to PPID, geriatric patients may also have additional significant age-related co-morbidities, including other endocrine, dental, musculoskeletal, respiratory, and cardiovascular disorders (Ireland 2016). These may serve as co-morbidities that require consideration for anesthetic management or they may be a primary presenting complaint requiring general anesthesia. A complete and detailed physical examination, supported by appropriate diagnostic testing, will assist in identifying these co-morbidities and allow for peri-anesthetic planning and improved post-anesthetic outcomes. For example, the addition of a CBC and serum biochemical analysis should be included in the pre-anesthetic work-up of all geriatric horses to provide information regarding general health and for evidence of co-morbidities that may not be evident on physical examination.

A thorough review of anesthesia in geriatric equine patients is beyond the scope of this chapter, and the reader is referred to other sources (Donaldson 2005).

Musculoskeletal and Lameness Anesthetic Considerations in Geriatric Horses

Musculoskeletal disease and lameness, specifically osteoarthritis, represent the second most frequent cause for referral and a major reason for euthanasia of geriatric horses (Ireland 2016). Laminitis is also a common lameness diagnosis in geriatric horses and has been reported in 24–82% of horses with PPID (Ireland 2016). Geriatric horses with lameness may present for advanced imaging, surgical intervention, or another primary complaint. Special care and attention should be taken with respect to proper positioning and padding, making sure that limbs are supported and that weight is evenly distributed. Use of multi-modal analgesia, even if the procedure itself is not painful (e.g. MRI), may help alleviate patient discomfort, pain, and disability during recovery. Assisted rope recovery may also be beneficial since painful osteoarthritis and/or laminitis may affect the ability of geriatric patients to stand during recovery.

Dental Anesthetic Considerations in Geriatric Horses

Dental disorders, including tooth loss, diastemata, periodontal disease, and wear abnormalities affect a high proportion of geriatric horses. These horses may require general anesthesia for advanced imaging (e.g. computed tomography) and/or dental extractions. Some procedures may be accomplished standing using combinations of an alpha-2 agonist, an opioid such as butorphanol or morphine, and locoregional anesthesia/analgesia (mental, inferior alveolar, infraorbital, and maxillary blocks). This multi-modal approach provides synergistic effects and enables the use of lower doses of each individual drug. This approach would be especially advantageous in geriatric horses since they may have increased sensitivity to sedative drugs and altered clearance. Further information on anesthesia and sedation for sinus and dental disease can be found in Chapter 1.

Gastrointestinal Anesthetic Considerations in Geriatric Horses

Colic is the most frequent reason for referral of horses ≥20 years old (Brosnahan and Paradis 2003; Silva and Furr 2013) and, depending on the study, is the most or second most common reason for euthanasia in geriatric horses (Ireland 2016; Miller et al. 2016). Geriatric horses referred to a surgical facility are more likely to have a surgical lesion compared to mature horses (Southwood et al. 2010). The etiologies of colic in geriatric horses tend to differ from those reported for younger horses. Geriatric horses have a higher frequency of cecal and large colon impactions which may be partly attributed to poor dentition (Ireland 2016). Horses ≥16 years of age are twice as likely to be diagnosed with a strangulating small intestinal lesion compared to

horses aged 4–15 years with strangulating pedunculated mesenteric lipoma being the most common diagnosis. Current studies indicate that there is no significant difference regarding complications or short-term survival between geriatric horses and mature horses (4–15 years) for small or large intestinal surgical lesions (Southwood et al. 2010; Gazzerro et al. 2015). For additional information on gastrointestinal disease, the reader is directed to the Chapter 10.

Respiratory Anesthetic Considerations in Geriatric Horses

Equine asthma or "heaves" is the most prevalent respiratory disease of geriatric horses (Ireland 2016; Marr 2016). Anesthetic management strategies of horses with equine asthma and other respiratory diseases are described in other chapters. It should be noted that PPID is an important predisposing cause of bronchopneumonia in older horses. Up to ~35% of PPID horses have opportunistic or secondary infections due to their inability to mount a satisfactory inflammatory response to pathogens. These infections may be recurrent and occult and not necessarily associated with obvious signs of respiratory disease; therefore, clinicians should adopt a high level of suspicion and pursue thorough physical examination and diagnostic tests such as cytological examination and microbiological culturing of airway fluid, thoracic radiography, and thoracic ultrasonography (Marr 2016).

Cardiac Anesthetic Considerations in Geriatric Horses

Cardiac murmurs are detected in ~20% of horses aged 15 years or older. Aortic valve degeneration is the most common of the valvular disorders and is associated with a pan-, holo-, or early diastolic, decrescendo murmur heard loudest over the aortic valve in the left fifth intercostal space and radiating toward the heart base (Marr 2016). Mitral regurgitation (MR) is also common in older horses and is associated with a systolic murmur heard loudest over the fifth intercostal space on the left side and radiating caudodorsally (Marr 2016). MR and AR are collectively referred to as left-sided valvular regurgitation (LSVR). The prevalence of LSVR increases with age; 13.5% in horses 15–23 years old and 14.8% in horses ≥24 years (Stevens et al. 2009). Clinically important tricuspid regurgitation is not as common (~5%) in geriatric horses and always occurs in conjunction with LSVR. Irregular cardiac rhythm consistent with atrial fibrillation (AF) was detected in 2% of horses ≥15 years of age and 4.4% of horses ≥30 years of age (Ireland et al. 2012) and is likely associated with underlying structural cardiac changes in geriatric horses. Anesthetic management of horses with cardiac disease is described in a separate chapter.

Neurological Anesthetic Considerations in Geriatric Horses

Neurologic impairment, including ataxia, blindness, seizures, and 'narcolepsy' (sleep deprivation) are more common in horses with PPID than aged horses without PPID (McFarlane 2011). Geriatric horses with PPID should be assessed for neurologic function prior to general anesthesia as neurological impediments may especially lead to serious complications during anesthetic recovery.

Equine Metabolic Syndrome/ Insulin Dysregulation

EMS or ID represents a clustering of risk factors for endocrinopathic laminitis. Emphasis should be placed on the early identification of EMS/ID-affected individuals that are at risk for laminitis and the institution of effective preventive measures because effective treatment of laminitis is often not possible. Endocrinopathic laminitis results directly from the influence of elevated circulating plasma insulin levels and any factor that might cause hyperinsulinemia likely increases the risk. Horses and ponies were traditionally characterized as being affected by EMS/ID when they had developed generalized obesity or regional adiposity, IR, and endocrinopathic laminitis. Other abnormalities that have also been identified in EMS/ID-affected equids include hypertriglyceridemia (hepatic lipidosis in Miniature Horses), estrous cycling abnormalities, and abnormalities in the concentrations of some circulating plasma adipocytokines (hyperleptinemia, hypoadiponectinemia).

Clinical Signs

EMS should be suspected in mature horses and ponies that develop either generalized obesity or regional adiposity. Regional adiposity refers to the gradual accumulation of subcutaneous adipose tissue deposits along the nuchal ligament and in proximity to the base of the tail. It should be emphasized that EMS/ID does not arise in all obese individuals and that EMS/ID is sometimes present in lean individuals. EMS/ID is regarded as the most common cause of laminitis in mature horses and ponies; thus, lameness is a common presenting complaint in EMS/ID-affected individuals. Other less well-characterized clinical manifestations include abnormalities of reproductive cycling in mature broodmares and seasonal hypertension. Recent studies further demonstrated that ponies with EMS/ID may be affected with myocardial hypertrophy (Heliczer et al. 2017). Insulin resistance is an important component of the hyperlipemia syndrome and hepatic lipidosis that develops in obese Miniature Horses and British pony breeds (and other breeds) when food intake has been diminished or discontinued.

Endocrine Tests for the Diagnostic Corroboration of EMS

Although diagnosis of EMS may be suspected based on consideration of a patient's breed, signalment, medical history, and results of physical/radiographic examination, corroborative endocrine testing should be undertaken to confirm the diagnosis and to establish a baseline characterization for future comparisons. The importance of endocrine testing is further appreciated when one considers that not all obese equids are affected by EMS/ID and that EMS/ID may develop in some relatively lean individuals. Diagnostic tests for EMS/ID may be categorized into those that evaluate the enteroinsular axis, those that evaluate IR, and those that evaluate related co-morbidities. For routine clinical practice, it is recommended that diagnosis of EMS/ID should be undertaken in a stepwise manner, beginning with measurement of baseline values of insulin and glucose. A complete review of the different testing methods for EMS/ID is beyond the scope of this chapter. Specific information on currently recommended testing methodologies can be found in the findings from the Equine Endocrinology Working Group. The reader is also directed to published reviews (Bertin and de Laat 2017).

Diagnostic Tests for IR

Demonstration of an elevated resting plasma insulin concentration (resting hyperinsulinemia) when being fed hay or during pasture grazing ($>50\,\mu U/ml$) is diagnostically supportive for EMS/ID. However, simply measuring plasma insulin concentration is an insensitive test for this condition as it produced many false negatives. Practical diagnosis of EMS/ID/IR is presently based on two applied dynamic tests, the oral sugar test (OST) and the insulin sensitivity test (IST). The OST consists of evaluating the plasma insulin concentration at 60 minutes following an oral dose of light corn Syrup (0.45 ml/kg of body weight). Diagnostic corroboration for EMS/ID is supported if the insulin concentration exceeds $63\,\mu U/ml$.

The IST presently specifically recommended for the purpose of establishing whether an equine patient is affected with IR (Bertin and Sojka-Kritchevsky 2013). Blood glucose concentration is measured before and at +30 minutes following IV administration of regular insulin (0.1 U/kg of body weight). In normal patients, the blood glucose concentration should decrease to below 50% of the baseline by 30 minutes. IR-affected patients fail to reduce blood glucose to less than 50% of the starting concentration under the influence of insulin.

Testing EMS/ID Candidates for PPID

In some instances, especially in older horses (>15 years of age), individuals may be affected by both EMS/ID and PPID. Although unproven, it has also been suggested that the presence of EMS/ID increases the likelihood that PPID will eventually develop. Currently, EMS/ID and PPID are regarded as independent conditions and the relationship between them is not fully understood. PPID-affected horses that are not affected with EMS/ID are thought to be less likely to be affected by clinical laminitis. However, PPID may carry its own risk regarding hyperinsulinemia (the melanocortin CLIP stimulates pancreatic insulin secretion). Since PPID is readily treated with pergolide, it is recommended that older horses (>15 years) and ponies affected by EMS/ID be evaluated for PPID. If PPID is present, the risk of laminitis may be mitigated by pergolide treatment.

Treatment and Management of EMS/ID

The principles of treatment for EMS/ID fall into the following categories:

1) Dietary recommendations intended to promote reversal of obesity (as needed) and to prevent significant post-prandial hyperglycemia and hyperinsulinemia.
2) Increased level of physical activity and exercise to the extent allowed depending on whether or not laminitis has occurred.
3) Pharmacological agents intended to improve insulin sensitivity, promote weight loss, and inhibit post-prandial hyperglycemia.
4) Management of laminitis.
5) Management of co-morbidities.

Strategies for Reversal of Obesity

As a defining component of EMS, obesity is associated with both IR and increased risk of laminitis. It is logical that the reversal of obesity should minimize the risk of laminitis and promote insulin sensitivity. Obese horses and ponies should not be "starved" for purposes of weight loss because severe calorie restriction leads to the activation of physiological mechanisms that promote worsening IR. Moreover, obese ponies, donkeys, and Miniature Horses are especially predisposed to hyperlipemia and hepatic lipidosis (potentially fatal) when subjected to a severely calorie restricted ration. Strategies intended to reverse obesity should include both increased physical activity and a reasonable, gradual restriction of dietary energy intake. Unfortunately, the development of painful laminitis in some EMS/ID-affected equids precludes the prescribed exercise for purposes of promoting weight reduction. In those patients, dietary adjustments and the specific management of laminitis, including pain management, must be undertaken to better address both obesity and EMS/ID. For detailed information on feeding strategies for weight loss in EMS/ID horses, readers are directed to veterinary nutrition resources.

Pharmacological Strategies for the Management of Refractory EMS/ID

In all cases, management of EMS/ID should be primarily centered on nutrition and exercise recommendations. Oral levothyroxine sodium appears to be helpful for the management of refractory cases of obesity and EMS/ID but should not be used as a lifelong management strategy. Levothyroxine sodium is usually administered daily (0.05–0.20 mg/kg, commonly 0.1 mg/kg) for a period of approximately three to six months. This treatment helps with initiation of weight loss in obese individuals and also promotes insulin sensitivity. The biguanide, metformin, is also recommended for treatment of EMS/ID (30 mg/kg, PO, q12 hours). In horses, metformin probably exerts a local pharmacological action at the epithelial lining of the small intestine and acts to inhibit glucose absorption, thus preventing both postprandial hyperglycemia and hyperinsulinemia. Orally administered metformin also promotes weight loss in obese equine patients. If the EMS/ID patient is concomitantly affected with PPID, treatment for PPID using pergolide mesylate (0.5–3.0 mg/day, PO, per 450 kg horse) should also be instituted. More recently, there has been increase in the use of sodium-glucose co-transporter 2 (SGLT2) inhibitors, such as velagliflozin, for the management of refractory cases of EMS/ID (Meier et al. 2018). SGLT2 inhibitors are showing promise as safe and effective drugs for the management of EMS/ID and prevention of laminitis by lessening hyperinsulinemic responses to dietary sugars and starch.

Implications for Anesthesia

Many horses and ponies afflicted with EMS/ID are also geriatric and may have concomitant PPID. The reader is referred to the above section which addresses the anesthetic concerns associated with these disorders and comorbidities. The primary remaining factor that has implications for general anesthesia is obesity. Several recent studies have documented the prevalence of obesity in horses in a variety of countries: 31.2% (Great Britain), 24% (Denmark), 24.5% (Australia), 28.6% (Canada) (Robin et al. 2015; Jensen et al. 2016; Potter et al. 2016; Kosolofski et al. 2017). Despite such a high prevalence of overweight/obesity in the horse populations of the world, there is little information regarding the implications or risk associated with anesthesia in these horses. Recently, a study suggested that a higher body mass index in horses may increase the risk for development of incisional complications (Hill et al. 2020). The veterinary literature regarding obesity and its relevance to anesthesia is in its infancy, and very little information is available even in small animal patients, despite an even higher prevalence of obesity of ~45% (Love and Cline 2015). Therefore, physiologic alterations and anesthetic management strategies are extrapolated from human and the few small animal references available. The reader is referred to comprehensive human texts for more complete review of the physiologic changes and anesthetic management of the obese anesthetic patient (Brodsky and Lemmens 2012; Leykin and Brodsky 2013).

Cardiovascular Effects of Obesity

Obesity increases metabolic oxygen requirements and one of the earliest changes to compensate for this is an increase in circulating blood volume caused by fluid and sodium retention. Hypervolemia leads to increased preload, stroke volume, and cardiac output. Increased left ventricular preload causes chamber dilation and, eventually, eccentric left ventricular hypertrophy. Activation of the renin-angiotensin-aldosterone system leads to systemic hypertension and the development of concentric left ventricular hypertrophy. Ventricular dysfunction progresses and may lead to congestive heart failure known as "obesity cardiomyopathy" in people. Tissue pathology associated with obesity cardiomyopathy includes myocardial fibrosis, fatty infiltration of the myocardium, and abnormal accumulation of free fatty acids and lipids in cardiac myocytes. Both hyperaldosteronism and type-2 DM predispose to fibrosis of the myocardial electrical conduction system leading to cardiac dysrhythmias.

The extent to which obese horses develop any of these cardiovascular abnormalities is presently unknown. However, it has been shown that obese ponies with chronic laminitis often develop systemic hypertension (Rugh et al. 1987). Therefore, an important first step when considering general anesthesia for obese equine patients is to identify cardiac or cardiovascular abnormalities if they exist. To this end, careful evaluation of the cardiovascular system is warranted in all obese (and geriatric) horses. Although not routinely performed preoperatively in horses, indirect blood pressure measurement may identify hypertension in

obese patients and may be a sentinel of cardiovascular dysfunction. Indirect blood pressure is readily measured using a blood pressure cuff placed around the tail or metatarsus (Garner et al. 1975; Olsen et al. 2016). Preoperative ECG assessment may also assist in identifying cardiac dysrhythmias.

Respiratory Effects of Obesity

Both ventilation and oxygenation are affected by obesity; as body weight increases so does oxygen consumption and carbon dioxide (CO_2) production. The work of breathing is increased because more energy must be expended while respiratory muscle efficiency is decreased. Accumulation of body fat in the chest wall and increased pulmonary blood flow decreases thoracic and pulmonary compliance, increases airway resistance and the mechanical work of breathing, and increases ventilation-perfusion mismatch. Functional residual capacity (FRC) is significantly decreased due to a reduction in expiratory reserve volume (ERV). As total lung capacity is reduced and FRC approaches residual volume, the airways may close during normal tidal ventilation. The decreased chest compliance and increased airway resistance results in a rapid, shallow breathing pattern. Obese humans and dogs have an increased respiratory rate in order to maintain minute ventilation and normal arterial CO_2 in the face of abnormal respiratory mechanics and increased work of breathing (Manens et al. 2014). Oxygenation variables (PaO_2, PaO_2/FiO_2, $PA-aO_2$) are poor in obese dogs under heavy sedation but improve following weight loss (Mosing et al. 2013).

Pre-anesthetic assessment of arterial blood gas with the patient breathing room air is recommended to establish a baseline and to guide management. In early obesity in humans, alveolar hyperventilation (P_aCO_2 30–35 mmHg) and mild hypoxemia (P_aO_2 70–90 mmHg) are present due to an increased ventilatory response to hypoxia. With increasing chronicity, chemoreceptor sensitivity to CO_2 decreases, resulting in a reduced ventilatory drive, thus increasing $PaCO_2$ and worsening of PaO_2 (Brodsky and Lemmens 2012).

In horses, it is well known that general anesthesia and recumbency have negative effects on ventilation and oxygenation, and the reader is referred to several recent reviews (Hubbell and Muir 2009; Moens 2013; Auckburally and Nyman 2017). Body mass (145–680 kg) significantly influences both arterial-alveolar carbon dioxide tension difference and alveolar dead space in anesthetized horses (Moens 1989). Additionally, larger abdomen or "round-bellied" horse can have a lower P_aO_2 and larger P_A-P_aO_2 gradient than flat-bellied horses (Moens et al. 1995) and lighter-weight, tall horses with larger thoracic circumference

maintain higher P_aO_2 during anesthesia than heavier, stockier horses with a narrower thoracic circumference (Mansel and Clutton 2008). Given the documented alterations in ventilation and oxygenation in obese people, it is likely that obesity would exacerbate the negative effects of general anesthesia and recumbency on oxygenation and ventilation in horses. A comprehensive review of optimization of ventilation/oxygenation in horses is beyond the scope of this article, and the reader is referred to recent review articles (Hubbell and Muir 2009; Moens 2013; Auckburally and Nyman 2017). However, some general strategies to address hypoxemia and hypoventilation are outlined in Table 11.1.

Table 11.1 Strategies to address hypoxemia and hypoventilation in overweight/obese horses that are to undergo general anesthesia.

Pre-oxygenation	Administration of oxygen via nasal cannula at 15 l/min for three minutes between sedation and induction. This is well tolerated by most horses and increases mean PaO_2 from 55 mmHg to 82.5 mmHg during anesthetic induction (van Oostrom et al. 2017).
Positive Pressure Ventilation	Administer positive pressure ventilation with an increased FiO_2 via a demand valve after intubation while positioning horse on the surgical table and moving to operating room.
Mechanical Ventilation	Institute intermittent positive pressure ventilation (IPPV) at the outset of general anesthesia.
Evaluate arterial blood gas status	Obtain an arterial blood gas at ~20 min after induction. Documents the PaO_2 and the $EtCO_2$-$PaCO_2$ difference. Repeated evaluations can be compared to these baseline values if patient status or ventilator parameter changes occur.
Increase tidal volume (V_T)	Use a minimum of 10–15 ml/kg V_T with a peak inspiratory pressure of 25–35 cmH$_2$O for adult horses.
Alveolar recruitment maneuvers (ARM)	1) Sustained increases in positive inspiratory pressure (PIP) to 40 cmH$_2$O for 40 s to open alveoli followed by positive end-expiratory pressure (PEEP) at 5–15 cmH$_2$O.
	Or
	2) Three consecutive breaths with PIP of 60, 80, and 60 cmH$_2$O followed by PEEP 10 cm H$_2$O.
	ARM may need to be repeated based on arterial blood gas results.
Positive end-expiratory pressure (PEEP)	5–15 cmH$_2$O.
Aerosolized albuterol	Administer 2 µg/kg inhaled via endotracheal tube.
Cardiac output	Increase cardiac output with IV fluids or inotropes (dobutamine) to improve lung perfusion.
Acepromazine	Add 0.02–0.035 mg/kg IV to recovery sedation plan to decrease V/Q mismatching by increasing blood flow to ventilated alveoli.

Pharmacologic Implications of Obesity

Determining the appropriate and safe dose for anesthetic drugs is a challenge in overweight/obese patients. Obesity alters the pharmacokinetics (drug distribution and clearance) and pharmacodynamics (drug effect) of some commonly employed anesthetic drugs. Obesity-associated pathophysiologic changes that are likely to affect drug distribution and elimination include: increased cardiac output, increased blood volume and extracellular fluid compartment, differences in regional blood flow, changes in renal clearance, and possible hepatic dysfunction (Brodsky and Lemmens 2012; Leykin and Brodsky 2013). Drug dosage recommendations are generally based on total body weight (TBW) in non-obese individuals. TBW is the patient's actual weight and includes two major components: lean body weight (LBW) and fat weight (FW). LBW includes muscle, bone, tendon, ligament, and body water while FW includes that contribution from adipose tissue. Humans are considered obese when the FW exceeds 30% of TBW. In dogs, an ideal body condition score (BCS) of 5/9 is approximately equal to a body fat percentage (BF%) of ~20–25% and each unit increase in BCS is associated with a ~5% increase in BF% (Love and Cline 2015). For obese humans, it has been recommended that drug dosage calculations be made on LBW, and calculations for estimating LBW have been published. Unfortunately, these relationships and their effect on pharmacokinetics (PK) in obese horses are not clear. The relationship between body mass and FW (for example, as assessed by body condition scoring) appears to be less straightforward in equine patients (Dugdale et al. 2010). To the authors' knowledge, there are currently no published recommendations for the scalar dosing for anesthetic agents in horses. Current recommendations for human and other animal species indicate that LBW may be the most appropriate scalar for sedatives, analgesics, and anesthetics including opioids, local anesthetics, and non-depolarizing neuromuscular blocking agents (Brodsky and Lemmens 2012; Leykin and Brodsky 2013; Love and Cline 2015).

Because of a horse's size, weight, and behavioral nature, under-dosing of sedatives and induction agents based on LBW is both challenging and potentially dangerous to personnel. Therefore, the authors recommend starting with premedication dosages according to LBW or at the low end of the dose range, and then adding additional drug as necessary to achieve the desired level of response and use induction agents at standard dosages. Dosages for intraoperative drug infusions may be based on LBW and increased as necessary according to patient status and pharmacodynamic effects.

Diabetes Mellitus

Overview

Diabetes mellitus (DM) is defined as a chronic disease in which the body's ability to produce or respond to the hormone insulin is inhibited. It results in abnormal carbohydrate metabolism, hyperglycemia, and glycosuria. Diabetes mellitus has been broadly characterized as either *type-1 or type-2*. In type-1, there is an absolute failure to produce insulin due to immune destruction of pancreatic beta cells. Type-2 diabetes is a state of peripheral tissue insensitivity to insulin ("insulin resistance") which initially causes increased insulin secretion (hyperinsulinemia) but may progress to impaired insulin production and secretion (pancreatic beta cell "burnout") and relative hypoinsulinemia. Overt DM, the situation in which hyperglycemia is accompanied by relative hypoinsulinemia, is rare in the equine species. In most instances, DM in equids develops as a complication of chronic peripheral IR associated with EMS/ID or PPID or both. These more commonly identified endocrinopathic conditions almost always represent states of "compensated" IR in which the blood glucose concentration is normal (normoglycemia) and pancreatic insulin secretion is elevated (hyperinsulinemia).

Overt DM should be considered in horses that have developed polyuria/polydipsia, lethargy, polyphagia, and weight loss. Diagnosis of DM is supported by laboratory results that demonstrate hyperglycemia, glycosuria, hypertriglyceridemia, and normal or low serum insulin concentrations. Identification of hyperglycemia with hyperinsulinemia is seen in EMS/ID. Other laboratory abnormalities that have been reported in horses affected with DM have included ketonemia, ketonuria, elevated serum fructosamine concentrations, and increased glycosylated hemoglobin (HbA1c) levels. Diagnosis of type-2 diabetes is further supported by the demonstration of an insulin resistant state as previously described.

Implications for Anesthesia

Typical DM, as experienced in humans and dogs, is rare in equine patients. The reader is referred to sections on PPID and EMS for anesthetic complications associated with hyperglycemia and concomitant abnormalities.

Pheochromocytoma (Sympathetic Paraganglioma)

Anatomy and Physiology of the Adrenal Gland

The paired adrenal glands are located in the retroperitoneal space near the cranial aspect of each kidney, measuring approximately 7×3 cm and weighing ~15–20 g each. Each adrenal gland is supplied by an adrenal artery which arises from the aorta or the renal artery (Toribio 2010). The histologic anatomy reflects the two different embryological origins and physiologic functions of the adrenal gland. The adrenal cortex is derived from mesodermal cells and is characterized by three zones: the outermost *zona glomerulosa* that secretes mineralocorticoids, the *zona fasciculata* that secretes glucocorticoids in

response to ACTH, and the *zona reticularis* that secretes sex hormones. The primary mineralocorticoid is aldosterone, which is important for regulation of blood pressure and fluid/electrolyte balance. Aldosterone is released in response to stimulation of the renin-angiotensin-aldosterone system and in reaction to hyperkalemia. Renin is produced in the kidney and converts circulating angiotensinogen to angiotensin I, which is then converted to angiotensin II by angiotensin converting enzyme (ACE) in the pulmonary circulation. Angiotensin II stimulates both the release of aldosterone and vasoconstriction. Aldosterone also stimulates excretion of potassium (kaliuresis) and the reabsorption of sodium, chloride, and water by the renal tubules. The primary function of glucocorticoids is regulation of metabolism including hepatic gluconeogenesis. Other effects include inhibition of glucose uptake and metabolism by peripheral tissues, inhibition of the action of insulin, stimulation of lipolysis, inhibition of protein synthesis, increased protein catabolism, increased glomerular filtration rate, inhibition of vasopressin, facilitation of the maintenance of vasomotor tone, stimulation of gastric acid secretion, and suppression of inflammation and immune responses. The adrenal medulla develops from neural crest ectoderm and consists of post-synaptic neurons that release epinephrine and norepinephrine into the circulation (Toribio 2010). Epinephrine is the major catecholamine secreted by the adrenal medulla in most mammals. Actions of catecholamines are mediated through alpha and beta-adrenergic receptors. Beta-1 receptors primarily affect the heart and beta-2 receptors affect metabolism and smooth muscle contraction. Epinephrine and norepinephrine stimulate beta receptors to increase cardiac contractility and heart rate. Norepinephrine causes vasoconstriction via stimulation of alpha receptors which results in increased vascular resistance and systolic blood pressure.

Pathophysiology

Most pheochromocytomas arise from the chromaffin cells of the adrenal medulla and secrete catecholamines independent of neural control causing uncontrolled stimulation of adrenergic receptors resulting in hypertension and tachyarrhythmias. Functionally competent pheochromocytomas are rare in horses, with only a few cases being reported in the literature. Most diagnostic confirmations of pheochromocytoma have been made at necropsy (Buckingham 1970; Gelberg et al. 1979; Frosher and Power 1982; Yovich and Ducharme 1983; Yovich et al. 1984; Johnson et al. 1995; Monahan and Craig 2016; Luethy et al. 2016).

Clinical Signs/Diagnosis

The age range of reported affected horses is 12–25 years (average 17 years) and one six-month-old foal. Horses with functional pheochromocytomas most commonly present with signs of colic or abdominal pain, likely resulting from either generalized ileus (marked adrenergic stimulation) or from pain associated with hemoabdomen due to tumor hemorrhage or rupture. Clinical signs of tachycardia, tachypnea, profuse sweating, and muscle tremors may be due to pain associated with colic, hypovolemic shock due to hemorrhage, and/or adrenergic stimulation from catecholamine release. Other signs may include cardiac arrhythmia, hypertension, anxiety, agitation, mydriasis, hyperthermia, weight loss, laminitis, respiratory disease, epistaxis, ascites, and ataxia. Affected horses often develop perirenal hemorrhage, hemoperitoneum, pale mucous membranes, and increased capillary refill time. In some cases, internal bleeding may be fatal. Other clinical abnormalities that have been attributed to the effects of a functional pheochromocytoma have included abortion, polyuria/polydipsia, and diarrhea. Abdominal palpation per rectum may reveal peri-renal/retroperitoneal swelling in the dorsal aspect of the abdomen (Johnson et al. 1995). Transcutaneous abdominal ultrasonography may identify intra-abdominal hemorrhage and/or a mass cranial or cranioventral to the kidney. Peritoneal fluid analysis will confirm hemorrhage. Catecholamine stimulation and myocardial degeneration/infarction may lead to cardiac arrhythmias such as ventricular tachycardia (Yovich et al. 1984; Luethy et al. 2016; Monahan and Craig 2016; Fouche et al. 2016). Results of routine laboratory evaluation tend to yield nonspecific abnormalities that are attributable to adrenergic stimulation and/or hemorrhage. Pheochromocytoma-associated hematological abnormalities may include hemoconcentration (due to splenic contraction or profuse sweating) and abnormalities in white blood cells (stress-associated leukocytosis, mature neutrophilia, and lymphocytosis). With acute hemorrhage, measurement of packed cell volume (PCV) is often normal or only slightly decreased and has limited value as a useful guide in estimating the volume of blood loss. This is due to the delay in extravascular fluid redistribution and concomitant splenic contraction. Plasma biochemical abnormalities include hyperglycemia, metabolic acidosis, azotemia, electrolyte disturbances (hyponatremia, hyperkalemia, hypocalcemia, and hyperphosphatemia) that are likely secondary to renal dysfunction, and elevated creatine kinase activity. Hyperlactatemia is often reported in cases of pheochromocytoma and attributed to the effects of decreased tissue oxygen delivery (vasoconstrictive ischemia or hemorrhagic shock) and increased sympathetic activity. Hyperglycemia can also be found in horses with functional pheochromocytoma. (Yovich and Ducharme 1983; Luethy et al. 2016). Analysis of urine may reveal glycosuria, and peritoneal fluid may be characterized by hemorrhage (Yovich et al. 1984; Luethy et al. 2016).

Definitive Diagnosis

Diagnosis in human patients is based on history, clinical signs, elevated plasma concentrations of metanephrine and norme-tanephrine, elevated urinary catecholamines, and advanced imaging. Measurement of uri-nary and plasma catecholamine metabolites, specifically normetanephrine, can contribute to diagnostic confirmation of pheochromocy-toma. Urine normetanephrine measurement was used to help confirm the only reported *ante mortem* diagnosis of pheochromocytoma in an equine patient (Fouche et al. 2016).

Treatment Options

Successful treatment of pheochromocytoma in horses has not been reported, and clinical signs resulting from a functional pheochromocy-toma have generally either caused death or led to euthanasia. Surgical removal via laparotomy or laparoscopy is recommended for humans and dogs with functional pheochromocyto-mas. Surgical removal of a pheochromocytoma in a horse has not been reported, although a technique for adrenalectomy in normal horses has been described (Slone et al. 1980). Diagnostic imaging to rule out bilateral tumors and/or metastasis should be performed prior to attempted surgical resection should be per-formed. These horses are commonly presented with abdominal pain and may be anesthetized for celiotomy due to intractable (colic) pain or in an attempt to identify and repair the source of intra-abdominal hemorrhage. High mortal-ity risk should be anticipated in horses with active abdominal hemorrhage that are hemo-dynamically unstable. It should be emphasized that anesthesia and/or surgery may also pro-voke an adrenergic surge and elicit life-threatening hypertension, hemorrhage, or cardiac arrhythmias.

Anesthetic Management

When planning anesthesia for a horse with a functional pheochromocytoma, initial prepa-ration should focus on restoring hemodynamic stability, pain management, and management of tachyarrhythmias.

Hemodynamic Stabilization

Initial treatment should be aimed at volume replacement with IV crystalloid fluids and/or blood transfusion. Colloids may be contraindicated due to their effects on platelet function, dilution of clotting factors, and destabilization of the fibrin clot. Antifibrinolytic drugs have been used to arrest ongoing hemorrhage in horses with hemoabdomen by inhibiting the breakdown of clots after formation. The lysine analogs aminocaproic acid (ACA) and tranexamic acid (TEA) inhibit plasminogen activator which decreases plasmin formation and stimulates the release of antiplasmin from endothelial cells. Current dosage recommen-dations for ACA are 3.5 mg/kg/min over 15 minutes followed by 0.25 mg/kg/min throughout the treatment period (Ross et al. 2007). Current dosing regimens for TEA (5–25 mg/kg, IV) in horses provided by the manufacturer are anecdotal and not sup-ported by pharmacokinetic studies. Both of these dosing regimens are based on human target plasma concentrations. *In vitro* study in horses suggests that the concentrations of ACA and TEA needed to inhibit fibrinolysis may only be 1/20th of the dose required in humans (Fletcher et al. 2013).

Pain Management

Analgesia can be provided with a multi-modal approach. Flunixin meglumine (1.1 mg/kg, IV q 12 hours) and lidocaine CRI (1.3 mg/kg, IV loading dose over 15 minutes, followed by 1.5 mg/kg/h OR 3.0 mg/kg/h for first hour, fol-lowed by 1.5 mg/kg/h thereafter) are com-monly used in horses with abdominal pain. Various opioids have also been used. Dexmedetomidine CRI 0.5–1.0 μg/kg/h can be used for adjunct analgesia and may also decrease the effects of norepinephrine through decreased sympathetic tone. Ketamine should be avoided for the anesthetic management of pheochromocytoma patients due to its stimu-latory effects on the sympathetic nerv-ous system.

Tachyarrhythmias

Accelerated ventricular rates and the presence of abnormal ventricular complexes can be treated with magnesium sulfate (2.2 mg/kg/min IV to effect up to a maximum of 25 g/450 kg horse, diluted in 1.0 l of 0.9% NaCl and administered over a 25-minute period) and/or lidocaine (0.1–0.5 mg/kg IV slowly q 5 minutes, up to a total dose of 1.5 mg/kg IV, followed by 50 μg/kg/min as a CRI) (Sleeper 2017). Other underlying etiologies of ventricular rhythm disturbance should also be considered and addressed, including pain, hypovolemia, shock, severe hypoxemia, acid/base and electrolyte abnormalities and concomitant myocardial degeneration and infarction due to the pheochromocytoma (Yovich et al. 1984).

Hyperglycemia

Protamine zinc insulin (0.1 IU/kg subcutaneous once) followed by an IV CRI of insulin (0.01–0.02 IU/kg/h) may be used to treat severe hyperglycemia due to catecholamines. Blood glucose concentrations should be monitored frequently (every 30–60 minutes depending on patient status) and the rate of CRI adjusted to maintain normoglycemia. This is especially important in horses under general anesthesia as detrimental effects of hypoglycemia (seizures, tachycardia, central nervous system (CNS) depression) are masked in the anesthetized patient.

General Anesthesia

Catecholamine release from pheochromocytomas is typically paroxysmal and hypertension may not be identified. This is the case in 50% of canine patients with pheochromocytoma and does not exclude the necessity for pre-anesthetic treatment using an alpha-adrenergic antagonist. Phenoxybenzamine (non-competitive, non-selective alpha-adrenergic antagonist) significantly decreases mortality in dogs (13 vs 48%). In a reported case in a Shetland pony, phenoxybenzamine dosage was extrapolated from canine dosages and progressively increased until the scheduled anesthesia

for diagnostic imaging (0.2 mg/kg PO q 24 hours for two days, then 0.3 mg/kg PO q 12 hours for two days, then 0.4 mg/kg PO q 12 hours for three days, then 0.5 mg/kg PO q 12 hours for eight days and then discontinued the evening prior to anesthesia) (Fouche et al. 2016). If present, persistent/severe sinus or supraventricular tachycardia may be treated using a beta-adrenergic antagonist such as propranolol (0.02–0.22 mg/kg IV q 12 hours, administer slowly over one minute) (Sleeper 2017).

Under ideal circumstances, surgical pheochromocytoma patients should be cross-matched to a suitable blood donor and compatible whole blood should be made available for transfusion. Heightened adrenergic influence also causes profound inhibition of renin-angiotensin activity, leading to excessive (urinary) fluid loss and hypovolemia. Therefore, the patient should be treated with IV crystalloid fluids throughout the night preceding anesthesia/surgery to correct fluid deficits and ongoing losses. Dexmedetomidine (1.0 μg/kg infused slowly over 10 minutes) has been shown to significantly suppress norepinephrine release in human beings with pheochromocytoma (Singh and Singh 2014), whereas the effects of xylazine or detomidine on catecholamine release are unknown. Ketamine use should be minimized due to its stimulatory effect on the sympathetic nervous system. Propofol, when used as a sole induction agent, is associated with a high incidence of excitement, paddling, and myotonus even when used with alpha-2-adrenergic agonist sedation. However, when guaifenesin (5%, 90 mg/kg) is administered prior to propofol (2–3.0 mg/kg IV), a smooth induction sequence should be anticipated (Brosnan et al. 2011). Inhalant anesthesia can be maintained using isoflurane or sevoflurane. Constant rate infusions of lidocaine (1.5 mg/kg/h) and dexmedetomidine (0.5–1.0 μg/kg/h) provide balanced anesthesia/analgesia along with prevention/treatment of tachyarrhythmias (lidocaine) and possible suppression of norepinephrine release (dexmedetomidine). Intraoperative monitoring should include ECG, direct blood pressure monitoring, pulse oximetry, capnometry, blood glucose concentration, and temperature. Hypercapnia can stimulate catecholamine release; therefore, horses should be placed on intermittent positive pressure ventilation (IPPV) immediately following induction. Capnography should be used to monitor end-tidal carbon dioxide (EtCO$_2$) but, due to the large EtCO$_2$-PaCO$_2$ difference in horses, blood gas analysis should be used to guide ventilatory adequacy. Tumor manipulation or even whole animal manipulation (induction/hoisting/positioning) may cause a catecholamine surge with severe hypertension and tachycardia, even in patients that have been premedicated with alpha-adrenergic blockade.

Anti-hypertensive and antiarrhythmic drugs should be readily available throughout the anesthetic period. Sodium nitroprusside, a potent arteriolar and venodilator, can be titrated to effect when administered as an infusion (diluted in 5% dextrose and titrated to effect at a dose of 0.1–0.3 μg/kg/min). Magnesium sulfate can be used to treat refractory ventricular arrhythmias and/or hypertension by direct inhibition of catecholamine release and arteriolar vasodilation. Ventricular arrhythmias should be treated if they are severe enough to result in signs of decreased cardiac output such as hypotension, which is more likely with heart rates >100 bpm in adult horses, but may occur at lower heart rates (HR) in anesthetized horses. Lidocaine is recommended for conversion of ventricular arrhythmias (0.1–0.5 mg/mg IV, administered slowly every five minutes up to a total dose of 1.3–1.5 mg/kg which can then be followed by a CRI of 0.05 mg/kg/min). Magnesium sulfate acts as a calcium channel blocker and has a slower onset of action than lidocaine but does not exert other significant cardiovascular effects. The recommended dose is 2.2 mg/kg/min to effect up to a maximum of 25 g/500 kg horse (Sleeper 2017). Once the tumor (source of catecholamines) has been removed, severe hypotension may ensue, especially if the horse has received pre-anesthetic alpha-adrenergic blockage. Continued volume replacement and use of dobutamine may be necessary to correct the subsequent hypotension.

Thyroid Disorders in Horses

Anatomy and Physiology

The thyroid gland of the horse has two lobes connected by a fibrous tissue isthmus. The thyroid lobes are palpable adjacent to the larynx in the dorsolateral aspect of the third-to-sixth tracheal rings. Although not usually readily palpable in healthy horses, one or both lobes may be more evident and/or readily palpable in older horses. The thyroid gland has a rich vascular supply (4–6 ml/min/g) provided by two major arteries that arise from the external carotid and subclavian arteries (Toribio 2010; Breuhaus 2011).

Thyroid hormone (TH) synthesis and secretion is regulated by a negative feedback system involving the hypothalamus, the pituitary gland, and the thyroid gland (the hypothalamic–pituitary-thyroid [HPT] axis). Iodothyronine synthesis and release by thyroid tissue is stimulated by TSH released from the anterior pituitary gland, which is, in turn, regulated by thyrotropin-releasing hormone (TRH) from the hypothalamus. TSH increases all aspects of thyroid synthesis including increasing synthesis of T3 and T4 hormones. Negative feedback regulation of TSH secretion is tightly controlled by circulating concentrations of unbound T3 and T4. Only the unbound fractions of THs are metabolically active.

THs, T3 and T4, are important for cell growth, differentiation, and metabolism in virtually all bodily tissues. TH receptors belong to a superfamily of nuclear receptors that act as nuclear transcription factors affecting gene expression that regulate cellular functions. T3, either directly transported into the cell or derived from

T4 intracellularly, is the principal effector hormone that interacts with TH receptors. Growth, thermogenesis, and energy metabolism are reliant on TH. THs stimulate protein synthesis and catabolism, regulate lipid metabolism, stimulate basal metabolic rate, and body heat production (Toribio 2010; Breuhaus 2011).

Hypothyroidism

Hypothyroidism (TH deficiency) may result from abnormalities in TRH or TSH (HPT axis abnormalities), decreased TH synthesis/release, alterations in deiodination of T4 to T3 in peripheral tissues, or changes in TH receptor sensitivity.

Hypothyroidism in adult horses is extremely rare and is not considered life-threatening. Surgically thyroidectomized horses exhibit decreased heart rates, respiratory rates, body temperatures, hypertriglyceridemia, and hypercholesterolemia. However, these indices tend to remain within normal limits for many years, making it difficult to identify these horses clinically. In a few reported cases, clinical signs of hypothyroidism included lethargy, exercise intolerance, and poor haircoat. It should be noted that, in many instances, historical clinical reporting of hypothyroidism was erroneously based simply on measurement of T3 and T4 because a validated equine TSH assay, as would be needed to establish the diagnosis, has not been made available to equine veterinary practitioners. Theoretically, TH concentrations would be reduced but TSH and TRH levels would be increased in horses truly affected with primary hypothyroidism (Toribio 2010; Breuhaus 2011).

Thyroid Tumors

Neoplasia is the most common cause of thyroid gland enlargement. Thyroid tumors have been classified as hyperplastic nodules, adenomas, adenocarcinomas, carcinomas, and C-cell tumors. Most thyroid tumors in horses are benign, do not seem to readily metastasize, and are reported to occur most frequently in horses >17 years of age (Breuhaus 2011). Horses are typically presented with thyroid gland enlargement but without clinical signs related to the enlargement (Figure 11.2). Most affected horses have normal circulating TH levels. Like hypothyroidism, hyperthyroidism is rare in horses; however, a few cases have been reported in horses >20 years of age. Signs associated with hyperthyroidism include weight loss despite ravenous appetite, tachycardia, tachypnea, hyperactive behavior, hyperhidrosis, polyuria/polydipsia, alopecia, and cachexia (Figures 11.2 and 11.3) (Toribio 2010; Breuhaus 2011; Troillet

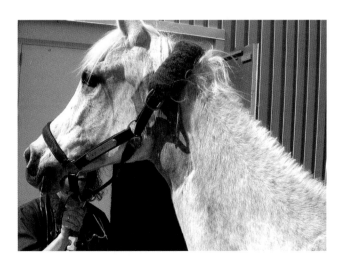

Figure 11.2 A 24-year-old horse with left-sided thyroid enlargement and hyperthyroidism resulting from thyroid adenocarcinoma.

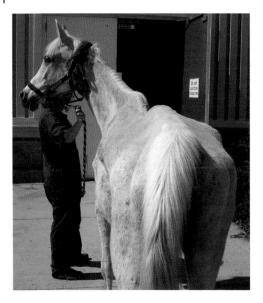

Figure 11.3 A 24-year-old horse with weight loss resulting from hyperthyroidism associated with thyroid adenocarcinoma.

et al. 2016). Serum TH concentrations (free T3, free T4, total T3, and total T4 concentrations) should be measured in horses with enlarged thyroid glands. Additional diagnostic characterizations may include ultrasonography, biopsy, T3 suppression testing, and nuclear scintigraphy.

Clinical pathology results may be normal or reveal co-existing disease in geriatric horses. A thorough medication history should be obtained since treatment of horses with phenylbutazone causes a significant decrease in total T4, free T4, and T3 (Morris and Garcia 1983; Ramirez et al. 1997). Upper airway endoscopy may reveal tracheal deviation/compression and decreased laryngeal function.

Surgical removal is not usually necessary when TH concentrations are normal and the enlarged glands are not interfering with swallowing or respiration. Horses affected with hyperthyroidism may be treated with oral propylthiouracil (PTU) to decrease circulating TH (Tan et al. 2008).

Rapid and pronounced cystic enlargement of the equine thyroid gland should be differentiated from neoplasia using ultrasonography and cytology. Thyroid enlargement as a result of a branchial remnant cyst can be successfully managed with surgical correction (Slovis et al. 2001; Nolen-Walston et al. 2009).

Hemithyroidectomy is the treatment of choice for horses that are experiencing rapid enlargement of the gland, have clinical signs associated with thyroid enlargement, or if the horse is affected with hyperthyroidism (Ramirez et al. 1998; Alberts et al. 2000; Elce et al. 2003).

Anesthetic Management

Pre-anesthesia and Induction

Physical examination should be performed to identify clinical abnormalities associated with thyroid enlargement. Thyroid tumors are most frequently encountered in geriatric horses and the patient should be thoroughly evaluated for geriatric co-morbidities. Horses presented with respiratory obstruction or distress may require temporary tracheostomy. Horses with upper airway noise or dyspnea should be pre-oxygenated. Horses that manifest upper airway clinical signs or tracheal deviation/compression may be more challenging to intubate. It may be necessary to place an endotracheal tube of smaller diameter than would normally be expected for the size of horse and so, a variety of sizes of endotracheal (ET) tubes should be readily available. Standard sedation, analgesic, and induction agents can be used in such cases.

Intraoperative Care

Intraoperative monitoring should include ECG, blood pressure, pulse oximetry, capnometry, and temperature. Direct arterial blood pressure assessment is recommended in horses. Blood gas analysis allows monitoring of acid–base, ventilation, oxygenation, and electrolyte status.

Surgery Associate Hemorrhage

Due to the high vascularization of the thyroid gland and the presence of large torturous vessels associated with thyroid tumors, significant intraoperative hemorrhage is a potential complication. Good communication with the surgical team and attention to precise dissection and hemostasis are required. In acute hemorrhage, it may require up to 12 hours for the PCV and total protein (TP) to reflect the severity because of the time required for fluid redistribution and the effects of splenic contraction. Therefore, estimation of blood loss during surgery is a useful guide for deciding if a patient requires a blood transfusion. Indications for blood transfusion for acute hemorrhage include: an estimated blood loss of ≥30%, a PCV ≤ 20%, blood lactate ≥4 mmol/l after fluid resuscitation, and an oxygen extraction ratio ≥ 50% (Mudge 2014).

Otherwise healthy horses usually readily compensate for up to a 10% blood loss (~5 l in a 500 kg horse) with crystalloid replacement of 3–4 times the volume of blood loss. Colloid (2–5 ml/kg) may be administered if losses approach 15–20% to provide oncotic support. Although intravenous fluids are needed to restore intravascular volume, they also dilute platelets and coagulation factors and may disrupt clot formation. Hydroxyethyl starch (HES) has also been associated with hypocoagulability in horses both *in vitro* and *in vivo*. HES is also potentially nephrotoxic, which is an important consideration in hypovolemic/hypotensive (blood loss) patients. Conservative fluid resuscitation is recommended until surgical hemostasis is achieved; however, this must be balanced with the risk of deleterious effects of prolonged hypotension during anesthesia. Blood loss >30%, along with clinical signs indicates requirement of transfusion. Clinical signs of tachycardia, pale mucous membranes, prolonged capillary refill time, decreasing plasma total solids, and hypotension are clinical indicators of the need for blood transfusion. However, heart rate often remains stable in anesthetized horses. Therefore, the anesthetist may need to rely on mucous membrane (MM) color, capillary refill time (CRT), blood pressure, and adequacy of arterial oxygenation as indicators for the need for transfusion (Wilson et al. 2003). Whole blood transfusion is indicated for acute blood loss since it restores blood volume as well as oxygen-carrying capacity, platelets, plasma proteins, and clotting factors (Mudge 2014).

Acute Thyrotoxicosis ("Thyroid Storm")

The overwhelming majority of horses presenting with thyroid tumors have normal TH levels. However, there are reports of hyperthyroidism and one report of a possible "thyroid storm" following hemithyroidectomy. Therefore, candidate patients should be assessed for serum TH levels and, if elevated, the anesthetist should be aware of this rare but life-threatening complication associated with thyrotoxicosis. Thyroid storm is associated with high mortality in human patients. The pathogenesis is not well understood; however, multiple factors seem to be involved in precipitating thyroid storm including elevated serum TH levels, rapid change in TH levels, nonthyroid illness, and activation of the sympathetic nervous system. Acute thyrotoxicosis has been most frequently encountered in hyperthyroid cats and dogs with functional thyroid tumors or following accidental overingestion of thyroid medication (Ward 2007). In humans, thyroid storm is often precipitated by an identifiable provocation such as infection, thyroid or non-thyroid surgery, radioactive iodine therapy, administration of iodinated contrast dyes, amiodarone therapy, withdrawal of anti-thyroid medication, vigorous palpation of the thyroid, and severe stress with nonthyroid illnesses. In humans, thyroid storm is a clinical diagnosis based on four major clinical manifestations: fever, CNS effects (ranging from agitation, seizures to coma), gastrointestinal/hepatic dysfunction (vomiting, diarrhea, abdominal pain, jaundice), and cardiovascular effects (sinus tachycardia, AF, congestive heart failure) (Ward 2007). Clinical signs associated with feline thyroid storm include: tachypnea and respiratory distress, tachycardia, cardiac murmur/arrhythmia, signs of congestive heart failure, severe hypertension, retinopathies due to hypertension, thromboembolic disease, neurologic abnormalities ranging from hyperexcitability to stupor, severe muscle weakness, and ventroflexion of the neck due to hypokalemia (Ward 2007).

Treatment of thyroid storm is aimed at reducing the production/secretion of THs, counteracting the peripheral effects of elevated THs, provision of systemic support, and identifying/eliminating any precipitating factors. Stress, surgery, and activation of the sympathetic nervous system are precipitating factors for thyroid storm. Therefore, in horses affected with hyperthyroidism, consideration should be given to reducing circulating TH levels prior to surgery. PTU has been used in horses as a relatively inexpensive and effective treatment to inhibit TH synthesis (Tan et al. 2008). PTU at an initial dose of 8.0 mg/kg orally once daily has been used successfully (Tan et al. 2008). Ketamine, currently the most widely used induction agent for equine general anesthesia, stimulates the sympathetic nervous system both directly and indirectly. Induction techniques that minimize ketamine use should therefore be considered.

Systemic support should focus on limiting the effects of elevated THs on the body. Rapid relief of the most detrimental peripheral effects (tachyarrhythmia) is provided by beta-adrenergic blockade using drugs such as propranolol and atenolol.

Recovery

Routine preparations and concerns for equine anesthetic recovery also apply to patients undergoing hemithyroidectomy. However, an additional concern for upper airway obstruction in horses undergoing hemithyroidectomy is post-operative laryngeal dysfunction/hemiplegia. Damage to the recurrent laryngeal nerve during surgery may result in laryngeal dysfunction with a risk of airway obstruction, particularly during the inspiratory phase of the ventilatory cycle. Options to maintain airway patency include maintenance of the orotracheal tube, placement of a nasotracheal tube, or temporary tracheostomy. The risk of orotracheal or nasotracheal tubes includes the potential for complete obstruction with development of negative pressure pulmonary edema.

Disorders of Calcium

Calcium Homeostasis

Calcium circulates in the plasma in three different states: bound to protein (principally, albumin), complexed with anions such as citrate and phosphate, and as (unbound) ionized calcium. Only ionized calcium is physiologically active and regulated through homeostatic mechanisms. Hypoproteinemia (especially, hypoalbuminemia) represent one of the most common explanations for total hypocalcemia in horses. Total hypocalcemia resulting from hypoalbuminemia is rarely associated with clinical signs because the ionized calcium concentration is usually maintained in the reference range in those cases.

Calcium availability in its ionized form is essential for numerous diverse physiological processes including hormone secretion, muscular contraction, enzyme activity, cell division, cell membrane stability, neuromuscular irritability, and hemostasis. Ionized calcium is also critical for many signal transduction pathways, vasoconstriction, and activation of protease enzymes. Circulating ionized calcium concentration is tightly regulated via mechanisms that collectively respond to changes in the plasma ionized calcium concentration. Regulation is distributed between the parathyroid glands, the thyroid glands, the alimentary tract, bone, and the kidneys. Parathyroid hormone (PTH) is secreted by chief cells in the parathyroid glands in response to ionized hypocalcemia or hyperphosphatemia and stimulates increased calcium resorption from bone and calcium resorption, inhibition of phosphate absorption, and elevated calcitriol (1,25-dihydroxycholecalciferol, or vitamin D3) synthesis in the kidney. Magnesium is essential for appropriate PTH secretion, and it should be emphasized that low magnesium status (hypomagnesemia) may lead to hypocalcemia (hypomagnesemia-associated calcium dysregulation). Elevated ionized calcium concentrations result in inhibited PTH release and stimulated secretion of thyrocalcitonin by the thyroid glands. Thyrocalcitonin acts to reduce renal resorption of both calcium and phosphate and to inhibit osteoclast activity.

The extent to which calcium is bound to plasma proteins (especially, albumin) versus circulating in its ionized form is significantly influenced by the presence of acidemia or alkalemia. Enhanced protein binding is promoted by alkalemic states such as those associated with exercise, hyperventilation (respiratory alkalosis), and chloride loss in sweat (metabolic hypochloremic alkalosis). Alkalosis also promotes magnesium binding to proteins (ionized hypomagnesemia) that may contribute to the pathogenesis and clinical manifestations of hypocalcemia.

Disorders Associated with Hypocalcemia

The most frequently identified clinical conditions in which hypocalcemia is identified include hypoalbuminemia (hypoproteinemia), anorexia, sepsis/endotoxemia, sweating (hyperhidrosis), gastrointestinal disease (colic), lactation (lactation or puerperal tetany), stressful long-distance transport (transit tetany), renal disease (both acute and chronic), cantharidin toxicity (blister beetle toxicosis), and nutritional secondary hyperparathyroidism. Less commonly, hypocalcemia may result from primary hypoparathyroidism, rhabdomyolysis, pancreatitis, hypomagnesemia, or following administration of various medications (sodium bicarbonate, furosemide, steroids, calcium-binding anti-coagulants, tetracycline antibiotics).

Clinical Signs Associated with Hypocalcemia

Clinical manifestations of acute hypocalcemia result from unavailable ionized calcium resulting in increased neuromuscular irritability and decreased smooth muscle contractility. Clinical signs of hypocalcemia include anxiety, tetany, lethargy, ataxia, muscle fasciculations, tremor, sweating, stiffness, tachypnea, dyspnea, dysphagia, ptyalism, seizures (convulsion), tachycardia/tachyarrhythmia (also bradycardia), and synchronous diaphragmatic flutter ("thumps"). Synchronous diaphragmatic flutter is recognized by the appearance of repetitive flank movements that coincide with heart contractions. Clinical signs of smooth muscle dysfunction during hypocalcemia include ileus, retention of fetal membranes, dystocia, and abnormal vascular tone (hypotension).

Disorders Associated with Hypercalcemia

Hypercalcemia is encountered infrequently in equine clinical practice. Primary hyperparathyroidism is a rare condition resulting from the excessive (unregulated) secretion of PTH by either hyperplastic or adenomatous parathyroid glands. Secondary hyperparathyroidism results from stimulated PTH secretion associated with either renal diseases in which hypovitaminosis D and hyperphosphatemia develop (renal secondary hyperparathyroidism) or from nutritional practices in which the daily ration is deficient in calcium or dietary calcium availability is inhibited by high concentrations of phosphorus or oxalate. However, hypercalcemia that develops in horses with chronic renal failure is usually more readily attributable to reduced renal calcium elimination than to secondary hyperparathyroidism.

Other conditions in which hypercalcemia has been reported include hypervitaminosis D, humoral hypercalcemia of malignancy (pseudohyperparathyroidism), idiopathic systemic granulomatous disease, systemic calcinosis, and following the oral or IV administration of calcium solutions for management of colic (iatrogenic).

Clinical Signs Associated with Hypercalcemia

Clinical abnormalities reported in horses affected with primary hyperparathyroidism include enlargement of facial bones and reduction of nasal passage diameter (*osteodystrophia fibrosa*), loss of body condition, lameness, and radiographic evidence of osteoporosis and attenuation of the dental lamina (including predisposition to fracture). Clinical signs associated with hypervitaminosis D are mainly attributable to the effects of hyperphosphatemia and include weight loss, inappetence, stiffness/lameness and reluctance to move (ligament calcification), and polyuria/polydipsia (renal failure resulting from renal calcinosis). In some cases, unexpected death may result from cardiovascular mineralization.

Diagnostic Testing for Disorders Associated with Hypocalcemia and Hypercalcemia

Diagnostic evaluation of calcium homeostasis in patients affected with hypocalcemia and hypercalcemia should include laboratory testing for plasma total protein (albumin) concentration, acid–base status, plasma total and ionized calcium concentrations, plasma total and ionized magnesium concentrations, plasma phosphate concentration, and urinary fractional excretions for calcium and phosphate. Further specialized diagnostic testing may include determination of plasma PTH, thyrocalcitonin, PTH-related protein, and vitamin D concentrations.

Implications for Anesthesia

Disorders of calcium may be acute or chronic and are often associated with concurrent abnormalities with phosphate and magnesium. Conditions in which the anesthetist is likely to encounter acute ionized hypocalcemia include colic, sepsis (foals), dystocia, retained placenta, lactation, long-distance transport, and rhabdomyolysis. Hypocalcemia in anesthetized horses may be caused by aggressive IV crystalloid, calcium-deficient fluid therapy, hypertonic saline, sodium bicarbonate, or blood products containing citrated anticoagulant. In studies evaluating ionized calcium in horses with surgically managed colic, 86–100% of horses were found to have concentrations below normal. Those with strangulating lesions had significantly lower ionized calcium than horse with nonstrangulating lesions (Dart et al. 1992; Garcia-Lopez et al. 2001).

Cardiovascular dysfunction in anesthetized horses may be observed. Acute/severe hypocalcemia may cause hypotension, decreased myocardial contractility, and bradycardia. ECG changes may include prolongation of the P-R, QRS, and QT intervals and bradycardia (Garcia-Lopez et al. 2001; Schenck et al. 2012). Inhalant anesthetics alter calcium effects in the myocardium by decreasing the rate of influx through the slow calcium channels in the myocardium, decreasing the uptake and release of calcium by the sarcoplasmic reticulum and decreasing the response of contractile proteins to calcium (Grubb et al. 1999). These effects contribute to the dose-dependent myocardial depression associated with inhalant anesthetics. Post-anesthetic myopathy has also been associated with intraoperative hypocalcemia (Grubb et al. 1999).

Many point-of-care analyzers provide ionized calcium measurement. Sample handling may have an effect on measurement, and a standard protocol for sample collection is recommended. Samples should be collected and processed anaerobically since exposure to air causes loss of CO_2 which increases pH and decreases the ionized calcium in the sample. Although ionized calcium can be measured in whole blood or in heparinized plasma, the type and amount of heparin may affect the accuracy of measurement. Zinc heparin may cause ionized calcium to be overestimated due to a decrease in pH which reduces protein binding of calcium whereas lithium heparin will cause ionized calcium to be underestimated. Syringes containing a premeasured amount of dry heparin are preferred to coating a syringe manually with an unknown or variable amount of liquid heparin (Schenck et al. 2012).

Treatment of hypocalcemia with 10% calcium chloride or calcium gluconate will help reverse depressed myocardial contractility associated with inhalant anesthetics. Calcium chloride (10%) contains 1.4 mEq/ml of ionized calcium, whereas calcium gluconate contains 0.45 mEq/ml. The dosage of standard calcium chloride is 5–10 ml/100 kg of body weight IV and can be very irritating to tissues if injected perivascularly. Calcium gluconate (23%) is dosed at 20 ml/100 kg of body weight whereas calcium borogluconate is dosed at 0.1–0.2 g/kg, IV (Hubbell and Muir 2009). The ECG should be carefully monitored during calcium infusion as first-degree atrioventricular (AV) block, sinus arrest, and AF have all been associated with calcium administration (Grubb et al. 1999).

Disorders of Magnesium

Magnesium Homeostasis

Less than 1% of the body's Mg content is present in the extracellular compartment. Magnesium is absorbed from the alimentary tract and excreted primarily via the kidneys. Magnesium is important for the maintenance of electrochemical gradients in excitable tissues, for oxidative phosphorylation, and is crucial for many diverse intracellular enzyme activities (particularly, generation and metabolism of adenosine triphosphate [ATP]).

Similar to calcium, Mg circulates in ionized, protein bound, and complexed forms, and concentrations are influenced by the plasma protein concentration and acid–base status (acidemia promotes ionization). Regulation of the extracellular concentration of Mg is principally dependent on the balance between gastrointestinal intake, renal excretion, and skeletal uptake. A dedicated endocrine system for Mg homeostasis does not exist. That said, several hormones (PTH, PTH-related protein, aldosterone, insulin, arginine vasopressin, and beta-adrenergic agonists) have been shown to promote renal magnesium resorption. Magnesium is protective against neurotoxicity, inflammation, free radical injury, and cardiotoxicity. Magnesium also causes bronchorelaxation (likely due to inhibition of calcium-mediated bronchoconstriction).

Disorders Associated with Hypomagnesemia

Conditions in which hypomagnesemia is identified are similar to those noted above that cause hypocalcemia. It is important to note that (ionized) Mg is essential for the normal production and secretion of PTH. Moreover, hypomagnesemia may contribute to hypocalcemia by inhibiting the effectiveness of PTH in peripheral tissues. Hypomagnesemia is more likely to develop during lactation, long-distance transport, strenuous exercise (sweating), following administration of furosemide, and in horses affected with either gastrointestinal or renal disease. The long-term use of proton pump inhibitors such as omeprazole may inhibit intestinal Mg absorption.

Clinical Signs Associated with Hypomagnesemia

Although severe whole-body Mg deficiency could lead to neuromuscular dysfunction, overt clinical signs referable to ionized hypomagnesemia are rare in horses. Clinical signs include paresis, ventricular arrhythmia, muscle fasciculations, convulsion, ataxia, and coma. Subclinical hypomagnesemia is likely more important in individuals affected with critical illness and it contributes to increased severity of systemic inflammation, cardiac arrhythmias, hypocalcemia, and hypokalemia. Hypomagnesemia causes elevated cytokine production and worsening inflammation in systemic inflammatory states, including endotoxemia in horses. Treatment of critical patients with Mg may improve clinical outcomes (including risk of death). It is common that both hypomagnesemia and hypocalcemia are identified as co-morbidities in horses with severe colic and, when present, will likely increase the risk for post-operative ileus and electrocardiographic disturbances.

Disorders Associated with Hypermagnesemia

Rarely reported, hypermagnesemia may result from iatrogenic factors (e.g. treatment with Epsom salt for management of colic, especially if co-administered with di-octyl sodium sulfosuccinate [DSS]), renal failure (reduced glomerular filtration), and extensive tissue damage (cellular release of Mg in conditions such as rhabdomyolysis or tumor lysis).

Clinical Signs Associated with Hypermagnesemia

Signs referable to hypermagnesemia include agitation, hyperhidrosis, muscle tremor, paresis/paralysis, tachypnea, and tachycardia.

Diagnostic Testing for Disorders Associated with Hypomagnesemia and Hypermagnesemia

Diagnostic evaluation of Mg homeostasis in patients affected with hypomagnesemia, hypermagnesemia, or for patients suspected to be affected with low total body Mg status may include laboratory testing for plasma total protein (albumin) concentration, acid–base status, plasma total and ionized Mg concentrations, and plasma total and ionized calcium concentrations.

Implications for Anesthesia

Calcium and magnesium homeostasis are intrinsically linked; therefore, horses that are hypocalcemic frequently have low magnesium. The majority (54%) of horses with surgically treated colic have low serum magnesium concentrations preoperatively (Garcia-Lopez et al. 2001). Horses with strangulating lesions

and those that developed post-operative ileus also had significantly lower magnesium concentrations levels than those with non-strangulating lesions and those that did not develop ileus (Garcia-Lopez et al. 2001).

Treatment of Hypomagnesemia

It is important to differentiate dosing with elemental Mg versus the Mg salt when supplementing Mg since miscalculation can lead to fatal overdose. Magnesium sulfate ($MgSO_4$) solution (9.7% Mg) provides 9.7 mg/kg of elemental Mg for a dose of 100 mg/kg. Magnesium chloride ($MgCl_2$, 25.5%) provides 25.5 mg/kg of elemental Mg for a dose of 100 mg/kg (Stewart 2011).

Daily dose rates for $MgSO_4$ in adult horses are 25–150 mg/kg/day which calculates to a dosage of 0.05–0.3 ml/kg of a 50% solution. This can be diluted into daily intravenous fluids and administered slowly. Magnesium has a relatively high safety index and has been infused at dosages as high as 29 mg/kg over two minutes (in 500 ml of isotonic fluids) for treatment of life-threatening arrhythmias associated with hypomagnesemia.

For treatment of refractory ventricular arrhythmias, for either awake or anesthetized horses, magnesium sulfate ($MgSO_4$) has been recommended at a dosage of 2–6 mg/kg/min (1.8–5.4 ml of 50% $MgSO_4$/450 kg horse/min) to effect for a maximal dose of 25 g (56 mg/kg). However, some authors indicate that up to 100 mg/kg of $MgSO_4$ can be administered safely to horses with only mild sedation as a side effect (Stewart 2011). Although Plasmalyte-A and Normosol-R both contain elemental Mg (3 mEq/l, 3.6 mg/dl), the amount is insufficient to provide the dose required to support patients with preoperative Mg deficits such as colic patients or post-operative patients with decreased feed intake. A 500 kg horse treated at a rate of 30 l/day (2.5 ml/kg/h) would receive 2.16 mg/kg/day of elemental Mg which is equivalent to 20 mg/kg of $MgSO_4$, leading to a daily deficit of 5.0–130 mg/kg (Stewart 2011).

References

Alberts, M.K., McCann, J.P., and Woods, P.R. (2000). Hemithyroidectomy in a horse with confirmed hyperthyroidism. *Journal of the American Veterinary Medical Association* 217: 1051–1054.

Auckburally, A. and Nyman, G. (2017). Review of hypoxaemia in anaesthetized horses: predisposing factors, consequences and management. *Veterinary Anaesthesia and Analgesia* 44: 397–408.

Berryhill, E.H., Thomasy, S.M., Kass, P.H. et al. (2017). Comparison of corneal degeneration and calcific band keratopathy from 2000 to 2013 in 69 horses. *Veterinary Ophthalmology* 20 (1): 16–26.

Bertin, F.R. and de Laat, M.A. (2017). The diagnosis of equine insulin dysregulation. *Equine Veterinary Journal* 49 (5): 570–576.

Bertin, F.R. and Sojka-Kritchevsky, J.E. (2013). Comparison of a 2-step insulin-response test to conventional insulin-sensitivity testing in horses. *Domestic Animal Endocrinology* 44 (1): 19–25.

Bidwell, L.A., Bramlage, L.R., and Rood, W.A. (2007). Equine perioperative fatalities associated with general anesthesia at a private practice – a retrospective case series. *Veterinary Anaesthesia and Analgesia* 34: 23–30.

Breuhaus, B.A. (2011). Disorders of the equine thyroid gland. *Veterinary Clinics of North America: Equine Practice* 27: 115–128.

Brodsky, J.B. and Lemmens, H.J.M. (2012). *Anesthetic Management of the Obese Surgical Patient*. Cambridge UK: Cambridge University Press.

Brosnahan, M.M. and Paradis, M.R. (2003). Demographic and clinical characteristics of geriatric horses: 467 cases (1989-1999). *Journal of the American Veterinary Medical Association* 223: 93–98.

Brosnan, R.J., Steffey, E.P., Escobar, A. et al. (2011). Anesthetic induction with guaifenesin and propofol in adult horses. *American Journal of Veterinary Research* 72: 1569–1575.

Buckingham, J.D. (1970). Case report. Pheochromocytoma in a mare. *Canadian Veterinary Journal* 11: 205–208.

Dart, A.J., Snyder, J.R., Spier, S.J. et al. (1992). Ionized calcium concentration in horses with surgically managed gastrointestinal disease: 147 cases (1988-1990). *Journal of the American Veterinary Medical Association* 201: 1244–1248.

Donaldson, L.L. (2005). Anesthetic considerations for the geriatric equine. In: *Equine Geriatric Medicine and Surgery* (ed. J.J. Bertone), 25–37. Philadelphia, PA, USA: Saunders Elsevier.

Dugdale, A.H.A., Curtis, G.C., Cripps, P. et al. (2010). Effect of dietary restriction on body condition, composition and welfare of overweight and obese pony mares. *Equine Veterinary Journal* 42 (7): 600–610.

Elce, T.A., Ross, M.W., Davidson, E.J. et al. (2003). Unilateral thyroidectomy in 6 horses. *Veterinary Surgery* 32: 187–190.

Fletcher, D.J., Brainard, B.M., Epstein, K. et al. (2013). Therapeutic plasma concentrations of epsilon aminocaproic acid and tranexamic acid in horses. *Journal of Veterinary Internal Medicine* 27: 1589–1595.

Fouche, N., Gerber, V., Gorgas, D. et al. (2016). Catecholamine metabolism in a Shetland Pony with suspected pheochromocytoma and pituitary *pars intermedia* dysfunction. *Journal of Veterinary Internal Medicine* 30: 1872–1878.

Frank, N. and Tadros, E.M. (2014). Insulin dysregulation. *Equine Veterinary Journal* 46: 103–112.

Frosher, B.G. and Power, H.T. (1982). Malignant pheochromocytoma in a foal. *Journal of the American Veterinary Medical Association* 181: 494–496.

Garcia-Lopez, J.M., Provost, P.J., Rush, J.E. et al. (2001). Prevalence and prognostic importance of hypomagnesemia and hypocalcemia in horses that have colic surgery. *American Journal of Veterinary Research* 62 (1): 7–12.

Garner, H.E., Coffman, J.R., Hahn, A.W. et al. (1975). Equine laminitis and associated hypertension: a review. *Journal of the*

American Veterinary Medical Association 166 (1): 56–57.

Gazzerro, D.M., Southwood, L.L., and Lindborg, S. (2015). Short-term complications after colic surgery in geriatric versus mature non-geriatric horses. *Veterinary Surgery* 44 (2): 256–264.

Gelberg, H., Cockerell, G.L., and Minor, R.R. (1979). A light and electron microscopic study of a normal adrenal medulla and a pheochromocytoma from a horse. *Veterinary Pathology* 16: 395–404.

Glover, C.M., Miller, L.M., Dybdal, N.O. et al. (2009). Extrapituitary and pituitary pathological findings in horses with pituitary pars intermedia dysfunction: a retrospective study. *Journal of Equine Veterinary Science* 29: 146–153.

Grubb, T.L., Benson, G.J., Foreman, J.H. et al. (1999). Hemodynamic effects of ionized calcium in horses anesthetized with halothane or isoflurane. *American Journal of Veterinary Research* 60: 1450–1435.

Helicer, N., Gerber, V., Bruckmaier, R. et al. (2017). Cardiovascular findings in ponies with equine metabolic syndrome. *Journal of the American Veterinary Medical Association* 250 (9): 1027–1035.

Hill, J.A., Tyma, J.T., Hayes, G.M. et al. (2020). Higher body mass index may increase the risk for the development of incisional complications in horses following emergency ventral midline celiotomy. *Equine Veterinary Journal* 52 (6): 799–804.

Hofberger, S., Gauff, F., and Licka, T. (2015). Suspensory ligament degeneration associated with pituitary *pars intermedia* dysfunction in horses. *Veterinary Journal* 203: 348–350.

Hubbell, J.A. and Muir, W.W. (2009). Anesthetic-associated complications. In: *Equine Anesthesia: Monitoring and Emergency Therapy*, 2e (eds. W.W. Muir and J.A. Hubbell), 397–417. St. Louis, MO: Saunders Elsevier.

Ireland, J.L. (2016). Demographics, management, preventive health care and disease in aged horses. *Veterinary Clinics of North America: Equine Practice* 32: 195–214.

Ireland, J.L. and McGowan, C.M. (2018). Epidemiology of pituitary *pars intermedia*

dysfunction: a systematic literature review of clinical presentation, disease prevalence and risk factors. *Veterinary Journal* 235: 22–33.

Ireland, J.L., McGowan, C.M., Clegg, P.D. et al. (2012). A survey of health care and disease in geriatric horses aged 30 years and older. *Veterinary Journal* 192: 57–64.

Jensen, R.B., Danielsen, S.H., and Tauson, A.H. (2016). Body condition score, morphometric measurements and estimation of body weight in mature Icelandic horses in *Denmark. Acta Veterinaria Scandinavica* 58 (Suppl 1): 59.

Johnson, P.J., Goetz, T.E., Foreman, J.H. et al. (1995). Pheochromocytoma in two horses. *Journal of the American Veterinary Medical Association* 206: 837–841.

Johnston, G.M., Taylor, P.M., Holmes, M.A. et al. (1995). Confidential enquiry of perioperative equine fatalities (CEFEF-1): preliminary results. *Equine Veterinary Journal* 27: 193–200.

Kadoi, Y. (2010a). Anesthetic considerations in diabetic patients. Part I: preoperative considerations of patients with diabetes mellitus. *Journal of Anesthesia* 24: 7369–7747.

Kadoi, Y. (2010b). Anesthetic considerations in diabetic patients. Part II: Intraoperative and postoperative management of patient with diabetes mellitus. *Journal of Anesthesia* 24: 748–756.

Kosolofski, H.R., Gow, S.P., and Robinson, K.A. (2017). Prevalence of obesity in the equine population of Saskatoon and surrounding area. *Canadian Veterinary Journal* 58 (9): 967–970.

Leykin, Y. and Brodsky, J.B. (2013). *Controversies in the Anesthetic Management of the Obese Surgical Patient*. Italy: Springer-Verlag.

Love, L. and Cline, M.G. (2015). Perioperative physiology and pharmacology in the obese small animal patient. *Veterinary Anaesthesia and Analgesia* 42: 119–132.

Luethy, D., Habecker, P., Murphy, B. et al. (2016). Clinical and pathological features of pheochromocytoma in the horse: a multi-center retrospective study of 37 cases (2007-2014). *Journal of Veterinary Internal Medicine* 30: 309–313.

Manens, J., Ricci, R., Damoiseaux, C. et al. (2014). Effect of body weight loss on cardiopulmonary function assessed by 6-minute walk test and arterial blood gas analysis in obese dogs. *Journal of Veterinary Internal Medicine* 28: 371–378.

Mansel, J.C. and Clutton, R. (2008). The influence of body mass and thoracic dimensions on arterial oxygenation in anaesthetized horses and ponies. *Veterinary Anaestheisa and Analgesia* 35: 392–399.

Marr, C.M. (2016). Cardiac and respiratory disease in aged horses. *Veterinary Clinics of North America: Equine Practice* 32: 283–300.

McFarlane, D. (2011). Equine pituitary *pars intermedia* dysfunction. *Veterinary Clinics of North America: Equine Practice* 27: 93–113.

McFarlane, D. and Toribio, R. (2010). Disorders of the endocrine system: pituitary *pars intermedia* dysfunction (equine Cushing's disease). In: *Equine Internal Medicine*, 3e (eds. S.M. Reed, W.M. Bayly and D.C. Sellon), 1262–1270. St. Louis, MO: Saunders/Elsevier.

McGowan, T.W., Pinchbeck, G.P., and McGowan, C.M. (2013). Prevalence, risk factors and clinical signs predictive from equine pituitary *pars intermedia* dysfunction in aged horses. *Equine Veterinary Journal* 45: 74–79.

Meier, A., Reiche, D., de Laat, M. et al. (2018). The sodium-glucose co-transporter 2 inhibitor velagliflozin reduces hyperinsulinemia and prevents laminitis in insulin-dysregulated ponies. *PLoS One* 13 (9): e0203655.

Miller, C., Utter, M.L., and Beech, J. (2013). Evaluation of the effects of age and pituitary *pars intermedia* dysfunction on corneal sensitivity in horses. *American Journal of Veterinary Research* 74 (7): 1030–1035.

Miller, M.A., Moore, G.E., Bertin, F.R. et al. (2016). What's new in old horses? Postmortem diagnoses in mature and aged equids. *Veterinary Pathology* 53 (2): 390–398.

Moens, Y. (1989). Arterial-alveolar carbon dioxide tension difference and alveolar dead space in halothane anaesthetized horses. *Equine Veterinary Journal* 21 (4): 282–284.

Moens, Y. (2013). Mechanical ventilation and respiratory mechanics during equine anesthesia. *Veterinary Clinics of North America: Equine Practice* 29: 51–67.

Moens, Y., Lagerweij, P., Gootjes, P. et al. (1995). Distribution of inspired gas to each lung in the anaesthetized horse and influence of body shape. *Equine Veterinary Journal* 27 (2): 110–116.

Monahan, C.F. and Craig, L.E. (2016). Pathology in practice. *Journal of the American Veterinary Medical Association* 248: 271–273.

Morris, D.D. and Garcia, M. (1983). Thyroid-stimulating hormone: response test in healthy horses, and effect of phenylbutazone on equine thyroid hormones. *American Journal of Veterinary Research* 44: 503–507.

Mosing, M., German, A.J., Holden, S.L. et al. (2013). Oxygenation and ventilation characteristics in obese sedated dogs before and after weight loss: a clinical trial. *Veterinary Journal* 198: 367–371.

Mudge, M.C. (2014). Acute hemorrhage and blood transfusions in horses. *Veterinary Clinics of North America: Equine Practice* 30: 427–436.

Niimura Del Barrio, M.C., David, F., Hughes, J.M.L. et al. (2018). A retrospective report (2003-2013) of the complications associated with the use of a one-man (head and tail) rope recovery system in horses following general anaesthesia. *Irish Veterinary Journal* 71: 6.

Nolen-Walston, R.D., Parente, E.J., Madigan, J.E. et al. (2009). Branchial remnant cysts of mature and juvenile horses. *Equine Veterinary Journal* 41 (9): 918–923.

Olsen, E., Pedersen, T.L.S., Robinson, R. et al. (2016). Accuracy and precision of oscillometric blood pressure in standing conscious horses. *Journal of Veterinary Emergency and Critical Care* 26 (1): 85–92.

Potter, S.J., Bamford, N.J., Harris, P.A. et al. (2016). Prevalence of obesity and owners' perceptions of body condition in pleasure horses and ponies in south-eastern Australia. *Australian Veterinary Journal* 94 (11): 427–432.

Ramirez, S., Wolfsheimer, K.J., Moore, R.M. et al. (1997). Duration of effects of phenylbutazone on serum total thyroxine and free thyroxine concentrations in horses. *Journal of Veterinary Internal Medicine* 11: 372–374.

Ramirez, S., McClure, J.J., Moore, R.M. et al. (1998). Hyperthyroidism associated with a thyroid adenocarcinoma in a 21-year-old gelding. *Journal of Veterinary Internal Medicine* 12: 475–477.

Robin, C.A., Ireland, J.L., Wylie, C.E. et al. (2015). Prevalence of and risk factors for equine obesity in Great Britain based on owner-reported body condition scores. *Equine Veterinary Journal* 47: 196–201.

Ross, J., Dallap, B.L., Dolente, B.A. et al. (2007). Pharmacokinetics and pharmacodynamics of epsilon-aminocaproic acid in horses. *American Journal of Veterinary Research* 68 (9): 1016–1021.

Rugh, K.S., Garner, H.E., Sprouse, R.F. et al. (1987). Left ventricular hypertrophy in chronically hypertensive ponies. *Laboratory Animal Science* 37 (3): 335–338.

Schenck, P.A., Chew, D.J., Nagode, L.A. et al. (2012). Disorders of calcium: hypercalcemia and hypocalcemia. In: *Fluid, Electrolyte, and Acid-Base Disorders in Small Animal Practice*, 4e (ed. S. Di Bartola), 120–194. St. Louis, MO, USA: Saunders Elsevier.

Silva, A.G. and Furr, M.O. (2013). Diagnoses, clinical pathology findings and treatment outcome of geriatric horses: 345 cases (2006–2010). *Journal of the American Veterinary Medical Association* 243: 1762–1768.

Singh, S. and Singh, A. (2014). Dexmedetomidine induced catecholamine suppression in pheochromocytoma. *Journal of Natural Science, Biology and Medicine* 5 (1): 182–183.

Sleeper, M.M. (2017). Equine cardiovascular therapeutics. *Veterinary Clinics of North America: Equine Practice* 33: 163–179.

Slone, D.E., Vaughan, J.F., Garrett, P.D. et al. (1980). Vascular anatomy and surgical technique for bilateral adrenalectomy in the equid. *American Journal of Veterinary Research* 41: 829–832.

Slovis, N.M., Watson, J.L., and Couto, S.S. (2001). Marsupialization and iodine sclerotherapy of a branchial cyst in a horse. *Journal of the American Veterinary Medical Association* 219 (3): 338–340.

Southwood, L.L., Gassert, T., and Lindborg, S. (2010). Colic in geriatric compared to mature non-geriatric horses. Part 2: treatment, diagnosis and short-term survival. *Equine Veterinary Journal* 42: 628–635.

Stevens, K.B., Marr, C.M., Horn, J.N. et al. (2009). Effect of left-sided valvular regurgitation of mortality and causes of death among a population of middle-aged and older horses. *Veterinary Record* 164: 6–10.

Stewart, A.J. (2011). Magnesium disorders in horses. *Veterinary Clinics of North America: Equine Practice* 27: 149–163.

Tan, R.H., Davies, S.E., Crisman, M.V. et al. (2008). Propylthiouracil for treatment of hyperthyroidism in a horse. *Journal of Veterinary Internal Medicine* 22: 1253–1258.

Toribio, R. (2010). Disorders of the endocrine system: thyroid gland. In: *Equine Internal Medicine*, 3e (eds. S.M. Reed, W.M. Bayly and D.C. Sellon), 1251–1260. St. Louis, MO: Saunders/Elsevier.

Troillet, A., Bottcher, D., Brehm, W. et al. (2016). Retrospective evaluation of hemithyroidectomy in 14 horses. *Veterinary Surgery* 45: 949–954.

Valverde, A. (2013). Balanced anesthesia and constant-rate infusions in horses. *Veterinary Clinics of North America: Equine Practice* 29: 89–122.

Van Oostrom, H., Schaap, M.W.H., and van Loon, J.P.A.M. (2017). Oxygen supplementation before induction of general anaesthesia in horses. *Equine Veterinary Journal* 49: 130–132.

Ward, C.R. (2007). Feline thyroid storm. *Veterinary Clinics of North America, Small Animal Practice* 37 (4): 745–754.

Wilson, D.V., Rondenay, Y., and Shance, P.U. (2003). The cardiopulmonary effects of severe blood loss in anesthetized horses. *Veterinary Anaesthesia and Analgesia* 30: 81–87.

Yovich, J.V. and Ducharme, N.G. (1983). Ruptured pheochromocytoma in a mare with colic. *Journal of the American Veterinary Medical Association* 183: 462–464.

Yovich, J.V., Hormey, F.D., and Hardee, G.E. (1984). Pheochromocytoma in the horse and measurement of norepinephrine levels in horses. *Canadian Veterinary Journal* 25: 21–25.

12

Anesthetic Management for Urogenital Interventions

Alexander Valverde[1], Valerie Moorman[2], and Kirsty Gallacher[3]

[1] *Department of Clinical Studies, Ontario Veterinary College, University of Guelph, 45 College Ave W, Guelph, Ontario, N1G 1R8, Canada*
[2] *Department of Large Animal Medicine, College of Veterinary Medicine, University of Georgia, 2200 College Station Road, Athens, GA, 30602, USA*
[3] *School of Animal and Veterinary Sciences, The University of Adelaide, 1454 Mudla Wirra Road, Roseworthy, South Australia, 5371, Australia*

Anatomy of Urogenital Systems, Male and Female

Several references are available and provide a comprehensive review of the anatomy of the male and female reproductive and urinary tracts in the horse. A brief summary is provided in the following text with focus on unique features in the horse that may be of benefit for clinical understanding.

The Female Reproductive Tract

The female reproductive tract comprises of bilateral ovaries and oviducts, and the uterus, cervix, vagina, and external genitalia. The equine ovaries are relatively large compared to other species and frequently described as "kidney-bean" shaped, but shape and size can be quite variable depending upon follicular content (range between $4 \times 2\,cm$ and $8 \times 5\,cm$). The ovaries and uterine tubes are the most cranial structures of the reproductive tract and may be found as far cranially as the third lumbar vertebrae or as far caudally as the fifth lumbar vertebrae. They are not as freely mobile as cows' ovaries, and, in non-pregnant animals, they are often located 5–10 cm directly cranial

to the upper third of the ipsilateral ileal shaft in the sublumbar region. The broad ligament, a peritoneal fold that attaches to the abdominal and pelvic walls, supports the reproductive tract. It consists of three regions (mesovarium, mesosalpinx, and mesometrium). The ovary is suspended by the mesovarium (the cranial border of this forms the suspensory ligament of the ovary). The mesosalpinx is a continuation of the mesovarium from its lateral border and suspends the uterine tube and forms the lateral proper ligament of the ovary, and the medial wall of the shallow ovarian bursa. The round ligament of the uterus extends from the uterine horn to the inguinal canal. The anatomy of the broad ligaments can be clinically relevant as exteriorization of the uterine horns or ovaries during surgical procedures is limited by the suspensory ligaments. The mesovarium is located for ecrasement and ligation during ovariectomy, and in standing animals, local anesthetics are applied to the mesovarium prior to performing these procedures.

The equine uterus is bicornuate, the uterine horns are moderately developed in the mare and are approximately 20–25 cm long, with the body being slightly shorter to almost equal in length. When viewed from above it is Y- or

T-shaped. The uterus is capable of wide variations in size, shape, and location based on stage of estrous cycle, seasonal influences, or pregnancy. The uterine horns are generally located in the abdominal cavity and in the non-pregnant mare the uterine body is found immediately in front of and frequently ventral to the cranial brim of the pelvis. It can also be partially located in the pelvic cavity where it is continuous caudally with the cervix. The cervix is approximately 6 cm long and lies in the pelvic cavity where it rests on the bladder and urethra.

The vagina of the mare is defined into two regions. The cranial vagina has only reproductive functions and extends from the cervix to the entrance of the urethra. The caudal region, the vestibule, extends from the urethral opening to the external vulva, and has both reproductive and urinary functions. A relatively distinct transverse fold (hymen) on the floor and sides of the vaginal wall is located immediately cranial to the external urethral orifice. Many texts refer only to the cranial region as the vagina and describe the vestibule region separately.

The Male Reproductive Tract

The male reproductive tract consists of bilateral testes, epididymides and ductus deferens, the accessory sex glands, and the penis. The scrotum protects and supports the testes and consists of four layers: skin, tunica dartos muscle, scrotal fascia, and parietal vaginal tunic. The scrotum of the stallion is located high in the inguinal region and is much less pendulous than in the ruminant species. The testicles of a normal stallion are palpable as two ellipsoidal structures and the long axes are horizontally positioned. Normal orientation of the testicle is determined by palpation of the tail of the epididymis and the ligament of the tail of the epididymis at the caudal pole of each testicle. There is a full complement of accessory genital glands in the horse, consisting of paired seminal vesicles, the prostate, the paired bulbourethral, and the paired ampullae of the ductus deferens. These are fully developed in the stallion and retain their juvenile status following castration in the gelding. The equine penis is of the musculo-cavernous type and consists of columns of erectile tissues. The cavernous spaces making up the erectile tissue of the penis are the corpus cavernosum, corpus spongiosum and corpus cavernosum glandis. Engorgement of these spaces with blood from branches of the external pudendal arteries and the obturator arteries is responsible for erection. The cavernous spaces within the penis are continuous with the veins responsible for drainage. When in a resting position, the penis measures about 50 cm with close to 20 cm being held within the prepuce. During maximal erection, it becomes three times as long. The prepuce in the horse is unique; the external lamina continues with the internal lamina at the level at which the preputial orifice is outlined, as in any other species, but the internal lamina makes an additional fold called the preputial fold. This fold allows for considerable lengthening of the penis on erection. The preputial fold separates the internal lamina from the free part of the penis and it also has both external and internal layers. The transition between the two layers outlines the preputial ring (entrance to the prepuce), which lies just within the preputial orifice. The preputial ring appears as a thick ring on the surface of the penis when it is protruded from the prepuce.

A combined summary of the arteries, veins, and nerves supplying the male and female urogenital tract is provided in Table 12.1. The veins of the pelvic cavity by and large are satellite to the arteries; deviations are noted in the table. The pelvis and pelvic organs have both a somatic and an autonomic component. While the somatic innervation is both sensory and motor in function and relates predominantly to the external genitalia and the pelvic floor, the autonomic innervation provides the sympathetic and parasympathetic nerve supply to the pelvic organs.

Physiological Considerations for Urogenital Interventions

The general considerations regarding anesthetic drug selection, delivery, and monitoring techniques in animals undergoing urogenital surgery using sedation or anesthesia are similar to those of the non-pregnant animal. However, changes in maternal physiology and concerns about fetal viability may further influence drug selection, patient positioning, and monitoring in pregnant mares.

Table 12.1   Summary of urogenital organs and their blood supply and innervation.

Organ	Innervation	Blood supply
Ovary	Sympathetic innervation through the renal and abdominal aortic plexuses	Ovarian artery (direct branch from the abdominal aorta)
Uterine tube	Same as ovary	Uterine branch of the ovarian artery and cranial branch of the uterine artery
Uterus	Parasympathetic innervation comes from the sacral outflow and reaches the genital tract via the pelvic nerves. Sympathetic innervation comes from the caudal mesenteric ganglion and plexus and goes to the organs via the hypogastric nerves and pelvic plexus	Uterine branch of the ovarian artery and cranial branch of the uterine artery supply the cranial uterine horn Uterine artery (branch of the external iliac artery) extends a caudal branch to anastomose with the uterine branch of the vaginal artery (from the internal pudendal artery) to supply remainder of horns and body of the uterus. Satellite veins accompany arteries, but the main venous drainage of the uterus is via the ovarian vein
Vagina	Nerves are derived through the sympathetic plexus and numerous ganglia are present in the adventia	Vaginal artery (branch of internal pudendal artery)
Vestibule and vulva	Pudendal (branches include – deep perineal and superficial perineal nerves) and caudal rectal nerves provide motor innervation to the muscles of the vestibule and vulva, and also sensory fibers to the mucous membrane of the vulva and the skin of the labia	Branches of internal pudendal artery (vestibular branch and ventral perineal artery) A second blood supply to this region, the obturator artery, terminates by entering the root of the clitoris
Perineum	Pudendal (S2–S4) and caudal rectal nerves (S4–S5)	Internal pudendal artery
Udder	Cutaneous innervation is divided between nerves of the flank and descending (mammary) branch of the pudendal nerve (S2–S4); iliohypogastric (L1), and the substance of the gland by the genitofemoral (L3–L4) nerves Sympathetic system caudal mesenteric plexus	External pudendal artery

Table 12.1 (Continued)

Organ	Innervation	Blood supply
Penis	Pudendal nerve (dorsal nerve of the penis) Deep perineal nerve supplies ischiocavernosus, bulbocavernosus, urethralis, retractor penis muscle Sympathetic fibers of the pelvic plexus supply the smooth muscle of the vessels and erectile tissue	External pudendal artery passes through the inguinal canal and supplies the cranial artery of the penis, which anastomoses on the dorsal surface of the penis with the middle artery of the penis (from the obturator) and dorsal artery of the penis (from the internal pudendal) The veins form an extensive plexus dorsal and lateral to the penis whose blood enters the accessory external pudendal vein but also the obturator and internal pudendal veins
Prepuce	Pudendal nerve Iliohypogastric nerve (medial branch) supplies skin on ventral abdomen, udder, and prepuce Genitofemoral nerve (genital branch) cremaster; vaginal tunic; skin of the prepuce, scrotum, and udder	External pudendal artery
Testis	Plexus of autonomic and visceral sensory nerves Nerves derived from the renal and caudal mesenteric plexuses, form the testicular plexus around the vessels, to which they are chiefly distributed	Testicular artery (from aorta) and its branch, the epididymal artery most of the vascular supply, some from the cremaster artery and the deferential artery also contribute to the testis (these three arteries are connected by numerous anastomosing vessels) Testicular veins divide and convolute to form the pampiniform plexus, which lies around the coiled testicular artery. The right testicular vein joins the caudal vena cava, and the left testicular vein joins the left renal vein
Scrotum	Genitofemoral nerve, pudendal nerve	Branch of external pudendal artery
Kidney	Sympathetic nerves to kidney are routed through the celiacomesenteric plexus. The vagus contributes to the parasympathetic supply	Renal artery which is a branch of the abdominal aorta. Veins are satellite and ultimately lead to the caudal vena cava
Bladder	Autonomic fibers – the sympathetic hypogastric and parasympathetic pelvic nerves. Sensory fibers are routed from the pudendal nerve	Vaginal (or prostatic artery) and also supplemented by the reduced umbilical arteries
Urethra	Pudendal nerve	Inferior vesicular artery, middle rectal artery, and internal pudendal vein

Data derived from: Sisson et al. (1975), Dyce et al. (1996), Budras et al. (2009), Auer and Stick (2012), Singh (2018).

Maternal Physiological Changes

The mare has a relatively long gestation period with the average length being approximately 340 days, and the range of normal gestation is considered to be 320–360 days (Rossdale 1993).

Pregnancy causes major adaptations in both physiology and anatomy and creates increased metabolic demands due to the growing fetal and uterine mass. Most of these adaptations influence anesthetic management of periparturient mare. Since almost all anesthetic agents depress cardiovascular and respiratory function, the physiological alterations occurring during pregnancy that have the most significant effect on anesthesia are those affecting these systems. The majority of the changes become more pronounced as gestation proceeds and in late gestation, can cause exacerbation of the cardiopulmonary changes associated with anesthesia and recumbency primarily because of decreases in respiratory reserve due to cranial displacement of the diaphragm.

There are limited studies on cardiopulmonary effects of pregnancy in the horse, but a number of references from other species, particularly women and sheep from which much of the information is extrapolated. Tidal volume and minute ventilation increase early in pregnancy in woman, with greater than 50% increases seen at term (McAuliffe et al. 2002). It has been well documented in humans that pregnancy reduces functional residual capacity (Bobrowski 2010), which reduces respiratory reserve. For the lungs to function as efficient gas exchangers, large mammals must avoid uneven distribution of ventilation and perfusion resulting from compression of the lung by the weight of the thoracic and abdominal viscera and changes in cardiac output. In the horse, the largest portion of the lung is in the dorsal aspect of the thorax with relatively little lung tissue lateral to the heart. In addition, the diaphragm slopes steeply ventral and cranial so in the nonpregnant horse the lungs lie dorsal to the abdominal cavity. As a result of this anatomical arrangement, the lungs are not compressed in the standing animal, and the weight of the abdominal viscera below the diaphragm typically aids lung expansion (Sorenson and Robinson 1980). However, has been shown in pregnant Shetland ponies in the standing position that as gestation advances, the ventral (dependent) lung regions are gradually less ventilated with a relative shift of regional ventilation toward dorsal (non-dependent) regions and that this situation reverses after foaling (Schramel et al. 2012). This could add to the respiratory compromise observed when horses are placed in dorsal recumbency during anesthesia.

During pregnancy in woman, the circulating blood volume increases but hemoglobin and plasma protein concentrations fall. Cardiac output increases throughout pregnancy, peripheral resistance decreases, but arterial blood pressure does not change (Robson et al. 1987). Near term, woman can become acutely hypotensive when placed on their backs due to aortocaval compression (McAuliffe et al. 2002). Aortocaval compression has not been specifically demonstrated in pregnant animals but heart rate, respiratory rate, and mean uterine artery blood pressure increased and arterial oxygenation decreased in cows during the third trimester of pregnancy, when positioned in dorsal recumbency (Dunlop et al. 1994), which suggests similar considerations exist in large animals.

Additionally, in the pregnant animal uterine blood flow is not subject to autoregulation and is directly proportional to perfusion pressure and inversely proportional to uterine vascular resistance. Anything leading to vasoconstriction, hypovolemia or a decrease in arterial blood pressure will therefore reduce uterine blood flow and consequently the supply of nutrients and oxygen to the fetus (Taylor 1997). Doppler sonographic studies in the horse have illustrated a decrease in the peripheral blood flow resistance in the first weeks of pregnancy and an increase in uterine blood flow volume (BFV), in the last trimester of pregnancy where BFV increased 50-fold in the uterine artery (2.5 ml/second at day 16 pregnancy to 124.4 ml/second near term). The diameter of the uterine artery was also shown to increase fourfold from 4 to 16 mm during gestation in mares. The distinct rise in uterine BFV in the last trimester is consistent with fetal growth as the metabolic demands of fetal tissues increase (Fowden et al. 2000a, Klewitz et al. 2015). Additional metabolic demand is met by increasing the supply of nutrients to the fetus from the placenta (Hay 1995).

The Equine Placenta

The horse's placenta is classified as diffuse because the fetus is in contact with the allantoamnion inside the chorioallantois and has a complete set of layers, including endometrial epithelium, maternal connective tissue, and maternal endothelial cells, therefore, classified as epitheliochorial with attachments to the entire endometrium (Furukawa et al. 2014). These three layers represent different levels of barriers to drug transfer prior to the three tissue layers also present in the fetus, namely fetal chorionic epithelial cells, fetal connective tissue, and endothelial cells. Many studies regarding drug transfer across the placenta for human application have been done in ruminants and pigs, who share the epitheliochorial arrangement of the placenta with the horse. However, ruminants have a cotyledonary placenta; the pig's is diffuse like the horse. The number of layers in the horse's placenta could delay drug transfer to the fetus, but focal thinning can occur which would counter that (Furukawa et al. 2014). Ultimately, it is placental blood flow that influences drug transfer (Mihaly and Morgan 1983).

The size of the uterus is governed by the size of the mare and in turn determines the available area for placentation and, hence, fetal growth (Allen et al. 2002). The placenta is a metabolically active organ and uses a range of substrates to meet its energy requirements which are higher than either the mare or the fetus (Hay 1991; Vaughan and Fowden 2016). Oxygen consumption by the combined uteroplacental tissues is similar to other species with epitheliochorial and hemochorial (humans) placentation and increases by 25–50% between mid-gestation and late gestation in the horse (Fowden et al. 2000b; Hay 2006; Vaughan and Fowden 2016). Glucose consumption per kg of combined uteroplacental tissues also increases between mid-gestation and late gestation in the horse (Fowden et al. 2000b). The equine uteroplacental tissues use 5 times more oxygen and 10 times more glucose than the fetus at both mid- and late gestation and are sensitive to changes in their nutrient supply producing prostaglandins in response to undernutrition (Fowden et al. 1994; Fowden et al. 2000b; Molina et al. 1991; Macdonald et al. 2000).

Drug Transfer Across the Placenta

Placental transfer of drugs is governed by the physicochemical properties of the drug and anatomical features of the placenta. The four main physicochemical properties of the drug are molecular size, protein binding in maternal blood, degree of ionization, and lipophilicity (Mihaly and Morgan 1983; Reynolds 1987, 1998), which provide a diffusion constant, unique to each drug. All four properties influence the behavior of the drug and cannot be considered individually, except for degree of ionization, which on its own can prevent placental crossing.

Transfer of drugs can occur by simple diffusion, facilitated diffusion via transport systems, active transport, and pinocytosis. Most drugs used in anesthesia have large diffusion constants – low molecular weights, high lipid solubility, and poor ionization – and diffuse rapidly across the placenta. The concentration of drug in the umbilical vein of a fetus however is not that to which the fetal target organs such as the heart and brain are exposed as most of the umbilical blood passes through the liver, where the drug may be metabolized or sequestered. The remainder of the umbilical blood passes through the ductus venous to the vena cava where it is diluted by drug-free blood from the hind end of the fetus. Thus, the fetal circulation protects vital tissues and organs from exposure to sudden high drug concentrations and when blood returns to the maternal circulation biotransformation and elimination is enhanced; therefore, the effects of anesthetic drugs in the fetus in utero could be considered more benign. Conversely, a neonate delivered under the effects of anesthetic drugs would need of its own biotransformation and elimination as soon as the placental unit is disrupted, and the effects of anesthetic drugs could be more profound given their underdeveloped systems.

Sedation and Analgesia for Standing Interventions

There are a number of surgical procedures in which standing surgical interventions are the procedure of choice. When making the decision to either perform a surgery standing or under general anesthesia, there are several factors to consider. The first and likely most important is the size and disposition of the horse as this will impact the safety of the horse and the personnel performing the procedure. Very small patients, such as miniature horses, may make the procedure more difficult for the surgeon to perform safely, as well as to maintain aseptic technique. Conversely, draft horses with a higher risk of post-operative complications compared to light breed horses following general anesthesia (Gleed and Short 1980; Olson 2002; Kraus et al. 2003) and good temperament may be better suited to standing interventions.

Debilitated horses may also be at higher risk of complications with general anesthesia and may be better candidates for standing procedures. In one report, several debilitated horses could not maintain appropriate blood pressures so general anesthesia was aborted and the procedure was performed standing at a later time (Arnold et al. 2010). Fractious horses

or those horses that do not respond appropriately to sedation may be patients that are not ideal candidates for standing surgical procedures. Appropriate facilities are also needed to safely perform standing surgical procedures and facilitate maintaining an aseptic surgical field and minimize contamination of the surgical site. The ability to provide appropriate analgesia to which might include both local analgesia and systemic medication is also a determinant of feasibility. In most cases of urogenital disease, the horse only displays mild discomfort and systemic analgesia can be provided with NSAIDs, in addition to medications utilized for sedation (alpha-2 adrenergic agonists and opioids). In situations where there is complete obstruction of the urinary tract (i.e. urethral obstruction) and the horse demonstrates moderate-to-severe signs of abdominal pain, a standing surgical procedure may be contraindicated (DeBowes 1988).

Patient Preparation for Standing Urogenital Procedures

In order for standing surgery to be performed optimally, appropriate patient restraint is critical. This typically involves the horse being contained in standing stocks, which limits the horse's ability to move (Figure 12.1). The stocks should be located in a quiet location, with minimal foot traffic, and a non-slippery flooring (Graham and Freeman 2014). These stocks ideally should be adjustable to accommodate differences in height and length of the horses; optimal stocks have padding and full rear door both for horse and surgeon safety (Beard 1991). In procedures where surgical access involves the flank, the height of the sides of the stocks needs to be adjusted so that the surgical field is not contaminated by the bars. Because of the location of the surgical site (either caudal abdomen or perineal location), the tail should be wrapped to prevent contamination of the surgical site and can be tied overhead to the stocks (Beard 1991). One additional benefit of the tail-tie is for additional support of the hindlimbs if

Figure 12.1 Standing surgery room. This set of stocks is contained within a dedicated room specifically for standing surgical procedures. The stocks have a non-slip flooring, have adjustable bars to accommodate different sized horses and that can be opened if a horse falls, have an overhead bar to tie the tail, and have padded forward and rear bars. Note that there is also a door at the front of the room, providing a secondary exit for personnel and the horse.

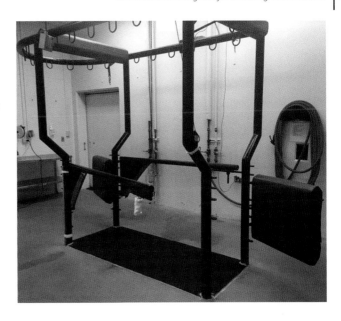

the horse develops hindlimb weakness following administration of epidural anesthetics (Beard 1991). For lengthy perineal surgical procedures in mares, placing and maintaining a urinary catheter can prevent surgical site contamination, especially since the use of alpha-2 adrenergic agonists results in diuresis (Thurmon et al. 1984; Tranquilli et al. 1984; Beard 1991; Alexander and Irvine 2000; Valverde 2010).

Sedation Protocols

For shorter length urogenital procedures (standing castration, perineal urethrotomy, partial phallectomy), sedation has been performed with intravenous xylazine hydrochloride (0.5–1.0 mg/kg) or detomidine hydrochloride (0.01–0.02 mg/kg) with or without the addition of butorphanol tartrate (0.05–0.01 mg/kg), although other alpha-2 agonists can also be used (Climent et al. 2009; Arnold et al. 2010; Adams and Hendrickson 2014). These doses can be re-administered as needed throughout the procedure. The use of an intravenous jugular catheter will allow quick and easy access for re-administration of medications (Graham and Freeman 2014).

For longer duration procedures or with horses that do not respond as expected to

typical doses of sedation, a variety of continuous rate infusions of alpha-2 adrenergic agonists, with or without the addition of opioids, can be utilized. One benefit of a continuous infusion includes reaching a constant plane of sedation without the peaks and troughs that can accompany bolus dosing (Vigani and Garcia-Pereira 2014). A number of these continuous rate infusions have been investigated in normal horses for their effects on sedation, ataxia, and analgesia (Solano et al. 2009; Ringer et al. 2012a, 2012b, 2013; Medeiros et al. 2017). Several other continuous rate infusions have been utilized for urogenital or other surgical procedures (Virgin et al. 2010; Adams and Hendrickson 2014; Seabaugh and Schumacher 2014; Potter et al. 2016). A number of reported combinations of alpha-2 adrenergic agonists and opioids used for continuous rate infusions are listed in Table 12.2.

Local Anesthesia/Analgesia

A variety of local anesthesia/analgesia techniques are utilized to facilitate standing urogenital procedures. Many of these techniques can also be utilized to provide supplemental analgesia in anesthetized patients. The most commonly utilized local anesthetics in horses

Table 12.2 Continuous rate infusions reported for standing sedation in horses.

Medication(s)	Loading dose (L) CRI dose (C)	Effects, Comments	Reported procedures	References
Dexmedetomidine	3.5 µg/kg (L) 5 µg/kg/h (C)	Significant decrease in head height during 90 minutes CRI, maximum ataxia was within first 15 minutes and then gradually decreased, significant decrease in tactile stimulation at 30 minutes and significant decrease in auditory stimulation up to 60 minutes after CRI started	None	Medeiros et al. (2017)
Dexmedetomidine + Butorphanol	3.5 µg/kg (L) 3.5 µg/kg/h (C) 20 µg/kg (L) 24 µg/kg/h (C)	Significant decrease in head height during 90 minutes CRI, maximum ataxia was within first 15 minutes and then gradually decreased, significant decrease in tactile and auditory stimulation at 30 minutes after CRI started	None	Medeiros et al. (2017)
Acepromazine + Detomidine + Buprenorphine	0.02 mg/kg (L) 10 µg/kg (L) ~0.6 µg/kg/min (C) 0.01 mg/kg (L)	CNS excitement (attributed to buprenorphine) Good degree of sedation	Dental and sinus procedures	Potter et al. (2016)
Acepromazine + Detomidine + Morphine	0.02 mg/kg (L) 10 µg/kg (L) ~0.6 µg/kg/min (C) 0.1 mg/kg (L)	Good degree of sedation	Dental and sinus procedures	Potter et al. (2016)
Romifidine	80 µg/kg (L) 30 µg/kg/h (C)	Good degree of sedation, ~ 1 hour recovery from sedation Redosing of romifidine required (20 µg/kg) for 5/11 dental procedures, 2/11 needed rescue analgesia (butorphanol)	None Dental or ophthalmologic procedures	Ringer et al. (2012b), Marly et al. (2014)

Drug/combination	Dose	Observations	Procedure	Reference
Romifidine + Butorphanol	80 µg/kg (L) 29 µg/kg/h (C) 18 µg/kg (L) 25 µg/kg/h (C)	Good degree of sedation, more ataxic than romifidine alone, ~1 hour recovery from sedation 1/10 needed bolus romifidine (20 µg/kg) for each a dentistry and ophthalmologic procedure, 0 needed rescue analgesia (butorphanol)	None Dental or ophthalmologic procedures	Ringer et al. (2012b), Marly et al. (2014)
Xylazine	1 mg/kg (L) 0.69 mg/kg/h (C)	Constant plasma concentrations of xylazine at 45 minutes	None	Ringer et al. (2012a)
Xylazine + Butorphanol	1 mg/kg (L) 0.65 mg/kg/h (C) 18 µg/kg (L) 25 µg/kg/h (C)	Constant plasma concentrations of xylazine at 45 minutes 3/10 horses fell (10–15 minutes after loading dose) 4/10 horses were insufficiently sedated (during second hour of sedation)	None	Ringer et al. (2012a)
Detomidine + Buprenorphine	10 µg/kg (L) 0.16 µg/kg/min (C) 6 µg/kg (L)	Good sedation for surgery	Laparoscopic sterilization	Van Dijk et al. (2003)
Xylazine Butorphanol Detomidine	0.33 mg/kg (L) 5 mg (L) 20 mg in 1 l polyionic fluids (titrate to effect) (C)	Total detomidine dose for the procedure 9–18 mg	Bilateral laparoscopic ovariectomy	Virgin et al. (2010)

are lidocaine, mepivacaine, ropivacaine, and bupivacaine. These anesthetics differ in their degree of lipid solubility, onset of activity, duration of activity, and toxicity. Each of these four local anesthetics has reported use for both peripheral and epidural anesthesia. In general, the duration of the procedure, as well as clinician familiarity with the anesthetic, often dictates which of these local anesthetics is chosen for a particular procedure.

While site of administration-dependent, in general terms, lidocaine and mepivacaine are similar in their duration (90–180 minutes and 120–180 minutes, respectively) of activity and have a relatively quick onset; bupivacaine has a longer onset and duration (180–500 minutes) of action (Skarda et al. 2009). One important side effect of bupivacaine is its cardiotoxicity which is magnified with inadvertent intravenous administration (Skarda et al. 2009). Ropivacaine has a quick onset of action and a longer duration of action (180–360 minutes) than lidocaine and mepivacaine and is reported to have less cardiotoxicity than bupivacaine (Skarda et al. 2009).

Infiltrative Blocks

Especially for surgical procedures performed in the flank region of the horse, infiltrative blocks can be especially useful. Methods of infiltration include the use of an inverted L block around the proposed surgical site or direct infiltration of local anesthetic at the surgical site (Seabaugh and Schumacher 2014). The technique is simple as there are no specific anatomic landmarks that have to be identified and relatively large volumes of local anesthetic may be safely administered (Skarda et al. 2009). However, local infiltrate at the line of surgical incision has been suggested to increase the risk of infection, and delay healing of the incision site (Moon and Suter 1993). Additionally, deeper tissues may only be partially desensitized especially in cases of flank laparotomy in obese horses (Skarda et al. 2009).

Infiltration of local anesthetic is commonly utilized for routine standing castration. Typically

for the adult horse (weighing 400–500 kg), 10–15 ml of either 2% lidocaine or 2% mepivacaine is infused either at the proposed incision lines on either side of the median raphe of the scrotum or as a ring block made surrounding the area of proposed incisions (Adams and Hendrickson 2014). Intratesticular administration may also be helpful to supplement this as noted in following text; the total dose should not exceed 2 mg/kg. Local anesthesia is also routinely used for perineal surgeries that are short in duration, including the Caslick's procedure. Again, approximately 10 ml of either 2% lidocaine or 2% mepivacaine (not to exceed 2 mg/kg) is used along the proposed incision line.

Infiltrative anesthesia can also be useful for anesthesia of visceral organs as for example to provide anesthesia of the testicle and spermatic cord during a routine standing castration (Adams and Hendrickson 2014). Intratesticular lidocaine diffuses into the spermatic cord and allows for appropriate anesthesia of the structures within the cord during emasculation. Additionally, partial phallectomy can be performed in the standing gelding or stallion by utilizing a local ring block at the level of the opening of the prepuce (i.e. proximal to the site of phallectomy) (Arnold et al. 2010; Adams and Hendrickson 2014). In mares, local infiltrate of anesthetic into the mesovarium is routinely performed for ovariectomies, whether they are removed via colpotomy, flank laparotomy, or laparoscopy (Virgin et al. 2010; Seabaugh and Schumacher 2014).

Paravertebral Blocks

While paravertebral anesthesia is most commonly performed in ruminant species, but may similarly be performed in horses. Blockade of the dorsal and ventral branches of spinal nerves T_{18}, L_1, and L_2 in the horse will provide flank desensitization, but because it can be technically more challenging, it is used less frequently (Moon and Suter 1993). That said, with knowledge of anatomical landmarks it can be readily performed (Delli-Rocili et al. 2020). The main benefits of this technique are that a smaller dose of local anesthetic are typically required and there are no direct impacts on the healing of the surgical incision site (Skarda et al. 2009). However, the landmarks can be difficult to palpate in heavily muscled horses, and if anesthetic is deposited inadvertently around the third lumbar nerve, there is a potential for motor deficits of the hindlimb (Skarda et al. 2009).

Epidural and Spinal Anesthesia and Analgesia

Anesthesia and analgesia can be accomplished by either epidural or subarachnoid injection (Natalini 2010). These techniques can be used to anesthetize the perineal or flank regions depending on where the anesthetic or analgesic medications are deposited. The most commonly used technique is the caudal epidural injection, but caudal subarachnoid injection, segmental dorsolumbar epidural injection, and thoracolumbar subarachnoid injection have also been reported (Skarda et al. 2009).

- *Caudal Epidural Injection*

   (Figure 12.2) Caudal epidural injection can be used to provide anesthesia and analgesia for surgical procedures of the urogenital tract, specifically for the perineal region, caudal reproductive tract (vulva, vestibule, vagina), and the caudal urogenital tract (urethra and bladder) (Natalini 2010). When properly performed, this technique should desensitize several nerves, including the caudal rectal, middle rectal, and pudendal nerves (Skarda et al. 2009). The goal of this technique is to desensitize the surgical site while allowing the horse to stand and maintain function of the hindlimbs (Natalini 2010).

   Most surgical procedures can be safely performed using a single injection into the sacrococcygeal or coccygeal epidural space. However, if a procedure is anticipated to be prolonged or if additional analgesics may be required in the peri-operative period, an epidural catheter may be placed. Placement of an epidural catheter can be used to allow repeated injection of anesthetic solution without the need for interruption of the surgical procedure to re-prep and re-administer anesthetics by a second epidural puncture (Green and Cooper 1984). Placement of an epidural catheter could also facilitate administration of analgesic medications post-operatively.

There are a number of anesthetics and analgesics that can be administered either on their own or in combination into the epidural space. These medications are commonly chosen based on clinician preference/familiarity and the desired length of anesthesia or analgesia desired. A list of commonly utilized medications, dosages, and anticipated duration of activity are listed in Table 12.3. In general, for surgical procedures, combination therapy with a local anesthetic and either an alpha-2 agonist or opioid is often utilized. Length of analgesia and anesthesia is typically longer than for the local anesthetic alone. Except for xylazine, most alpha-2 agonists or opioids do not provide sufficient local anesthesia to be able to perform surgery. As a group, alpha-2 agonists block C-fiber conduction through the blockade of substance P (Riedl et al. 2009; Valverde 2010). Additionally, xylazine blocks A-delta fibers with a more profound effect than other alpha-2 agonists, giving it the ability to work as an anesthetic (Valverde 2010). Combinations of alpha-2 agonists and local anesthetics can cause substantial ataxia and occasionally recumbency can result (Robinson and Natalini 2002). This most commonly occurs when too large a volume is used and paralysis is induced from cranial spread of the anesthetic. If there is only partial paralysis, the horse can be supported using a tail-tie, but if the horse becomes recumbent and distressed, inducing and maintaining anesthesia until the motor effects dissipate may be beneficial (Robinson and Natalini 2002).

Alpha-2 agonists, such as detomidine and xylazine, also cause additional side effects, including perineal edema, perineal sweating, bradycardia, second-degree atrioventricular blockade, significant sedation, and/or ataxia (Robinson and Natalini 2002). In horses where multiple epidural injections have been

(a)

(b)

(c)

(d)

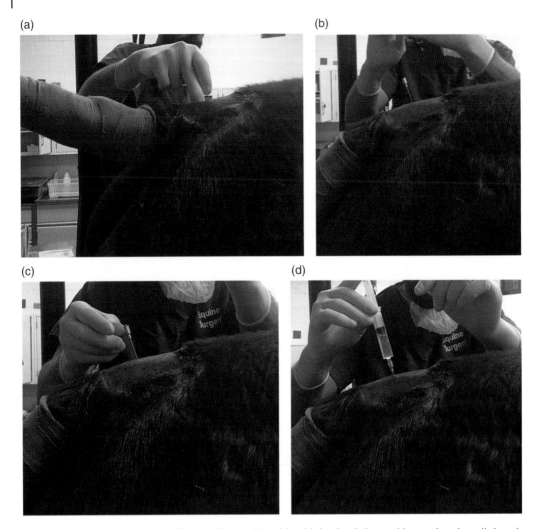

Figure 12.2   Caudal epidural. (a) The site for caudal epidural injection is located by moving the tail dorsal and ventral, to locate the sacrococcygeal or first intercoccygeal space. (b) A 20- or 18-gauge 3.8 cm hypodermic or spinal needle is placed through the skin at the site of the first coccygeal space. (c) 0.9% saline has been placed in the hub of the needle prior to advancement into the epidural space. (d) Once the 0.9% saline has been aspirated into the epidural space by the negative pressure present in the epidural space, the medication volume is injected. There should be no resistance to injection, which can be tested by placing a small air bubble within the syringe.

performed, incomplete blockade can occur, which may be secondary to presence of fibrous tissue, adhesions, or inability to inject due to changes in anatomy (Natalini 2010).

Opioids may also be administered via caudal epidural injection. Methadone, hydromorphone, meperidine and morphine have been used and providing varying onset and duration of effect. Meperidine has been associated with motor weakness whereas morphine is associated with pruritis, which is thought to be related to the local release of histamine (Robinson and Natalini 2002).

- ***Caudal Subarachnoid Injection***

This technique is performed by placing a Huber-point Tuohy needle with a stylet (17 gauge, 19.5 cm) with the bevel directed caudally into the lumbosacral intervertebral space (Skarda et al. 2009). This space is located at the most proximal place in the gluteal

Table 12.3   Commonly utilized drugs for epidural anesthesia ± analgesia. In general, alpha-2 agonists (xylazine, detomidine, medetomidine) produce variable anesthesia and are best used in combination with local anesthetics.

Drug(s)	Dose (mg/kg)	Dose (ml) – typical 450 kg horse	Duration (min)	Remarks
Lidocaine 2%	0.22–0.35	5–8	45–180	Higher doses can result in severe ataxia and/or recumbency
Mepivacaine 2%		5–8	90–180	
Ropivacaine (0.1–0.5%)		5–10	180–480	Minimal sedation and ataxia
Bupivacaine (0.1–0.5%)	0.06	5–8	180–480	
Xylazine	0.17–0.25		60–180	
Detomidine	0.02–0.06		120–240	Can result in systemic sedation, higher doses may be needed for sufficient analgesia
Medetomidine	0.002–0.005		240–360	
Lidocaine 2% + xylazine	0.22 (L) + 0.17 (X)		240–360	Ataxia and/recumbency are possible
Lidocaine 2% + morphine	0.22 (L) + (0.1–0.2 (M))		240–360	
Bupivacaine 0.125% + morphine	0.02 (B) + (0.1–0.2 (M))		480–720	
Lidocaine 2% + Neostigmine	0.2 (L) + 0.5 −2 µg/kg (N)		120–150	More prolonged analgesia and ataxia then lidocaine alone, potential decrease in HR and blood pressure
Lidocaine 2% + Tramadol	0.2 (L) + 0.5 (T)		210	More prolonged analgesia and ataxia then lidocaine alone

From Robinson and Natalini (2002), Skarda (1996), Skarda et al. (2009), Natalini (2010), Seabaugh and Schumacher (2014), Vigani and Garcia-Pereira (2014), DeRossi et al. (2012).

region, and a divot can be identified between the last lumbar vertebrae (L6) and the sacral vertebrae with digital palpation. The subarachnoid space is approximately 10–15 cm deep and is positively identified by aspirating cerebrospinal fluid through the needle following removal of the stylet. A catheter is fed through the needle to the terminal aspect of the subarachnoid space, which is located near the third sacral vertebra (approximately 10 cm) (Skarda and Muir 1994; Skarda et al. 2009). Smaller volumes of local anesthetics (one third that of caudal epidural administration) are effective for caudal anesthesia

using this technique compared to caudal epidural injection (Skarda et al. 2009). Additional advantages of this technique over caudal epidural anesthesia include quicker time to onset and easier desensitization of spinal nerves since they are not covered with dura within the subarachnoid space (Skarda et al. 2009). However, this technique is more difficult, and the duration of action is reported to be shorter than caudal epidural (Skarda and Muir 1994; Skarda et al. 2009).

- ***Segmental Dorsolumbar Epidural Injection***
This technique requires placement of a Huber-point Tuohy needle with a stylet into the

epidural space at the lumbosacral space and then advancing the catheter to the level of T18–L1. Injecting local anesthetic (4 ml) in this location can desensitize the spinal nerves T18 to L2, which can provide appropriate anesthesia of both flank regions (Skarda et al. 2009). If the catheter kinks or curls and does not feed cranially, there is the risk of inadvertent anesthesia of the femoral nerve, which can result in temporary hind limb paralysis (Skarda et al. 2009). Because the difficulty performing this technique, it is not commonly utilized.

- ***Thoracolumbar Subarachnoid Injection***
This technique is similar to the segmental dorsolumbar epidural technique, as the site of needle puncture is at the lumbosacral space, but the needle is placed into the subarachnoid space (confirmed by the presence of cerebrospinal fluid) and a catheter is inserted to the level of T18–L1. A small volume (1.5–2 ml) of local anesthetic (2% mepivacaine) is injected to anesthetize the spinal cord from approximately T14 to L3, which allows desensitization of the flank region (Skarda et al. 2009). Benefits of this technique are similar to caudal subarachnoid injection, which include quick onset to action and direct access of the local anesthetic to nerve roots (Skarda et al. 2009).

Peri-neural Anesthesia: Pudendal, Perineal, Caudal Rectal Nerves

For certain procedures of the urogenital tract, specific nerve blocks can be utilized to improve local anesthesia during the surgical procedure and to potentially improve pain management post-operatively (Gallacher et al. 2016). This may be especially helpful in horses that have received repeated caudal epidural injections and have as a consequence, are less responsive to further caudal epidurals, or have developed fibrous tissue or adhesions (Schumacher et al. 1985; Gallacher et al. 2016). For surgical procedures of the anus, perineum, and vestibule in the mare and anus, perineum, glans penis and lamina interna of the prepuce (area distal to the preputial ring) in the male, anesthesia of the pudendal, caudal rectal, and superficial perineal nerves can be used to provide surgical anesthesia (Schumacher et al. 1985; Gallacher et al. 2016).

Several approaches to blocking these nerves has been described. These nerves can be accessed by passing a 15 cm 18 gauge spinal needle dorsolateral to the anus, using transrectal palpation to identify a foramen where the caudal rectal artery and vein exit medially along the sacrosciatic ligament (Schumacher et al. 1985). More recently, another technique has been described using electric stimulation to identify the pudendal nerve. A 10 cm needle is placed proximal to the tuber ischia, lateral to the anus and/or vulva externally, and medial to the sacrosciatic ligament, using a gloved hand within the vestibule of mares to guide the needle away from the wall of the rectum and vestibule (Gallacher et al. 2016). Both the right and left nerves should be anesthetized, and 10–20 ml of 2% lidocaine or mepivacaine per site was found to be sufficient to provide surgical anesthesia (Gallacher et al. 2016). Potential complications of both techniques to anesthetize the pudendal nerve are inadvertent needle penetration into the rectum or vagina and puncture of vasculature, resulting in hematoma (Schumacher et al. 1985; Gallacher et al. 2016).

In male horses, standing partial phallectomy with penile retroversion can be facilitated with caudal epidural anesthesia and anesthesia of the dorsal nerves of the penis, either by placing local anesthetic around the pudendal nerves or by instilling local anesthetic around the superficial and deep dorsal nerves of the penis at the level of the tuber ischii (Perkins et al. 2003). The location for injection of the superficial branches is 2 cm to the right and left of the median raphe at the level of the ischial arch using approximately 5 ml of mepivacaine 2%, subcutaneously. For blockade of the deep branches, the same location is used and a 3.75 cm 20 gauge hypodermic needle is directed toward midline from both the left and right sides (Perkins et al. 2003).

General Anesthesia

Several factors need to be considered when general anesthesia is planned for urogenital interventions. Foremost, the risk of general anesthesia to the patient needs to be considered in procedures that can be readily performed in the horse standing with proper sedation. Urogenital interventions include elective and emergency conditions; therefore, the health status of the patient varies. The nature of the condition can affect the behavior of the patient (e.g. aggressive males or females) due to hormonal influence, and can also induce physiological changes (e.g. pregnancy).

In dealing with pregnant patients, consideration for both the mare and fetus/neonate safety and survival is necessary, and in case of general anesthesia, there is no universal optimal anesthetic technique; more important is the familiarity and conditions in which the surgical and anesthesia team perform at their best. The homeostasis of the fetus can be affected by the health condition of the mother, the risks associated with recumbency and anesthetic drugs that may impede proper blood flow to the placenta and fetus, and the manipulation of the abdomen that potentially causes mechanical interference and local inflammation (Reitman and Flood 2011).

The use of anesthetics, sedatives, and analgesic drugs in pregnant individuals can potentially affect cellular differentiation and organogenesis in early fetal development, through interference with second messenger systems between cells, signaling, mitosis, and DNA synthesis (Sturrock and Nunn 1975; Kress 1995; Langmoen et al. 1995; Reitman and Flood 2011). However, clinical observational studies of human fetal development and studies in laboratory animals have not found a direct correlation between drugs used routinely during the administration of anesthesia and teratogenicity (Shepard and Lemire 2010; Reitman and Flood 2011), with the exception of exposure to nitrous oxide during early pregnancy, which may result in pregnancy loss and reduced fertility (Rowland et al. 1992; Rowland et al. 1995). Presently, nitrous oxide is uncommonly used in equine anesthesia.

Risk of General Anesthesia

Mortality Considerations

For procedures that must be performed under general anesthesia, factors that contribute to an increased risk of morbidity/mortality must be addressed to improve outcomes. This includes the size (weight), age and behavior of the horse, positioning and proper padding on the surgery table or floor, duration of the procedure, effects of anesthetic drugs, health status (e.g. ASA classification), and expertise of the personnel.

Equine mortality from general anesthesia is higher than for other commonly anesthetized domestic species. Overall mortality is estimated anywhere between 0.24 and 1.9% (Young and Taylor 1993; Mee et al. 1998a, 1998b; Johnston et al. 2002, 2004; Bidwell et al. 2007; Senior 2013) and has traditionally included occurrence for up to seven-days from the anesthetic event. Both the intra-operative and recovery period are considered high risk, due to cardiovascular collapse in the former circumstance and the added risk of accidental trauma (fractures, myopathy, and neuropathies) in the latter. Up to 30% of mortality rate can occur in recovery from fractures (23–26%) and myopathy/neuropathy (7%) (Johnston et al. 2002, 2004). When critical and emergency cases are considered, including cases classified for anesthetic risk as ASA > 3 (severe systemic disease), mortality rate increases several fold (4–10 times) (Mee et al. 1998a, 1998b; Johnston et al. 2002, 2004; Bidwell et al. 2007; Rioja et al. 2012; Senior 2013). Mortality can be particularly high in emergency cesarean sections (C-sections) due to the nature of the procedure and confounding factors such as dehydration, electrolyte and acid–base imbalances, the added weight from the foal and interference with cardiovascular function (hypotension, low cardiac output) in a mare positioned in dorsal recumbency for surgery, intra-operative bleeding, and pain and weakness in recovery (Johnston et al. 2002; Rioja et al. 2012). Mortality rates of 9–21.5% during or after general anesthesia have been reported in emergency C-sections due to dystocia (Freeman et al. 1999; Byron et al. 2002; Maaskant et al. 2010; Rioja et al. 2012); whereas survival rate can reach 100% in elective C-sections (Freeman et al. 1999). For mares undergoing controlled vaginal delivery under general anesthesia, survival rates of 71–94% have been reported (Byron et al. 2002; Maaskant et al. 2010).

Mortality of the Fetus/Neonate

There is a lack of equine-specific information about the risk of using drugs during gestation, which makes it challenging when selecting an anesthetic protocols for anesthesia in a pregnant patient for obstetric or non-obstetric surgery. In addition to other conditions, in both circumstances there should be minimal interference with uterine contractility and fetal vitality.

For non-obstetric surgery (e.g. for colic) in pregnant mares, it is important to avoid drugs that might result in fetal abnormalities or conditions that contribute to abortion. The biggest risk factors for abortion are long anesthetic time and intra-operative hypotension with mares with an anesthetic time ≥ 3 hours being six times more likely to abort (Chenier and Whitehead 2009). In that same study, there was also no difference in the foaling rate for mares that received progestin supplementation versus those that had not (Chenier and Whitehead 2009). Hypoxemic conditions during colic surgery in the last 60 days of pregnancy were also linked to abortion or severely compromised foals at delivery that did not survive (Santschi et al. 1991).

Abortion rate has been reported in one study as (46.2%) for mares undergoing colic surgery versus mares treated medically for colic (21.8%), and may result from secondary complications, such as placentitis that create an unfavorable environment (Chenier and Whitehead 2009). In another study, there was no significant difference found but perhaps a clinically relevant difference between the abortion rate of surgical (20.5%) and medical (10.8%) colic cases (Boening and Leendertse 1993). Positioning in dorsal recumbency during colic surgery may contaminate the vagina with air and debris due to relaxation and opening of the vulvar lips. Mares with poor perineal conformation, impairment of the vestibulo-vaginal sphincter, or cervical compromise may be at increased risk. Therefore, pregnant mares admitted for non-obstetric surgeries may potentially benefit from placement of a vulvar suture or staples (Caslick's surgery) prior to anesthesia.

Foals are normally delivered within 20–30 minutes of chorioallantoic rupture (stage 2 labor) (Youngquist 1988). Dystocia in the mare is considered a true emergency and can have profound effect on survival of the foal. It is uncommon to deliver a live foal from a dystocia mare after 60–90 minutes from the start of the second stage of labor (Embertson 1999). The presentation and positioning of the foal and level of engagement with the birth canal will have a direct effect on the potential length of time a foal may have to survive, due to umbilical cord compression or placental separation. Rapid dystocia resolution corresponds to improved fetal outcome (Byron et al. 2002; Norton et al. 2007). For each 10 minute increase in Stage 2 duration above 30 minutes, there is a 10% increased risk of the fetus being dead at delivery and a 16% increased risk of the fetus not surviving to discharge. Another study showed that there was only a 13.6 minute time difference between the total mean dystocia duration for foals that lived and those that did not survive. It has been demonstrated that employing a coordinated dystocia management protocol can significantly decrease time from hospital arrival to dystocia resolution for referred emergency cases (Norton et al. 2007). It is important to approach dystocias with a consistent plan aimed at delivering the foal in the shortest possible time while minimizing complications in the mare. There are typically four procedures used to resolve dystocia in the mare: (i) assisted vaginal delivery, in which the mare is conscious (potentially sedated) and manually assisted in vaginal delivery of an intact foal; (ii) controlled vaginal delivery, in which the mare is anesthetized and the clinician is in control of vaginal delivery of an intact foal; (iii) fetotomy, in which the dead fetus is reduced to two or more parts and removed vaginally in the awake, sedated or anesthetized mare; and (iv) cesarean section, in which the fetus is removed through a uterine incision by celiotomy. The choice of restraint, positioning, and drug selection therefore varies.

Morbidity Considerations

- ### Position

  While dorsal recumbency is preferred for most urogenital procedures in anesthetized horses, occasionally a horse may be maintained in lateral recumbency. In both circumstances there are significant changes to distribution of blood flow notably to muscle and lung. Lateral recumbency can affect dependent muscles by compression of vessels and which along with increases in vascular resistance decrease blood flow. This is exacerbated by low blood pressure and/or cardiac output predisposing to anaerobic conditions (Raisis 2005). Non-dependent muscles can also have decreased blood flow from changes in vascular tone and decreased blood pressure.

  Dorsal recumbency can result in the same adverse effects to muscles and although dependent back muscles are more affected, horses seem to cope better during recovery as compared to myopathy occurring in lateral recumbency. Dorsal recumbency however causes more compromise to ventilation resulting in hypercapnia and ventilation and perfusion ratios – V/Q causing hypoxemia and may influence venous return and consequently cardiac output (Hall 1981; Nyman and Hedenstierna 1989). Mechanical ventilation can further compromise circulation and in the pregnant mare, the gravid uterus

potentially exerts aorto-caval compression to further exacerbates the negative effects of positioning on cardiac output.

For some urogenital procedures, the Trendelenburg position is recommended to improve surgical access. This involves positioning the head lower than the pelvis, while in dorsal recumbency, at an angle of 30–45°. This position can be combined with insufflation of the abdomen with CO_2 to perform laparoscopic urogenital surgery, including cryptorchidectomy, inguinal herniorrhaphy, ovariectomy, tissue biopsies, and abdominal exploratories (Hofmeister et al. 2008), or without insufflation to facilitate procedures while displacing abdominal viscera forward to access the bladder or difficult to reach structures such as the ventral aspect of the cervix (O'Leary et al. 2013). Insufflation of the abdomen in horses undergoing colopexy without Trendelenburg position also demonstrated hypercapnia and increased mean arterial pressure, in addition to an increase in cardiac output and a decrease in vascular resistance; the latter effects were induced by the stimulatory effects of hypercapnia (Donaldson et al. 1998). For additional information on management of horses undergoing laparoscopic procedures, please refer to Chapter 9.

- ### Pain and Stress

  In pregnancy, uterine blood flow is significantly affected by pain and uterine contractions (Greiss 1972). The pressure generated by uterine contractions can exceed the perfusion pressure and impede adequate uterine blood flow, despite increases in systemic cardiac output and blood pressure from sympathetic stimulation caused by pain in the mother (Greiss 1972; Shnider et al. 1979); therefore, an appropriate plane of anesthesia may help offset these effects.

  Uterine blood flow is highly dependent on a low vascular resistance (Datta et al. 2010) and episodes of vasoconstriction induced by endogenous catecholamines (norepinephrine), in conditions of stress and pain, have been shown to impair uterine blood flow for brief periods of time (<3 minutes) in animal models subjected to a noxious stimulus or stressful situations (loud noises and sudden movements of personnel) (Shnider et al. 1979). In addition, hyperventilation and hypocapnia are common under conditions of stress and pain. Decreases in $PaCO_2$ by 45–48% from control values can induce vasoconstriction and decrease in uterine blood flow by 25–43% in several animal models that included rabbits, sheep, and rhesus monkeys (Behrman et al. 1967; Leduc 1972; Levison et al. 1974). Conversely, induced hypercapnia ($PaCO_2 > 61$ mmHg), increased uterine blood flow by 117%, through vasodilation and increases in blood pressure in pigs (Hanka et al. 1975), and smaller changes in $PaCO_2$ (46 mmHg) did no change placental blood flow in rabbits (Leduc 1972). The effect of positive intrathoracic pressure ventilation alone can significantly reduce venous return and cardiac output (Steffey and Howland, 1980; Hodgson et al. 1986; Khanna et al. 1995) and result in decreased uterine perfusion. In addition, overzealous positive intrathoracic pressure ventilation can result in hyperventilation and hypocapnia and further decrease uterine perfusion (Levison et al. 1974). To avoid fluctuations in uterine blood flow and fetal perfusion is best to maintain $PaCO_2$ within normal to slightly elevated values described for horses.

- ***Anesthetic Drugs***

  Morbidity and mortality studies in anesthetized horses point out that the use of balanced techniques (combination of inhalational anesthesia with injectable anesthetics throughout the maintenance period) and total inhalational anesthesia, results in higher risk than the use of total intravenous anesthesia (Johnston et al. 2002). However, several confounding factors, from health status to complexity of the surgery, make the risk higher in critical cases, not just the choice of anesthetic technique.

  In general, considering the four main drug properties that facilitate placental transfer (e.g. molecular size, protein binding, degree of ionization, and lipophilicity) all anesthetic drugs can potentially reach the fetus because their molecular weight is <500 Da (Griffiths and Campbell 2014). Unbound drug diffuses, based on a concentration gradient, with ease, due to the lipophilic non-ionized nature of the drug; conversely, highly protein bound drugs (e.g. diazepam at 98%) form a large hydrophilic molecule, poorly permeable to the placenta (Reynolds 1987, 1998; Griffiths and Campbell 2014), compared to drugs with low protein binding (e.g. ketamine at 48%). Some drugs can reach higher fetal (versus maternal) concentrations, dictated by high volumes of distribution of the drug (e.g. ketamine), whereas others may behave the opposite (e.g. benzodiazepines, opioids, propofol, alpha-2 agonists, local anesthetics) (Conklin et al. 1980; Reynolds 1987, 1998; Dailland et al. 1989; Griffiths and Campbell 2014; Yu et al. 2015). However, the health status of both mare and fetus should be considered as this may shift the transfer and drug concentrations between them. For example, studies in pregnant pony mares show that, compared to the dam, the fetus had lower blood oxygen tension and higher blood carbon dioxide tension and lower pH (pH 7.44 in the dam, 7.35 in the fetus). All three of these conditions were shown to be exacerbated in the foal during anesthesia compared to the dam being awake (Taylor et al. 1992); the lower fetal pH may cause drugs, like detomidine, that are weak bases to accumulate.

Note that adjuvant drugs, such as neuromuscular blocking agents and the anticholinergic glycopyrrolate, which are highly ionized, cross the placenta poorly, and do not impact the neonate (Reynolds 1998; Griffiths and Campbell 2014).

Effects of Inhalational Anesthetics

In general, inhalational anesthetics are ideal drugs for urogenital procedures because they provide excellent muscle relaxation and a titratable anesthetic depth. However, cardiorespiratory depression from current inhalational anesthetics (isoflurane, sevoflurane, desflurane) is dose dependent and manifests by low blood pressure, low cardiac output, low systemic vascular resistance, and low stroke volume (Steffey and Howland 1980; Grosenbaugh and Muir 1998). Horses maintained under spontaneous ventilation show better cardiovascular function because of co-existing arterial hypercapnia (55–85 mmHg) and sympathetic effects from it, and avoidance of positive intrathoracic pressure, which interferes with venous return (Steffey and Howland 1980; Hodgson et al. 1986; Khanna et al. 1995). However, positive pressure ventilation is often used in horses to maintain normocapnia and improve arterial oxygenation, and cardiovascular support is provided with use of inotropic drugs, such as dobutamine.

Although general anesthesia is frequently combined with a regional anesthetic technique in other species, caution is advised in horses since some of the regional techniques can affect locomotor function (e.g. epidural local anesthesia), which in the standing sedated horse may be counteracted by the stay apparatus that ensures limb stabilization in a non-ambulatory horse placed in a chute. Conversely, a horse recovering from anesthesia with impaired locomotor function is at high risk of injury. Assisted recoveries (e.g. head and tail ropes), to improve outcomes, should be considered in horses where a regional technique with the potential to influence hind limb function was used to facilitate the procedure, but where general anesthesia was also performed.

The effects of inhalational anesthetics in pregnant animals deserve special comments. Most studies have been carried out in other species (human, sheep) and extrapolated to the rest of species, including the horse. Inhalational anesthetics can maintain uterine blood flow at concentrations close to the minimum alveolar concentration (MAC), despite the decrease in vascular resistance (observed in human subjects)

and blood pressure associated with them. Uterine blood flow is ideal under conditions of low vascular resistance (Datta et al. 2010) and for this reason in people blood flow remains constant with inhalational anesthetics, unless there is marked hypotension (Palahniuk and Shnider 1974). The effects on uterine blood flow in horses are largely unknown. The increased affinity of fetal hemoglobin for oxygen (left shift) and the higher hemoglobin concentration in fetal blood than the mother (15 g/dl versus 12 g/dl) allow the fetus to withstand reductions in oxygen delivery during decreased placental blood flow, due to more efficient oxygen extraction and higher oxygen-carrying capacity (Wilkening and Meschia 1983; Datta et al. 2010). The administration of inhalational anesthetics with an enriched fraction of inspired oxygen favors a higher partial pressure of oxygen and oxygen content in blood and uptake by the fetus.

Of special concern is positioning of the mare in dorsal recumbency because of the potential for aortocaval compression caused by the gravid uterus and its effect on venous return and cardiac output, which results in hypotension and decreased uterine blood flow. If blood loss and/or dehydration is also present, this further reduces uterine blood flow as do anesthetic concentrations > 1.5 MAC (Palahniuk and Shnider 1974).

It is noteworthy that the MAC for inhalational anesthetics is reduced by 25–40% in pregnant ewes. This is, related to high progesterone levels that can induce a sedative effect (Palahniuk et al. 1974). Mares have no circulating levels of progesterone after 200 days of gestation, but it is present in the placenta and fetal circulation, and progestagens are found in the mare close to the time of parturition (Silver 1994). MAC determinations have not been carried out in pregnant mares so it remains unclear if there is an effect of these hormones on anesthetic dose. It is interesting that in rats, gestational MAC reduction is not related to progesterone levels (Grota and Eik-Nes 1967; Strout and Nahrwold 1981).

Isoflurane decreases urine production and promotes fluid retention by increasing interstitial fluid volume (Connolly et al. 2003; Valverde et al. 2012). This effect is at least in part thought to be mediated due to the increased secretion of vasopressin (Adams et al. 1994). In addition, inhalant anesthetics decrease glomerular filtration rate and renal blood flow, reducing urine production (Burchardi and Kaczmarczyk 1994). Because of concomitant use of other drugs, such as alpha-2 agonists, urine production may not be reduced, due to opposite effects of the latter drugs (see below). Inhalation anesthetics also inhibit the micturition reflex by suppressing detrusor contractions (Baldini et al. 2009), which ultimately will result in an increased transfer of fluid from the interstitial space to the bladder, once the inhalational anesthetic is discontinued, which predisposes to distended bladders in the recovery period. The effects of anesthetics on urine production should be considered for urogenital surgery, to avoid overdistention of the bladder, interference with the surgical procedure (constant micturition in standing animals), and the risk of micturition or discomfort from a full bladder that may affect the quality of recovery.

Effects of Injectable Anesthetics

Acepromazine

Acepromazine is mostly used for its tranquilizing effect through central dopamine D2 receptor blockade. Peripherally, it blocks alpha receptors in vascular smooth muscle and reduces vascular resistance, leading to potential hypotension; however, in a recent survey, it was shown that hypotension from acepromazine used at low doses does not appear to be significant and is readily treated with standard measures, such as sympathomimetics and light plane of anesthesia (Driessen et al. 2011). The vasodilatory effects of acepromazine also affect minimally uterine blood flow in other species (Hodgson et al. 2002).

The use of acepromazine in male horses (geldings or stallions) should be cautious because of reported cases of penile protrusion that can progress to paraphimosis (inability to reposition the penis within the prepuce)

(Driessen et al. 2011) and lead to devastating consequences especially in a breeding stallion. The risk of permanent penile dysfunction from acepromazine use in anesthetized horses is however very low ($\leq$1 in 10 000 cases) (Driessen et al. 2011). Mechanistically, blockade of alpha receptors is at least partially responsible for causing motor interference of the retractor penis *in vitro* in horses (Ambache and Killick 1978). Similarly, the use of alpha-1 blockers in people is associated with vasodilation by blocking the effects of norepinephrine on the smooth muscle of corpus cavernosum and cavernosal arteries, increasing blood flow to the penis and causing tumescence (Traish et al. 2000), which facilitates penile protrusion. Acepromazine is not absolutely contraindicated in male horses, but proper monitoring and immediate management is imperative if penile protrusion is observed.

Alpha-2 Agonists

Alpha-2 agonists are routinely used for sedation, prior to induction of anesthesia. These drugs increase systemic vascular resistance and blood pressure, which induces reflex bradycardia and often atrioventricular blocks, resulting in a decrease in cardiac output (Bettschart-Wolfensberger et al. 2005; Solano et al. 2009; Valverde 2010; Schauvliege et al. 2011; Gozalo-Marcilla et al. 2012).

The use of alpha-2 agonists for urogenital procedures have two adverse effects that need to be considered. First, these drugs increase urine production from reduced arginine vasopressin secretion with a possible secondary influence through hyperglycemia due to an inhibitory action on the secretion of insulin from pancreatic cells (Thurmon et al. 1984; Tranquilli et al. 1984; Alexander and Irvine 2000; Peterhoff et al. 2003). Urine production of up to 8 ml/kg/h was measured in horses anesthetized for approximately three hours and also received a medetomidine infusion and isotonic fluid rate of <6 mL/kg/h, compared to 3 mL/kg/h of urine in horses not receiving the infusion (Valverde et al. 2010). This fluid loss is tolerated by normovolemic and non-compromised horses, but it should be considered in critical animals or those where water intake is restricted. In addition, alpha agonists, including sympathomimetics and alpha-2 sedative agonists, can bind to alpha-1 receptors of the internal sphincter of the urethra, increasing its tone and prevent voiding of the bladder, leading to urinary retention (Verhamme et al. 2008; Baldini et al. 2009). Therefore, it is recommended to catheterize the bladder in horses receiving infusions of alpha-2 agonists, to prevent bladder distention and discomfort or leakage during recovery (Valverde et al. 2010).

The second concern from alpha-2 agonist administration is the effect of these drugs on increasing intrauterine pressure through increased uterine contractions, for up to 30 minutes post-administration (Schatzmann et al. 1994). Despite this effect, administration throughout the pregnancy period has demonstrated no interference with pregnancy (Katila and Oijala 1988; Jedruch et al. 1989; Luukkanen et al. 1997) and uterine blood flow is well preserved (Araujo and Ginther 2009).

Opioids

Opioids are often administered for analgesia, and appear to have no adverse effects on uterine blood flow. While reports on analgesic efficacy are mixed, it is postulated that they can help preserve uterine blood flow by avoiding sympathetic stimulation resulting from noxious stimulation. While there has been limited study of opioids in pregnant horses, side effects such as respiratory depression often mentioned in human anesthesia may be of lesser consequence in the horse. Lipophilicity which has an impact on placental transfer to the neonate should be considered. Buprenorphine, Butorphanol, and Fentanyl (Reynolds 1987) are among the more lipophilic opioids used in clinical practice. Morphine conversely has a low lipid solubility (Reynolds 1987) and has a molecular weight greater than 100 Da (at 285 Da) which retards the movement of hydrophilic passage (Reynolds 1987). If used in the dam during

anesthetic management, the neonate should be evaluated and if deemed necessary, naloxone may be used to reverse side effects.

Benzodiazepines

Benzodiazepines (diazepam, midazolam) are used frequently in equine anesthesia. In people, chronic use of benzodiazepines has been associated with urinary retention and impaired micturition through their muscle relaxation properties on the detrusor muscle (Verhamme et al. 2008; Baldini et al. 2009). This effect is probably less likely to occur after single dosing in horses. The main concern with benzodiazepines is their ability to cross the placenta readily, due to their high lipid solubility and unionized form, and although cardiovascular effects tend to be minimal, their use in pregnant animals for delivery/cesarean section can result in excessive muscle relaxation in the neonate (hypotonicity and low Apgar scores), especially with diazepam (Conklin et al. 1980). This may require antagonism with flumazenil. While the potential for transfer exists, midazolam showed lower fetal to maternal plasma concentrations than diazepam, (Conklin et al. 1980).

Guaifenesin

Guaifenesin (glyceryl guaiacolate) is often used in the induction phase to facilitate a smooth induction or as part of total intravenous anesthesia, due to its strong skeletal muscle relaxation properties (Hubbell et al. 1980). This drug causes a decrease in vascular resistance and hypotension. Neonatal foal plasma concentrations of approximately 30% of corresponding maternal plasma concentrations measured after its use for induction in two mares for cesarean section (Hubbell et al. 1980). In the author's experience, it appears that, despite this, foals are not depressed when the mare has received guaifenesin.

Lidocaine

Lidocaine is frequently used intravenously (IV) as part of balanced techniques in horses (Valverde et al. 2005, 2010; Valverde 2013), and has been shown to provide antinociceptive effects in ponies undergoing castration under halothane anesthesia (Murrell et al. 2003, 2005). It has minimal cardiovascular effects at recommended doses and does not affect uterine blood flow (Biehl et al. 1977). Additional information of its effects during pregnancy and C-section are not known.

Induction Drugs

Induction agents can often cause a decrease in vascular resistance and hypotension, which must be considered in pregnant animals due to the impact of this effect on placental blood flow. Ketamine, propofol, alfaxalone, and etomidate can all result in hypotension from varying degrees of myocardial depression and vasodilation (Hubbell et al. 1980; Bettschart-Wolfensberger et al. 2003; Umar et al. 2007; Wakuno et al. 2017). These effects tend to be transient in healthy horses, but can be significant and persistent in compromised horses. In general, broad-based studies in animals have shown that uterine blood flow is well maintained with most of these induction agents (Craft et al. 1983; Alon et al. 1993; Fresno et al. 2008). In current practice, it is most common that ketamine or combinations of ketamine and propofol are used for equine anesthesia induction following appropriate premedication and with concurrent use of centrally acting muscle relaxants.

Sympathomimetics

Sympathomimetics used for blood pressure and cardiac output support should be considered for their effects on uterine blood flow. Drugs with beta-1 effects are preferred to maintain uterine blood flow over drugs with alpha-1 effects; therefore, drugs such as dobutamine, dopamine, and ephedrine, in which beta effects can be elicited by titrating the dose, are recommended (Grünberger and Szalay 1983; Butler et al. 2001; Erkinaro et al. 2004). Dobutamine lacks strong alpha

effects *in vivo* and instead can decrease or not change vascular resistance (Robie et al. 1974; Ohta et al. 2013; Dancker et al. 2018), but will increase blood pressure by increasing cardiac output in normovolemic circumstances. As in sheep (Butler et al. 2001), studies in horses and foals administered dobutamine have shown increases in hemoglobin concentrations (Valverde et al. 2006; Schier et al. 2016) and so may benefit oxygen delivery through this mechanism as well. Conversely, drugs that provide only alpha-agonistic actions (phenylephrine) increase blood pressure through increases in vascular resistance, and can decrease uterine blood flow (Cottle et al. 1982; Erkinaro et al. 2004). Drugs with strong alpha- and beta effects, such as epinephrine and norepinephrine can cause maternal placental vasoconstriction (Leduc 1972; Hood et al. 1986), despite increases in blood pressure and cardiac output.

Hence, dobutamine is suggested as the first-line therapy of hypotension in pregnant horses to avoid interference with uterine blood flow. Muscle blood flow is also better preserved with dobutamine than with drugs that have alpha-vasoconstrictor effects, which is highly relevant in horses (Raisis 2005; Schier et al. 2016).

Anticholinergics

Atropine and glycopyrrolate can cause urinary retention by blocking the parasympathetic fibers that help with contraction of the detrusor muscle and relaxation of the neck of the bladder (Verhamme et al. 2008; Baldini et al. 2009). These drugs are not used frequently in horses due to their muscarinic effects also causing decreases in gastrointestinal motility (Ducharme and Fubini 1983; Singh et al. 1997). In pregnant mares, atropine is lipid soluble and will cross the placental and may induce tachycardia in the fetus, unlike glycopyrrolate, which has poor placental transfer (Reynolds 1998; Griffiths and Campbell 2014). The effects of buscopan in similar circumstances of use have not been elucidated.

References

Adams, A. and Hendrickson, D.A. (2014). Standing male equine urogenital surgery. *The Veterinary Clinics of North America. Equine Practice* 30: 169–190.

Adams, H.A., Schmitz, C.S., and Baltes-Gotz, B. (1994). Endocrine stress reaction, hemodynamics and recovery in total intravenous and inhalation anesthesia: propofol versus isoflurane. *Anaesthesist* 43: 730–737.

Alexander, S.L. and Irvine, C.H.G. (2000). The effect of the alpha-2-adrenergic agonist, clonidine, on secretion patterns and rates of adrenocorticotropic hormone and its secretagogues in the horse. *Journal of Neuroendocrinology* 12: 874–880.

Allen, W.R., Wilsher, S., Turnbull, C. et al. (2002). Influence of maternal size on placental, fetal and postnatal growth in the horse. Development in utero. *Reproduction* 123: 445–453.

Alon, E., Ball, R.H., Gillie, M.H. et al. (1993). Effects of propofol and thiopental on maternal and fetal cardiovascular and acid-base variables in the pregnant ewe. *Anesthesiology* 78: 562–576.

Ambache, N. and Killick, S.W. (1978). Species differences in postganglionic motor transmission to the retractor penis muscle. *British Journal of Pharmacology* 63: 25–34.

Araujo, R.R. and Ginther, O.J. (2009). Vascular perfusion of reproductive organs in pony mares and heifers during sedation with detomidine or xylazine. *American Journal of Veterinary Research* 70: 141–148.

Arnold, C.E., Brinsko, S.P., Love, C.C., and Varner, D.D. (2010). Use of a modified Vinsot technique for partial phallectomy in 11 standing horses. *Journal of the American Veterinary Medical Association* 237: 82–86.

Baldini, G., Bagry, H., Aprikian, A., and Carli, F. (2009). Postoperative urinary retention. *Anesthesiology* 110: 1139–1157.

Beard, W. (1991). Standing urogenital surgery. *The Veterinary Clinics of North America. Equine Practice* 7: 669–684.

Behrman, R.E., Parer, J.T., and Novy, M.J. (1967). Acute maternal respiratory alkalosis (hyperventilation) in the pregnant rhesus monkey. *Pediatric Research* 1: 354–363.

Bettschart-Wolfensberger, R., Bowen, I.M., Freeman, S.L. et al. (2003). Medetomidine-ketamine anaesthesia induction followed by medetomidine-propofol in ponies: infusion rates and cardiopulmonary side effects. *Equine Veterinary Journal* 35: 308–313.

Bettschart-Wolfensberger, R., Freeman, S.L., Bowen, I.M. et al. (2005). Cardiopulmonary effects and pharmacokinetics of I.V. dexmedetomidine in ponies. *Equine Veterinary Journal* 37: 60–64.

Bidwell, L.A., Bramlage, L.R., and Rood, W.A. (2007). Equine perioperative fatalities associated with general anaesthesia at a private practice: a retrospective case series. *Veterinary Anaesthesia and Analgesia* 34: 23–30.

Biehl, D., Shnider, S.M., Levinson, G., and Callender, K. (1977). The direct effects of circulating lidocaine on uterine blood flow and foetal well-being in the pregnant ewe. *Canadian Anaesthetists' Society Journal* 24: 445–451.

Bobrowski, R.A. (2010). Pulmonary physiology in pregnancy. *Clinical Obstetrics and Gynecology* 53: 285–300.

Boening, K.J. and Leendertse, I.P. (1993). Review of 115 cases of colic in the pregnant mare. *Equine Veterinary Journal* 25: 518–521.

Budras, K., Sack, W., and Rock, S. (2009). *Anatomy of the Horse*, 5e. Hannover, Germany: Schlütersche.

Burchardi, H. and Kaczmarczyk, G. (1994). The effect of anaesthesia on renal function. *European Journal of Anaesthesiology* 11: 163–168.

Butler, E.C., Moon, P.F., Gleed, R.D. et al. (2001). The effects of maternal plasma dobutamine levels on fetal oxygenation in anaesthetized sheep. *Veterinary Anaesthesia and Analgesia* 28: 34–41.

Byron, C.R., Embertson, R.M., Bernard, W.V. et al. (2002). Dystocia in a referral hospital setting: approach and results. *Equine Veterinary Journal* 35: 82–85.

Chenier, T.S. and Whitehead, A.E. (2009). Foaling rates and risk factors for abortion in pregnant mares presented for medical or surgical treatment of colic: 153 cases (1993–2005). *The Canadian Veterinary Journal* 50: 481–485.

Climent, F., Ribera, T., Arguelles, D. et al. (2009). Modified technique for the repair of third-degree rectovaginal lacerations in mares. *The Veterinary Record* 164: 393–396.

Conklin, K.A., Graham, C.W., Murad, S. et al. (1980). Midazolam and diazepam: maternal and fetal effects in the pregnant ewe. *Obstetrics and Gynecology* 56: 471–474.

Connolly, C.M., Kramer, G.C., Hahn, R.G. et al. (2003). Isoflurane but not mechanical ventilation promotes extravascular fluid accumulation during crystalloid volume loading. *Anesthesiology* 98: 670–681.

Cottle, M.K.W., Van Petten, G.R., and van Muyden, P. (1982). Effects of phenylephrine and sodium salicylate on maternal and fetal cardiovascular indices and blood oxygenation in sheep. *American Journal of Obstetrics and Gynecology* 143: 170–176.

Craft, J.B. Jr., Coaldrake, L.A., Yonekura, M.L. et al. (1983). Ketamine, catecholamines, and uterine tone in pregnant ewes. *American Journal of Obstetrics and Gynecology* 146: 429–434.

Dailland, P., Cockshott, I.D., Lirzin, J.D. et al. (1989). Intravenous propofol during cesarean section: placental transfer, concentrations in breast milk, and neonatal effects. A preliminary study. *Anesthesiology* 71: 827–834.

Dancker, C., Hopster, K., Rohn, K., and Kästner, S.B. (2018). Effects of dobutamine, dopamine, phenylephrine and noradrenaline on systemic haemodynamics and intestinal perfusion in isoflurane anaesthetised horses. *Equine Veterinary Journal* 50: 104–110.

Datta, S., Kodali, B.S., and Segal, S. (2010). Uteroplacental blood flow. In: *Obstetric Anesthesia Handbook*, 5e, 59–71. New York: Springer Science+Business Media.

DeBowes, R.M. (1988). Surgical management of urolithiasis. *The Veterinary Clinics of North America. Equine Practice* 4: 461–471.

Delli-Rocili, M.M., Cribb, N.C., Trout, D.R. et al. (2020). Effectiveness of a paravertebral nerve block versus local portal blocks for laparoscopic closure of the nephrosplenic space: a pilot study. *Veterinary Surgery* 49: 1007–1014.

DeRossi, R., Maciel, F.B., Modolo, T.J.C., and Pagliosa, R.C. (2012). Efficacy of concurrent epidural administration of neostigmine and lidocaine for perineal analgesia in geldings. *American Journal of Veterinary Research* 73: 1356–1362.

Donaldson, L.L., Trostle, S.S., and White, N.A. (1998). Cardiopulmonary changes associated with abdominal insufflation of carbon dioxide in mechanically ventilated, dorsally recumbent, halothane anaesthetised horses. *Equine Veterinary Journal* 30: 144–151.

Driessen, B., Zarucco, L., Kalir, B., and Bertolotti, L. (2011). Contemporary use of acepromazine in the anaesthetic management of male horses and ponies: a retrospective study and opinion poll. *Equine Veterinary Journal* 43: 88–98.

Ducharme, N.G. and Fubini, S.L. (1983). Gastrointestinal complications associated with the use of atropine in horses. *Journal of the American Veterinary Medical Association* 182: 229–231.

Dunlop, C.I., Hodgson, D.S., Smith, J.A. et al. (1994). Cardiopulmonary effects of positioning pregnant cows in dorsal recumbency during the 3rd trimester. *American Journal of Veterinary Research* 55: 147–151.

Dyce, K.M., Sack, W.O., and Wensing, C.J.G. (1996). The abdomen of the horse. In: *Textbook of Veterinary Anatomy*, 2e (eds. K.M. Dyce, W.O. Sack and C.J.G. Wensing), 529–549. Philadelphia: WB Saunders.

Embertson, R.M. (1999). Dystocia and caesarean sections: the importance of duration and good judgement. *Equine Veterinary Journal* 31: 179–180.

Erkinaro, T., Mäkikallio, K., Kavasmaa, T. et al. (2004). Effects of ephedrine and phenylephrine on uterine and placental circulations and fetal outcome following fetal hypoxaemia and epidural-induced hypotension in a sheep model. *British Journal of Anaesthesia* 93: 825–832.

Fowden, A.L., Ralph, M.M., and Silver, M. (1994). Nutritional regulation of uteroplacental prostaglandin production and metabolism in pregnant ewes and mares during late-gestation. *Experimental and Clinical Endocrinology* 102: 212–221.

Fowden, A.L., Taylor, P.M., White, K.L., and Forhead, A.J. (2000a). Ontogenic and nutritionally induced changes in fetal metabolism in the horse. *The Journal of Physiology* 528: 209–219.

Fowden, A.L., Forhead, A.J., White, K.L., and Taylor, P.M. (2000b). Equine uteroplacental metabolism at mid- and late gestation. *Experimental Physiology* 85: 539–545.

Freeman, D.E., Hungerford, L.L., Schaeffer, D. et al. (1999). Caesarean section and other methods for assisted delivery: comparison of effects on mare mortality and complications. *Equine Veterinary Journal* 31: 203–207.

Fresno, L., Andaluz, A., Moll, X., and García, F. (2008). The effects on maternal and fetal cardiovascular and acid-base variables after the administration of etomidate in the pregnant ewe. *Veterinary Journal* 177: 94–103.

Furukawa, S., Kuroda, Y., and Sugiyama, A. (2014). A comparison of the histological structure of the placenta in experimental animals. *Journal of Toxicologic Pathology* 27: 11–28.

Gallacher, K., Santos, L.C., Campoy, L. et al. (2016). Development of a peripheral nerve stimulator-guided technique for equine pudendal nerve blockade. *Veterinary Journal* 217: 72–77.

Gleed, R. and Short, C.E. (1980). A retrospective study of the anesthetic management of adult draft horses. *Veterinary Medicine, Small Animal Clinician* 75: 1409–1414.

Gozalo-Marcilla, M., Schauvliege, S., Segaert, S. et al. (2012). Influence of a constant rate infusion of dexmedetomidine on cardiopulmonary function and recovery quality in isoflurane anaesthetized horses. *Veterinary Anaesthesia and Analgesia* 39: 49–58.

Graham, S. and Freeman, D. (2014). Standing diagnostic and therapeutic equine abdominal surgery. *The Veterinary Clinics of North America. Equine Practice* 30: 143–168.

Green, E.M. and Cooper, R.C. (1984). Continuous caudal epidural anesthesia in the horse. *Journal of the American Veterinary Medical Association* 184: 971–974.

Greiss, F.C. (1972). Uterine blood flow during pregnancy. *Medical College of Virginia Quaterly* 8: 52–60.

Griffiths, S.K. and Campbell, J.P. (2014). Placental structure, function and drug transfer. *Continuing Education in Anesthesia, Critical Care and Pain* 15: 84–89.

Grosenbaugh, D.A. and Muir, W.W. (1998). Cardiorespiratory effects of sevoflurane, isoflurane, and halothane anesthesia in horses. *American Journal of Veterinary Research* 59: 101–106.

Grota, L.J. and Eik-Nes, K.B. (1967). Plasma progesterone concentrations during pregnancy and lactation in the rat. *Journal of Reproduction and Fertility* 13: 83–91.

Grünberger, W. and Szalay, S. (1983). Uterine and systemic vascular responses to dopamine in pregnant ewes. *Archives of Gynecology* 233: 259–262.

Hall, L.W. (1981). General anesthesia. Fundamental considerations. *The Veterinary Clinics of North America. Large Animal Practice* 3: 3–15.

Hanka, R., Lawn, L., Mills, I.H. et al. (1975). The effects of maternal hypercapnia on foetal oxygenation and uterine blood flow in the pig. *The Journal of Physiology* 247: 447–460.

Hay, W.W. (1991). Energy and substrate requirements of the placenta and fetus. *The Proceedings of the Nutrition Society* 50: 321–336.

Hay, W.W. (1995). Regulation of placental metabolism by glucose supply. *Reproduction, Fertility, and Development* 7: 365–375.

Hay, W.W. (2006). Placental-fetal glucose exchange and fetal glucose metabolism.

Transactions of the American Clinical and Climatological Association 117: 321–340.

Hodgson, D.S., Steffey, E.P., Grandy, J.L., and Woliner, M.J. (1986). Effects of spontaneous, assisted and controlled ventilatory modes in halothane-anesthetized geldings. *American Journal of Veterinary Research* 47: 992–996.

Hodgson, D.S., Dunlop, C.I., Chapman, P.L., and Smith, J.A. (2002). Cardiopulmonary effects of xylazine and acepromazine in pregnant cows in late gestation. *American Journal of Veterinary Research* 63: 1695–1699.

Hofmeister, E., Peroni, J.F., and Fisher, A.T. (2008). Effects of carbon dioxide insufflation and body position on blood gas values in horses anesthetized for laparoscopy. *Journal of Equine Veterinary Science* 28: 549–553.

Hood, D.D., Dewan, D.M., and James, F.M. (1986). Maternal and fetal effects of epinephrine in gravid ewes. *Anesthesiology* 64: 610–613.

Hubbell, J.A., Muir, W.W., and Sams, R.A. (1980). Guaifenesin: cardiopulmonary effects and plasma concentrations in horses. *American Journal of Veterinary Research* 41: 1751–1755.

Jedruch, J., Gajewski, Z., and Kuussaari, J. (1989). The effect of detomidine hydrochloride on the electrical activity of uterus in pregnant mares. *Acta Veterinaria Scandinavica* 30: 307–311.

Johnston, G.M., Eastment, J.K., Wood, J.L., and Taylor, P.M. (2002). The confidential enquiry into perioperative equine fatalities (CEPEF): mortality results of phases 1 and 2. *Veterinary Anaesthesia and Analgesia* 29: 159–170.

Johnston, G.M., Eastment, J.K., Taylor, P.M., and Wood, J.L. (2004). Is isoflurane safer than halothane in equine anaesthesia? Results from a prospective multicentre randomized controlled trial. *Equine Veterinary Journal* 36: 64–71.

Katila, T. and Oijala, M. (1988). The effect of detomidine (Domosedan) on the maintenance of equine pregnancy and foetal development: ten cases. *Equine Veterinary Journal* 20: 323–326.

Khanna, A.K., McDonell, W.N., Dyson, D.H., and Taylor, P.M. (1995). Cardiopulmonary effects of hypercapnia during controlled intermittent positive pressure ventilation in the horse. *Canadian Journal of Veterinary Research* 59: 213–221.

Klewitz, J., Struebing, C., Rohn, K. et al. (2015). Effects of age, parity, and pregnancy abnormalities on foal birth weight and uterine blood flow in the mare. *Theriogenology* 83: 721–729.

Kraus, B.M., Parente, E.J., and Tulleners, E.P. (2003). Laryngoplasty with ventriculectomy or ventriculocordectomy in 104 draft horses (1992–2000). *Veterinary Surgery* 32: 530–538.

Kress, H.G. (1995). Effects of general anaesthetics on second messenger systems. *European Journal of Anaesthesiology* 12: 83–97.

Langmoen, I.A., Larsen, M., and Berg-Johnsen, J. (1995). Volatile anaesthetics: cellular mechanisms of action. *European Journal of Anaesthesiology* 12: 51–58.

Leduc, B. (1972). The effect of hyperventilation on maternal placental blood flow in pregnant rabbits. *The Journal of Physiology* 225: 339–348.

Levison, G., Shnider, S.M., deLorimier, A.A., and Steffenson, J.L. (1974). Effects of maternal hyperventilation on uterine blood flow and fetal oxygenation and acid-base status. *Anesthesiology* 40: 340–347.

Luukkanen, L., Katila, T., and Koskinen, E. (1997). Some effects of multiple administration of detomidine during the last trimester of equine pregnancy. *Equine Veterinary Journal* 29: 400–402.

Maaskant, A., De Bruijn, C.M., Schutrups, A.H., and Stout, T.A.E. (2010). Dystocia in Friesian mares: prevalence, causes and outcome following caesarean section. *Equine Veterinary Education* 22: 190–195.

Macdonald, A.A., Chavatte, P., and Fowden, A.L. (2000). Scanning electron microscopy of the microcotyledonary placenta of the horse (*Equus caballus*) in the latter half of gestation. *Placenta* 21: 565–574.

Marly, C., Bettschart-Wolfensberger, R., Nussbaumer, P. et al. (2014). Evaluation of a romifidine constant rate infusion protocol with or without butorphanol for dentistry and ophthalmologic procedures in standing horses. *Veterinary Anaesthesia and Analgesia* 41: 491–497.

McAuliffe, F., Kametas, N., Costello, J. et al. (2002). Respiratory function in singleton and twin pregnancy. *BJOG* 109: 765–769.

Medeiros, L.Q., Gozalo-Marcilla, M., Taylor, P.M. et al. (2017). Sedative and cardiopulmonary effects of dexmedetomidine infusions randomly receiving, or not, butorphanol in standing horses. *The Veterinary Record* 181: 402. https://doi.org/10.1136/vr.104359.

Mee, A.M., Cripps, P.J., and Jones, R.S. (1998a). A retrospective study of mortality associated with general anaesthesia in horses: emergency procedures. *The Veterinary Record* 142: 307–309.

Mee, A.M., Cripps, P.J., and Jones, R.S. (1998b). A retrospective study of mortality associated with general anaesthesia in horses: elective procedures. *The Veterinary Record* 14: 275–276.

Mihaly, G.W. and Morgan, D.J. (1983). Placental drug transfer: effects of gestational age and species. *Pharmacology & Therapeutics* 23: 253–266.

Molina, R.D., Meschia, G., Battaglia, F.C., and Hay, W.W. (1991). Gestational maturation of placental glucose transfer capacity in sheep. *The American Journal of Physiology* 261: R697–R704.

Moon, P.E. and Suter, C.M. (1993). Paravertebral thoracolumbar anesthesia in 10 horses. *Equine Veterinary Journal* 25: 304–308.

Murrell, J.C., Johnson, C.B., White, K.L. et al. (2003). Changes in the EEG during castration in horses and ponies anaesthetized with halothane. *Veterinary Anaesthesia and Analgesia* 30: 138–146.

Murrell, J.C., White, K.L., Johnson, C.B. et al. (2005). Investigation of the EEG effects of intravenous lidocaine during halothane anaesthesia in ponies. *Veterinary Anaesthesia and Analgesia* 32: 212–221.

Natalini, C.C. (2010). Spinal anesthetics and analgesics in the horse. *The Veterinary Clinics of North America. Equine Practice* 26: 551–564.

Norton, J.L., Dallap, B.L., Johnston, J.K. et al. (2007). Retrospective study of dystocia in mares at a referral hospital. *Equine Veterinary Journal* 39: 37–41.

Nyman, G. and Hedenstierna, G. (1989). Ventilation-perfusion relationships in the anaesthetised horse. *Equine Veterinary Journal* 21: 274–281.

Ohta, M., Kurimoto, S., Ishikawa, Y. et al. (2013). Cardiovascular effects of dobutamine and phenylephrine infusion in sevoflurane-anesthetized thoroughbred horses. *The Journal of Veterinary Medical Science* 75: 1443–1448.

O'Leary, J.M., Rodgerson, D., Spirito, M., and Gomez, J. (2013). Foaling rates after surgical repair of ventral cervical lacerations using a Trendelenburg position in 18 anesthetized mares. *Veterinary Surgery* 42: 716–720.

Olson, K.N. (2002). Anesthesia for laryngoplasty with or without sacculectomy in 85 draft horses: comparison with 322 thoroughbreds. *Veterinary Anaesthesia and Analgesia* 29: 105–106.

Palahniuk, R.J. and Shnider, S.M. (1974). Maternal and fetal cardiovascular and acid-base changes during halothane and isoflurane anesthesia in the pregnant ewe. *Anesthesiology* 41: 462–472.

Palahniuk, R.J., Shnider, S.M., and Eger, E.I. (1974). Pregnancy decreases the requirement for inhaled anesthetic agents. *Anesthesiology* 41: 82–83.

Perkins, J.D., Schumacher, J., Waguespack, R.W., and Hanrath, M. (2003). Penile retroversion and partial phallectomy performed in a standing horse. *The Veterinary Record* 153: 184–185.

Peterhoff, M., Sieg, A., Brede, M. et al. (2003). Inhibition of insulin secretion via distinct signalling pathways in α2-adrenoceptor knockout mice. *European Journal of Endocrinology* 149: 343–350.

Potter, J.J., MacFarlane, P.D., Love, E.J. et al. (2016). Preliminary investigation comparing a detomidine continuous rate infusion combined with either morphine or buprenorphine for standing sedation in horses. *Veterinary Anaesthesia and Analgesia* 43: 189–194.

Raisis, A.L. (2005). Skeletal muscle blood flow in anaesthetized horses. Part II: effects of anaesthetics and vasoactive agents. *Veterinary Anaesthesia and Analgesia* 32: 331–337.

Reitman, E. and Flood, P. (2011). Anaesthetic considerations for non-obstetric surgery during pregnancy. *British Journal of Anaesthesia* 107: i72–i78.

Reynolds, F. (1987). Placental transfer of opioids. *Baillieres Clinical Anaesthesiology* 4: 859–881.

Reynolds, F. (1998). Drug transfer across the term placenta. *Trophoblast Research* 12: 239–255.

Riedl, M.S., Schnell, S.A., Overland, A.C. et al. (2009). Coexpression of alpha 2A-adrenergic and delta-opioid receptors in substance P-containing terminals in rat dorsal horn. *The Journal of Comparative Neurology* 513: 385–398.

Ringer, S.K., Portier, K.G., Fourel, I., and Bettschart-Wolfensberger, R. (2012a). Development of a xylazine constant rate infusion with or without butorphanol for standing sedation of horses. *Veterinary Anaesthesia and Analgesia* 39: 1–11.

Ringer, S.K., Portier, K.G., Fourel, I., and Bettschart-Wolfensberger, R. (2012b). Development of a romifidine constant rate infusion with or without butorphanol for standing sedation of horses. *Veterinary Anaesthesia and Analgesia* 39: 12–20.

Ringer, S.K., Portier, K., Torgerson, P.R. et al. (2013). The effects of a loading dose followed by constant rate infusion of xylazine compared with romifidine on sedation, ataxia and response to stimuli in horses. *Veterinary Anaesthesia and Analgesia* 40: 157–165.

Rioja, E., Cernicchiaro, N., Costa, M.C., and Valverde, A. (2012). Perioperative risk factors for mortality and length of hospitalization in mares with dystocia undergoing general anesthesia: a retrospective study. *The Canadian Veterinary Journal* 53: 502–510.

Robie, N.W., Nutter, D.O., Moody, C., and McNay, J.L. (1974). in vivo analysis of adrenergic receptor activity of dobutamine. *Circulation Research* 34: 663–671.

Robinson, E.P. and Natalini, C.C. (2002). Epidural anesthesia and analgesia in horses. *The Veterinary Clinics of North America. Equine Practice* 18: 61–82.

Robson, S.C., Hunter, S., Moore, M., and Dunlop, W. (1987). Hemodynamic changes during the puerperium: a Doppler and M-mode echocardiographic study. *British Journal of Obstetrics and Gynaecology* 94: 1028–1039.

Rossdale, P.D. (1993). Clinical view of disturbances in equine foetal maturation. *Equine Veterinary Journal. Supplement* 14: 3–7.

Rowland, A.S., Baird, D.D., Weinberg, C.R. et al. (1992). Reduced fertility among women employed as dental assistants exposed to high levels of nitrous oxide. *The New England Journal of Medicine* 327: 993–997.

Rowland, A.S., Baird, D.D., Shore, D.L. et al. (1995). Nitrous oxide and spontaneous abortion in female dental assistants. *American Journal of Epidemiology* 141: 531–538.

Santschi, E.M., Slone, D.E., Gronwall, R. et al. (1991). Types of colic and frequency of postcolic abortion in pregnant mares – 105 cases (1984–1988). *Journal of the American Veterinary Medical Association* 199: 374–377.

Schatzmann, U., Jozzfck, H., Stauffer, J.L. et al. (1994). Effects of alpha 2-agonists on intrauterine pressure and sedation in horses: comparison between detomidine, romifidine and xylazine. *Zentralblatt für Veterinärmedizin. Reihe A* 41: 523–529.

Schauvliege, S., Gozalo-Marcilla, M., Verryken, K. et al. (2011). Effects of a constant rate infusion of detomidine on cardiovascular function, isoflurane requirements and recovery quality in horses. *Veterinary Anaesthesia and Analgesia* 38: 544–554.

Schier, M.F., Raisis, A.L., Secombe, C.J. et al. (2016). Effects of dobutamine hydrochloride on cardiovascular function in horses anesthetized with isoflurane with or without acepromazine maleate premedication. *American Journal of Veterinary Research* 77: 1318–1324.

Schramel, J., Nagel, C., Auer, U. et al. (2012). Distribution of ventilation in pregnant Shetland ponies Shetland ponies measured by electrical impedance tomography. *Respiratory Physiology & Neurobiology* 180: 258–262.

Schumacher, J., Bratton, G.R., and Williams, J.W. (1985). Pudendal and caudal rectal nerve blocks in the horse-an anesthetic procedure for reproductive surgery. *Theriogenology* 24: 457–464.

Seabaugh, K.A. and Schumacher, J. (2014). Urogenital surgery performed with the mare standing. *The Veterinary Clinics of North America. Equine Practice* 30: 191–209.

Senior, J.M. (2013). Morbidity, mortality, and risk of general anesthesia in horses. *The Veterinary Clinics of North America. Equine Practice* 29: 1–18.

Shepard, T.H. and Lemire, R.J. (2010). *Catalog of Teratogenic Agents*, 13e. Baltimore: Johns Hopkins University Press.

Shnider, S.M., Wright, R.G., Levinson, G. et al. (1979). Uterine blood flow and plasma norepinephrine changes during maternal stress in the pregnant ewe. *Anesthesiology* 50: 524–527.

Silver, M. (1994). Placental progestagens in the sheep and horse and the changes leading to parturition. *Experimental and Clinical Endocrinology* 102: 203–211.

Singh, B. Dyce, K.M. (2018). Dyce, Sack, and Wensing's textbook of veterinary anatomy. In: *The pelvis and reproductive organs of the horse*, 5e (B. Singh and K.M. Dyce), 552. St. Louis, Missouri: Elsevier.

Singh, S., McDonell, W., Young, S., and Dyson, D. (1997). The effect of glycopyrrolate on heart rate and intestinal motility in conscious horses. *Journal of Veterinary Anaesthesia* 24: 14–19.

Sisson, S., Grossman, J.D., and Getty, R. (1975). *Sisson and Grossman's the Anatomy of the Domestic Animals*, 5e. Philadelphia, USA: WB Saunders.

Skarda, R.T. (1996). Comparison of antinociceptive, cardiovascular, and respiratory effects, head ptosis, and position of pelvic limbs in mares after caudal epidural administration of xylazine and detomidine hydrochloride solution. *American Journal of Veterinary Research* 57: 1338–1345.

Skarda, R.T. and Muir, W.W. (1994). Caudal analgesia induced by epidural or subarachnoid administration of detomidine hydrochloride solution in mares. *American Journal of Veterinary Research* 55: 670–680.

Skarda, R.T., Muir, W.W., and JAE, H. (2009). Local anesthetic drugs and techniques. In: *Equine Anesthesia: Monitoring and Emergency Therapy*, 2e (eds. W.W. Muir and H. JAE), 210–242. St. Louis: Saunders/Elsevier.

Solano, A.M., Valverde, A., Desrocher, A. et al. (2009). Behavioural and cardiorespiratory effects of a constant rate infusion of medetomidine and morphine for sedation during standing laparoscopy in horses. *Equine Veterinary Journal* 41: 153–159.

Sorenson, P.R. and Robinson, N.E. (1980). Postural effects on lung-volumes and asynchronous ventilation in anesthetized horses. *Journal of Applied Physiology* 48: 97–103.

Steffey, E.P. and Howland, D. Jr. (1980). Comparison of circulatory and respiratory effects of isoflurane and halothane anesthesia in horses. *American Journal of Veterinary Research* 41: 821–825.

Strout, C.D. and Nahrwold, M.L. (1981). Halothane requirement during pregnancy and lactation in rats. *Anesthesiology* 55: 322–323.

Sturrock, J.E. and Nunn, J.F. (1975). Mitosis in mammalian cells during exposure to anesthetics. *Anesthesiology* 43: 21–33.

Taylor, P.M. (1997). Anesthesia for pregnant animals. *Equine Veterinary Journal. Supplement* 24: 1–9.

Taylor, P.M., Silver, M., and Fowden, A.L. (1992). Intravenous catheterization of fetus and mare in late pregnancy – management and respiratory, circulatory and metabolic effects. *Equine Veterinary Journal* 24: 391–396.

Thurmon, J.C., Steffey, E.P., Zinkl, J.G. et al. (1984). Xylazine causes transient dose-related hyperglycemia and increased urine volumes in mares. *American Journal of Veterinary Research* 45: 224–227.

Traish, A., Kim, N.N., Moreland, R.B., and Godlstein, I. (2000). Role of alpha adrenergic receptors in erectile function. *International Journal of Impotence Research* 12: 248–263.

Tranquilli, W.J., Thurmon, J.C., Neff-Davis, C.A. et al. (1984). Hyperglycemia and hypoinsulinemia during xylazine-ketamine anesthesia in thoroughbred horses. *American Journal of Veterinary Research* 45: 11–14.

Umar, M.A., Yamashita, K., Kushiro, T., and Muir, W.W. III (2007). Evaluation of cardiovascular effects of total intravenous anesthesia with propofol or a combination of ketamine-medetomidine-propofol in horses. *American Journal of Veterinary Research* 68: 121–127.

Valverde, A. (2010). Alpha-2 agonists for pain therapy in horses. *The Veterinary Clinics of North America. Equine Practice* 26: 515–532.

Valverde, A. (2013). Balanced anesthesia and constant rate infusions. *The Veterinary Clinics of North America. Equine Practice* 29: 89–122.

Valverde, A., Gunkel, C., Doherty, T.J. et al. (2005). Effect of a constant rate infusion of lidocaine on the quality of recovery from sevoflurane or isoflurane general anaesthesia in horses. *Equine Veterinary Journal* 37: 559–564.

Valverde, A., Giguère, S., Sánchez, L.C. et al. (2006). Effects of dobutamine, norepinephrine and vasopressin on cardiovascular function in anesthetized neonatal foals with induced hypotension. *American Journal of Veterinary Research* 67: 1730–1737.

Valverde, A., Rickey, E., Sinclair, M. et al. (2010). Comparison of cardiovascular function and quality of recovery in isoflurane-anaesthetised horses administered a constant rate infusion of lidocaine or lidocaine and medetomidine during elective surgery. *Equine Veterinary Journal* 42: 192–199.

Valverde, A., Gianotti, G., Rioja-Garcia, E., and Hathway, A. (2012). Effects of high-volume, rapid-fluid therapy on cardiovascular function and hematological values during isoflurane-induced hypotension in healthy dogs. *Canadian Journal of Veterinary Research* 76: 99–108.

Van Dijk, P., Lankveld, D.P.K., Rijenhuizen, A.B.M., and Jonker, F.H. (2003). Hormonal, metabolic and physiological effects of laparoscopic surgery using a detomidine-buprenorphine combination in standing horses. *Veterinary Anaesthesia and Analgesia* 30: 71–79.

Vaughan, O.R. and Fowden, A.L. (2016). Placental metabolism: substrate requirements and the response to stress. *Reproduction in Domestic Animals* 51: 25–35.

Verhamme, K.M., Sturkenboom, M.C., Stricker, B.H., and Bosch, R. (2008). Drug-induced urinary retention: incidence, management and prevention. *Drug Safety* 31: 373–388.

Vigani, A. and Garcia-Pereira, F.L. (2014). Anesthesia and analgesia for standing equine surgery. *The Veterinary Clinics of North America. Equine Practice* 30: 1–17.

Virgin, J., Hendrickson, D., Wallis, T., and Rao, S. (2010). Comparison of intraoperative behavioral and hormonal responses to noxious stimuli between mares sedated with caudal epidural detomidine hydrochloride or a continuous intravenous infusion of detomidine hydrochloride for standing laparoscopic ovariectomy. *Veterinary Surgery* 39: 754–760.

Wakuno, A., Aoki, M., Kushiro, A. et al. (2017). Comparison of alfaxalone, ketamine and thiopental for anaesthetic induction and recovery in thoroughbred horses premedicated with medetomidine and midazolam. *Equine Veterinary Journal* 49: 94–98.

Wilkening, R.B. and Meschia, G. (1983). Fetal oxygen uptake, oxygenation, and acid-base balance as a function of uterine blood flow. *The American Journal of Physiology* 13: H749–H755.

Young, S.S. and Taylor, P.M. (1993). Factors influencing the outcome of equine anaesthesia: a review of 1,314 cases. *Equine Veterinary Journal* 25: 147–151.

Youngquist, R.S. (1988). Equine referral hospital dystocias. In: *Proceedings of the American Society of Theriogenologists*, pp. 73–79.

Yu, M., Han, C., Jiang, X. et al. (2015). Effect and placental transfer of dexmedetomidine during caesarean section under general anaesthesia. *Basic & Clinical Pharmacology & Toxicology* 117: 204–208.

13

Anesthetic Management of Foals

Kara Lascola and Stuart Clark-Price

Department of Clinical Sciences, College of Veterinary Medicine, Auburn University, 1220 Wire Road, Auburn, AL, 36849, USA

Introduction

The neonatal foal presenting for general anesthesia is a unique challenge in the equine species. Several reviews of anesthesia for the equine neonate have been previously published, and the reader is directed to those for a global overview of anesthesia of the neonate (Tranquilli and Thurmon 1990; Dunlop 1994; Hubbell and Muir 2009; Fischer and Clark-Price 2015). This chapter will serve to provide an update to current practices and provide focused information on specific techniques and conditions related to anesthesia of the neonatal foal while still covering some general information.

Physiology of the Neonate

The neonatal period is generally classified as the first four weeks of life and is a period of very rapid physiologic change and adaptation, particularly in the cardiovascular, respiratory, immune, and neurologic systems. Accordingly, these systems function at a reduced capacity to tolerate stresses and disease states can tip the balance into uncompensated illness. Providing anesthesia for these patients thus requires an understanding of the differences in physiology of the neonate from mature horses so that

anesthetic plans are tailored to this unique subset of horses. While an exhaustive description of neonatal physiology is beyond the scope of this chapter, aspects of cardiovascular and respiratory physiology that can impact clinical anesthetic management will be discussed. Much of the information provided in this chapter comes from studies in human neonates, as comparatively, literature on anesthesia of the equine neonate is sparse.

Cardiovascular Physiology

As the equine fetus nears term, heart rate decreases from 120 beats per minute to 80 beats per minute. This is a result of a baroreceptor reflex from an increase in fetal blood pressure. This indicates a response to increased plasma concentrations of catecholamines, angiotensin converting enzyme, and vasopressin as the fetus readies for birth (Fowden et al. 2020). Interestingly, cardiac baroreceptors sensitivity decreases during the last trimester which suggests that central "resetting" of baroreceptor response occurs after birth in the neonatal period and is thus often described as immature. In the first few moments after birth, a transition from fetal to neonatal (transitional) circulation occurs. Pulmonary vascular resistance is very high in the fetus so that most of the blood ejected from the right ventricle bypasses the lungs and enters the aorta and then systemic circulation. Upon birth, inflation of the lungs causes a drop in pulmonary vascular resistance and blood flows from the right ventricle into the pulmonary circulation causing a pressure drop and a narrowing of the ductus arteriosus. Left atrial pressure rises and right and left heart volume and ventricular output equalize causing closure of the foramen ovale. The ductus arteriosus further constricts as oxygen tension increases and placental-derived prostaglandins decrease (Marr 2015; Saikia and Mahanta 2019). In horses, the ductus arteriosus may be patent in normal healthy foals up to one week of life (Fries et al. 2020). A rise in pulmonary vascular resistance (pulmonary hypertension) in foals can cause the transitional circulation to revert to fetal circulation and result in tissue hypoxia (Cottrill et al. 1987).

The neonatal heart contracts at near maximal effort because of a large release of catecholamines and thyroid hormone late in gestation and at birth. Neonates need a larger cardiac output relative to the adult horse to provide oxygen and nutrients to growing tissues with very high metabolic demands. As a result, stroke volume remains relatively constant and cardiac output is mainly a product of changes in heart rate (Saikia and Mahanta 2019). Therefore, there is very little cardiac reserve in myocardial performance and small decreases in heart rate can produce large reductions in cardiac output. Sedative, anesthetic, and analgesic drugs that decrease heart rate can therefore have clinically relevant effects on the cardiovascular system and may alter patient management (see the following text).

Respiratory Physiology

Neonatal lung physiology and pulmonary mechanics are different from older foals and adult horses (Neumann and von Ungern-Sternberg 2014). Immaturity of the respiratory center in the brain stem and peripheral and central chemoreceptor responses lead to irregular breathing patterns that can present anywhere from tachypnea to long periods of apnea. This results from an inefficient and easily impaired response to blood pH and carbon dioxide and oxygen tensions ($PaCO_2$ and PaO_2). The response to hypercapnia can be attenuated without an appropriate increase in tidal volume and/or ventilation rate while a biphasic response to hypoxia can be seen with an initial increase in ventilation rate and a subsequent decrease that may progress to apnea. The addition of sedative and anesthetic drugs can further blunt these responses (Kurth et al. 1987). Additionally, neonates can have an exaggerated Hering-Breuer inflation reflex in that activation of stretch receptors in the lungs and airways can result in vagal inhibition of the respiratory centers of the brain stem (Stocks et al. 1996). Anatomically, compliance of the pharynx, larynx, trachea, and bronchial tree is greater in neonates and can lead to dynamic airway collapse, particularly during inspiration (Neumann and von Ungern-Sternberg 2014). Because of small airways, luminal material such as blood or secretions can greatly increase the work of breathing which can be more difficult on neonates due to a highly compliant chest wall compared to older horses. Newborn foals have fewer alveoli and alveolar surface area compared to one-month-old foals and adult horses (Johnson et al. 2014). As such, neonates can develop atelectasis more easily in dependent lung regions than more mature horses. Additionally, ill foals may have reduced production of pulmonary surfactant, which can further affect alveolar opening. A compliant and deformable chest wall result in a larger portion of the energy generated from diaphragmatic contraction to be wasted on thoracic distortion (Neumann and von Ungern-Sternberg 2014). Immaturity and weakness of the diaphragm and intercostal muscles also contribute to the potential for respiratory insufficiency, and this can be further potentiated with the addition of sedative and anesthetic agents. Functional residual capacity (FRC) is lower in neonates than in adults. This can lead to reduced oxygen reserves and higher chance of hypoxemia. Additionally, due to lower elastic properties of lungs, closing volume in neonates can be less than FRC resulting in terminal closure of airway (Mansell et al. 1972).

Anesthetized neonatal foals may require assisted or mechanical ventilation due to an inability to maintain appropriate PaO_2 and $PaCO_2$. Lung-protective strategies for ventilation of neonatal lungs are recommended to minimize the possibility of ventilator-induced lung injury (VILI) (Neumann and von Ungern-Sternberg 2014) (see the following text).

General Considerations for Anesthesia of Foals

Anesthesia of a foal is not simply anesthesia of a small horse. Physiologic and immunologic immaturity, unique disease conditions and responses to illness, and size differences can make general anesthesia more challenging. Indeed, horses less than one month of age have an increased risk of dying in the peri-operative period (within seven days after surgical procedure) compared to young adult horses (Johnston et al. 2002). This may be because of a lack of familiarity with providing anesthesia for foals, lack of pharmacokinetics and pharmacodynamics information of drugs used in neonates, and that neonates are most commonly anesthetized for correction of serious illnesses. Appropriate planning, preparation, and equipment are key factors for increasing the odds of successful outcomes.

Pre-anesthetic Evaluation and Preparation

Knowledge of signalment, history, results of diagnostic tests, medications administered, and a thorough physical examination are the mainstay of pre-anesthetic evaluation of foals

and are critical when formulating an anesthetic plan.

The breed of the foal is important as genetic disease in familial lines may help identify foals that are potentially at higher risk for anesthetic complications. An inclusive list of genetic disorders that may clinically manifest in foals is beyond the scope of this chapter. However, some examples include hyperkalemic periodic paralysis in Quarter horses, fragile foal syndrome in Warmbloods, glycogen branching enzyme deficiency in Quarter horse and Paint breeds, polysaccharide storage myopathy, and malignant hyperthermia (Traub-Dargatz et al. 1992; Finno et al. 2009; Martin et al. 2020).

Inquiring about the mare's health during pregnancy, primiparous or multiparous status, lactation, the foal's gestational age, birth location and delivery, and immediate post-partum activity should be routine to determine if developmental delays and/or failure of passive transfer may have occurred. It is also important to determine if any medications have been administered prior to the foal presenting for anesthesia. Previously administered antimicrobial, sedative, or analgesic drugs may negatively interact with drugs in an anesthetic plan and may require adjustments.

Sample collection for clinical pathological diagnostic tests to assess immune function and status, hydration and nutrition, acid–base and electrolyte balance should be performed to establish baselines and repeated at necessary intervals to monitor health status. A complete blood count, biochemistry panel, electrolyte analysis, and arterial blood gas may be necessary to assess function of various physiologic systems. Additionally, samples for blood culture should be acquired before initiating antimicrobial therapy if septicemia is suspected. Quantification of plasma IgG concentration should be assessed for status of passive transfer of immunoglobulins from colostrum. Thoracic and abdominal radiographs and ultrasound can be utilized to assess for rib fracture, pneumonia, abscesses formation, free fluid (samples should be collected for diagnostic tests), or structural abnormalities that may require advances therapeutic techniques.

Physical examination of a foal should be through and systematic with a focus on the neurologic, cardiovascular, respiratory, and urinary systems. Select normal physical exam and clinical pathology parameters can be found in Table 13.1. Abnormalities detected during physical examination should be investigated for identification of underlying cause and corrective or stabilizing therapies employed to the greatest extent possible prior to an anesthetic event.

Neonatal foals usually present with their dam and separation for anesthesia and surgery can be a stressful event for the mare, foal, and personnel. Some mares will become agitated and potentially dangerous when foals are handled and/or removed from the mare's line of sight. Facility procedures and protocols that maximize personnel safety should be followed at all times when working around a mare and foal pair. If the foal is ambulatory, then walking the mare and allowing the foal to follow to the induction area prior to premedication may minimize stress and anxiety. If the foal is not ambulatory, premedication in the stall will sedate the foal and allow for transportation on a gurney without flailing. Sedation of the mare is frequently necessary to minimize vocalization, agitation, aggressive behavior, and stall walking and can be done with a combination of xylazine or detomidine with acepromazine for immediate sedation and longer duration tranquilization during the period the foal is absent. Separation should be held off as long as possible until right before premedication and induction and the foal should be allowed to nurse up until just before sedation to minimize to potential for hypoglycemia. Once sedative medications are administered, foals should be prevented from nursing to reduce the risk of aspiration of milk. After induction of the foal, the sedated mare can be returned to the stall.

Table 13.1 Select normal reference ranges for various physiologic and clinical pathology parameters in neonatal foals (7–12 days of age).

Parameter	Range
Physiologic parameters	
Heart rate (beats/min)	80–100
Respiratory rate (breaths/min)	20–40
Temperature (°F/°C)	99–102/37–39
Parameter	**Mean ± SD**
Arterial blood gas (FiO$_2$ = 0.21)	
pH	7.442 ± 0.015
PaO$_2$ (mmHg)	78.4 ± 5.9
PaCO$_2$ (mmHg)	38.5 ± 2.4
HCO$_3$ (mEq/l)	27.6 ± 0.7
Lactate (mmol/l)	1.4 ± 0.2
Complete blood count	
RBC (×10^6/μl)	9.26 ± 0.8
Hemoglobin (g/dl)	13.2 ± 1.2
Packed cell volume (%)	36.5 ± 3.1
Total protein (g/dl)	6.4 ± 0.6
Fibrinogen (mg/dl)	310 ± 90
Total white blood cells (WBC) (cells/dl)	9000 ± 2200
Neutrophils (cells/dl)	6500 ± 2000
Bands (cells/dl)	<50
Lymphocytes (cells/dl)	2200 ± 575
Monocytes (cells/dl)	300 ± 135
Eosinophils (cells/dl)	20 ± 4
Basophils (cells/dl)	17 ± 2
Serum biochemistry	
Sodium (mEq/l)	140 ± 4.2
Chloride (mEq/l)	101 ± 4.0
Potassium (mEq/l)	4.5 ± 0.4
Calcium (mg/dl)	11.4 ± 0.8
Magnesium (mg/dl)	2.7 ± 0.15
Glucose (mg/dl)	150 ± 30
Blood urea nitrogen (mg/dl)	13.5 ± 5.5
Creatinine (mg/dl)	1.3 ± 0.3
Albumin (g/dl)	3.1 ± 0.5
Globulin (g/dl)	3.2 ± 0.5
Albumin : Globulin ratio	1.1 ± 0.4

Anesthetic/Analgesic Drugs

Commonly used sedative, analgesic, and anesthetic agents can have a clinically relevant impact on physiologic systems and can lead to an increase in morbidity and mortality in equine patients. In healthy, mature horses, there are adequate physiologic reserves to allow for safe compensation of these effects. However, the equine neonate can be particularly susceptible to adverse anesthetic events because of immaturity in physiologic systems and thus requires careful titration of dosages and intensive monitoring for physiologic parameter deviations. Statements can be found in literature suggesting that the neonatal blood–brain barrier is immature, leaky, or even absent in the neonate and thus is more permeable to anesthetic/sedative agents. However, more recent evidence suggests that this barrier is impermeable and that tight junctions are formed very early in fetal life (Ek et al. 2006; Saunders et al. 2019). There is little doubt that a developing brain is more vulnerable to drugs and toxins than an adult brain, but this appears to be related to a higher transport capacity of transporter proteins in the central nervous system (Saunders et al. 2019). Perinatal hypoxic–ischemic-related brain injury is associated with pathologic disruption of the blood–brain barrier (Disdier and Stonestreet 2020). Thus, foals with perinatal asphyxia syndrome (PAS) should be treated as though they have disruption of the blood–brain barrier with further considerations of risk versus benefit and dosages for drug selection. Common sense implies that reduced dosages and use "to effect" should be applied to anesthetic/sedative drug administration to neonatal foals. Dosages of various sedative, analgesic, and anesthetic agents used in neonatal foals can be found in Table 13.2.

Sedatives and Tranquilizers

In adult horses, reliable, fast acting sedation is necessary to improve handling and the quality of anesthesia. However, with neonatal foals, many of the commonly used sedatives can have detrimental effects on an immature cardiovascular system. The most commonly used classes of sedative in horses are alpha-2 agonists and phenothiazines.

The alpha-2 agonists, xylazine, detomidine, and romifidine, are favored in adult horses because of their reliable, quick acting sedation and analgesia (Sanchez and Robertson 2014; Moorman et al. 2019). However, drugs in this category can have profound effects through alpha-receptor agonism. In healthy foals up to 28 days of age, xylazine administration can result in bradycardia, hypertension and then hypotension, upper airway obstruction, ventilatory stridor, decreased minute ventilation, marked ataxia, and recumbency (Carter et al. 1990). A reduction in cardiac output associated with alpha-2 agonist use is well known and likely to be more profound in foals as their cardiac output is more heart rate dependent than mature horse. Alpha-2 agonists in horses may negatively affect gastrointestinal motility and perfusion and increase post-glomerular diuresis that may be detrimental to fluid and electrolyte balance, particularly in compromised patients (Rutkowski et al. 1991; Sutton et al. 2002; Nuñez et al. 2004; Zullian et al. 2011). Due to the immature cardiovascular status of neonatal foals and the likelihood of clinically relevant disease, minimizing the use of alpha-2 agonist drugs, whenever possible, is recommended.

Acepromazine, a phenothiazine, is a centrally acting dopamine receptor antagonist that is useful as a tranquilizer in horses. Onset of action is up to approximately 20 minutes and has a dose-dependent duration of action of 1–2.5 hours in horses (Marroum et al. 1994). Additionally, packed cell volume is reduced by up to 20% and blood pressure significantly decreases (Marroum et al. 1994). Due to its long duration of action, lack of a reversal agent, and actions on the circulatory system, acepromazine has not gained wide popularity for sedation in neonatal foals.

Benzodiazepines have centrally acting muscle relaxation and sedative effects through

Table 13.2 Dosages of sedative, analgesic, anesthetic, and adjunctive drugs for use in neonatal foals.

Drug	Dosage	Comments
Sedative drugs		
Diazepam	0.05–0.2 mg/kg, IV	May cause excitement in healthy foals over two weeks of age. Propylene glycol vehicle may cause vascular irritation
Midazolam	0.05–0.2 mg/kg, IV	May cause excitement in healthy foals over two weeks of age
Xylazine	0.5–1.0 mg/kg, IV	Can have profound cardiovascular side effects. Avoid in sick foals and foals less than two weeks of age
Detomidine	0.005–0.015 mg/kg, IV	Can have profound cardiovascular side effects. Avoid in sick foals and foals less than two weeks of age
Dexmedetomidine	0.003–0.007 mg/kg, IV 0.001 mg/kg/h constant rate infusion (CRI), IV	Can have profound cardiovascular side effects. Avoid in sick foals and foals less than two weeks of age CRI will reduce MAC of inhalant
Acepromazine	n/a	Not recommended for use in foals due to a long duration of effect, associated hypotension, and lack of reversal agent
Analgesic drugs		
Butorphanol (opioid)	0.1–0.2 mg/kg, IV	Agonist–antagonist profile and may provide less analgesia than other opioids
Morphine (opioid)	0.1–0.5 mg/kg, IV	Higher dosages may cause excitement
Hydromorphone (opioid)	0.025–0.05 mg/kg, IV	Dosages described are for adult horses
Fentanyl (opioid)	0.002–0.004 mg/kg, IV 1–2 µg/kg/h, IV	Higher dosages may cause excitement and increased locomotor activity
Buprenorphine (opioid)	0.01–0.02 mg/kg, IV	Longer duration of action and not reversible
Flunixin meglumine (NSAID)	0.25–1.1 mg/kg, IV	Risk of GI ulceration
Meloxicam (NSAID)	0.2–0.6 mg/kg, IV	Risk of GI ulceration
Firocoxib (NSAID)	0.1 mg/kg	May cause less GI upset than other NSAIDs
Lidocaine (local anesthetic)	1–2 mg/kg total dose for local anesthesia techniques 1 mg/kg, IV followed by 25 µg/kg/min CRI	CRI provides MAC reduction
Mepivacaine (local anesthetic)	1–2 mg/kg total dose for local anesthetic techniques	Cardiotoxic and should not be administered IV
Bupivacaine (local anesthetic)	1–2 mg/kg total dose for local anesthetic techniques	Cardiotoxic and should not be administered IV

(Continued)

Table 13.2 (Continued)

Drug	Dosage	Comments
Anesthetic drugs		
Ketamine	1.0–2.0 mg/kg, IV	Combine with a benzodiazepine for muscle relaxation
Propofol	2.0–4.0 mg/kg, IV	Administer to effect slowly
		Dose and rate-dependent hypotension and respiratory depression
		Smooth recovery
Ketamine/propofol combination ("ketofol")	0.5 mg/kg, IV ketamine 2.0 mg/kg, IV propofol	Administer ketamine first and then administer propofol to effect
Alfaxalone	2 mg/kg, IV 6 mg/kg/h CRI, IV	Muscle rigidity and rough recovery possible
Isoflurane	MAC = 1.31	Value is for adult horses and is likely lower for neonatal foals
Sevoflurane	MAC = 2.84	Value is for adult horses and is likely lower for neonatal foals
Adjunctive drugs		
Atropine	0.02–0.04 mg/kg, IV	
Glycopyrrolate	0.005–0.01 mg/kg, IV	
Dobutamine	3–10 μg/kg/min, IV	Inotropic support
Norepinephrine	0.1–1.0 μg/kg/min, IV	Vasopressor support
Vasopressin	0.1–1.0 mU/kg/min, IV	May reduce splanchnic circulation
Atipamezole	0.05–0.1 mg/kg, intramuscular (IM)	Used for reversal of α2 agonist drugs
		IM use only
		Severe hypotension can result if administered IV
Flumazenil	0.01–0.05 mg/kg, IV	Reversal of benzodiazepines
Naloxone	0.005–0.05 mg/kg, IV	Reversal of opioids
		Repeat dosage until desired effect achieved
Mannitol	0.25–1.0 g/kg, IV	May be useful in foals with PAS. Administer over 15–30 min through a filter
Regular insulin	0.25–0.5 U/kg, IV	Check serum glucose 20 min after administration and as needed afterward to monitor for hypoglycemia or hyperglycemia
Polymyxin B	2000–5000 U/kg, IV	Treatment for endotoxemia. Higher doses can be ototoxic and nephrotoxic
Dextrose	In IV fluids as 1–5% solution	Solutions greater than 5% can result in red blood cell damage/lysis

enhancing the effects of the inhibitory neuro-transmitter γ aminobutyric acid (GABA) on chloride and other ion channels. Benzodiazepines have minimal clinically relevant effects on cardiovascular or ventilatory performance. Additionally, drugs in this class have potent anticonvulsive activity which may be helpful in foals with neonatal asphyxia (Johne et al. 2021). Traditionally, benzodiazepines such as midazolam and diazepam are combined with ketamine for their muscle relaxant properties during induction of anesthesia in horses. In adult horses, benzodiazepines provide little to no sedation but can produce ataxia, anxious, agitated, or aggressive behavior and are not recommended as a single therapy (Muir 2009; Fischer and Clark-Price 2015). However, in foals less than two to four weeks of age, benzodiazepines can produce profound sedation, relaxation, and recumbency (Fischer and Clark-Price 2015). Midazolam may be preferred over diazepam due to formulation differences. Diazepam is not water-soluble and is therefore found with propylene glycol as a carrier agent. At high doses, propylene glycol can be tissue irritating and cause necrosis, hemolysis, and cardiac arrhythmias (Lim et al. 2014). Midazolam gives the benefit of being water-soluble and thus formulations are made without propylene glycol. Midazolam can be administered intramuscularly if intravenous access is limited. Additionally, intranasal midazolam is reported to be effective for seizure control in dogs (Charalambous et al. 2017) and though not published, anecdotal reports suggest similar anti-seizure and sedative effects when administered intranasal in foals. The pharmacokinetics of midazolam have been well described in adult horses at dosages of 0.05 and 0.1 mg/kg (Hubbell et al. 2013). However, the pharmacokinetics have not been described in juvenile or neonatal horses. Neonatal foals presenting for anesthesia frequently have disease that may have an immunological component (i.e. failure of passive transfer, sepsis). Midazolam has been shown to suppress phagocytosis and oxidative burst, essential functions of the innate immune system, in equine neutrophils, and macrophages; however, it is unknown if this has any clinical implications (Massoco and Palermo-Neto 2003).

Opioid Analgesics

It is important to recognize that, at birth, animals have a developing nociceptive system. Although not completely mature, neonatal animals are able to process and interpret pain sensations. In fact, the ability to "feel" pain occurs early in the second half of gestation (Bellieni 2020). The central nervous system is quite plastic at birth, and structural and functional "fine-tuning" of the nociceptive system continues as the animal develops. The spinal circuitry is activity dependent and therefore there can be long-term detrimental consequences to untreated pain (van den Hoogen et al. 2019). Untreated pain can lead to neurotoxicity, alterations in spinal neuronal circuits, and apoptosis of developing neuronal brain cells (van den Hoogen et al. 2019). Questions continue to surround the use of opioids as analgesics in horses with behavioral changes (aggression, sedation), gastrointestinal stasis, and respiratory depression during anesthesia being main points of contention. Butorphanol, a κ agonist – μ antagonist, is the most commonly used opioid in horses. Butorphanol has been evaluated in healthy neonatal foals at 0.05 mg/kg and although the pharmacokinetics are different from adult horses (greater volume of distribution and faster clearance in neonates), it appears to be well tolerated with minimal effects on vital parameters (Arguedas et al. 2008). Clinical signs of sedation and increased nursing behaviors can be expected to occur. Of the numerous μ agonist opioids available for clinical use, there is little published data in neonatal foals. Anecdotal use of morphine suggests that it provides clinically relevant sedation when combination with midazolam as a premedication prior to surgery. Fentanyl, a μ agonist opioid, is considered 100 times more potent than morphine and is used commonly as an infusion during anesthesia for surgery in small animal patients. Fentanyl has been studied in healthy foals in a dose escalation manner (Knych et al. 2015). At dosages greater than 4 μg/kg, foals develop ataxia, muscle rigidity, and may head press. Foals become heavily sedated and recumbent at 32 μg/kg. It is important to note that efficacy studies with opioids have not been performed in neonatal foals and clinical use is frequently based on clinical experience and extrapolation from adult horses and other species. Local use of opioids, particularly intra-articular use of preservative free morphine, may allow for a reduced dosage and minimizing systemic effects while still benefiting from the analgesic properties. In the authors' opinion, μ agonist opioids should be considered for routine use in anesthetized neonatal foals that are undergoing invasive, painful procedures as the negative effects of pain outweigh the potential negative effects of opioid use.

Induction Agents

Ketamine continues to be the induction agent used most commonly in adult horses as it provides rapid unconsciousness, can be administered in a reasonable volume, and provides for a smooth and controlled induction. However, in neonatal foals, the concern about controlling a large body mass during induction is not as problematic as an adult horse and therefore allows for more options for induction.

When inducting a neonatal foal for anesthesia, quick control of the airway is essential to provide oxygen and ventilatory support as hypoxemia can rapidly occur. In human infants, hypoxemia during anesthesia is recognized as a critical factor that increases morbidity and mortality (Disma et al. 2021). Intubation can be quickly accomplished with the use of inhalants, ketamine, propofol, or alfaxalone in neonatal foals.

Inhalant anesthetics has been used for induction of anesthesia in foals (Steffey et al. 1991). A facemask with an airtight seal can be applied over the nose of a foal for induction, but in depressed or gently restrained foals, nasotracheal intubation can be performed in the awake animal. This requires use of a long, straight, silicone endotracheal tube with an internal diameter of 6–14 mm depending on the size of the foal (Figure 13.1). Soaking the endotracheal tube in warm water to soften and applying water-based lubricant to the outer surface will facilitate insertion. Additionally, desensitizing the nasal mucosa with lidocaine may improve compliance from the foal. Once placed, the endotracheal tube can be attached to a breathing circuit on an anesthesia machine, and oxygen and inhalant anesthetic can be administered for induction. Inhalant anesthetics cause dose-dependent vasodilation and decreased cardiac output through reduced stroke volume in adult horses and similar changes should be expected in foals (Steffey and Howland 1980; Steffey et al. 2005). Careful titration of the dose of inhalant anesthetic during induction and maintenance of anesthesia while minimizing side effects can be achieved through attentive physiologic parameter monitoring of the foal.

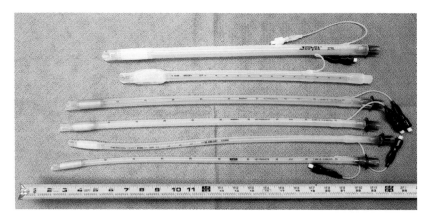

Figure 13.1 Various sized silicone tubes that can be utilized for nasotracheal or endotracheal intubation in neonatal foals.

Ketamine, a dissociative anesthetic, induces anesthesia through non-competitive interaction with N-methyl-D-aspartate receptors in the central nervous system. Ketamine administration results in maintenance or even elevation of heart rate and blood pressure through increased release and inhibition of reuptake of endogenous catecholamines like epinephrine. After a relatively small volume for injection, a predictable pattern of induction is observed in adult horses. However, ketamine use, particularly in short procedures can result in excitement and dysphoria during the recovery period and more recently, research in laboratory animals suggests that ketamine can increase neuronal apoptosis in developing brains and produce long-term cognitive impairment, even after a single dose (Blaise 2015; Sampaio et al. 2018). To date, no research has been published in equine neonates, so it is unknown how ketamine effects the developing foal brain.

Propofol is a unique phenolic anesthetic agent in that it is structurally distinct from all other injectable anesthetic drugs. It acts as an agonist at the GABA complex resulting in cell hyperpolarization. Propofol has the favorable properties of a rapid, smooth induction and a short, delirium free recovery. Propofol has administration rate and dose-dependent adverse effects on spontaneous ventilation and blood pressure. Slow infusion at the lowest dosage necessary for intubation can minimize hypoventilation and hypotension. While research in adult horses is available, published studies on use of propofol in neonatal foals is limited. Anecdotal reports indicate that veterinarians are using propofol as an induction agent for foals more commonly. However, similar to ketamine, studies in laboratory animals suggest that propofol may have toxic effects in a developing brain. Repeated injections but not a single injection of propofol in neonatal mice resulted in long-term motor and behavioral learning impairment (Zhou et al. 2021).

The combination of ketamine and propofol ("ketofol") has been described for use in human neonates and healthy adult dogs (Martinez-Taboada and Leece 2014; Hayes et al. 2021). In human neonates, the combination may result in a small reduction in the risk of hypotension, bradycardia, and apnea, with a slight increase in tachycardia. In adult dogs, ketofol induction resulted in a higher pulse rate and mean arterial pressure with a quality of induction and ease of intubation greater than propofol alone. The authors have used this combination to induce anesthesia in foals, and clinical impression is that it achieves a smooth induction and a stable plane of anesthesia.

Alfaxalone is a steroidal anesthetic agent with a physical structure similar to progesterone. Alfaxalone is thought to work through interaction with GABA. Alfaxalone has been used as an induction agent in adult horses with an induction time shorter than ketamine but with a more prolonged recovery time (Wakuno et al. 2017). Total intravenous anesthesia with alfaxalone has been reported in healthy foals and one donkey foal (Jones et al. 2019; Loomes 2020). Prolonged recovery was noted. Pharmacodynamic data in foals suggests clinically acceptable heart rate and blood pressures during anesthesia after a single injection; however, oxygen supplementation may be required to prevent hypoxemia (Goodwin et al. 2012). Alfaxalone is not approved for use in humans, and there are currently no studies available assessing neurotoxicity in developing brains.

Maintenance Agents

For short procedures (<30 minutes), maintenance of anesthesia may be provided with additional doses of injectable anesthetics such as propofol or alfaxalone. Oxygen/ventilatory support may be necessary due to the respiratory depressant effects of the drugs combined with the foal's physiologic immaturity. For major surgical procedures or the need for prolonged anesthesia (>30 minutes), inhalant anesthetics isoflurane and sevoflurane are the mainstay. This requires tracheal intubation and the use of an anesthesia machine. Many of the large animal anesthesia machines that are commonly used for adult horses are not suitable for anesthesia of foals weighing less than 330 lbs. (150 kg). The large volume of the breathing circuit in these machines makes quick adjustment of anesthetic vapor concentration nearly impossible and the larger one-way valves may result in clinically relevant resistance to breathing. Additionally, for foals that require mechanical ventilation, large animal anesthesia machine bellows may not safely accommodate smaller tidal volumes, flow rates, and pressures necessary to prevent lung injury. Standard small animal anesthesia machines and mechanical ventilators can be utilized for safe delivery of anesthetic. More recently, an electronic large animal anesthesia machine with a precision motor piston driven ventilator became available on the veterinary market (Tafonius, Hallowell Engineering and Manufacturing Corporation). With the use of a "foal circuit," very precise ventilation utilizing various modes of ventilation can be applied for use in foals. The minimum alveolar concentration (MAC), common use, and side effects of isoflurane (MAC = 1.31) and sevoflurane (MAC = 2.84) have been well described in adult horses (Steffey et al. 1977, 2005; Brosnan 2013). MAC values of isoflurane and sevoflurane in foals have not been reported. However, MAC values of inhalant anesthetics are decreased in human term neonates less than one month of age and even further decreased in human pre-term neonates (LeDez and Lerman 1987). Thus, neonatal foals likely require lower concentrations of isoflurane and sevoflurane similarly and practitioners are advised to adjust vaporizers downward in neonatal foals during anesthesia to minimize excessive anesthetic depth. Previously mentioned, cardiovascular side effects of vasodilation and decreased stroke volume can be problematic and techniques (use of supplemental analgesic drugs) that allow for a reduced concentration of inhalant to be administered should be considered. Ventilatory changes can also be expected to occur in neonatal foals during inhalant anesthesia.

Hypoventilation progressing to apnea should be expected as inhalant dose increases. The neonatal brain has an altered response to elevations in carbon dioxide resulting in irregular breathing patterns (Neumann and von Ungern-Sternberg 2014). Further blunted by inhalant anesthetics, a weak respiratory drive frequently results in the need for assisted or mechanical ventilation of foals.

In 2016, the United States Food and Drug Administration issued a warning that repeated or lengthy (>3 hours) general anesthesia in children less than three years of age may affect the development of the child's brain (Olutoye et al. 2018). This statement was made due to mounting evidence of anesthetic toxicity in the developing brains of research animals. Drugs in two classes of sedative/anesthetic agents were implicated: GABA agonists (e.g. inhalant anesthetics, benzodiazepines, and propofol) and N-methyl-D-aspartate (NMDA) antagonists (e.g. ketamine). Neuronal anesthetic toxicity can lead to structural, functional, and compensatory changes in sensory and learning systems (Aksenov et al. 2020). Neurotoxicity of inhalant anesthetics appears to be through enhancement of apoptosis in various parts of the brain that can lead to cognitive deficits (Jevtovic-Todorovic et al. 2003). This phenomenon appears to occur only in developing brains, as inhalants do not have similar effects in mature brains (Stratmann et al. 2010). To date, there is no information on the effect of anesthetic drugs on the development of the equine brain. However, in light of the recommendations in human neonates, it seems prudent that practitioners should limit the duration and number of anesthetic episodes and the dosages of sedative and anesthetic drugs used in foals as much as possible.

Monitoring and Support During Anesthesia

Depending on the physical condition of the foal, the anticipated length of the anesthetic event and the procedure for which it is being anesthetized for, the level of intensity of monitoring and support varies. It should be stressed that regardless of the procedure, physical assessment of the foal should be performed at regular intervals as physical status of neonatal foals can change rapidly. This included thoracic auscultation of the heart and lungs, palpation of pulse quality, mucous membrane color, and capillary refill time. For procedures or diagnostic of less than 15 minutes, nasal insufflation of oxygen, and the addition of pulse oximetry to physical assessment may be all that is required. For longer or invasive procedures, use of a vital parameter monitor including electrocardiogram, end-tidal gas analysis, pulse oximetry, and direct arterial blood pressure measurement should be considered.

Cardiovascular Monitoring and Support

The goal of cardiovascular monitoring is assessing the adequacy of circulation and tissue perfusion. Heart rate and rhythm (ECG), mucous membrane color and capillary refill time, peripheral temperature, arterial blood pressure, and blood lactate concentration are useful tools for assessment. Dark mucous membranes, prolonged capillary refill times, cool extremities, and elevated lactate concentrations can all suggest poor perfusion and indicate the need for intervention. Likewise,

decreases in heart rate and blood pressure can indicate depressed pump function. Resting values for heart rate and blood pressure change during the first few weeks of a foal's life as physiologic growth and maturity progress. Foals can be expected to have higher heart rates and lower blood pressure in the first week as compared to the second week, and younger foals have a decreased corrective response to anesthetic-induced hypotension (O'Connor et al. 2005). Vital signs should be interpreted based on the foal's age, and more aggressive therapies to combat hypotension may be necessary in younger foal. Arterial blood pressure can be measured via indirect methods with an appropriately sized cuff placed around the base of the tail. However, similar to other species, indirect blood pressure measurement is likely not suitable for decision making after a single measurement and only useful for detecting trends over time. However, as the cardiovascular status of anesthetized foals can change quickly, the authors recommend direct blood pressure measurement from an arterial catheter for systemically ill foals or any foal undergoing general anesthesia for more than 30 minutes. Arterial catheters can be placed in the transverse facial, lateral metatarsal, lingual, or femoral arteries (Figure 13.2) (Fischer and Clark-Price 2015). In adult horses, a target

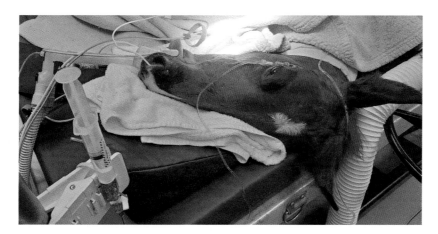

Figure 13.2 Cannulation of the facial artery in a foal during anesthesia for direct measurement of arterial blood pressure.

value for mean arterial blood pressure of 70 mmHg or greater has been associated with a decrease in morbidity and mortality, particularly associated with equine peri-anesthetic myopathy (Schauvliege and Gasthuys 2013). Neonatal foals likely do not need to maintain mean arterial blood pressures of 70 mmHg or greater. Cardiovascular studies in foals for recommendation of arterial blood pressure are not available. However, in anesthetized human neonates, a 20% reduction in systolic blood pressure compared to awake baseline resulted in a less than 10% chance of cerebral desaturation (Michelet et al. 2015). When awake neonatal foal blood pressure is considered, the human study suggests that mean arterial blood pressure of >50 mmHg may be acceptable in anesthetized foals.

Cardiac output monitoring is not routinely performed in clinical veterinary patients. However, more recently, an ultrasound dilution (UDCO) method has been developed for human infants that utilizes a peripheral venous and arterial catheter. Invasive heart catheterization or loss of blood that is necessary for other methods is not needed for UDCO. This method has been validated for use in foals to assess cardiac function and has the advantage of being useful in awake and anesthetized foals (Shih et al. 2009; Fries et al. 2020). For critically ill foals, measurement of cardiac function with UDCO before, during, and after anesthesia may help detect cardiac performance changes early and guide goal-directed therapy.

Hypotension during anesthesia may be related to vasodilation, hypovolemia, bradycardia, and/or decreased contractility (decreased stroke volume). Treatment aimed at hypotension should be directed at an identified underlying cause and not "shot gun" therapy aimed at improving a number on a vital signs monitor. As previously stated, foals have minimal cardiovascular reserve and thus heavy-handed administration of corrective therapies may result in further worsening of cardiovascular function and patient health status. Hypotension may be simply related to the anesthetic agents used, and decreasing the plane of anesthesia may allow for acceptable correction of parameters. Hemodynamic instability related to shock may be observed in any anesthetized foal as most anesthetic episodes are related to correction of diseases that have systemic impact. Shock in neonates is most commonly diagnosed only after the onset of the hypotensive phase which indicates serious disease progression. Early identification and intervention is key to successful management (Singh et al. 2018). Ideally, identification of potential or the onset of shock occurs early on and the foal is stabilized prior to anesthesia (see sepsis in the following text). Once meaningful hypotension is identified, a systematic examination for cause should be performed. A combination of physical parameters (anesthetic depth, capillary refill time, mucous membrane color, extremity temperature), vital sign monitor parameters (heart rate and rhythm, pulse oximetry, end-tidal CO_2) and clinical pathology findings (blood gas, electrolyte, lactate, and hematocrit) should be utilized for determining course of action. While anticholinergic drugs (atropine, glycopyrrolate) have traditionally been avoided for use in adult horses due to concerns surrounding gastrointestinal stasis, use to accelerate heart rate in foals may be sufficient to counter anesthetic-induced bradycardia. Hypovolemia should be corrected with intravenous fluid therapy to correct losses. However, overaggressive use of fluids may result in fluid overload and hypernatremia (Fielding and Magdesian 2015). Fluid boluses of 20 ml/kg have been suggested and should be repeated up to three times (Fielding and Magdesian 2015). Goals for fluid therapy are a blood lactate concentration less than 4 mmol/l, normalization of perfusion parameters, and urine production. If hypotension persists after fluid therapy, infusion of inotropic and/or vasopressors should be instituted. Dobutamine is used for inotropic support, and norepinephrine is used for vasopressor support (Hollis et al. 2006; Valverde et al. 2006; Fielding and Magdesian 2015). The combined use of dobutamine and norepinephrine in foals has been described and has been used by the authors for cardiovascular support in severely ill foals that did not have adequate response to single therapy (Hollis et al. 2006). Vasopressin increases vascular resistance and blood pressure in anesthetized foals; however, splanchnic circulation is decreased resulting in a potential decrease in gastric mucosal perfusion (Valverde et al. 2006).

Ventilatory Monitoring and Support

The unique respiratory physiology of the neonatal foal and the depressant effects of sedative, analgesic, and anesthetic drugs, often necessitate the use of assisted or mechanical ventilation during anesthesia. Adequacy of ventilation in the anesthetized foal can be assessed with a combination of pulse oximetry, end-tidal gas determination, and arterial blood gas analysis. Hypercapnia ($PaCO_2 > 55$ mmHg, $pH \leq 7.25$) is usually an indicator of hypoventilation while hypoxemia is usually an indicator of a reduced gas diffusion across the alveolar-capillary barrier. Some indications for mechanical ventilation during general anesthesia in the neonatal foal include persistence of hypoxemia and/or hypercapnia, use of neuromuscular blocking agents, thoracic procedures or

imaging studies, irregular ventilator pattern that impedes uptake and maintenance of inhalant anesthetic, and spontaneous movements of the thoracic wall or abdomen that impedes a surgical procedure.

Due to the immaturity of a foal's lungs, lung-protective strategies that minimize VILI should be considered. VILI can result from excessively high tidal volume (volutrauma), higher pressures during ventilation (barotrauma), shear forces damaging lung that is insufficiently opened (atelectotrauma), subsequent release of pro-inflammatory cytokines, and high levels of oxygen resulting in oxidative stress (oxygen toxicity) (Neumann and von Ungern-Sternberg 2014). Lung-protective ventilation strategies that avoid high tidal volume and airway pressure, use of recruitment maneuvers, and preventing repetitive opening and closing of alveoli through use of positive end-expiratory pressure are recommended (Table 13.3).

Fluid and Electrolyte Monitoring and Therapy

Fluid, electrolyte, and acid–base status is monitored via analysis of blood samples. Shifts in parameters can happen rapidly and frequent sampling can allow for identification and initiation of therapies aimed at correction and

Table 13.3 Lung-protective mechanical ventilator strategies for neonatal foals.

Aim	Means
Maintain normal functional residual capacity	• Use positive end-expiratory pressure of 4–6 cm H_2O and adjust as needed
Optimize tidal volume	• Use volume-targeted ventilation to avoid over-distension or under-inflation of alveoli (set target V_T at 10–15 ml/kg) • Adjust V_T by adjusting peak inspiratory pressure (PIP < 15 cm H_2O)
Maintain normocapnia (ETCO$_2$ 30–45 mmHg; PaCO$_2$ 35–45 mmHg;	• Adjust V_T within recommended limits • Adjust respiratory rate between 20 and 40 breaths/min • Control inspiratory and expiratory times to avoid under-inflation and inadvertent positive end-expiratory pressure (PEEP)
Optimize oxygenation	• Avoid SPO$_2$ values <92% or PaO$_2$ values <80 mmHg

Source: Adapted from Neumann and von Ungern-Sternberg (2014).

balance. Derangements in sodium, chloride, and potassium are common in sick foals and fluid and electrolyte balance may vary depending on the disease (see below for treatment recommendations for specific diseases and conditions). Correction of fluid deficits and electrolyte imbalance should take place prior to inducing anesthesia whenever possible. While foals have a higher percentage of total body water than adult horses (10%), foals have a lower colloidal oncotic pressure, that, when accompanied with excessive exogenously administered fluids, can result in rapid development of edema (Magdesian 2013). Therefore, high volumes of fluids (other than fluid boluses needed for hypotension) should not be administered during anesthesia. If daily maintenance fluids are being administered as part of a treatment plan, those can be continued at a similar rate, or if maintenance fluids are not being administered, fluid rates of 2–5 ml/kg/h can be administered during anesthesia. While initial replacement fluids should utilize isotonic fluids such as lactate Ringer's solution, maintenance fluids before and during anesthesia should be comprised of hypotonic fluid solutions. Hypotonic fluids with supplementation of potassium (based on serum potassium concentrations) and dextrose (based on serum glucose concentrations) are thought to be more appropriate than isotonic fluids (Dathan and Sundaram 2021; Fielding and Magdesian 2015). Daily sodium requirements are quickly met with oral and intravenous fluid therapy in foals; thus, the use of isotonic fluids results in sodium retention secondary to a foal's inability to excrete large amounts of sodium quickly. Commercial maintenance fluids are hypotonic (approximately 110 mOsmol/l) and can be utilized or standard isotonic crystalloid fluids (approximately 295 mOsmol/l) can be diluted with sterile water to make a hypotonic solution similar to commercial products. If potassium supplementation is required, potassium phosphate may be used to supplement the maintenance fluids instead of potassium chloride to minimize hyperchloremia. For older healthy foals (>2 weeks), standard isotonic solutions can be utilized.

Dextrose support will likely be needed during anesthesia of neonatal foals, as glycogen storage is not sufficient to maintain appropriate blood glucose levels. Blood glucose should be checked at regular intervals (30–60 minutes) during anesthesia and adjustments made to intravenous fluid dextrose concentrations to maintain blood glucose concentrations between 150 and 250 mg/dl during anesthesia. Blood glucose in awake foals should be maintained at approximately 150 mg/dl. Dextrose can be added to the intravenous fluids to achieve a concentration of 1–5%. Solutions greater than 5% can be hyperosmolar and result in hyperglycemia, lysis of red blood cells, and osmotic diuresis, and should be avoided.

Plasma can be utilized for foals with a low oncotic pressure and/or hypoalbuminemia. In adult horses, plasma can be cost prohibitive for colloidal support but in foals, 20–40 ml/kg of fresh frozen plasma may be feasible. In cases of failure of passive transfer, hyperimmune plasma may be used for immunoglobulin replacement and immune therapy. However, failure of passive transfer should be corrected well before anesthesia and surgery is considered as these foals are at high risk for infections and sepsis.

Body Temperature Monitoring and Thermal Support

Inadvertent peri-anesthetic hypothermia (IPH) is one of the more common adverse events associated with general anesthesia. IPH is associated with delayed recovery, poor wound healing, increased risk of infection, altered coagulation, and hypotension (Clark-Price 2015). Neonatal foals have a larger surface area to body mass ration than older horses and have less skeletal muscle mass, thus they lose body heat more rapidly and have less capacity to generate heat. Additionally, hypothermia is further exacerbated by the impairment of thermoregulatory centers in the brain stem (Sessler 2015). Monitoring the body temperature of foals is therefore an essential part of an anesthetic plan. Aggressive heat support is necessary throughout the anesthetic period and during recovery. During anesthesia, use of active warming techniques (circulating warm water pads, force warm air blankets, resistive polymer electric blankets) that cover as much of the foal as possible can help reduce the temperature gradient from the foal to the environment and minimize hypothermia. Similarly in recovery, use of active warming as well as covering the foal in pre-warmed blankets can be used to reduce recovery time and complication.

Recovery

The goal of the recovery period is to transition the foal to an awake and standing state as quickly as possible. This will allow the foal to be returned to the mare and nursing to maintain blood glucose. Recovery of a foal can be done in either a dedicated recovery stall or in a stall with the mare nearby. Recovery in a stall with the mare is not recommended to prevent injury to personnel and the foal by an agitated mare. The authors prefer to recovery foals in a warm, quiet, and padded recovery stall and then bring the mare to the foal once the foal is standing. The mare and foal can be walked back to the wards once the foal is standing and has nursed. Foals should be placed in sternal recumbency to promote resolution of atelectasis. As stated previously, warming the foal will help reduce recovery time; however, reversal of sedative drugs may be necessary if recovery is prolonged. In general, foals should be fully recovered within one hour after discontinuing inhalation anesthetics. Intravenous fluids for electrolyte and glucose support can be continued during recovery and supplemental oxygen via nasal insufflation can be utilized to maintain SPO_2 values greater than 92%. Neonatal foals can be manually restrained during the recovery period by having control of the head and keeping the nose pointed upward. This minimizes struggling and the potential for injury. When the foal demonstrates vigorous attempts to stand, assistance to stand can be performed by grasping the base of the tail and giving firm support while the foal moves to a standing position.

Pain Management of the Foal

Neonates are a special population when it comes to pain management, as there is a fine balance between optimal pain relief and adverse drug effects (Maitra et al. 2014). As previously mentioned, untreated pain can have short- and long-term negative consequences to a foal. Pain management can not only alleviate pain, it can lower anesthetic requirements during anesthesia and improve recovery afterward. In humans, opioid use in neonates undergoing surgery is associated with a blunted stress response and improved outcomes (Anand et al. 1987; Anand and Hickey 1992). The stress response initiates protein, fat, and carbohydrate catabolism and can cause metabolic acidosis, hypoglycemia, hyperglycemia, and electrolyte abnormalities that can increase morbidity and mortality (Goldman and Koren 2002). Opioids are the mainstay of analgesia in neonates; however, local and regional anesthetic techniques should be considered whenever possible. While many of the commonly used techniques in adult horses have not been described in neonates, anatomical landmarks are similar facilitating use. Care should be taken to reduce the dosage of local anesthetics utilized due to increased risk of toxicity in the neonate. Non-steroidal anti-inflammatory drugs (NSAIDs) are utilized in neonates; however, publications on their use in equine neonates is lacking and their use should be done with caution and close monitoring of renal and gastrointestinal function.

Anesthetic Considerations of Neonatal Foals with Specific Conditions/Diseases

Stabilization prior to administration of any sedative or anesthetic agents is critical for improving the odds of a successful outcome.

Foals with many of the following conditions present as medical emergencies and not surgical emergencies. Therapies aimed at normalizing fluid volume, electrolyte, acid/base, and immunological status should be considered prior to surgical planning. Waiting for a period of time (in some cases, just a few hours) for correction of imbalances will result in a foal much more suitable for anesthesia and surgery.

Sepsis and Sepsis Associated Localized Infections

Sepsis is one of the most common medical conditions affecting neonatal foals (≤14 days of age) and is a leading cause of morbidity and mortality in this age group. The financial burden to owners is significant particularly when the prognosis for recovery is often uncertain (Weber et al. 2015; Sheats 2019; Furr and McKenzie 2020). The reported prevalence of sepsis in neonatal foals is approximately 25–60% of cases presenting for intensive care to tertiary veterinary hospitals (Weber et al. 2015; Wong and Wilkins 2015; Giguère et al. 2017; Wong et al. 2018; Furr and McKenzie 2020). Survival varies significantly (26–81%) with more recent reports demonstrating improvements in outcome (Gayle et al. 1998; Corley et al. 2005; Sanchez et al. 2008; Wong et al. 2018; Sheats 2019; Furr and McKenzie 2020). Sepsis in hospitalized humans, including pediatrics, also represents a leading cause of morbidity and mortality (Hall et al. 2013) and much of the criteria used in veterinary medicine for defining sepsis and the related condition systemic inflammatory response syndrome (SIRS) are derived from human medicine with modifications as needed for species-specific differences in disease pathophysiology and diagnostic criteria.

Sepsis is defined as life-threatening organ dysfunction secondary to a dysregulated host response to infection (Singer et al. 2016). SIRS is defined as an overwhelming and dysregulated systemic inflammatory response to various infectious and noninfectious triggers, one of which may be sepsis (Bone et al. 1992). In uncontrolled disease, sepsis can progress to septic shock which includes circulatory, cellular, and metabolic derangements and ultimately multiorgan dysfunction (MODS) in the face of appropriate and aggressive treatment. These definitions and accompanying scoring systems for sepsis and SIRS have been developed in an attempt to provide clinically relevant criteria to improve early recognition in at-risk human and equine neonatal patients (Brewer et al. 1988; Brewer and Koterba 1988; Bone et al. 1992; Corley et al. 2005). More recently, these definitions and scoring systems have been modified to account for physiologic and maturational differences among different age groups of foals, and the reader is referred to the associated references for further details (Wong and Wilkins 2015; Wong et al. 2018; Wilkins 2018).

The pathophysiology of sepsis and accompanying SIRS is multifactorial and complex and influenced according to the site of infection and the bacterial pathogens involved. In neonatal foals, the understanding of the pathophysiology is further complicated by potential variability in transfer of maternal cytokines in the colostrum, genetic factors, and immaturity of the immune system (Wong and Wilkins 2015; Perkins and Wagner 2015; McKenzie 2018). Regardless, involvement of the immune, hemostatic, cardiovascular, nervous, and endocrine systems is likely. Under normal immunologic conditions, recognition of bacterial infection initiates a controlled and protective inflammatory response. Recruitment of inflammatory cells (macrophages, neutrophils) triggers the staged production and release of primary inflammatory mediators including cytokines (TNFa, IL-6, IL-1B), enzymes (COX-2, iNOS), and adhesion molecules, and the subsequent release of secondary mediators (acute phase proteins, prostaglandins, leukotrienes, reactive oxygen species). These pro-inflammatory events are balanced by cytokine-mediated counter-regulatory anti-inflammatory responses. In sepsis (and SIRS), exaggeration of the pro-inflammatory response and dysregulation of the anti-inflammatory response occurs, resulting in a cascade of events associated with excessive and uncontrolled systemic inflammation and tissue damage. Widespread endothelial activation, vasoactive-mediated vascular abnormalities, and increased vascular permeability are common and may be accompanied by alterations in platelet function and hemostasis. If unchecked, vascular and hemostatic dysfunction, including disseminated intravascular coagulopathy, hypotension that may become refractory, tissue perfusion impairment and injury, cellular dysfunction, and ultimately damage to multiple organ systems are all possible.

Sepsis represents one of the most significant causes of SIRS in neonatal foals. Other potential triggers include viral infection, trauma, hemorrhage, PAS, localized infection, and non-septic inflammatory events (Wong and Wilkins 2015). Numerous risk factors have been proposed for the development of sepsis in foals (Taylor 2015; Wong and Wilkins 2015; McKenzie 2018; Furr and McKenzie 2020). Maternal factors include placentitis, uterine infection, dystocia, and maternal illness in late gestation. Failure of passive transfer (FPT) of immunity is considered a major risk factor particularly when accompanied by poor management practices (Taylor 2015; McKenzie 2018). Specific conditions that foals may present for separately, but that may also predispose them to or occur secondary to sepsis, include PAS, wounds, and localized infection associated with pneumonia, enterocolitis, omphalophlebitis, meningoencephalitis, or arthritis (Taylor 2015; McKenzie 2018; Furr and McKenzie 2020). The gastrointestinal tract and umbilicus have been considered the most common sites for bacterial infection associated with sepsis (Hollis et al. 2008; Taylor 2015; Furr and McKenzie 2020).

While the clinical manifestation and diagnosis of sepsis in neonatal foals is largely based on established diagnostic criteria for SIRS, in many foals initial clinical signs are vague or nonspecific and influenced by other comorbidities, administration of medications, or the duration of illness (Taylor 2015; McKenzie 2018). General findings on physical examination may include depression, lethargy, and decreased nursing. Changes in heart and respiratory rate are common, but not specific for sepsis, and hyper- or hypothermia are considered more sensitive indicators (Wong and Wilkins 2015; Wong et al. 2018). Ultrasound can be a useful diagnostic tool particularly for evaluating the pulmonary, gastrointestinal, and urogenital systems and umbilical structures. Characteristic cytologic abnormalities include presence of band cells and changes in white blood cell count. Other hematologic abnormalities are variable and may include azotemia, hypoxemia, acidosis, altered electrolytes, reductions in protein or glucose, hyperlactatemia, and changes in acute phase proteins, among others. Blood culture is ideal for confirming the diagnosis of sepsis and for directing antimicrobial therapy; however, a negative result does not rule out sepsis particularly in the face of evidence supporting localized or systemic infection and clinical signs of SIRS (Taylor 2015; Wong and Wilkins 2015; McKenzie 2018). Blood culture has relatively poor sensitivity and specificity. Positive results are obtained in only 25–36% of cases and previous administration of antimicrobials interferes with results (Taylor 2015; Wong and Wilkins 2015; Giguère et al. 2017). Gram-negative organisms predominate, but the prevalence of gram-positive organisms has increased in recent years (Marsh and Palmer 2001; Russell et al. 2008; Theelen et al. 2014; Toombs-Ruane et al. 2016; Furr and McKenzie 2020).

Prompt and aggressive treatment is essential, particularly with respect to instituting broad-spectrum antimicrobial therapy with parenterally administered bactericidal drugs. Combination therapy with aminoglycosides and a penicillin or a third-generation cephalosporin is most common and antimicrobials such as metronidazole can be added when anaerobic infection is a concern. Excellent nursing care is critical especially in recumbent foals where complications such as a ruptured bladder or pressure sores can easily develop. Additional medical therapy will vary according to the severity and duration of disease and typically includes fluid resuscitation and support, blood pressure support, and anti-inflammatory therapy. Hyperimmune plasma is administered to address FPT and to provide additional colloidal support. When tissue perfusion is not achieved with appropriate fluid resuscitation, inopressor therapy may be required. Inopressor agents include dobutamine, vasopressin, norepinephrine, dopamine, and epinephrine. Flunixin meglumine or other non-steroidals can provide anti-inflammatory support but should be administered judiciously in neonatal foals. The use of corticosteroids for the treatment of sepsis is controversial but may be of use if critical illness-related corticosteroid insufficiency (CIRCI) is suspected (McKenzie 2018). Targeted therapy at focal sites of infection, such as the umbilicus, urogenital tract, or joints may also be warranted and may necessitate surgical intervention. Additional therapy is instituted according to individual needs of the patient and may include nutritional support, intranasal oxygen insufflation, gastroprotectants, or other supportive care. Serial monitoring of vital and hematological parameters (e.g. lactate, glucose, electrolytes) can help direct treatment and assess response to therapy.

Anesthesia of Foals with Sepsis

Anesthesia of the septic foal can be of particular challenge due to the potential for severe systemic derangements. It must be stressed again that most conditions associated with sepsis are medical and not surgical emergencies. Stabilization of the foal with goal-directed therapy as previously described for normalization of physiologic and biochemical parameters is a must. This may require the procedure to be postponed hours to days. However, this delay will result in a more stable anesthetic patient and a higher likelihood for an optimal outcome. Once stabilized, anesthesia can proceed as described above. Extreme care should be taken to not expose the immunocompromised foal to additional potential sources of infectious agents, and the use of aseptic techniques and equipment should be implemented. Surgical tables, padding, and recovery areas should be thoroughly cleaned before and after use. Gloves should be worn at all times when handling the foal or equipment that will come in contact with the foal. Use of sterilized endotracheal tubes and meticulously cleaned anesthetic delivery and monitoring equipment should be standard practice. Placement of venous or arterial catheters should be done with appropriate skin preparation and the use of sterile gloves. Hypervigilant monitoring with a focus on cardiovascular parameters and body temperature should occur throughout the anesthetic period as rapid changes may occur. During surgery where release of endotoxin from Gram-negative bacteria is possible (umbilical resection, gastrointestinal surgical manipulation, septic arthritis), pretreatment with hyperimmune plasma or polymyxin B may help mitigate the inflammatory response. Antimicrobial therapy and use of anti-inflammatory medications during anesthesia and throughout the recovery period should be considered.

Perinatal Asphyxia Syndrome

The term PAS refers to a clinical syndrome recognized in human and equine neonates that develops in response to oxygen deprivation to the fetus or newborn during the perinatal period. PAS can be triggered by events that impede blood flow or gas exchange to or from the fetus (Ahearne et al. 2016). The resultant hypoxia can lead to significant multisystemic effects of which neurologic dysfunction is the most commonly recognized clinical manifestation. While a variety of terms are used to describe this condition, PAS is often preferred because it recognizes the likelihood that multiple organ systems are affected. Within PAS, neurologic disease is specifically referred to as hypoxic–ischemic encephalopathy (HIE) or neonatal encephalopathy (NE). Other organ systems with high oxygen demand are particularly sensitive to hypoxic or ischemic events, and in human infants various cardiopulmonary, renal, endocrine, and gastrointestinal abnormalities can be identified in up to 50% of PAS cases (Fattuoni et al. 2015). The incidence of PAS in humans is estimated at 2–10 per 1000 live births with a mortality of 15–60% depending on access to and quality of maternal and neonatal care (Lee et al. 2013; Ahearne et al. 2016). Significant long-term neurologic deficits are recognized in approximately 25% of surviving infants with HIE (Ballet 2010; Ahearne et al. 2016).

In foals, HIE was first described a century ago in neonatal thoroughbreds demonstrating neurologic abnormalities including seizures, loss of affinity for the dam, loss of suckle, and central blindness (Reynolds 1930). Since then, it has become recognized as the most common neurologic disorder affecting neonatal foals with incidence estimated at 1–2% of all foals born (Rossdale and Leadon 1975; Bernard et al. 1995; Gold 2015). Additional terms used to describe this condition include NE, neonatal maladjustment syndrome (NMS), dummy foals, wanderers or barkers, among others. Currently, NE and NMS are used to refer to the neurologic condition in foals. In affected foals, clinical presentation varies widely and overall mortality is approximated at 20% (Bernard et al. 1995; Wong et al. 2011; Lyle-Dugas et al. 2016). Foals with multiple co-morbidities (e.g. sepsis, pneumonia), severe ischemic neurologic disease, or multiorgan failure, or seizure activity are less likely to survive (Gold et al. 2016; Lyle-Dugas et al. 2016). Long-term outcome for surviving foals is good. As with PAS in human neonates, abnormalities involving other organ systems are often recognized in affected foals. Risk factors include maternal

(hemorrhage, anemia, systemic disease, placental abnormalities) or fetal (dystocia, umbilical cord compression, sepsis, meconium aspiration) problems (Gold 2015; Toribio 2019) While perinatal hypoxic events most likely contribute to the development of PAS and NE in many foals, there is greater recognition that impaired transition from intrauterine to extrauterine life plays a role in disease pathogenesis in a subset of foals and explains the variability in clinical manifestation of disease (Aleman et al. 2017, 2019; Toribio 2019).

The pathogenesis of the cellular and molecular events that occur in response to hypoxic damage to the central nervous system (CNS) has been reviewed in detail (Dickey et al. 2011; Douglas-Escobar and Weiss 2015; Wong and Wilkins 2015; McKenzie 2018; Toribio 2019). Much of what is known about this complex process in foals is extrapolated from other species and remains incompletely understood. Damage occurs in two phases over a period of hours to days and ultimately results in neuronal cell death by necrosis or apoptosis. In the acute phase, oxygen and glucose deprivation, reduced adenosine triphosphate (ATP) availability, and subsequent failure of neuronal cell ATP-dependent Na/K pumps promotes intracellular influx of Na, H_2O, and Cl resulting in cellular swelling and necrosis. Intracellular Na influx also increases cell membrane depolarization. In response, excess release and impaired metabolism of glutamate, the major excitatory neurotransmitter of the CNS, occurs. The second phase occurs hours to days later and may explain the delay in onset or worsening of clinical signs demonstrated by some foals. Continued stimulation of NMDA and other glutamate receptors causes increased intracellular Ca^{2+} influx and activity, mitochondrial dysfunction, reperfusion injury, oxidative damage, excitotoxicity, microglial mediated neuro-inflammation, and ultimately cellular apoptosis.

A link between persistence of increased neurosteroid concentrations and impaired transition from intra- to extrauterine life has been proposed in the pathogenesis of NE particularly for foals with no identifiable hypoxic events and who are otherwise clinically healthy (Aleman et al. 2013; Diesch and Mellor 2013; Aleman et al. 2017; Toribio 2019). Neurosteroids are synthesized within the CNS and play a role in modulating neuronal activity and CNS development. During gestation, neurosteroids such as allopregnanolone and pregnenolone suppress fetal arousal and activity primarily through modulation of the GABAa receptors (Reddy 2009; Giatti et al. 2015). In healthy term babies, concentrations of these steroids decrease rapidly within 48 hours of birth. Failure to decrease is associated with maladaptation to extrauterine life and clinical signs of NE. Increased plasma concentrations of neurosteroids have been identified in foals diagnosed with NE (Holtan et al. 1991; Houghton et al. 1991; Aleman et al. 2013) and in two healthy foals, experimentally administered allopregnanolone induced transient clinical signs mimicking NE (Madigan et al. 2012). The reason for why neurosteroid concentrations remain increased in otherwise healthy foals is not known but it has been theorized that pressure during transition through the birth canal is important (Aleman et al. 2017). The role of neurosteroids is likely complex, and alterations in neurosteroid concentrations are also observed in response to hypoxic insults in foals with NE as well as sepsis (Swink et al. 2021).

Clinical signs of PAS in foals vary in type, time of onset, progression, and severity. A definitive diagnosis is challenging as clinical signs of PAS can occur with other diseases and a history of a precipitating event may be unknown. While some foals appear abnormal at the time of, or very shortly after, birth, for most foals the onset of clinical abnormalities occurs within 12–72 hours of birth (Tennent-Brown et al. 2015; McKenzie 2018). Disease is frequently progressive. Neurologic abnormalities are most often referable to the cerebrum but can also be consistent with brainstem or spinal cord dysfunction. Abnormalities include weakness, loss of suckle reflex, altered responsiveness (depression or hyperexcitability), disorientation relative to the udder, loss of tongue coordination, abnormal vocalizations ("barker foal"), lack of affinity for the dam, central blindness, abnormal respiratory patterns, vestibular signs, changes in muscle tone, and in severe cases seizure, coma, or death (Gold 2015; Tennent-Brown et al. 2015; Toribio 2019). Concurrent renal and gastrointestinal abnormalities are common and may include azotemia, reduced urine output, colic, ileus, enterocolitis, gastric reflux, abdominal distension, and dysphagia. More rarely, metabolic, endocrine, and cardiopulmonary dysfunction is identified. Specific diagnostics should focus on ruling out other causes of neurologic disease and identifying systemic disease or problems in other organ systems.

Most foals recover with good nursing and supportive care with treatment adjusted according to clinical manifestation of disease. Therapeutic hypothermia, which has shown promise in reducing death or long-term disability in human infants with HIE (Wassink et al. 2019), is currently not available to neonatal foals. In foals that are otherwise healthy and demonstrating mild signs, application of targeted physical compression over the thorax ("Madigan Squeeze") may hasten recovery (Aleman et al. 2017). Other specific elements of therapy include ensuring adequate nutrition (enteral or intravenous), glucose regulation, intranasal insufflation of humidified oxygen, intravenous fluid support, or antimicrobial coverage when sepsis or bacterial infection is confirmed. Neuroprotectants such as thiamine, magnesium sulfide, or mannitol may be administered in foals with more significant neurologic signs, but little evidence exists that they improve outcome. Similarly, respiratory stimulants such as caffeine or doxapram hydrochloride are used in foals with respiratory compromise but are of questionable efficacy (Giguère et al. 2008). Control of seizures is important in these foals in order to prevent exacerbation of glutamate neuroexcitatory activity. Administration of benzodiazepines (diazepam, midazolam) or phenobarbital is common, with the administration of levetiracetam (Keppra) being more recently evaluated in foals (MacDonald et al. 2018). Additional therapy should be directed toward addressing co-morbidities or identified abnormalities with specific organ systems.

Anesthesia of Foals with Perinatal Asphyxia Syndrome

Foals with PAS may require anesthesia for diagnostics or surgical procedures for other conditions. These foals can be extremely challenging to anesthetize as they often require continuation of advanced supportive therapy during anesthesia. Oxygen, glucose, fluid, and electrolyte support should be continued throughout the anesthetic and recovery period. Hypoxemia should not be allowed to occur and insufflation with oxygen should be provided anytime the foal is not intubated and administered oxygen from an anesthesia machine. Intravenous (IV) fluid therapy should be titrated to needs and not be excessive as organ and cerebral edema can occur. Drug protocols that offer neuronal protection should be considered and include the use of benzodiazepines and propofol. In particular, the use of propofol for induction and maintenance of anesthesia instead of inhalants such as isoflurane may have a protective effect on brain stem functions in animals that suffer from PAS (Smit et al. 2013). The use of ketamine is controversial in human neonates with PAS as it may both initiate or inhibit seizure activity. Ketamine has been used as a treatment for seizures that are unresponsive to other therapies in older children and adults. However, the potential for ketamine-mediated neurotoxicity in the damaged neonatal brain is still unclear and more research is needed before it can be recommended (Huntsman et al. 2020). For seizure control in foals prior to anesthesia, levetiracetam may be useful. The pharmacokinetics have been described in neonatal foals and a dose of 32 mg/kg PO or IV q12–24 hours has been described (MacDonald et al. 2018).

During anesthesia, blood glucose, electrolyte, and blood gas analysis at regular intervals should be performed to allow for educated adjustments to therapies. The use of mannitol and naloxone during recovery may improve recovery parameters and shorten time to standing.

Conditions of the Respiratory Tract

In equine neonates, respiratory disease is one of the most common contributors to patient morbidity and mortality (Beech 1985; Freeman and Paradis 1992; Bedenice et al. 2003; Wilkins 2003; Wilkins et al. 2007; Reuss and Cohen 2015). Causes may include congenital problems, primary pulmonary disease, and thoracic trauma. Diagnosis of respiratory disease can often be challenging as overt clinical signs may not be obvious and can vary according to the nature and severity of disease and the presence of co-morbidities. Prompt recognition and treatment of these conditions is important for successful patient outcome.

Congenital defects involving the respiratory system are rare and primarily affect the extrathoracic airways. Congenital conditions, such as choanal atresia and epiglottic or pharyngeal cysts, may result in overt respiratory signs soon after birth or can cause dysphagia, thus predisposing foals to aspiration pneumonia. Choanal atresia represents a failure of the bucconasal membrane to rupture in the developing fetus, causing complete obstruction of the involved nasal passage (Aylor et al. 1984; Hogan et al. 1995; James et al. 2006; Bienert-Zeit and Ohnesorge 2011). When bilateral, respiratory distress is noted at birth, a tracheotomy is required to secure a patent airway. Pharyngeal and epiglottic cysts occur most often in the subepiglottic region but can also involve the dorsal nasopharynx or soft palate (Koch and Tate 1978; Stick and Boles 1980; Gutierrez-Nibeyro 2020). The cysts are thought to be embryonic remnants of the thyroglossal or craniopharyngeal ducts but may also represent inflammation affecting pharyngeal mucous glands. Clinical presentation varies from asymptomatic to more obvious signs of respiratory distress, cough, dysphagia with milk reflux, and aspiration pneumonia. Surgical correction is required for both conditions and may include laser ablation, resection, or fenestration of the buccopharyngeal membrane.

Pneumonia is the leading cause of pulmonary disease in neonatal foals with concurrent conditions such as sepsis or SIRS contributing to patient morbidity and mortality (Wilkins 2003; Wilkins et al. 2007; Reuss and Cohen 2015). The etiology of pneumonia in neonatal foals is complex, and many factors can influence disease severity. Viral pneumonia secondary to *Equine herpesvirus-1* or *Equine arteritis virus* infection, is very rarely reported and almost always fatal (Wilkins 2003). Bacterial pneumonia is by far the most common cause of pneumonia in neonates, occurring secondary to sepsis or as primary aspiration pneumonia (Wilkins 2003; Reuss and Cohen 2015). In septic foals, progression to the severe condition of equine neonatal acute respiratory distress syndrome (ARDS) is a significant risk and carries a poorer prognosis (Bedenice et al. 2003; Wilkins 2003).

The prevalence of bacterial pneumonia in septic neonatal foals is reported to be 19–50% (Freeman and Paradis 1992; Stewart et al. 2002; Sanchez et al. 2008). Bacterial infection causing sepsis can occur in utero, at parturition, or shortly after birth, and can localize to specific organ systems including the lung. Bacterial organisms identified with septic pneumonia are similar to those most commonly isolated on blood culture from septic foals (Reuss and Cohen 2015). Gram-negative infection predominates, with *Escherichia coli*, *Klebsiella* spp. and *Actinobacillus* spp. commonly isolated. In mixed bacterial infections, additional organisms include *Streptococcus* spp., *Staphylococcus* spp., and *Enterococcus* spp. (Hoffman et al. 1993; Marsh and Palmer 2001;

Reuss and Cohen 2015). Clinical signs of SIRS and infection to other organ systems accompany those of pneumonia, complicating the clinical presentation.

Aspiration of milk is an important cause of primary bacterial pneumonia in neonatal foals. Common predisposing causes include weakness, dysphagia, and an uncoordinated or poor suckle reflex secondary to sepsis, PAS, or dysmaturity. Congenital problems associated with aspiration include cleft palate or elongated soft palate, pharyngeal dysfunction, subepiglottic cysts, or esophageal abnormalities. Finally, iatrogenic causes include improper bottle feeding, improper placement of naso-esophageal or nasogastric feeding tubes, or improper position of foal when feeding through the tube (Wilkins 2003; Reuss and Cohen 2015). Mixed bacterial infection affecting the caudoventral lung is typical.

ARDS causes rapidly progressive respiratory failure and is associated with high mortality in affected patients. ARDS develops when a primary disease or injury triggers acute, overwhelming, and uncontrolled inflammation in the lung and the subsequent hallmark features of ARDS: severe pulmonary damage and edema, respiratory dysfunction, and profound hypoxemia. The classification of ARDS is based on the degree of hypoxemia (PaO_2/FiO_2 ratio) and in humans is categorized as mild (PaO_2/FiO_2 >200 and ≤300 mmHg), moderate (PaO_2/FiO_2 >100 and ≤200 mmHg), and severe (PaO_2/FiO_2 ≤100 mmHg) (Ranieri et al. 2012). In veterinary species, the distinction between acute lung injury (ALI; PaO_2/FiO_2 ≤300 mmHg) and ARDS (PaO_2/FiO_2 ≤200 mmHg) is still made. In neonatal foals, pneumonia and bacterial sepsis represent the most likely risk factors for ARDS. Because of the relative hypoxemia of normal neonatal foals compared to adults during the first week of life, separate PaO_2/FiO_2 cut-offs exist to define these conditions in this age group (Table 13.4) (Wilkins et al. 2007; Wilkins and Lascola 2015). It is important to remember that ARDS (and ALI) in neonatal

Table 13.4 Cut-off values (mmHg) used to define acute lung injury (ALI) and acute respiratory distress syndrome (ARDS) by age in neonatal foals. These values were obtained from foals breathing room air in lateral recumbency.

Postnatal Age	Normal PaO_2/FiO_2	ALI PaO_2/FiO_2	ARDS PaO_2/FiO_2
60 minutes	>300	<175	<115
12 hours	>350	<200	<140
24 hours	>350	<200	<140
48 hours	>350	<200	<140
4 days	>400	<250	<160
7 days	>430	<280	<190

Source: Adapted from Wilkins et al. (2007).

foals is distinguished from neonatal equine respiratory distress syndrome which is a distinct clinical syndrome resulting from primary surfactant deficiency in premature foals <24 hours of age. (Wilkins et al. 2007)

Other rarer causes of pulmonary disease in the neonatal foal include meconium aspiration and persistent pulmonary hypertension of the newborn (PPHN). Meconium aspiration occurs in response to fetal distress in utero or at the time of parturition, and although rarely reported, can cause devastating pulmonary disease. Meconium causes a chemical pneumonitis, marked surfactant dysfunction, and obstruction of the alveoli and airways with meconium, edema fluid, inflammatory cells, and other debris (Wilkins 2003; Reuss and Cohen 2015). In response, marked ventilation and perfusion mismatch and severe hypoxemia is noted. This condition carries a grave prognosis. PPHN has been experimentally induced and only rarely suspected in neonatal foals (Cottrill et al. 1987; Lester et al. 1999). This condition represents a reversion to fetal circulatory patterns and is characterized by increased postnatal pulmonary vascular resistance. The majority of PPHN cases develop secondary to severe respiratory disease in the immediate post-partum period. Other causes may include congenital cardiac disease or in utero hypoxemic stress. Neonates are at greatest risk in the first 48–72 hours of life when the

final transition from fetal to extrauterine circulation occurs. In foals, the condition can be difficult to differentiate from other causes of hypoxemia and is characterized by persistent or worsening hypercapnic hypoxemia.

Diagnosis and characterization of pulmonary disease in neonatal foals is challenging. Overt clinical signs of respiratory disease, such as dyspnea, paradoxical chest wall motion, cough, or nasal discharge, are variable and may be subtle or absent (Wilkins 2003; Lester and Lester 2001). Thoracic auscultation may also be unrewarding even in foals with significant pulmonary disease. In most cases additional diagnostics are essential in order to characterize the nature and severity of disease. Arterial blood gas analysis is important to determine the degree of respiratory compromise. Hematologic analysis (complete blood count, biochemistry) is useful in cases where infectious or inflammatory conditions such as SIRS or sepsis are suspected. Foals with significant respiratory compromise may not be stable enough for procedures such as tracheobronchial fluid aspiration; however, in cases of septic pneumonia, blood culture can be used to direct antimicrobial therapy.

Diagnostic imaging, such as ultrasound, radiography, or computed tomography (CT), play a critical role in the diagnosis of respiratory disease in equine neonates, and detailed descriptions of their use in neonatal foals are available (Lester and Lester 2001; Bedenice et al. 2003; Kutasi et al. 2009; Lascola and Joslyn 2015; Marr 2015). In certain foals, CT may allow for more accurate anatomic and morphologic characterization of pulmonary disease and may also provide more accurate evaluation of non-lung thoracic structures (Lascola and Joslyn 2015). Radiographic or ultrasonographic images can frequently be acquired stall-side and without the need for sedation in standing or recumbent neonatal foals. Sedation or general anesthesia is required for CT-imaging in foals (Figure 13.3). Midazolam and butorphanol, and if needed, propofol, usually provide sufficient sedation for imaging of spontaneously breathing healthy and sick neonatal foals (Lascola et al. 2013; Lascola and Joslyn 2015). The use of anesthesia with or without mechanical ventilation allows for delivery of lung recruitment maneuvers and may be more suitable when imaging of multiple sites is required or when additional procedures are required. Regardless of the modality chosen for imaging, atelectasis represents one of the most commonly identified artifacts (Lascola et al. 2013; Lascola and Joslyn 2015; Schliewert et al. 2015; Lascola et al. 2016). Atelectasis can be identified within minutes even in healthy neonatal foals undergoing thoracic radiography or CT-imaging and may interfere with image interpretation. Lung recruitment maneuvers with inspiratory pressures of 30 cm H_2O may be necessary to distinguish atelectasis from pulmonary disease in thoracic CT.

Thoracic trauma is a relatively common occurrence in neonatal foals that may be present without any outward clinical abnormalities. In one field study, rib fractures and costochondral dislocations were identified in 20% of otherwise clinically normal Thoroughbred foals <3 days of age (Jean et al. 1999). Fractures may also contribute significantly to morbidity and mortality in foals. In separate studies involving neonatal foals hospitalized for other conditions, the prevalence of fractures was almost 20% and fractures contributed significantly to mortality in almost 30% of cases (Sprayberry et al. 2001; Schambourg et al. 2003). It is possible that increased handling of hospitalized and often recumbent foals may result in displacement or other complications associated with fractures and this risk must be considered when working with this age group (Sprayberry 2015). Rib fractures are identified most often on the left side of the thorax at the costochondral junction and when limited to single nondisplaced fractures or laterally displaced fractures, may remain subclinical (Jean et al. 1999; Marr 2015; Sprayberry 2015). Multiple fractures or medially displaced fractures carry the greatest risk

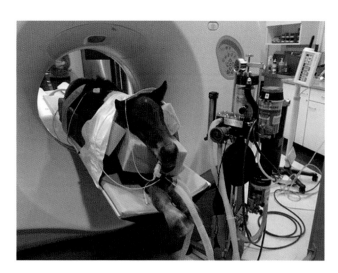

Figure 13.3 Anesthesia of a neonatal foal for CT evaluation of lower respiratory diseases. Alveolar recruitment maneuvers up to 30 cm H_2O may be necessary to distinguish between atelectasis and primary pulmonary diseases.

for complications particularly when they occur over the heart (ribs 4–7) or the mid-thoracic region (Marr 2015; Sprayberry 2015). Laceration of the intercostal blood vessels or parietal pleura may result in significant hemothorax. Lung contusions and pericardial or myocardial trauma are also possible, and laceration of the diaphragm can result in herniation of bowel segments into the thoracic cavity.

Clinical signs associated with rib fractures can range from asymptomatic, to mild tachycardia associated with pain, to more severe signs including respiratory distress, flail chest, or those indicating cardiac or gastrointestinal compromise (Marr 2015). Careful palpation over the thorax may identify asymmetry or edema over fractures or can elicit signs of discomfort and represent an important component of any physical examination in a neonatal foal. While radiography can be utilized to detect fractures, ultrasonography is more sensitive and allows for more thorough evaluation of the thoracic structures (Jean et al. 2007). In complicated cases requiring surgical intervention, CT may provide added information (Marr 2015). Foals that are otherwise healthy can be managed conservatively with exercise restriction and analgesics as needed. In recumbent and medically compromised foals without complications associated with fractures, supportive care, close monitoring and attention to positioning, and handling techniques is critical. In foals with multiple fractures and at increased risk for complications, surgical stabilization is necessary (Marr 2015).

Anesthesia of the Foal with Respiratory Tract Disorders

Foals with upper airway diseases may present for surgical correction and may require intubation through a tracheotomy to facilitate surgical access. If the foal presents with a tracheotomy in place, intubation through the tracheotomy after induction is relatively simple and transition to maintenance of anesthesia is usually smooth (see Chapter 3 on airway diseases).

All neonatal foals presenting for anesthesia should be assumed to have lower airway disease unless proven otherwise. Subclinical pneumonia is often a sequela to other diseases as previously described. Blood gas analysis before, during, and after anesthesia can be helpful in assessing the degree in which oxygenation may be impaired and lung-protective strategies as previously described should be employed as lung tissue may already be damaged. When possible, humidification of oxygen used for insufflation or for delivery of anesthesia may improve mucociliary clearance and maintenance of a liquid layer on airway epithelium consistent with normal physiologic conditions (Schiffmann 2006).

Anesthesia for foals presenting for surgical correction of rib fractures presents a unique challenge as there may be compromises to cardiac tissue, lung tissue, hemothorax, pneumothorax, and chest wall trauma. Aspiration of blood or air from the thoracic cavity may be necessary to allow for lung expansion and should be performed prior to induction of anesthesia if possible. Blood loss may be severe enough to warrant blood transfusion. Whole blood can be acquired from the mare if donor animals are not available. For displaced fractures, care must be taken during induction and movement of the induced foal to prevent puncture of deep structures by the fractured ends of the rib(s). Likewise, mechanical ventilation may need to be initially avoided until the rib ends can be stabilized to prevent lung trauma. One lung ventilation of the non-affected side may be advisable in foals with very severe unilateral fractures. The authors have performed one lung intubation in anesthetized foals with the use of long silicone endotracheal tube (see Figure 13.1) directed into the non-affected lung with use of an endoscope as a stylet. Intercostal local anesthetic blocks of the affected ribs should be considered for analgesia. The intercostal nerves course just caudal to the ribs and have significant overlap of adjacent intercostal spaces. Thus, not only does the intercostal space of the affected rib need to be blocked, but two intercostal spaces cranial and caudal to rib for a total of five intercostal nerves require blockade for complete anesthesia.

Umbilical Disorders

The internal structures of the umbilicus include the umbilical vein, paired umbilical arteries, and the urachus. In the fetus, these structures play a critical role in the exchange of oxygen and nutrients with the placenta and in the excretion of urine from the fetal bladder to the allantoic cavity. In the normal newborn, the umbilical cord should break spontaneously at a few centimeters from the body wall of the foal shortly after birth (Morresey 2011; Morresey 2014; McKenzie 2018). Blood loss associated with cord separation is typically mild and transient but can become severe if separation of the umbilicus is premature, associated with trauma, or if the cord is manually torn or cut. Immediately after birth, a considerable portion of the foal's blood volume is still circulating within the attached placenta. With early or traumatic separation, hemorrhage or subcutaneous rupture of the urachus and urine accumulation within the abdominal wall are both possible (McKenzie 2018).

Regression and atrophy of the internal umbilical structures begins within days of birth and progresses over several weeks (McCoy et al. 2020). The umbilical vein, which courses to the liver, becomes incorporated into the falciform ligament. The paired right and left umbilical arteries, which travel along either side of the bladder to the aorta, regress to form the round ligaments of the bladder. The urachus, which exists as a potential space between the umbilical arteries, connects the bladder to the allantoic cavity and becomes the median ligament of the bladder (Sprayberry 2008; McCoy et al. 2020). Age-related ultrasonographic changes in size and appearance of these structures have been described for normal foals (Reef and

Collatos 1988; Reef et al. 1989; Reef 1991; McCoy et al. 2020). Disease or disorders affecting the structures of the umbilical remnant are common in neonatal foals with a reported morbidity across breeds of 5% (Linford 2011; Codina et al. 2019; McCoy et al. 2020). The most common umbilical disorders include patent urachus and infection of umbilical remnants.

Patent urachus occurs when the urachal remnant does not close, and urine continues to be voided externally. In most foals, functional closure of the urachus occurs at parturition, allowing the bladder to distend and triggering the appropriate neurologic reflexes and posturing associated with normal micturition. Anatomical closure of the urachus occurs over several weeks as the umbilical remnants regress (McCoy et al. 2020). Although a simple patent urachus can develop at the time of umbilical cord separation, it more often occurs a few days after birth. In foals straining to defecate because of meconium impaction or constipation, increased intra-abdominal pressure may cause reopening of the urachal space (Sprayberry 2008; McKenzie 2018). Patent urachus can also be seen in foals with umbilical remnant infections or in recumbent foals with systemic illness. Standing foals often still demonstrate normal posturing and passage of urine through the urethra, but urine dribbling or streaming from the umbilical stump is also observed. In recumbent foals, excess moisture associated with the external umbilical remnants and urine scald along the abdominal wall or inside the hindlimbs may be noted, and the external umbilical stump may appear macerated (McKenzie 2018).

A diagnosis of a patent urachus can usually be made based on clinical signs, especially in foals that are not recumbent. Foals without concurrent disease or infection associated with the remnants should otherwise appear healthy. Ultrasound can confirm the diagnosis and is important for evaluating the internal umbilical structures for other abnormalities or signs of infection (Sprayberry 2008). Treatment options for patent urachus and umbilical infection include medical management or surgical excision of the remnants. For the majority of cases, medical management should be attempted first and is usually successful but may require one to two weeks of therapy. A simple patent urachus often resolves within several days with close monitoring and keeping the area clean and dry. Chemical cautery using silver nitrate sticks should be done with care as tissue necrosis and infection can develop (McKenzie 2018).

Administration of broad-spectrum antimicrobials is often the mainstay of medical management, especially when there is evidence of or a high risk for infection, as in recumbent foals or foals with systemic illness. In cases where surgical correction is necessary, stabilization prior to surgery is essential. This is particularly true for critically ill neonates as they are at greater risk for adverse events associated with anesthesia and for post-operative complications (Fischer and Clark-Price 2015).

Infection of the umbilical remnants may be limited to focal abscess formation of the external umbilical remnant. Infection of any (or all) of the internal structures including the urachus (urachitis), arteries (omphaloarteritis), and vein (omphalophlebitis) is also possible (McKenzie 2018). External bacterial contamination of the umbilicus and ascending infection is one possible route of infection. Bacteremia associated with generalized septicemia or with inflammation or infection at another site is also possible. Along with gastrointestinal tract disease, umbilical infections represent one of the most common sources of bacteremia (Furr and McKenzie 2020) with reported secondary complications including septic arthritis, physitis, and osteomyelitis, sepsis, pneumonia, diarrhea, distal aortic aneurysm, and abdominal adhesions (Magata et al. 2010; Archer et al. 2012; Nogradi et al. 2013; Giguère et al. 2017; Oreff et al. 2017; McKenzie 2018; Codina et al. 2019).

The clinical presentation of foals with umbilical remnant infections varies according to location, severity, and the presence of other co-morbidities. Recognizable abnormalities associated with focal infections of the external remnant include palpable swelling, heat, and pain. Discharge is often noted from the umbilicus. With severe infections, fever or hematologic indicators of inflammation are identified and cellulitis affecting the adjacent body wall occasionally develops (Reef et al. 1989; McKenzie 2018). Internal infections can present occultly with no palpable or visible abnormalities, and ultrasonographic evaluation is required (Sprayberry 2008). Foals often demonstrate signs of systemic inflammation. Increases in liver enzymes in foals with infection of the umbilical vein suggest secondary hepatitis. A patent urachus or clinical indicators of uroperitoneum may also be identified. Ultrasonographic evaluation of the umbilical remnants is important for both external and internal infections. With internal remnant infections, it is essential for definitive diagnosis, for identifying which internal structures are involved, for determining the extent of infection, and for treatment planning and monitoring response to therapy.

For most foals with umbilical infection, medical management should be attempted prior to surgical treatment. Close monitoring and administration of broad-spectrum antimicrobials remains the mainstay of medical therapy. Resolution may take several weeks. External abscesses can sometimes be drained and lavaged (McKenzie 2018). Surgery is considered in infections refractory to medical treatment, with evidence of worsening infection, or with patient debilitation. In all cases, the risks of general anesthesia and potential for post-operative complications should be considered and patients stabilized prior to anesthesia.

Surgical correction primarily involves resection of the umbilical remnants through a midline approach. Laparoscopic resection has been described as has marsupialization and lavage of the umbilical vein (Edwards and Fubini 1995; Fischer 1998). Reported survival after surgical resection is 66–91% with higher mortality associated with umbilical vein infections (Edwards and Fubini 1995; Reef et al. 1989; Giguère et al. 2017; Oreff et al. 2017; Codina et al. 2019). Septic arthritis, azotemia, younger age, co-morbidities, and post-operative complications have been reported to negatively impact short-term outcome (Oreff et al. 2017; Codina et al. 2019). In a recent study by Codina et al., post-operative complications were identified in 40% of foals undergoing surgical resection of umbilical remnants. Of these, 19% were anesthesia related and primarily attributed to prolonged recovery or trauma in recovery. Both longer anesthesia time and FPT of immunoglobulins were associated with increased risk for complications. While more complicated resections necessitated longer anesthesia, surgeons often performed multiple procedures under the same anesthetic event.

Anesthesia of the Foal with Umbilical Disorders

Anesthesia of foals with patent urachus is usually uneventful. This condition is not a surgical emergency, and thus foals should be stabilized and any other co-morbidity addressed and treated prior to anesthesia. Pain management and an uneventful recovery are of primary concerns to ensure the foal is returned to the mare and nursing as quickly as possible. Anesthesia of foals with umbilical infections can be more challenging. Depending on the degree of infection, the foal may be less stable due to systemic sepsis. Deeper infections that involve the umbilical vein may require greater surgical access and involvement of the liver. Longer procedure times and hemorrhage are possible. Anesthetic plans for theses foals should include the possible need of cardiovascular support and blood products. Anesthetist's knowledge of any pre-anesthetic diagnostic imaging findings can be helpful in estimating procedure length and difficulty. An ultrasound-guided subcostal transversus abdominis plane (TAP) block has been described in foals and may be useful for foals undergoing anesthesia for abdominal procedures (Freitag et al. 2021). If a TAP block is not feasible, bupivacaine applied to the linea alba during abdominal closure may provide some degree of analgesia (Jones et al. 2019). Total intravenous anesthesia with alfaxalone, dexmedetomidine, and remifentanil provides acceptable anesthesia for abdominal surgery in health foals (Jones et al. 2019). Use in systemically ill foals should be done with caution as cardiac index and stroke volume index decline over time. Additionally, recovery with this protocol can be prolonged with some foals not reaching standing position until after 90 minutes.

Uroperitoneum

Uroperitoneum is reported to occur in 2.5% of hospitalized neonatal foals and is the most common urogenital disorder affecting this age group (Kablack et al. 2000). Rupture to the dorsal wall of the bladder represents the most common cause of uroperitoneum, with urachal rupture being the second most common cause. Ureteral and urethral ruptures have been rarely reported. Most primary cases of bladder rupture occur secondary to trauma sustained during or after parturition and dystocia is considered a risk factor. In hospitalized foals, prolonged recumbency, sepsis, and disruption of normal neurologic control of micturition, as with PAS, represent important predisposing causes. Presentation is usually within a few days to a week of life and while there is no sex predilection in hospitalized or older foal, colts appear to be over-represented in primary cases presenting within one to two days of birth (Behr et al. 1981; Richardson and Kohn 1983; Dunkel et al. 2005; McKenzie 2018). Urachal rupture presents with more subtle clinical signs and is not always accompanied by a patent urachus. Concurrent infection, ischemia, or necrosis of the urachus, hospitalization for another primary disease, prolonged recumbency, and bladder distention are all risk factors (McKenzie 2018).

During parturition, high pressures can be exerted on the bladder and cause a rupture particularly when the bladder is full. In colts, the longer urethra and smaller internal pelvic diameter increase urethral resistance and predisposes them to rupture under these conditions. Other sources of stress that can cause a primary rupture include trauma, often associated with parturition, and umbilical cord torsion. In hospitalized foals, iatrogenic bladder rupture can occur during inappropriate handling of recumbent foals with full bladders. In septic foals, focal necrosis or infection of the wall of the bladder can also cause rupture.

Prompt recognition and identification of associated hematologic abnormalities is important in foals with uroperitoneum. It is important to realize that clinical signs can differ between hospitalized foals with comorbidities and in foals presenting with a primary rupture (Kablack et al. 2000; Dunkel et al. 2005). Classic clinical signs associated with primary rupture include stranguria, urine dribbling, and frequent posturing to attempt to urinate. These clinical signs can sometimes be confused with foals straining to defecate, and meconium impaction is an important early differential. As uroperitoneum progresses, abdominal distention can develop, and foals can become increasingly depressed and lose interest in nursing. Ventral edema can be observed and may represent subcutaneous urine accumulation. In hospitalized foals, especially those that are recumbent, clinical manifestation of uroperitoneum can be more subtle and may be masked by clinical signs associated with concurrent disease (Kablack et al. 2000). In these cases, reduced frequency of urination or volume of urine, and inappropriate weight gain may be all that is noted.

As with clinical signs, laboratory abnormalities associated with uroperitoneum vary depending on duration and whether the case is a primary referral or hospitalized foal. Azotemia, electrolyte derangements of hyperkalemia, hyponatremia, and hypochloremia, and metabolic acidosis represent the classic abnormalities. In foals with respiratory compromise secondary to abdominal distention, hypoxemia and hypercapnia can develop. Azotemia, characterized by increased creatinine, is typically secondary to post-renal causes, but acute kidney injury can also develop. Classic electrolyte abnormalities are usually not as prominent in hospitalized foals maintained on intravenous fluid support and not on a milk diet (Kablack et al. 2000; Dunkel et al. 2005). Mare's milk, and subsequently the urine of a nursing foal, are relatively high in potassium and free water, and low in sodium and chloride (Vaala 2015). Thus, with uroperitoneum, the equilibration of urine electrolytes and water with serum across the peritoneal membrane creates the classic electrolyte derangements in nursing foals with uroperitoneum.

Additional diagnostics that can confirm uroperitoneum include abdominal ultrasound and abdominocentesis. Free, nonechogenic abdominal fluid may be noted. Complete evaluation of the urinary tract should be performed. Large tears can occasionally be visualized in the bladder or urachus (Sprayberry 2008). Contrast radiography and CT can be helpful for locating urine leakage from other parts of the urinary system. Abdominocentesis provides definitive confirmation of uroperitoneum through measurement of peritoneal creatinine concentration that is as least twice that of serum creatinine concentration (McKenzie 2018). Concurrent peritonitis carries a more guarded prognosis and thus cytology, protein concentration, specific gravity, and possibly culture and sensitivity should also be obtained from peritoneal fluid.

While surgical repair is ultimately required, uroperitoneum represents a medical emergency and initial treatment should focus on stabilization of the foal and addressing azotemia, electrolyte derangements and volume deficits, correcting abdominal distension, and treating any concurrent illness. Hyperkalemia, especially $\geq 6\,mEq/l$, is life-threatening and necessitates immediate attention. Cardiac derangements include depression of atrial, atrial-ventricular, and ventricular conduction, shortened ventricular repolarization, and increased action potential threshold. Foals with hyperkalemia should be monitored with an ECG. Findings on ECG can include peaked T-waves and shortened QT intervals that progress to prolonged P-R intervals, flattening of the P wave, and widening of the QRS intervals (Love 2011). Third-degree atrioventricular (AV) block, ventricular premature contractions (VPC's), and ventricular fibrillation are possible and in severe cases asystole and cardiac arrest occur. When possible, abdominal drainage to remove accumulated urine is recommended as this reduces whole-body potassium stores. Drainage serves the dual purpose of decreasing pressure on the diaphragm and thoracic cavity and thus can also help resolve respiratory compromise (McKenzie 2018). Treatment for hyperkalemia should also include administration IV fluids as well as calcium gluconate to inhibit action of potassium on cell membranes, and insulin and dextrose or Na-HCO$_3$ to promote intracellular uptake of potassium (Love 2011).

The prognosis for foals with uncomplicated uroperitoneum is generally good. Concurrent illness carries a more guarded prognosis (Kablack et al. 2000; Dunkel et al. 2005). Reported complications in foals with uroperitoneum can include peritonitis, sepsis, re-rupture, and respiratory disorders ranging from transient post-operative oxygen dependency to more significant problems of pneumonia or ARDS. Prompt recognition of uroperitoneum and adequate pre-surgical stabilization is important to minimize adverse events during anesthesia and development of post-operative complications.

Anesthesia of Foals with Uroperitoneum

Uroperitoneum is a medical emergency and not a surgical emergency. Correction of electrolyte imbalances and acid–base status must be performed prior to induction of anesthesia for surgical correction. Foals with serum potassium >5.5 mEq/l should not be anesthetized. Anesthesia should be postponed until serum potassium is corrected. This can be achieved in a short period of time (frequently less than two hours) with aggressive therapy. Acid–base shifts and thus potassium shifts can occur rapidly after induction of anesthesia and critically elevated serum potassium (>6.0 mEq/l) with subsequent arrhythmias occurring prior to the initiation of vital parameter monitoring. Thus life-threatening abnormalities may occur immediately after induction and not recognized until an ECG is attached to the patient well after the event has started. During anesthesia, serum electrolytes should continue to be monitored. Respiratory acidemia may further exacerbate hyperkalemia. Mechanical ventilation and monitoring of end-tidal carbon dioxide can be extremely helpful in these cases. Serum pH can be rapidly manipulated with changes in ventilation and PaCO$_2$. An acute increase in PaCO$_2$ of 10 mmHg decreases pH by 0.05 units. Whereas an acute decrease in PaCO$_2$ of 10 mmHg increases pH by 0.1 units. Since potassium is exchanged with hydrogen ions, increasing pH will cause cells to exchange free potassium with hydrogen ions to maintain electroneutrality. Hyperventilation of anesthetized foals, in conjunction with standard therapies, can be used to treat hyperkalemia.

Intestinal Accidents

Colic is a common presenting complaint in neonatal foals (Bryant and Gaughan 2005; Ryan and Sanchez 2005; MacKinnon et al. 2013; McKenzie 2018). While non-gastrointestinal problems, such as uroperitoneum or peritonitis, represent important differentials for foals presenting with signs of abdominal discomfort, this discussion will focus on causes of colic that are of gastrointestinal origin.

Diagnosing the underlying cause of colic in neonatal foals is often challenging. While distinguishing between primary medical and surgical problems is a critical diagnostic step, it is also important to remember that progressive pain that is unresponsive to analgesic therapy and medical conditions that do not resolve with appropriate medical therapy can warrant surgical exploration regardless of the suspected underlying cause. While many foals are very demonstrative in showing signs of abdominal pain, clinical signs are often variable or non-specific and can be complicated by underlying co-morbidities. In one study, 63% of foals presenting for evaluation of colic had concurrent disease affecting another body system (MacKinnon et al. 2013). Furthermore, conditions such as sepsis or PAS can both predispose foals to gastrointestinal disease and can also impact treatment decisions as well as prognosis (Bryant and Gaughan 2005; MacKinnon et al. 2013; McKenzie 2018).

Classic clinical signs of abdominal discomfort in foals include decreased nursing, "tail flagging," tenesmus, abdominal distension, rolling, and lying in dorsal recumbency. Passage of a nasogastric tube is performed to check for reflux and external abdominal or digital rectal palpation can sometimes identify obstructions. Diagnostic evaluation should include thorough abdominal ultrasound to evaluate intestinal motility, distension, and wall thickness. The presence of free abdominal fluid should be noted, and all other abdominal structures evaluated. Abdominocentesis can be of use when free fluid is identified, to rule out peritonitis or uroperitoneum, and for detection of ischemic intestinal compromise. Abdominal radiographs may be of use in certain obstructive or congenital conditions. Other diagnostics, such as hematologic analysis, can help refine diagnosis and are important for detecting other co-morbidities and determining the overall systemic health of the neonate. These should be tailored to the specific needs of the patient.

The most common medical gastrointestinal conditions associated with signs of colic include meconium impaction, enterocolitis, and "colic of unknown origin" (Magdesian 2005; Ryan and Sanchez 2005; Palmer 2012;

MacKinnon et al. 2013). Other less common causes may include secondary ileus in foals with sepsis or PAS and equine gastric ulcer disease in sick hospitalized foals (McKenzie 2018). When compared to surgical problems, outcome for medically treated gastrointestinal conditions is generally considered more favorable, but this may be influenced by the nature of the problem and the presence of other medical co-morbidities (MacKinnon et al. 2013). Regardless of the cause, supportive care is important for these conditions and may depend on the severity and specific cause of disease.

Meconium is comprised of mucus, bile, glandular secretions, cells, and digested amniotic fluid. In most foals, it is passed within a few hours of birth, after ingestion of colostrum (Palmer 2012; McKenzie 2018). The risk for impaction increases if the meconium is not passed within 12 hours of birth and represents the most common cause of intestinal obstruction in neonatal foals (Pusterla et al. 2004; Palmer 2012; McKenzie 2018). The small colon and the pelvic inlet are the most common sites of impaction (Knottenbelt et al. 2004; Pusterla et al. 2004). Clinical signs of colic develop secondary to intestinal gas distension. Abdominal distension and frequent posturing or straining to defecate can be observed. Enemas (warm-soapy water; sodium phosphate; acetylcysteine retention) are of diagnostic and therapeutic benefit and represent the first line of treatment for this condition (Ryan and Sanchez 2005; Pusterla et al. 2004; McKenzie 2018). Intravenous fluids, nutritional support, and analgesic therapy with opioids or judicious administration of NSAIDs are often provided. In rare cases, surgical correction may be warranted for non-resolving impactions.

Enterocolitis represents the most common gastrointestinal disorder in neonatal foals and is typically accompanied by diarrhea (Ryan and Sanchez 2005; MacKinnon et al. 2013). Signs of abdominal discomfort are common, and enterocolitis should always be included as a differential when evaluating a foal with colic.

Treatment is primarily medical and can often be intensive; however, in severe cases, such as with necrotizing enterocolitis, unrelenting pain may necessitate exploratory celiotomy (MacKinnon et al. 2013). Furthermore, ileus and gas distension associated with enterocolitis increase a foal's risk for developing intestinal volvulus or intussusception, both of which are surgical emergencies (Adams et al. 1998; Cable et al. 1997; Stephen et al. 2004; Bryant and Gaughan 2005). Rotavirus represents the most common infectious cause of enterocolitis in neonatal foals with other important infectious agents including *Clostridium difficile* and *C. perfringens*, *Salmonella* sp., *E. coli*, *Enterococcus* sp., and, more rarely *Aeromonas* sp. and *Cryptosporidium* (Mair et al. 1990; Magdesian 2005; Frederick et al. 2009; MacKinnon et al. 2013; Slovis et al. 2014; McKenzie 2018). PAS associated gastrointestinal dysfunction and necrotizing enterocolitis are identified more sporadically as causes of enterocolitis in foals and may or may not be associated with infectious agents (Cudd and Pauly 1987; Jones et al. 1988; McKenzie 2018).

The most common surgical gastrointestinal problems in neonatal foals include small intestinal strangulating lesions, nonreducible inguinal hernias, and congenital defects (Bryant and Gaughan 2005; MacKinnon et al. 2013). Thorough evaluation of a foal presenting with surgical colic is critical, and medical stabilization should be attempted whenever possible. Furthermore, co-morbidities such as sepsis, enterocolitis, or PAS should be considered in the decision to pursue surgical intervention as they can impact prognosis and suitability for surgery. Additional concerns for neonates can include cardiovascular consequences associated with anesthesia or those directly related to surgery such as hypothermia, blood loss, incisional infections, and abdominal adhesion formation (Beck et al. 2017). Foals are thought to be prone to the development of intra-abdominal adhesions because of more prolific fibrin deposition at sites of serosal injury (Southwood and Baxter 1997; Cable et al. 1997;

Singer and Livesey 1997; Bryant and Gaughan 2005). Adhesion formation can result in secondary gastrointestinal (GI) obstruction and thus may impact short- and long-term outcome (Bryant and Gaughan 2005).

Neonatal foal survival associated with gastrointestinal surgery has often been considered lower than that of mature horses but the evidence for this is somewhat conflicting (Bryant and Gaughan 2005; MacKinnon et al. 2013). Outcome for foals requiring surgery varies according to lesion type and location, age group of foals evaluated, duration of the problem, and co-morbidities (Cable et al. 1997; Santschi et al. 2000; Bryant and Gaughan 2005; MacKinnon et al. 2013). In most studies, strangulating or primary small intestinal lesions carry a poor prognosis for survival (Cable et al. 1997; Singer and Livesey 1997; Adams et al. 1998; Santschi et al. 2000; MacKinnon et al. 2013).

Small intestinal strangulating obstructions represent one of the most common causes of surgical colic in neonatal foals and carry the poorest prognosis for survival particularly when there is a delay in presentation for evaluation (Cable et al. 1997; Bryant and Gaughan 2005; MacKinnon et al. 2013). Foals with these conditions generally present with acute onset and progressive abdominal pain that is nonresponsive to analgesic therapy. Delay in recognition and correction of the problem can result in significant cardiovascular derangements, electrolyte disturbances, and SIRS which all impact survival. Small intestinal volvulus develops when the intestine rotates around the mesenteric route and is often a complication of segmental ileus and associated gas distension of the bowel (Greet 1992; Bryant and Gaughan 2005). As mentioned, sepsis, PAS, and enterocolitis are all risk factors in neonatal foals. Regardless of the underlying cause, severe intestinal compromise can develop. Intussusceptions most often involve invagination of the small intestine within the jejunum or at the ileocecal junction (Bryant and Gaughan 2005).

Jejunal-jejunal intussusceptions are more often acute in nature while ileocecal intussusceptions can have a more chronic progression (Cable et al. 1997; Singer and Livesey 1997; Adams et al. 1998). Although not always identified, the "bulls-eye" lesion is a classic ultrasonographic finding associated with intussusception and represents the edematous inner wall of the intussusceptum surrounded by the thin outer wall of the intussuscipiens (Reef 1998).

Inguinal hernias most commonly present as easily reducible and asymptomatic conditions in neonatal foals (Bryant and Gaughan 2005). These are identified within the first one to two days of birth as soft, unilateral swellings adjacent to the scrotal area. Rarely, bilateral swellings can be appreciated. Reducible hernias develop in response to delayed closure of the internal inguinal ring. Medical management involving manual reduction or use of truss bandages is typically successful but may take several weeks to a few months. More rarely, foals may present with nonreducible and direct inguinal hernias which are considered surgical emergencies (Gaughan 1998; Bryant and Gaughan 2005). Nonreducible hernias develop when there is a rupture of the vaginal tunic, and bowel becomes entrapped in subcutaneous tissue. In these circumstances, pronounced scrotal and preputial swelling and edema are appreciated as are signs of colic and systemic inflammation proportional to the degree of intestinal compromise.

Congenital defects of the gastrointestinal tract include atresia of the colon, rectum, or anus. Very rarely, congenital aganglionosis of the distal small or large intestine (Overo lethal white syndrome) is encountered in Overo–Overo-bred Paint horses. These conditions are rare and often fatal and early recognition is important particularly as they should be ruled out when considering surgical intervention. Clinical signs associated with these conditions present within the first several hours of life and initially resemble those associated with meconium impaction but progress in severity.

Administration of an enema does not yield meconium or meconium staining in expelled enema fluid (Ryan and Sanchez 2005). Diagnosis involves digital or visual examination of the anus (atresia ani) as well as contrast radiography (Atresia recti or coli) with exploratory celiotomy required for definitive diagnosis of atresia coli (Epstein 2014). Atresia ani has a favorable response to surgical correction but may be accompanied by other congenital defects, such as hypospadias (Epstein 2014; Nelson et al. 2015; McKenzie 2018). Atresia recti and coli are generally considered fatal as outcome is poor with surgical correction, and they are often accompanied by other neurologic or gastrointestinal motility problems (Bryant and Gaughan 2005; Epstein 2014; McKenzie 2018).

Anesthesia for Foals with Intestinal Accidents

While medical stabilization prior to anesthesia of foals with any disorder is important, foals presenting for acute, often strangulating, lesions of the intestinal tract may not allow for prolonged stabilization. Thus, foals with intestinal accidents typically are some of the most unstable patients presenting for anesthesia. Intractable pain and endotoxemia and sepsis associated with a compromised bowel may further make pre-anesthetic stabilization difficult. Rapid induction to unconsciousness may be necessary to alleviate discomfort. Diagnostic procedures and collection of samples for clinical pathology may occur after induction. Thus, some degree of physiologic stabilization may need to occur during anesthesia. Correction of blood gas, fluid, and electrolyte imbalances can occur in relatively short period of time setting up the foal to be more stable during the remaining anesthetic period. Techniques for reduction of MAC may be particularly helpful as hypotension and cardiovascular depression is common. Infusions of lidocaine and/or opioids (fentanyl) may be of particular use. Additionally, the use of previously mentioned TAP block can be used for analgesia of the abdominal wall and MAC reduction.

Vigilant monitoring of vital signs can help with early recognition of complications, as previously mentioned, foals presenting for abdominal surgery often have co-morbidities. Blood gas and electrolyte analysis will help guide ventilation support and electrolyte and glucose supplementation. Blood pressure monitoring will identify hypotension and the need for exogenous cardiovascular support should be anticipated (dobutamine, norepinephrine, etc.). Although volume replacement and ongoing fluid therapy should be initiated, monitoring fluid input to prevent edema formation, especially in foals that have dysfunction of the capillary beds, is critically important. These foals may benefit from colloidal support in the form of plasma.

Intensive support may need to continue through the recovery period and transition to intensive care post-operatively.

Conclusion

Anesthesia of the neonatal foal is not simply anesthesia of a small horse. Adaptation and transition from in utero development to mature physiology takes place over a period of time during early life. Thus, it is necessary for those providing anesthesia to have an understanding of the changes occurring as well as unique aspects of disease conditions that affect neonatal foals. Developing anesthetic plans that account for developmental physiology, pathophysiology of disease and co-morbidities, expected complications and corrective measures, use of appropriate medications, and proper analgesia in neonatal foals can improve chances for successful outcomes.

References

Adams, R., Koterba, A.M., and Brown, M.P. (1998). Exploratory celiotomy for gastrointestinal disease in neonatal foals: a review of 20 cases. *Equine Veterinary Journal* 20 (1): 9–12.

Ahearne, C.E., Boylan, G.B., and Murray, D.M. (2016). Short and long term prognosis in perinatal asphyxia: an update. *World Journal of Clinical Pediatrics* 5 (1): 67–74.

Aksenov, D.P., Miller, M.J., Dixon, C.M. et al. (2020). Impact of anesthesia exposure in early development on learning and sensory functions. *Developmental Psychobiology* 62 (5): 559–572.

Aleman, M., Pickles, K.J., Conley, A. et al. (2013). Abnormal plasma neuroactive progestagen derivatives in ill, neonatal foals presented to the neonatal intensive care unit. *Equine Veterinary Journal* 45: 661–665.

Aleman, M., Weich, K.M., and Madigan, J.E. (2017). Survey of veterinarians using a novel physical compression squeeze procedure in the management of neonatal maladjustment syndrome in foals. *Animals: An Open Access Journal From MDPI* 7 (9): 69.

Aleman, M., McCue, P.M., Chigerwe, M. et al. (2019). Plasma concentrations of steroid precursors, steroids, neuroactive steroids, and neurosteroids in healthy neonatal foals from birth to 7 days of age. *Journal of Veterinary Internal Medicine* 33 (5): 2286–2293.

Anand, K.J. and Hickey, P.R. (1992). Halothane-morphine compared with high-dose sufentanil for anesthesia and postoperative analgesia in neonatal cardiac surgery. *New England Journal of Medicine* 326 (1): 1–9.

Anand, K.J., Sippell, W.G., and Aynsley-Green, A. (1987). Randomized trial of fentanyl anaesthesia in preterm babies undergoing surgery: effects on the stress response. *Lancet* 1 (8527): 243–248.

Archer, R.M., Gordon, S.J., Carslake, H.B. et al. (2012). Distal aortic aneurysm presumed to be secondary to an infected umbilical artery in a foal. *New Zealand Veterinary Journal* 60 (1): 65–68.

Arguedas, M.G., Hines, M.T., Papich, M.G. et al. (2008). Pharmacokinetics of butorphanol and evaluation of physiologic and behavioral effects after intravenous and intramuscular administration to neonatal foals. *Journal of Veterinary Internal Medicine* 22 (6): 1417–1426.

Aylor, M.K., Campbell, M.L., Goring, R.L. et al. (1984). Congenital bilateral choanal atresia in a Standardbred foal. *Equine Veterinary Journal* 16 (4): 396–398.

Ballet, D.E. (2010). Cooling for newborns with hypoxic ischemic encephalopathy: RHL commentary: The WHO Reproductive Health Library. World Health Organization, Geneva. http://apps.who.int/rhl newborn/cd00331_ballotde_com/en/

Beck, J., Loron, G., Masson, C. et al. (2017). Monitoring cerebral and renal oxygenation status during neonatal digestive surgeries using near infrared spectroscopy. *Frontiers in Pediatrics* 5 https://doi.org/10.3389/fped.2017.00140.

Bedenice, D., Heuwieser, W., Solano, M. et al. (2003). Risk factors and prognostic variables for survival of foals with radiographic evidence of pulmonary disease. *Journal of Veterinary Internal Medicine* 17 (6): 868–875.

Beech, J. (1985). Respiratory problems in foals. *Veterinary Clinics of North America. Equine Practice* 1 (1): 131–149.

Behr, M.J., Hackett, R.P., Bentinck-Smith, J. et al. (1981). Metabolic abnormalities associated with rupture of the urinary bladder in neonatal foals. *Journal of the American Veterinary Medical Association* 178: 263–266.

Bellieni, C.V. (2020). Analgesia for fetal pain during prenatal surgery: 10 years of progress. *Pediatric Research* https://doi.org/10.1038/s41390-020-01170-2.

Bernard, W.V., Reimer, J.M., and Cudd, T. (1995). Historical factors, clinicopathologic findings, clinical features, and outcome of equine neonates presenting with or developing signs of central nervous system disease. *Proceedings of the American Association of Equine Practitioners* 41: 222–224.

Bienert-Zeit, A. and Ohnesorge, B. (2011). Congenital bilateral choanal stenosis in a warmblood foal. *Veterinary Record* 169 (9): 232b.

Blaise, G.A. (2015). Ketamine. In: *Faust's Anesthesiology Review*, 4e (eds. M.J. Murray, B.A. Harrison, J.T. Mueller, et al.), 166–167. Philadelphia, PA: Elsevier Saunders.

Bone, R.C., Balk, R.A., Cerra, F.B. et al. (1992). Definitions for sepsis and organ failure and guidelines for the use of innovative therapies in sepsis. The ACCP/SCCM Consensus Conference Committee. American College of Chest Physicians/Society of Critical Care Medicine. *Chest* 101 (6): 1644–1655.

Brewer, B.D. and Koterba, A.M. (1988). Development of a scoring system for the early diagnosis of equine neonatal sepsis. *Equine Veterinary Journal* 20 (1): 18–22.

Brewer, B.D., Koterba, A.M., Carter, R.L. et al. (1988). Comparison of empirically developed sepsis score with a computer generated and weighted scoring system for the identification of sepsis in the equine neonate. *Equine Veterinary Journal* 20 (1): 23–24.

Brosnan, R.J. (2013). Inhaled anesthetic in horses. *Veterinary Clinics of North America. Equine Practice* 29 (1): 69–87.

Bryant, J.E. and Gaughan, E.M. (2005). Abdominal surgery in neonatal foals. *Veterinary Clinics of North America. Equine Practice* 21 (2): 511–535.

Cable, C.S., Fubini, S.L., Erb, H.N. et al. (1997). Abdominal surgery in foals: a review of 119 cases (1877–1994). *Equine Veterinary Journal* 29 (4): 257–261.

Carter, S.W., Robertson, S.A., Steel, C.J. et al. (1990). Cardiopulmonary effects of xylazine sedation in the foal. *Equine Veterinary Journal* 22 (6): 384–388.

Charalambous, M., Bhatti, S.F.M., Van Ham, L. et al. (2017). Intranasal midazolam versus rectal diazepam for the management of canine status epilepticus: a multicenter randomized parallel-group clinical trial. *Journal of Veterinary Internal Medicine* 31 (4): 1149–1158.

Clark-Price, S. (2015). Inadvertent perianesthetic hypothermia in small animal patients. *The Veterinary Clinics of North America. Small Animal Practice* 45 (5): 983–994.

Codina, L.R., Were, S.R., and Brown, J.A. (2019). Short-term outcome and risk factors for post-operative complications following umbilical resection in 82 foals (2004-2016). *Equine Veterinary Journal* 51: 323–328.

Corley, K.T., Donaldson, L.L., and Furr, M.O. (2005). Arterial lactate concentration, hospital survival, sepsis and SIRS in critically ill neonatal foals. *Equine Veterinary Journal* 37 (1): 53–59.

Cottrill, C.M., O'Connor, W.N., Cudd, T. et al. (1987). Persistence of foetal circulatory pathways in a newborn foal. *Equine Veterinary Journal* 19 (3): 252–255.

Cudd, T. and Pauly, T.H. (1987). Necrotizing enterocolitis in two equine neonates. *Compendium of Continuing Education Veterinary* 9: 88–88.

Dathan, K. and Sundaram, M. (2021). Comparison of isotonic versus hypotonic intravenous fluid for maintenance fluid therapy in neonates more than or equal to 34 weeks of gestational age – a randomized clinical trial. *Journal of Maternal-Fetal and Neonatal Medicine*: 1–8. https://doi.org/10.1080/14767058.2021.1911998.

Dickey, E.J., Long, S.N., and Hunt, R.W. (2011). Hypoxic ischemic encephalopathy— what can we learn from humans? *Journal of Veterinary Internal Medicine* 25: 1231–1240.

Diesch, T.J. and Mellor, D.J. (2013). Birth transitions: pathophysiology, the onset of consciousness and possible implications for neonatal maladjustment syndrome in the foal. *Equine Veterinary Journal* 45: 656–660.

Disdier, C. and Stonestreet, B.S. (2020). Hypoxic-ischemic-related cerebrovascular changes and potential therapeutic strategies in the neonatal brain. *Journal of Neuroscience Research* 98 (7): 1468–1484.

Disma, N., Veyckemans, F., Virag, K. et al. (2021). Morbidity and mortality after anaesthesia in early life: results of the European prospective multicentre observational study, neonate and children audit of anaesthesia practice in Europe (NECTARINE). *British Journal of Anaesthesia* 126 https://doi.org/10.1016/j.bja.2021.02.016.

Douglas-Escobar, M. and Weiss, M.D. (2015). Hypoxic-ischemic encephalopathy: a review for the clinician. *Journal of American Medical Association Pediatrics* 169: 397–403.

Dunkel, B., Palmer, J.E., Olson, K.N. et al. (2005). Uroperitoneum in 32 foals: influence of intravenous fluid therapy, infection, and sepsis. *Journal of Veterinary Internal Medicine* 19: 889–893.

Dunlop, C.I. (1994). Anesthesia and sedation of foals. *Veterinary Clinics of North America. Equine Practice* 10 (1): 67–85.

Edwards, R.B. 3rd. and Fubini, S.L. (1995). A one-stage marsupialization procedure for management of infected umbilical vein remnants in calves and foals. *Veterinary Surgery* 24 (1): 32–35.

Ek, C.J., Dziegielewska, K.M., Stolp, H. et al. (2006). Functional effectiveness of the blood-brain barrier to small water-soluble molecules in developing and adult opossum (*Monodelphis domestica*). *Journal of Comparative Neurology* 496 (1): 13–26.

Epstein, K.L. (2014). Congenital causes of gastrointestinal disease. *Equine Veterinary Education* 26: 345–346.

Fattuoni, C., Palmas, F., Noto, A. et al. (2015). Perinatal asphyxia: a review from a metabolomics perspective. *Molecules* 20: 7000–7016.

Fielding, C.L. and Magdesian, K.G. (2015). Sepsis and septic shock in the equine neonate. *Veterinary Clinics of North America. Equine Practice* 31 (3): 483–496.

Finno, C.J., Spier, S.J., and Valberg, S.J. (2009). Equine diseases caused by known genetic mutations. *Veterinary Journal* 179 (3): 336–347.

Fischer, B. and Clark-Price, S. (2015). Anesthesia of the equine neonate in health and disease. *Veterinary Clinics of North America. Equine Practice* 31 (3): 567–585.

Fischer, A.T. Jr. (1998). Laparoscopically assisted resection of umbilical structures in foals. *Journal of the American Veterinary Medical Association* 214 (12): 1813–1816.

Fowden, A.L., Giussani, D.A., and Forhead, A.J. (2020). Physiological development of the equine fetus during late gestation. *Equine Veterinary Journal* 52 (2): 165–173.

Frederick, J., Giguere, S., and Sanchez, L.C. (2009). Infectious agents detected in the feces of diarrheic foals: a retrospective study of 233 cases (2003-2008). *Journal of Veterinary Internal Medicine* 23: 1254–1260.

Freeman, L., Paradis, M.R. (1992) Evaluating the effectiveness of equine neonatal care. Veterinary Medicine USA. http://agris.fao.org/agris-search/search.do?recordID=US9306437.

Freitag, F.A., Amora, D.S. Jr., Muehlbauer, E. et al. (2021). Ultrasound-guided modified subcostal transversus abdominis plane block and influence of recumbency position on dye spread in equine cadavers. *Veterinary Anaestheisa and Analgesia* 48 (4): 596–602.

Fries, R.C., Clark-Price, S.C., Kadotani, S. et al. (2020). Quantitative assessment of left ventricular volume and function by transthoracic and transesophageal echocardiography, ultrasound velocity dilution, and gated magnetic resonance imaging in healthy foals. *American Journal of Veterinary Research* 81 (12): 930–939.

Furr, M. and McKenzie, H. 3rd. (2020). Factors associated with the risk of positive blood culture in neonatal foals presented to a referral center (2000-2014). *Journal of Veterinary Internal Medicine* 34 (6): 2738–2750.

Gaughan, E.M. (1998). Inguinal hernias in horses. *Compendium of Continuing Education* 20 (9): 1057–1059.

Gayle, J.M., Cohen, N.D., and Chaffin, M.K. (1998). Factors associated with survival in septicemic foals: 65 cases (1988-1995). *Journal of Veterinary Internal Medicine* 12 (3): 140–146.

Giatti, S., Garcia-Segura, L.M., and Melcangi, R.C. (2015). New steps forward in the neuroactive steroid field. *Journal of Steroid Biochemistry and Molecular Biology* 153: 127–134.

Giguère, S., Slade, J.K., and Sanchez, L.C. (2008). Retrospective comparison of caffeine and doxapram for the treatment of hypercapnia in foals with hypoxic-ischemic encephalopathy. *Journal of Veterinary Internal Medicine* 22 (2): 401–405.

Giguère, S., Weber, E.J., and Sanchez, L.C. (2017). Factors associated with outcome and gradual improvement in survival over time in 1065 equine neonates admitted to an intensive care unit. *Equine Veterinary Journal* 49 (1): 45–50.

Gold, J.R. (2015). Perinatal asphyxia syndrome. *Equine Veterinary Education* 29 (3): 158–164.

Gold, J., Chaffin, M.K., Burgess, B.A. et al. (2016). Factors associated with non-survival in foals diagnosed with perinatal asphyxia syndrome. *Journal of Equine Veterinary Science* 38: 82–86.

Goldman, R.D. and Koren, G. (2002). Biologic markers of pain in the vulnerable infant. *Clinics in Perinatology* 29 (3): 415–425.

Goodwin, W., Keates, H., Pasloske, K. et al. (2012). Plasma pharmacokinetics and pharmacodynamics of alfaxalone in neonatal foals after an intravenous bolus of alfaxalone following premedication with butorphanol tartrate. *Veterinary Anaesthesia and Analgesia* 39 (5): 503–510.

Greet, T.R. (1992). Ileal intussusception in 16 young thoroughbreds. *Equine Veterinary Journal* 24 (2): 81–83.

Gutierrez-Nibeyro, S.D. (2020). Pharyngeal cysts in horses. In: *Large Animal Internal Medicine*, 6e (eds. B.P. Smith, D.C. Van Metre and N. Pusterla), 630–631. St. Louis, MO: Elsevier.

Hall, M.J., Levant, S., and DeFrances, C.J. (2013). Trends in inpatient hospital deaths: National Hospital Discharge Survey, 2000-2010. *NCHS Data Brief* 118: 1–8.

Hayes, J.A., Alijuhani, T., De Oliveira, K. et al. (2021). Safety and efficacy of the combination of propofol and ketamine for procedural sedation/anesthesia in the pediatric population: a systematic review and meta-analysis. *Anesthesia and Analgesia* 132 (4): 979–992.

Hoffman, A.M., Viel, L., Prescott, J.F. et al. (1993). Association of microbiologic flora with clinical, endoscopic, and pulmonary cytologic findings in foals with distal respiratory tract infection. *American Journal of Veterinary Research* 54 (10): 1615–1622.

Hogan, P.M., Embertson, R.M., and Hunt, R.J. (1995). Unilateral choanal atresia in a foal. *Journal of the American Veterinary Medical Association* 207 (4): 471–473.

Hollis, A.R., Ousey, J.C., Palmer, L. et al. (2006). Effects of norepinephrine and a combined norepinephrine and dobutamine infusion on systemic hemodynamics and indices of renal function in normotensive neonatal thoroughbred foals. *Journal of Veterinary Internal Medicine* 20 (6): 1437–1442.

Hollis, A.R., Wilkins, P.A., Palmer, J.E. et al. (2008). Bacteremia in equine neonatal diarrhea: a retrospective study (1990-2007). *Journal of Veterinary Internal Medicine* 22: 1203–1209.

Holtan, D.W., Houghton, E., Silver, M. et al. (1991). Plasma progestagens in the mare, fetus and newborn foal. *Journal of Reproduction and Fertility* 44: S517–S528.

van den Hoogen, N.J., de Kort, A.R., Allegaert, K.M. et al. (2019). Developmental neurobiology as a guide for pharmacological management of pain in neonates. *Seminars in Fetal and Neonatal Medicine* 24 (4) https://doi.org/10.1016/j.siny.2019.05.004.

Houghton, E., Holtan, D.W., Grainger, L. et al. (1991). Plasma progestogen concentrations in the normal and dysmature newborn foal. *Journal of Reproduction and Fertility* 44: S609–S617.

Hubbell, J.A.E., Kelly, E.M., Aarnes, T.K. et al. (2013). Pharmacokinetics of midazolam after intravenous administration to horses. *Equine Veterinary Journal* 45 (6): 721–725.

Hubbell, J.A.E. and Muir, W.W. (2009). Anesthetic protocols and techniques for specific procedures. In: *Equine Anesthesia Monitoring and Emergency Therapy*, 2e (eds. W.W. Muir and J.A.E. Hubbell), 430–438. St. Louis, MO: Saunders Elsevier.

Huntsman, R.J., Strueby, L., and Bingham, W. (2020). Are ketamine infusion a viable option for refractory neonatal seizures? *Pediatric Neurology* 103: 8–11.

James, F.M., Parente, E.J., and Palmer, J.E. (2006). Management of bilateral choanal atresia in a foal. *Journal of the American Veterinary Medical Association* 229 (11): 1784–1789.

Jean, D., Laverty, S., Halley, J. et al. (1999). Thoracic trauma in newborn foals. *Equine Veterinary Journal* 31: 149–152.

Jean, D., Picandet, V., Macieira, S. et al. (2007). Detection of rib trauma in newborn foals in an equine critical care unit: a comparison of ultrasonography, radiography and physical examination. *Equine Veterinary Journal* 39 (2): 158–163.

Jevtovic-Todorovic, V., Hartman, R.E., Izumi, Y. et al. (2003). Early exposure to common anesthetic agents causes widespread neurodegeneration in the developing rat brain and persistent learning deficits. *Journal of Neuroscience* 23 (3): 876–882.

Johne, M., Römermann, K., Hampel, P. et al. (2021). Phenobarbital and midazolam suppress neonatal seizures in a noninvasive rat model of birth asphyxia, whereas bumetanide is ineffective. *Epilepsia* 62 (4): 920–934.

Johnson, L., Montgomery, J.B., Schneider, J.P. et al. (2014). Morphometric examination of the equine adult and foal lung. *Anatomical Record* 297 (10): 1950–1962.

Johnston, G.M., Eastment, J.K., Wood, J.L.N. et al. (2002). The confidential enquiry into perioperative equine fatalities (CEPEF): mortality results of Phase 1 and 2. *Veterinary Anaesthesia and Analgesia* 29 (4): 159–170.

Jones, R.L., Adney, W.S., Alexander, A.F. et al. (1988). Hemorrhagic necrotizing enterocolitis associated with Clostridium difficile infection in four foals. *Journal of the American Veterinary Medical Association* 193: 76–79.

Jones, T., Bracamonte, J.L., Ambros, B. et al. (2019). Total intravenous anesthesia with alfaxalone, dexmedetomidine and remifentanil in healthy foals undergoing abdominal surgery. *Veterinary Anaesthesia and Analgesia* 46 (3): 315–324.

Kablack, K.A., Embertson, R.M., Bernard, W.V. et al. (2000). Uroperitoneum in the hospitalised equine neonate: retrospective study of 31 cases, 1988-1997. *Equine Veterinary Journal* 32: 505–508.

Knottenbelt, D.C., Holdstock, N., and Madigan, J.E. (2004). *Equine Neonatology: Medicine and Surgery*. Edinburgh: Saunders.

Knych, H.K., Steffey, E.P., Casbeer, H.C. et al. (2015). Disposition, behavioural and physiological effects of escalating doses of intravenously administered fentanyl to young foals. *Equine Veterinary Journal* 47 (5): 592–598.

Koch, D.B. and Tate, L.P. Jr. (1978). Pharyngeal cysts in horses. *Journal of the American Veterinary Medical Association* 173: 860–862.

Kurth, C.D., Spitezer, A.R., Broennle, A.M. et al. (1987). Postoperative apnea in preterm infants. *Anesthesiology* 66 (4): 483–488.

Kutasi, O., Horvath, A., Harnos, A. et al. (2009). Radiographic assessment of pulmonary fluid clearance in healthy neonatal foals. *Veterinary Radiology & Ultrasound* 50 (6): 584–588.

Lascola, K.M. and Joslyn, S. (2015). Diagnostic imaging of the lower respiratory tract in neonatal foals: radiography and computed tomography. *The Veterinary Clinics of North America. Equine Practice* 31 (3): 497–514.

Lascola, K.M., O'Brien, R.T., Wilkins, P.A. et al. (2013). Qualitative and quantitative interpretation of computed tomography of the lungs in healthy neonatal foals. *American Journal of Veterinary Research* 74 (9): 1239–1246.

Lascola, K.M., Clark-Price, S.C., Joslyn, S.K. et al. (2016). Use of manual alveolar recruitment maneuvers to eliminate atelectasis artifacts identified during thoracic computed tomography of healthy neonatal foals. *American Journal of Veterinary Research* 77 (11): 1276–1287.

LeDez, K.M. and Lerman, J. (1987). The minimum alveolar concentration (MAC) or isoflurane in preterm neonates. *Anesthesiology* 76 (3): 301–307.

Lee, A.C., Kozuki, N., Blencowe, H. et al. (2013). Intrapartum-related neonatal encephalopathy incidence and impairment at regional and global levels for 2010 with trends from 1990. *Pediatric Research* 74 (Suppl 1): 50–72.

Lester, G.D. and Lester, N.V. (2001). Abdominal and thoracic radiography in the neonate. *The Veterinary Clinics of North America. Equine Practice* 17 (1): 19–46.

Lester, G.D., DeMarco, V.G., and Norman, W.M. (1999). Effect of inhaled nitric oxide on experimentally induced pulmonary hypertension in neonatal foals. *American Journal of Veterinary Research* 60 (10): 1207–1212.

Lim, T.Y., Poole, R.L., and Pageler, N.M. (2014). Propylene glycol toxicity in children. *Journal of Pediatric Pharmacology and Therapeutics* 19 (4): 277–282.

Linford, R.L. (2011). Disorders of the bladder, urachus, and umbilicus in the neonatal foal. In: Western Veterinary Conference, Las Vegas, NV.

Loomes, K. (2020). Alfaxalone total intravenous anaesthesia in a donkey foal. *Veterinary Anaesthesia and Analgesia* 47 (5): 733–734.

Love, E.J. (2011). Anaesthesia in foals with uroperitoneum. *Equine Veterinary Education* 23: 508–511.

Lyle-Dugas, J., Giguere, S., Mallicote, M.F. et al. (2016). Factors associated with outcome in 94 hospitalised foals diagnosed with neonatal encephalopathy. *Equine Veterinary Journal* 49: 207–210.

MacDonald, K.D., Hart, K.A., Davis, J.L. et al. (2018). Pharmacokinetics of the anticonvulsant levetiracetam in neonatal foals. *Equine Veterinary Journal* 50 (4): 532–536.

Mackinnon, M.C., Southwood, L.L., Burke, M.J. et al. (2013). Colic in equine neonates: 137 cases (2000-2010). *Journal of the American Veterinary Medical Association* 243 (11): 1586–1595.

Madigan, J.E., Haggett, E.F., Pickles, K.J. et al. (2012). Allopregnanolone infusion induced neurobehavioral alterations in a neonatal foal: is this a clue to the pathogenesis of neonatal maladjustment syndrome? *Equine Veterinary Journal* 44: S109–S112.

Magata, F., Ishii, M., Oikawa, E. et al. (2010). Purulent necrotic dislocation of the hip joint associated with umbilical infection in a foal. *Journal of Equine Science* 21 (2): 17–20.

Magdesian, K.G. (2005). Neonatal foal diarrhea. *Veterinary Clinics of North America. Equine Practice* 21: 295–312.

Magdesian, G. (2013). Fluid and electrolyte balance. In: *Manual of Equine Neonatal Medicine*, 4e (ed. J.E. Madigan), 98–110. Woodland, CA: Live Oak Publishing.

Mair, T.S., Taylor, F.G., Harbour, D.A. et al. (1990). Concurrent cryptosporidium and coronavirus infections in an Arabian foal with combined immunodeficiency syndrome. *Veterinary Record* 126: 127–130.

Maitra, S., Baidya, D.K., Khanna, P. et al. (2014). Acute perioperative pain in neonates: An evidence-based review of neurophysiology and management. *Acta Anaesthesiologica Taiwanica* 52 (1): 30–37.

Mansell, A., Bryan, C., and Levison, H. (1972). Airway closure in children. *Journal of Applied Physiology* 33 (6): 711–714.

Marr, C.M. (2015). The equine neonatal cardiovascular system in health and disease. *Veterinary Clinics of North America. Equine Practice* 31 (3): 545–565.

Marroum, P.J., Webb, A.I., Aeschbacher, G. et al. (1994). Pharmacokinetics and pharmacodynamics of acepromazine in horses. *American Journal of Veterinary Research* 55 (10): 1428–1433.

Marsh, P.S. and Palmer, J.E. (2001). Bacterial isolates from blood and their susceptibility patterns in critically ill foals: 543 cases (1991-1998). *Journal of the American Veterinary Medical Association* 218 (10): 1608–1610.

Martin, K., Brooks, S., Vierra, M. et al. (2020). Fragile foal syndrome (PLOD1 c.2032G>A) occurs across diverse horse populations. *Animal Genetics* 52 (1): 137–138.

Martinez-Taboada, F. and Leece, E.A. (2014). Comparison of propofol with ketofol, a propofol-ketamine admixture, for induction of anaesthesia in healthy dogs. *Veterinary Anaesthesia and Analgesia* 41 (6): 575–582.

Massoco, C. and Palermo-Neto, J. (2003). Effects of midazolam on equine innate immune response: a flow cytometric study. *Veterinary Immunology and Immunopathology* 95 (1–2): 11–19.

McCoy, A.M., Lopp, C.T., Kooy, S. et al. (2020). Normal regression of the internal umbilical remnant structures in Standardbred foals. *Equine Veterinary Journal* 52 (6): 876–883.

McKenzie, H.C. III (2018). Disorders of foals. In: *Equine Internal Medicine* (eds. S.M. Reed, W.M. Bayly and D.C. Sellon), 1365–1459. St. Louis, MO: Elsevier.

Michelet, D., Arslan, O., Hilly, J. et al. (2015). Intraoperative changes in blood pressure associated with cerebral desaturation in infants. *Paediatric Anaesthesia* 25 (7): 681–688.

Moorman, V.J., Bass, L., and King, M.R. (2019). Evaluation of the effects of commonly used α2-adrenergic receptor agonists alone and in combination with butorphanol tartrate on objective measurements of lameness in horses. *American Journal of Veterinary Research* 80 (9): 868–877.

Morresey, P.R. (2011). The placenta. In: *Equine Reproduction*, 2e (eds. A.O. McKinnon, E.L. Squires, W.E. Vaala, et al.), 18–21. Ames, IA: Wiley-Blackwell.

Morresey, P.R. (2014) Umbilical Problems, AAEP Focus on the first year of life, pp. 18-21.

Muir, W.W. (2009). Anxiolytics, nonopioid sedative-analgesics, and opioid analgesics. In: *Equine Anesthesia Monitoring and Emergency Therapy*, 2e (eds. W.W. Muir and J.A.E. Hubbell), 185–209. St. Louis, MO: Saunders Elsevier.

Nelson, B.B., Ferris, R.A., McCue, P.M. et al. (2015). Surgical management of atresia ani and perineal hypospadias in a miniature donkey foal. *Equine Veterinary Education* 27: 525–529.

Neumann, R.P. and von Ungern-Sternberg, B.S. (2014). The neonatal lung – physiology and ventilation. *Paediatric Anaesthesia* 24 (1): 10–21.

Nogradi, N., Magdesian, K.G., Whitcomb, M.B. et al. (2013). Imaging diagnosis-aortic aneurysm and ureteral obstruction secondary to umbilical artery abscessation in a 5-week-old foal. *Veterinary Radiology & Ultrasound* 54 (4): 384–389.

Nuñez, E., Steffey, E.P., Ocampo, L. et al. (2004). Effects of alpha2-adrenergic receptor agonists on urine production in horses deprived of food and water. *American Journal of Veterinary Research* 65 (10): 1342–1346.

O'Connor, S.J., Gardner, D.S., Ousey, J.C. et al. (2005). Development of baroreflex and endocrine responses to hypothesive stress in newborn foals and lambs. *Pflügers Archiv* 450 (5): 298–306.

Olutoye, O.A., Baker, B.W., Belfort, M.A. et al. (2018). Food and Drug Administration warning on anesthesia and brain development: implications for obstetric and fetal surgery. *American Journal of Obstetrics and Gynecology* 218 (1): 98–102.

Oreff, G.L., Tatz, A.J., Dahan, R. et al. (2017). Surgical management and long-term outcome of umbilical infection in 65 foals (2010-2015). *Veterinary Surgery* 46 (7): 962–970.

Palmer, J.E. (2012). Colic and diaphragmatic hernias in neonatal foals. *Equine Veterinary Education* 24: 340–342.

Perkins, G.A. and Wagner, B. (2015). The development of equine immunity: current knowledge on immunology in the young horse. *Equine Veterinary Journal* 47 (3): 267–274.

Pusterla, N., Magdesian, K.G., Maleski, K. et al. (2004). Retrospective evaluation of the use of acetylcysteine enemas in the treatment of meconium retention in foals: 44 cases (1987-2002). *Equine Veterinary Education* 16: 133–136.

Ranieri, V.M., Rubenfeld, G.D., Thompson, B.T. et al. (2012). Acute respiratory distress syndrome: the Berlin Definition. *Journal if the American Medical Association* 307 (23): 2526–2533.

Reddy, D.S. (2009). The role of neurosteroids in the pathophysiology and treatment of catamenial epilepsy. *Epilepsy Research* 85: 1–30.

Reef, V.B. (1991). Advances in diagnostic ultrasonography. *The Veterinary Clinics of North America. Equine Practice* 7 (2): 451–466.

Reef, V.B. (1998). Pediatric abdominal ultrasonography. In: *Equine Diagnostic Ultrasound*, 1e (ed. V.B. Reef), 364–403. Philadelphia, PA: WB Saunders.

Reef, V.B. and Collatos, C. (1988). Ultrasonography of umbilical structures in clinically normal foals. *American Journal of Veterinary Research* 49 (12): 2143–2146.

Reef, V.B., Collatos, C., Spencer, P.A. et al. (1989). Clinical, ultrasonographic, and surgical findings in foals with umbilical remnant infections. *Journal of the American Veterinary Medical Association* 195 (1): 69–72.

Reuss, S.M. and Cohen, N.D. (2015). Update on bacterial pneumonia in the foal and weanling. *The Veterinary Clinics of North America. Equine Practice* 31 (1): 121–135.

Reynolds, E.B. (1930). Clinical notes on some conditions met within the mare following parturition and in the newly born foal. *Veterinary Record* 10: 277.

Richardson, D.W. and Kohn, C.W. (1983). Uroperitoneum in the foal. *Journal of the American Veterinary Medical Association* 182: 267–271.

Rossdale, P.D. and Leadon, D.P. (1975). Equine neonatal disease: a review. *Journal of Reproduction and Fertility* 23: 658–661.

Russell, C.M., Axon, J.E., Blishen, A. et al. (2008). Blood culture isolates and antimicrobial sensitivities from 427 critically ill neonatal foals. *Australian Veterinary Journal* 86 (7): 266–271.

Rutkowski, J.A., Eadesm, S.C., and Moore, J.N. (1991). Effects of xylazine butorphanol on cecal arterial blood flow, cecal mechanical activity, and systemic hemodynamics in horses. *American Journal of Veterinary Research* 52 (7): 1153–1158.

Ryan, C.A. and Sanchez, L.C. (2005). Nondiarrheal disorders of the gastrointestinal tract in neonatal foals. *Veterinary Clinics of North America. Equine Practice* 21 (2): 313–332.

Saikia, D. and Mahanta, B. (2019). Cardiovascular and respiratory physiology in children. *Indian Journal of Anaesthesia* 63 (9): 690–697.

Sampaio, T.B., de Oliveira, L.F., Constantino, L.C. et al. (2018). Long-term neurobehavioral consequences of a single ketamine neonatal exposure in rats: effects on cellular viability and glutamate transport in frontal cortex and hippocampus. *Neurotoxicity Research* 34 (3): 649–659.

Sanchez, L.C. and Robertson, S.A. (2014). Pain control in horses: what do we really know? *Equine Veterinary Journal* 46: 517–523.

Sanchez, L.C., Giguère, S., and Lester, G.D. (2008). Factors associated with survival of neonatal foals with bacteremia and racing performance of surviving Thoroughbreds: 423 cases (1982-2007). *Journal of the American Veterinary Medical Association* 233: 1446–1452.

Santschi, E.M., Slone, D.E., Embertson, R.M. et al. (2000). Colic surgery in 206 juvenile thoroughbreds: survival and racing results. *Equine Veterinary Journal* 32: 32–36.

Saunders, N.R., Dziegielewska, K.M., Møllgård, K. et al. (2019). Recent developments in understanding barrier mechanisms in the developing brain: drugs and drug transporters in pregnancy, susceptibility or protection in the fetal brain? *Annual Review of Pharmacology and Toxicology* 59: 487–505.

Schambourg, M.A., Laverty, S., Mullim, S. et al. (2003). Thoracic trauma in foals: post mortem findings. *Equine Veterinary Journal* 35 (1): 78–81.

Schauvliege, S. and Gasthuys, F. (2013). Drugs for cardiovascular support in anesthetized horses. *Veterinary Clinics of North America. Equine Practice* 29 (1): 19–49.

Schiffmann, H. (2006). Humidification of respired gases in neonates and infants. *Respiratory Care Clinics of North America* 12 (2): 321–336.

Schliewert, E.C., Lascola, K.M., O'Brien, R.T. et al. (2015). Comparison of radiographic and computed tomographic images of the lungs in healthy neonatal foals. *American Journal of Veterinary Research* 76 (1): 42–52.

Sessler, D.I. (2015). Temperature regulation and monitoring. In: *Miller's Anesthesia*, 8e (eds. R.D. Miller, N.H. Cohen, L.I. Eriksson, et al.), 1622–1646. St. Louis, MO: Saunder Elsevier.

Sheats, M.K. (2019). A comparative review of equine SIRS, sepsis, and neutrophils. *Frontiers in Veterinary Science* 12 (6): 69.

Shih, A., Giguère, S., Sanchez, L.C. et al. (2009). Determination of cardiac output in neonatal foals by ultrasound velocity dilution and its comparison to the lithium dilution method. *Journal of Veterinary Emergency and Critical Care* 19 (5): 438–443.

Singer, E.R. and Livesey, M.A. (1997). Evaluation of exploratory laparotomy in young horses: 102 cases (1987–1992). *Journal of the American Veterinary Medical Association* 211 (9): 1158–1162.

Singer, M., Deutschman, C.S., Seymour, C.W. et al. (2016). The third international consensus definitions for sepsis and septic shock (Sepsis-3). *Journal of the American Medical Association* 315 (8): 801–810.

Singh, Y., Katheria, A.C., and Vora, F. (2018). Advances in diagnosis and management of hemodynamic instability in neonatal shock. *Frontiers in Pediatrics* 6 https://doi.org/10.3389/fped.2018.00002.

Slovis, N.M., Elam, J., Estrada, M. et al. (2014). Infectious agents associated with diarrhoea in neonatal foals in central Kentucky: a comprehensive molecular study. *Equine Veterinary Journal* 46: 311–316.

Smit, A.L., Seehase, M., Stokroos, R.J. et al. (2013). Functional impairment of the auditory pathway after perinatal asphyxia and the short-term effect of perinatal propofol anesthesia in lambs. *Pediatric Research* 74 (1): 34–38.

Southwood, L.L. and Baxter, G.M. (1997). Current concepts in management of abdominal adhesions. *Veterinary Clinics of North America. Equine Practice* 13 (2): 415–435.

Sprayberry, K.A. (2008). The urinary system. In: *Color Atlas of Diseases and Disorders of the Foal* (eds. S.B. McAuliffe and N.M. Slovis), 167–188. New York, Edinburgh: Elsevier Saunders.

Sprayberry, K.A. (2015). Ultrasonographic Examination of the Equine Neonate: Thorax and Abdomen. *The Veterinary Clinics of North America. Equine Practice* 31 (3): 515–543.

Sprayberry, K.A., Bain, F.T., Seahorn, T.L. et al. (2001). 56 cases of rib fractures in neonatal foals hospitalized in a referral center intensive care unit from 1997-2001. *Proceedings of the American Association of Equine Practitioners* 47: 395–399.

Steffey, E.P. and Howland, D. (1980). Comparison of circulatory and respiratory effects of isoflurane and halothane anesthesia in horses. *American Journal of Veterinary Research* 41 (5): 821–825.

Steffey, E.P., Howland, D., Giri, S. et al. (1977). Enflurane, halothane, and isoflurane potency in horses. *American Journal of Veterinary Research* 38 (7): 1037–1039.

Steffey, E.P., Willits, N., Wong, P. et al. (1991). Clinical investigations of halothane and isoflurane for induction and maintenance of foal anesthesia. *Journal of Veterinary Pharmacology and Therapeutics* 14 (3): 300–309.

Steffey, E.P., Mama, K.R., Galey, F.D. et al. (2005). Effects of sevoflurane dose and mode of ventilation on cardiopulmonary function and blood biochemical variable in horses. *American Journal of Veterinary Research* 66 (4): 669–677.

Stephen, J.O., Corley, K.T., Johnston, J.K. et al. (2004). Small intestinal volvulus in 115 horses: 1988–2000. *Veterinary Surgery* 33 (4): 333–339.

Stewart, A.J., Hinchcliff, K.W., Saville, W.J. et al. (2002). Actinobacillus sp bacteremia in foals: clinical signs and prognosis. *Journal of Veterinary Internal Medicine* 16: 464–471.

Stick, J.A. and Boles, C. (1980). Subepiglottic cyst in three foals. *Journal of the American Veterinary Medical Association* 177: 62–64.

Stocks, J., Dezateux, C., Hoo, A.F. et al. (1996). Delayed maturation of Hering-Breuer inflation reflex activity in preterm infants. *American Journal of Respiratory and Critical Care Medicine* 154 (5): 1411–1417.

Stratmann, G., Sall, J.W., Bell, J.S. et al. (2010). Isoflurane does not affect brain cell death, hippocampal neurogenesis, or long-term neurocognitive outcome in aged rats. *Anesthesiology* 112 (2): 305–315.

Sutton, D.G.M., Preston, T., Christley, R.M. et al. (2002). The effects of xylazine, detomidine, acepromazine and butorphanol on equine solid phase gastric emptying rate. *Equine Veterinary Journal* 34 (5): 486–492.

Swink, J.M., Rings, L.M., Snyder, H.A. et al. (2021). Dynamics of androgens in healthy and hospitalized newborn foals. *Journal of Veterinary Internal Medicine* 35 (1): 538–549.

Taylor, S. (2015). A review of equine sepsis. *Equine Veterinary Education* 27 (2): 99–109.

Tennent-Brown, B.S., Morrice, A.V., and Reed, S. (2015). The equine neonatal central nervous system: development and diseases. *Veterinary Clinics of North America. Equine Practice* 31: 587–600.

Theelen, M.J., Wilson, W.D., Edman, J.M. et al. (2014). Temporal trends in in vitro antimicrobial susceptibility patterns of bacteria isolated from foals with sepsis: 1979-2010. *Equine Veterinary Journal* 46 (2): 161–168.

Toombs-Ruane, L.J., Riley, C.B., Kendall, A.T. et al. (2016). Antimicrobial susceptibility of bacteria isolated from neonatal foal samples submitted to a New Zealand veterinary pathology laboratory (2004 to 2013). *New Zealand Veterinary Journal* 64 (2): 107–111.

Toribio, R.E. (2019). Equine neonatal encephalopathy: facts, evidence and opinions. *Veterinary Clinics of North America. Equine Practice* 35: 363–378.

Tranquilli, W.J. and Thurmon, J.C. (1990). Management of anesthesia in the foal. *Veterinary Clinics of North America. Equine Practice* 6 (3): 651–663.

Traub-Dargatz, J.L., Ingram, J.T., Stashak, T.S. et al. (1992). Respiratory stridor associated with polymyopathy suspected to be hyperkalemic periodic paralysis in four quarter horse foals. *Journal of the American Veterinary Medical Association* 201 (1): 85–89.

Vaala, W. (2015). Manifestations and management of disease in foals: distended and/or painful abdomen. In: *Large Animal Internal Medicine*, 5e (ed. G. Lester), 273–278. St. Louis: Elsevier Mosby.

Valverde, A., Giguère, S., Sanchez, L.C. et al. (2006). Effects of dobutamine, norepinephrine, and vasopressin on cardiovascular function in anesthetized neonatal foals with induced hypotension. *American Journal of Veterinary Research* 67 (10): 1730–1737.

Wakuno, A., Aoki, M., Kushiro, A. et al. (2017). Comparison of alfaxalone, ketamine and thiopental for anaesthetic induction and recovery in Thoroughbred horses premedicated with medetomidine and midazolam. *Equine Veterinary Journal* 49 (1): 94–98.

Wassink, G., Davidson, J.O., Dhillon, S.K. et al. (2019). Therapeutic hypothermia in neonatal hypoxic-ischemic encephalopathy. *Current Neurology and Neuroscience Reports* 19 (2): 2.

Weber, E.J., Sanchez, L.C., and Giguère, S. (2015). Re-evaluation of the sepsis score in equine neonates. *Equine Veterinary Journal* 47 (3): 275–278.

Wilkins, P.A. (2003). Lower respiratory problems of the neonate. *The Veterinary Clinics of North America. Equine Practice* 19 (1): 19–33.

Wilkins, P.A. (2018). What's in a word? The need for SIRS and sepsis definitions in equine medicine and surgery. *Equine Veterinary Journal* 50 (1): 7–9.

Wilkins, P.A. and Lascola, K.M. (2015). Update on interstitial pneumonia. *The Veterinary Clinics of North America. Equine Practice* 31 (1): 137–157.

Wilkins, P.A., Otto, C.M., Baumgardner, J.E. et al. (2007). Acute lung injury and acute respiratory distress syndromes in veterinary medicine: consensus definitions: The Dorothy Russell Havemeyer Working Group on ALI and ARDS in Veterinary Medicine. *Journal of Veterinary Emergency and Critical Care* 17 (4): 333–339.

Wong, D.M. and Wilkins, P.A. (2015). Defining the systemic inflammatory response syndrome in equine neonates. *The Veterinary Clinics of North America. Equine Practice* 31 (3): 463–481.

Wong, D., Wilkins, P.A., Bain, F.T. et al. (2011). Neonatal encephalopathy in foals. *Compendium of Continuing Education Veterinary* 33: E5.

Wong, D.M., Ruby, R.E., Dembek, K.A. et al. (2018). Evaluation of updated sepsis scoring systems and systemic inflammatory response syndrome criteria and their association with sepsis in equine neonates. *Journal of Veterinary Internal Medicine* 32 (3): 1185–1193.

Zhou, H., Xie, Z., Brambrink, A.M. et al. (2021). Behavioural impairments after exposure of neonatal mice to propofol are accompanied by reductions in neuronal activity in cortical circuitry. *British Journal of Anesthesia* 126 https://doi.org/10.1016/j.bja.2021.01.017.

Zullian, C., Menozzi, A., Pozzoli, C. et al. (2011). Effects of α2-adrenergic drugs on small intestinal motility in the horse: an in vitro study. *Veterinary Journal* 187 (3): 342–346.

14

Anesthetic Management of Other Domesticated and Non-Domesticated Equids

Sathya Chinnadurai[1] and Nora Matthews[2,3]

[1] *Saint Louis Zoo, 1 Government Drive, Saint Louis, MO, 63110, USA*
[2] *Department of Small Animal Clinical Sciences, College of Veterinary Medicine & Biomedical Sciences, Texas A&M University, 408 Raymond Stotzer Pkwy, College Station, TX, 77845, USA*
[3] *Department of Clinical Sciences, College of Veterinary Medicine, Cornell University, 930 Campus Road, Ithaca, NY, 14853, USA*

Introduction

Animals discussed in this section can fall into four broad categories, domesticated donkeys and mules, domesticated horses, that by nature and training are not able to be handled in a routine manner (rodeo horses), feral horses (mustangs), and truly wild species (e.g. zebra). Working with any of these animals requires a special understand of unique aspects of physiology, pharmacology, and handling that are distinct from other horses.

will freeze until it has had a chance to assess the risk associated with it. Attempts to push or scare the donkey forward (commonly used in horses) are generally unsuccessful; however, time is generally effective. Numerous publications have appeared that discuss differences in pharmacokinetics of anesthetics and analgesics (Coakley et al. 1999; Mealy et al. 2004; Sinclair et al. 2006; Taylor et al. 2008; Matthews and Thiemann 2015), while at the same time, much of the available knowledge on donkeys is from clinical experience and does not come from scientific research.

Domesticated Donkeys and Mules

Previous articles (Matthews et al. 2005) and book chapters (Matthews 2009) have covered some of the differences in physiology, behavior, and pharmacology which exist between donkeys and horses. These species-related differences have numerous implications for anesthetic and analgesic strategies in donkeys. For instance, the donkey's relative lack of flight response contributes to its reputation for stubbornness; when confronted with an unknown and unevaluated obstacle, a donkey

Pre-anesthetic Evaluation and Patient Preparation

Preoperative evaluation of the donkey should be as thorough as it would be for a horse, including an accurate estimate of body weight (Appendix 3: Heart Girth Nomogram, *The Professional Handbook of the Donkey, 4e*, 2008). It is critically important to recognize that normal parameters for temperature, respiratory, and heart rates as well as hematological and biochemical parameters (Appendix 1, *The Professional Handbook of the Donkey, 4e*, 2008) may be significantly different than in horses.

Equine Anesthesia and Co-Existing Disease, First Edition. Stuart Clark-Price and Khursheed Mama.
© 2022 John Wiley & Sons, Inc. Published 2022 by John Wiley & Sons, Inc.

Normal values for adrenocorticotropic hormone (ACTH) and insulin are significantly different for donkeys as compared to horses, while other values (e.g. cortisol) are not different (Dugat et al. 2010). Many normal values for mules have not been established, so caution should be used when interpreting blood work.

Preoperative assessment and treatment of pain should also be diligent; donkeys may not exhibit pain as openly as horses, so severe pain may be present which should be treated prior to anesthesia (Regan et al. 2016). In the author's experience (NM), failure to adequately treat pain preoperatively may lead to cardiovascular decompensation after induction of anesthesia. Appropriate use of non-steroidal anti-inflammatory drugs (NSAID's) are well reviewed in other sources (Grosenbaugh et al. 2011). In general, NSAIDs are very effective in donkeys, but dosing intervals should be shorter as most are metabolized more rapidly in donkeys than in horses. Although some differences between sizes/breeds of donkeys have been documented for analgesics such as phenylbutazone, as well as injectable anesthetics (Matthews et al. 2001), there is really very little information about many other breeds of donkeys throughout the world. Comparative studies of drugs such as tramadol, which has been shown to have low bioavailability in Italian donkeys (Giorgi et al. 2009) might show differences in other breeds. Donkeys are also more likely to be hyperlipemic when stressed or ill; hyperlipemia needs to be treated as early as possible to ensure survival of the patient.

Intravenous Catheterization and Premedication

Jugular catheterization is facilitated by use of good restraint; a donkey or mule should be tied short to an unmovable object. When necessary, restraint with ropes, hobbles, or squeeze gate can be used similar to what might be used with cattle. Donkeys and mules are much less likely to fight restraint (although they will try it out), allowing procedures to be performed with less

trauma to all. An intravenous catheter must be long enough (the author prefers at least 9 cm or more) to penetrate the thicker skin and fascia of the donkey while still remaining within the vein. Although the jugular vein is in the same location as in the horse, it is covered by the cutaneous colli muscle, which is thicker than in the horse (Herman 2009) as well as a fascial layer. This may make it more difficult to visualize the vein, and the catheter may need to be introduced at a slightly different angle compared to the horse. Use of a lidocaine "bleb," placed subcutaneously over the vein, is recommended for increased tolerance to catheter placement. Transdermal lidocaine can be used for donkeys (or mules) which are "needle shy," 20–30 minutes must be allowed for sufficient transdermal absorption to anesthetize the skin.

Choices for sedation and premedication were previously reported (Matthews et al. 2005). Since that publication, an additional report has described the pharmacokinetics of xylazine in mules compared to horses (Latzel 2012). The half-life of xylazine in mules was 15 minutes shorter than in the horse, and the horse dose did not provide sufficient sedation. It is recommended that the dosage of xylazine for mules should be 1.5 times greater than the dosage needed in horses. This is consistent with the authors' experience with sedation of mules, but not required for donkeys. The recent introduction of detomidine oral gel has been found to be very useful for donkeys and mules which are difficult to inject (NM, personal observation); the label dose appears to provide good sedation in donkeys when adequate time (40 minutes) is allowed for absorption.

Induction and Maintenance with Injectable Anesthetics

Numerous drug combinations have been used for induction and maintenance of donkeys and mules with injectable drugs (Matthews et al. 2005). Intermittent boluses of xylazine and ketamine can be used, but may need to be given more frequently than in horses; approximately every 10 minutes, compared to 15–20 minutes in horses particularly for donkeys since they metabolize ketamine more rapidly. One study evaluated various combinations of guaifenesin with xylazine and ketamine (Taylor et al. 2008) and found that GKX (guaifenesin 50 mg/ml, ketamine 2 mg/ml, xylazine 0.5 mg/ml) produced satisfactory anesthesia following premedication with 1.1 mg/kg xylazine. Induction was accomplished by rapid gravity administration of the mixture until the donkey became recumbent, then the infusion was slowed and maintained as indicated by monitoring anesthetic depth (approximately 1.5 ml/kg/h). For larger donkeys and mules, where restraint of the patient during induction might be difficult, a xylazine/ketamine induction can be used, and then the GKX mixture started for maintenance. This mixture can be used when transport of the patient is required.

Thiopental has been described for induction (7 mg/kg intravenous [IV]) and maintenance (8 mg/kg) of anesthesia in donkeys for 100 minutes after premedication with atropine, acepromazine, and xylazine (Emami et al. 2006). Induction and maintenance quality were reported to be good, but recovery was slow; standing time was 92 minutes after anesthesia was concluded. Propofol has been reported for use as an induction agent in donkeys (Matthews et al. 2005). An additional report compared propofol bolus (2 mg/kg) to thiopental bolus (10 mg/kg) after premedication with xylazine (1.0 mg/kg) (Abd-Almaseeh 2008). Induction time was slightly faster and of better quality with thiopental, but recovery was considered to be better with propofol. Apnea was observed with thiopental, but not with propofol. Propofol (1 mg/kg) combined with ketamine (2 mg/kg) and compared to ketamine alone (3 mg/kg) after premedication with xylazine (1.0 mg/kg) has been described (Abass et al. 2007). The combination of ketamine and propofol produced a smoother induction, better muscle relaxation, longer anesthesia time, and smoother recoveries than ketamine alone.

Maintenance with Inhalational Anesthetics, Support, and Monitoring

Maintenance with inhalational anesthesia is recommended for longer procedures (>60 minutes) and for older or sicker patients. Endotracheal intubation can usually be achieved blindly, although it may be slightly more difficult than in horses, due to anatomical differences in the donkey (Herman 2009). Halothane, isoflurane, or sevoflurane can be used; no apparent differences in minimum alveolar concentrations have been noted between horses and donkeys. Heart and respiratory rates, blood pressure, eye signs, and muscle relaxation should all be monitored. Respiratory rates are usually higher in anesthetized donkeys than in horses and respiratory depression seen with isoflurane in horses does not appear to be as great a problem in donkeys, i.e. the "breath-holding" seen in horses during isoflurane anesthesia does not prohibit the use of isoflurane in donkeys.

Blood pressure appears to be the most reliable indicator of depth of anesthesia in donkeys; rapid increase usually indicates the patient is light and likely to move. Blood pressure can be measured indirectly using a cuff or directly using an arterial catheter attached to an aneroid manometer or transducer. Percutaneous placement of the arterial catheter is facilitated by cutting through the skin with a sterile needle before introducing the catheter to prevent "burring" of the catheter by the thick skin and fascia. A branch of the maxillary artery or lateral metatarsal artery is easiest to catheterize, but large auricular arteries are also available. Administration of intravenous fluids (such as lactated Ringer's solution) is recommended at 5–10 ml/kg/h, especially during inhalational anesthesia, to support blood pressure. Appropriate positioning to protect radial and peroneal nerves and padding to prevent myositis is also recommended. Myositis appears to be less of a concern in donkeys than in horses (presumably because of smaller muscle mass), but prevention is still wise (especially in larger draft mules).

Peri-operative Analgesics

Butorphanol (0.02–0.04 mg/kg/h), ketamine (0.4–0.6 mg/kg/h) or lidocaine (1.5 mg/kg/h) can be used to provide intraoperative analgesia when needed, but there is no information specific to the use of these drugs in donkeys compared to horses; clinical judgment must be used. Local blocks (with lidocaine or bupivacaine) can also be used for specific procedures (e.g. pastern arthrodesis, castration) to achieve analgesia. Transdermal fentanyl patches have been used on donkeys and may be effective for some types of pain; however, information specific to analgesia in donkeys is greatly needed. The pharmacokinetics of tramadol have been reported, but no information about efficacy is available (Giorgi et al. 2009). In general, there is a lack of information on the use of analgesics, especially opioids, in the donkey.

Recovery

Donkeys usually recover well from anesthesia, but often take longer to attempt standing than horses. As with horses, attention must be paid to ensure a patent airway; "snoring" noises may indicate partial airway obstruction which can be relieved by straightening the donkey's head and neck or passing a small nasogastric tube into the upper airway. Lack of analgesia can produce a rough recovery, but donkeys are not prone to becoming hysterical in recovery as horses are. Many donkeys will require assistance to stand by lifting on the tail and some may rise hind end first similar to a bovid while others will rise in the same manner as a horse. As might be expected, mules can follow either their donkey or horse lineage when recovering; therefore, it is difficult to predict how an individual animal will rise during recovery.

Local Anesthetic Techniques

Local anesthetic techniques can be beneficial in a modern multi-modal anesthetic approach

(Lamont 2008). Both during general anesthesia and in standing surgical procedures, these techniques can be a valuable addition. Local anesthetic techniques similar to those used in horses will likely be successful; however, minimal research has been performed evaluating most of them.

Epidural Anesthesia

Epidural anesthesia has been described in the donkey (Shoukry et al. 1975). Most common indications include rectal or vaginal prolapse or to treat melanomas in the tail and perineal region, but it can also be used for long-term analgesia after hindlimb surgery or with painful conditions in the hindlimb like septic arthritis. A thorough description of the anatomy of the sacral and coccygeal vertebrae of the donkey is available (Burnham 2002). The first intercoccygeal space in the donkey is narrower than the second and, therefore, the latter is more suited for caudal epidural puncture. The needle can be directed at an angle of 30° from the horizontal and can be introduced into the vertebral canal, because there are no large tail muscles. The spinal processes of the sacral and coccygeal segments are more easily palpated in the donkey compared to the horse (Burnham 2002).

Standing Surgery in Donkeys and Mules

In order to perform standing surgery in donkeys, proper sedation is a first requisite. Sedative and analgesic effects of detomidine have been described in donkeys (Mostafa et al. 1995). Detomidine at 5–10 mcg/kg provides adequate sedation whereas increasing the dosage to 20–40 mcg/kg provides sedation and strong analgesia. While donkeys seem to have similar clinical effects to alpha-2 agonists, mules require approximately 50% more xylazine, compared to donkeys and horses (Matthews et al. 1997). Higher requirements for romifidine were also reported in untamed mules (Alves et al. 1999).

Protocols for standing surgery can be composed of sedatives in constant rate infusions (CRI), combined with systemic opioids and local anesthetic techniques. Protocols used in horses have been used successfully in donkeys as well (Van Dijk et al. 2003). For example, laparoscopic ovariectomy in standing donkeys using xylazine sedation and local infiltration of the laparoscopic portal sides with lidocaine has been described (Aziz et al. 2008). This protocol could also be combined with epidural morphine (0.1 mg/kg) for additional analgesia, a technique that is described for horses (Van Hoogmoed and Galuppo 2005). Adding epidural morphine to this standing anesthesia protocol led to decreased surgical time, improved patient comfort, and reduced the sedation needed to perform ovariectomy.

Feral, Less Domesticated, and Wild Equids

Although, not handled in the conventional horseman's manner, rodeo horses are used to being around humans, wearing halters, are extensively transported and used to standing in cattle chutes (Figure 14.1).

Depending on the equipment available, it is possible to sedate them intramuscularly or intravenously with an alpha-2 agent (e.g. xylazine or detomidine) in a chute. Doses for sedation depend on route of administration and are generally larger than would be used for a more handled horse. One author (NM) has seen and sedated rodeo horses with twice normal doses of xylazine or detomidine; induction is then possible in the chute with IV diazepam-ketamine at normal doses. The horse's head can be controlled during induction with a halter rope and intravenous catheter placed immediately after induction (Figure 14.2).

The horse can then be transported to surgical area using "triple-drip" for maintenance of anesthesia and a horse-slide (or movable table). This process is reversed when surgery is completed; the horse is transported to a recovery area, or pen adjacent to the chute, or stall from which the horse can be returned to handling areas after recovery.

Mustangs and other feral horses, while from a similar lineage as the domestic horse breeds, have not been managed or trained for working and can behave similar to a wild equid. Numerous references exist for darting feral horses with more modern drug combinations (Hampton et al. 2016; Matthews and Myers 1993; Woolnough et al. 2012; Zabek et al. 2014).

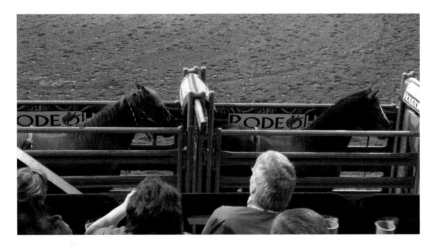

Figure 14.1 Bucking horses standing in chutes.

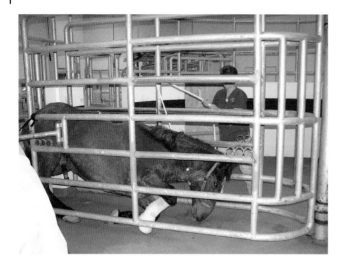

Figure 14.2 A bucking horse being induced in a cattle chute.

Truly wild species, such as zebras, wild asses, and Przewalski's horses, belong to the genus *Equus*, similar to the domestic horse, but do not have a history of domestication by humans and have not been purpose-bred for qualities befitting a working or pleasure horse. Wild equids are only naturally found in Africa (zebra and African wild ass) and Asia (Przewalski's horse and Asiatic wild ass). While the anatomy and physiology of these species is very similar to the domestic horse, there are special safety consideration for handling the animals and the drugs needed for anesthesia. Capture and anesthesia-related morbidity and mortality is inherent with any species, especially with wild animals (Arnemo et al. 2006). Physical or mechanical restraint can be stressful to non-domesticated species, and sedation can reduce stress in the animal and decrease risk of injury to the animal and humans (Cattet et al. 2006). In the case of invasive procedures, restraint without consideration for analgesia may be inappropriate and anesthesia or local analgesia should be used.

Special Logistical and Safety Considerations

Human safety, ease of patient access, and restraint techniques must all be considered when planning to anesthetize non-domestic horses. For these species, a combination of behavioral, physical, mechanical, or chemical restraint may be used. The clinician supervising the procedures should assume responsibility for life and safety of animal and personnel. That clinician will need to have proper facilities, for both chemical and mechanical restraint and understand the tools needed for each type of restraint. The authors advise clinicians to learn from the experiences of others and consult experienced zoo or wildlife veterinarians before getting their initial experience with rare or dangerous species.

As these species are not accustomed to human contact, routine restraint techniques are not usually feasible. Confinement and physical barriers provide protection for the human staff but also limit access to the unsedated animals. It is highly advised to have some form of restraint available (e.g. pen, chute, corral, or movable panels) as horses can travel large distances while becoming sedated. Such physical barriers limit the routes of drug administration to remote or distance injection. Administration of drugs can be achieved by dart or pole syringe. Commercial pole syringes can be either manual or spring-loaded and are useful for short-range delivery of drugs. The practitioner does need to get fairly close to animal, usually within 3–6 ft (1–2 m). These devices can be fairly startling to the animal and

Figure 14.3 A Przewalski's horse with a remotely delivered dart in the hip.

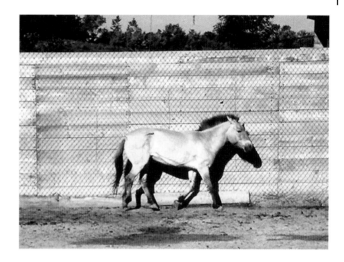

have the potential to be traumatic to both the animal and the clinician. When the practitioner cannot physically enter the same space as the animals, remote projection should be considered (Figure 14.3).

A variety of remote delivery devices can be used. Blowpipes can be very accurate and relatively atraumatic. It is often difficult to penetrate thick equid skin or cover long distances with a blowpipe. Carbon dioxide–powered pistols are useful for short range (0–15 m). Gas- and powder-charged rifles are used for long range (up to 100 m) (Figure 14.4).

Any darting episode has the potential for equipment failure, including broken needles or darts, poor dart charging resulting in partial drug discharge. Insufficient gun charge resulting in the dart not reaching the animal, dropping too much and hitting a target below the intended target or failing to fully penetrate the skin leading to subcutaneous or intradermal discharge can result in failure. Conversely, excessive charge can result in trauma to the animal or excessive recoil and the dart could bounce back out of the animal (Isaza 2014).

Highly regulated compounds, such as ultrapotent opioids and concentrated drug formulations, are often used for non-domestic equids. Human safety concerns are paramount for these drugs and are discussed below. In the US, ultrapotent opioids and compounded concentrated formulations of midazolam, butorphanol, and

Figure 14.4 A feral horse darted in an unrestrained area.

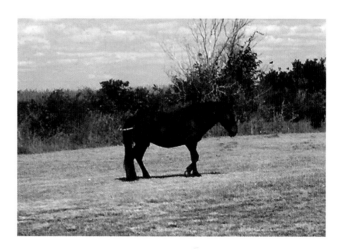

ketamine can only be purchased and used under a special permit and are only available from one supplier (Zoopharm, Wildlife Pharmaceuticals, Ft. Collins, CO). This additional paperwork and licensing may make use of these drugs impractical for most practitioners.

Many long-acting tranquilizers that may be used in zoo species are strictly regulated due to concerns over misuse in performance horses (Baird et al. 2006). Veterinarians looking to purchase and use these drugs must be acutely aware of the risks associated with them and the likely legal ramifications should any of these drugs be detected in a performance horse. Butyrophenones are not commonly available in the United States and must be purchased from compounding pharmacies.

Types of Anesthetic Protocols for Wild and Feral Equids

Examples of anesthetic protocols are listed in Table 14.1. The principal drugs for wild equid anesthesia are the ultrapotent opioids. Etorphine (M99) is the original ultrapotent opioid and was first synthesized in 1963 and used for wild equids since at least 1985 (Plotka et al. 1987). Etorphine has activity at μ-, δ-, and κ- opioid receptors and is 1000–4000 times more potent than morphine. Commonly reported side effects of etorphine are apnea, rigidity, and hypertension. Two other commonly used ultrapotent opioids are carfentanil and thiafentanil (A3080), both are analogs of fentanyl. Carfentanil is 100 times more potent than fentanyl and 10000 times more than morphine. Thiafentanil (A3080) is slightly less potent than carfentanil, with a shorter duration of action. The primary benefit of thiafentanil over carfentanil in non-domestic ruminants is reduced respiratory depression and lower likelihood of renarcotization, though neither drug has been widely evaluated in equids. Carfentanil has been used successfully in Przewalski's horses, with no reported complications (Allen 1992), though multiple reports of unsatisfactory induction with carfentanil in zebra lead to investigation of anesthetic protocols that did not require

ultrapotent opioids (Allen 1992; Klein and Citino 1995).

All ultrapotent opioids are potentially lethal to humans. The drugs can be absorbed via inhalation, injection, broken skin, or through mucous membranes. A single immobilization dose for an animal can contain 10–200 lethal human doses. Personal safety is of the utmost importance, and veterinary staff needs to use proper protective clothing, including long-sleeves and long pants, gloves, and face shields (Figure 14.5). Reversal agents (opioid antagonists) should always be drawn up and ready before handling any ultrapotent opioid.

The opioid antagonists, naloxone and naltrexone, work by competitive antagonism of the opioid receptors. Given alone, these drugs can cause some central nervous system (CNS) stimulation, with minimal cardiovascular effects. Naltrexone has over twice the potency of naloxone. Though naloxone is less potent and has a shorter duration, it is the only drug approved for human use in the case of accidental exposure. As the duration of action of naloxone is shorter than the ultrapotent opioids, renarcotization is possible. One should remember that when opioid sedation is reversed, opioid-induced analgesia is also reversed. To reverse etorphine, 25 mg of naltrexone for every 1 mg of etorphine can be used.

Supplemental drugs, such as tranquilizers and muscle relaxants, are often used in conjunction with opioids. These combination protocols may improve muscle relaxation and reduce the amount of opioid needed for anesthesia. Acepromazine or alpha-2 agonists, such as xylazine and detomidine, are easily available and commonly used in combination with ultrapotent opioids. Alpha-2 agonist/dissociative combinations are among the most common induction protocols for domestic horses and can also be utilized with wild horses, especially when access to etorphine is difficult or deemed too high of a risk (Woolnough et al. 2012). Medetomidine and ketamine induction with atipamezole reversal has been used successfully

Table 14.1 Examples of anesthetic protocols for wild equids.

Type of protocol	Induction agents	Reversal agents	Species	Comments	Reference
Ultrapotent opioid combination	Detomidine (0.08 mg/kg) followed by induction with: Midazolam (0.05 mg/kg) Ketamine (0.5 mg/kg) Etorphine (0.015 mg/kg)	Naltrexone	Zebra		Authors' unpublished data
	Etorphine (0.018 mg/kg) Acepromazine (0.075 mg/kg) and xylazine (0.16 mg/kg)	0.045 mg/kg diprenorphine	Przewalski's horse		Walzer 2014
	Carfentanil (0.02 mg/kg)	Naltrexone 1.0 mg/kg	Przewalski's horse	No renarcotization reported	Allen 1992
Alpha-2/dissociative combinations	Medetomidine (0.07–0.1 mg/kg) Ketamine (1.8–2.6 mg/kg)	Atipamezole (0.2 mg/kg)	Przewalski's horse	Insufficient in 3/14 animals	Matthews et al. 2010
Standing sedation	Detomidine (0.1 mg/kg) followed 10 minutes later by butorphanol (0.13 mg/kg)		Zebra	Can be supplemented with etorphine for recumbency	Hoyer et al. 2012

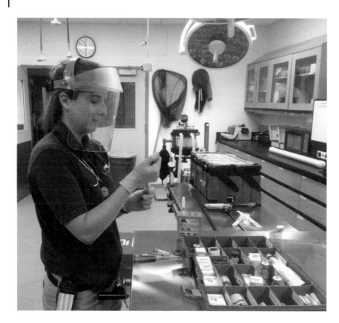

Figure 14.5 Proper handling of ultrapotent opioids while preparing a dart.

in Przewalski's horses. This combination resulted in rapid induction and recovery in most horses studied though 3/11 horses did not become sufficiently anesthetized for examination and hoof trimming (Matthews et al. 2010). Similarly, combinations of medetomidine with tiletamine and zolazepam have provided satisfactory inductions and recoveries for feral horses in a field setting (Zabek et al. 2014).

Standing sedation has been described in Grevy's zebras. Remote administration of detomidine (0.1 mg/kg) and followed 10 minutes later by butorphanol (0.13 mg/kg) has produced heavy standing sedation in both Grevy's and Burchell's zebra. In this study, animals that needed additional supplementation were provided etorphine and acepromazine (Hoyer et al. 2012). It should be noted that standing sedation does put the staff of increased risk of injury if the animal becomes reactive. When performed safely, standing sedation may reduce the risk of myopathy and maintains the animal's body in a more appropriate physiologic position for normal ventilation.

Historically, neuromuscular blockade has been used as a sole immobilization agent in wild and feral horses (Berger et al. 1983). Drugs such as succinylcholine can provide rapid immobilization, but are not appropriate as sole agent for painful or stressful procedures. As such, the authors cannot recommend these drugs in this chapter. Use of succinylcholine as a sole agent for painful procedures, such as castration is considered unethical and should be universally discouraged. While the immobilization technique has been used extensively for decades with non-domestic equids, the potential adverse effects on animal welfare make this technique outmoded and it has been effectively replaced with sedation and anesthesia.

Long-acting neuroleptic drugs, such as butyrophenone and phenothiazine tranquilizers, have been widely used to facilitate transport and housing of equids (Walzer 2014). Shorter acting butyrophenones, such as azaperone may last four to six hours, while longer acting formulations, such as the decanoate formulation of haloperidol may last up to three weeks (Ebedes and Raath 1999; Read 2002). Extrapyramidal side effects have been reported in equids, especially with long-acting phenothiazines, such as fluphenazine (Baird et al. 2006; Brewer et al. 1990; Kauffman et al. 1989). Clinical signs of overdose include muscle rigidity, Parkinsonian-like tremoring, and pacing, wandering, excitability, dystonia (abnormal face and body movement), and tardive dyskinesia (involuntary rhythmic movement of tongue, face, and jaw). Neither butyrophenones nor phenothiazines are reversible and treatment of these untoward side effects is symptomatic (Read 2002). Given the extended duration of action of some formulations, these side effects can last weeks and are potentially life-threatening.

Planning the Anesthetic Episode

The anesthetic protocol design needs to account for the animal, type of restraint, and the intended procedure (including degree and duration of pain) as well as the environmental conditions at the capture and work sites. Many non-domesticated equids can be flighty and the stress of confinement and separation from the herd or surprise of a dart injection can result in self-trauma, collisions, fracture, or myopathy. The anesthetist must be able to safely deliver the chosen drug combination in the field situation. In many situations, remote delivery of drugs to an unrestrained animal is faster and less stressful to the animal than physical restraint (Cattet et al. 2003, 2006; Hampton et al. 2016). Extended chasing or long restraint

can cause increases in lactate and increase risk of self-injury. Terrain and capture conditions play an important role if an anesthetic protocol involves a slow induction or recovery. A slow induction protocol increases the chance of over-exertion and myopathy as well as increasing the likelihood of escape or injury from environmental hazards (Arnemo et al. 2006). Environmental conditions such as heat, cold, rain, wind, and snow can contribute to hypothermia or hyperthermia associated with capture and the procedure. Performing general anesthesia in the field may be technically challenging when equipment designed for a single location, e.g. hospital use, must be modified for use in remote locations with limited access to electrical power and oxygen. There is the additional challenge of having sufficient supplies transported to and stored at a field site (Chinnadurai et al. 2016). Capture and anesthesia-related morbidity and mortality may occur with field immobilizations, regardless of anesthetic protocols (Arnemo et al. 2006; DelGiudice et al. 2005). Within a zoo setting, procedures performed in a stall or enclosed space may allow for more extensive monitoring of an animal's vital parameters (Figure 14.6). Additionally, anesthetic recovery in an enclosed padded stall will allow for observation during the recovery period (Figure 14.7).

Figure 14.6 Evaluating an anesthetized zebra in a padded stall. The zebra is ventilated with a demand valve and vital parameters are monitored with capnography, pulse oximetry, electrocardiogram, and non-invasive blood pressure measurements.

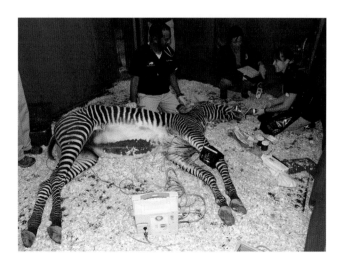

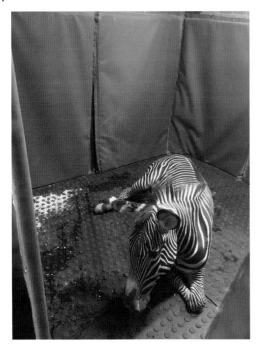

Figure 14.7 A zebra stallion recovering from anesthesia unassisted in a padded recovery stall.

Behavior of the individual species and animal will affect the logistics of the procedures. As a prey species, equids will react to an approaching threat. That flight distance varies by species and for the individual animal. Visual barriers may decrease flight distance and allow the darter closer access to the animals. With training and acclimation, an animal's comfort with human handler can increase, allowing closer access. When the individual's flight distance is violated, the animal may choose to flee, potentially with reckless abandon.

Anesthetic Consequences and Complications

Opioid side effects in animals can include excitement, aimless wandering, myopathy, respiratory depression, hypertension, bradycardia, muscle rigidity, and renarcotization. Renarcotization is recurrence of sedation after apparent recovery and can occur when the duration of action of reversal is shorter than the opioid agonist. Renarcotization has been reported after reversing etorphine or carfentanil with naltrexone in equids (Allen 1992, 1990). When the animal is anesthetized in a captive setting, a second dose of reversal agent can be administered. Chances of renarcotization could be lowered by using shorter acting opioids or reducing dose of opioid needed by adding an alpha-2 agonist or ketamine.

When working in a field setting, there is the risk of injury, especially fractures associated with turbulent inductions and a recoveries without the benefit of a confined space such as a recovery stall. Outdoor captures carry the risk of drowning and hypothermia or hyperthermia, depending on ambient conditions. Remote drug delivery equipment such as dart projectors carry intrinsic risk of injury to the animal. Such devices should only be used by trained personnel familiar with the terrain and species at hand.

Exertional myopathy can occur due to rapid changes in perfusion and tissue pH with exertion or restraint. Metabolic disturbances result from hyperlactatemia and myolysis with rapid release of intracellular potassium. Factors such as stress, hyperthermia, use of ultrapotent opioids, and hypoperfusion have been implicated. Exertional myopathy is described in terms of distinct forms or syndromes. The peracute form will present as shock or sudden death, often with no gross lesions. The most commonly recognized form is acute and can occur shortly after or during recovery and is initially characterized by ataxia. This condition may progress in the hours to days after the immobilization, and the animal may develop myoglobinuria secondary to myolysis. Animals with myoglobinuria may succumb to acute renal failure, due to pigment nephropathy. Treatment consists of fluid diuresis, diligent monitoring, and correction of electrolyte disorders and analgesia. Anti-inflammatories, antioxidants, and muscle relaxants may limit further damage (Arnemo et al. 2006; Paterson 2014).

One must also consider social factors, such as herd reintegration. When removing an animal from the herd or band of horses that it is part of, there is a risk of failure to reintegrate that animal back into the group. This could be due to frightening of the group during the capture of the target individual as well as delayed recovery and residual sedation or ataxia which might impart the anesthetized individual from being successfully reintegrated. In some wild horses, disruption of the herd structure can lead to poor reproductive success over time (Berger et al. 1983).

Many of the anesthetic protocols utilized in domestic horses for field anesthesia and monitoring can be modified for less tractable equids, though the handling and drug delivery techniques can be quite different (Walzer 2014). When choosing a method of capture or restraint, pain, animal stress, and both human and animal safety must be considered. It is essential that the veterinarian evaluate all aspects of the protocol, including species, terrain, and capture and restraint methodology, to minimize animal risk.

References

Abass, B.T., Al-Hyani, O.H., and Al-Jobory, A.K.H. (2007). Anesthesia in xylazine premedicated donkeys with ketamine and ketamine-propofol mixture: a comparative study. *Iraqi Journal of Veterinary Sciences* 21: 117–123.

Abd-Almaseeh, Z.T. (2008). Comparative anesthetic protocols: propofol and thiopental in xylazine premedicated donkeys. *Journal of Animal and Veterinary Advances* 7: 1563–1567.

Allen, J.L. (1990). Renarcotization following etorphine immobilization of nondomestic equidae. *Journal of Zoo and Wildlife Medicine* 21 (3): 292–294.

Allen, J.L. (1992). Immobilization of Mongolian wild horses (*Equus przewalskii przewalskii*) with carfentanil and antagonism with naltrexone. *Journal of Zoo and Wildlife Medicine* 23 (234): 422–425.

Alves, G.E.S., Faleiros, R.R., Gheller, V.A., and Vieria, M.M. (1999). Sedative effect of romifidine in untamed mules. *Ciência Rural* 29: 51–55.

Arnemo, J.M., Ahlqvist, P., Andersen, R. et al. (2006). Risk of capture-related mortality in large free-ranging mammals: experiences from Scandinavia. *Wildlife Biology* 12 (1): 109–113.

Aziz, D.M., Al-Badrany, M.S., and Taha, M.B. (2008). Laparoscopic ovariectomy in standing donkeys by using a new instrument. *Animal Reproduction Science* 107: 107–114.

Baird, J., Arroyo, L., and Vengust, M. (2006). Adverse extrapyramidal effects in four horse given fluphenazine decanoate. *Journal of the American Veterinary Medical Association* 229 (1): 104–110.

Berger, J., Kock, M., Cunnigham, C. et al. (1983). Chemical restraint of wild horses: effects on reproduction and social structure. *Journal of Wildlife Diseases* 19 (3): 265–268.

Brewer, B., Hines, M., and Stewart, J. (1990). Fluphenazine induced Parkinson-like syndrome in a horse. *Equine Veterinary Journal* 22 (2): 136–137.

Burnham, S.L. (2002). Anatomical differences of the donkey and mule. *AAEP Proceedings* 48: 102–109.

Cattet, M.R., Christison, K., Caulkett, N.A., and Stenhouse, G.B. (2003). Physiologic responses of grizzly bears to different methods of capture. *Journal of Wildlife Diseases* 39 (3): 649–654.

Cattet, M.R.L., Bourque, A., Elkin, B.T. et al. (2006). Evaluation of the potential for injury with remote drug-delivery systems. *Wildlife Society Bulletin* 34 (3): 741–749.

Chinnadurai, S.K., Strahl-Heldreth, D., Fiorello, C.V., and Harms, C.A. (2016). Best-practice guidelines for field-based surgery and anesthesia of free-ranging wildlife. I. Anesthesia and analgesia. *Journal of Wildlife Diseases* 52 (2s): S14–S27.

Coakley, M., Peck, K.E., Taylor, T.S. et al. (1999). Pharmacokinetics of flunixin meglumine in donkeys, mules and horses. *American Journal of Veterinary Research* 60: 1441–1444.

DelGiudice, G.D., Sampson, B.A., Kuehn, D.W. et al. (2005). Understanding margins of safe capture, chemical immobilization, and handling of free-ranging white-tailed deer. *Wildlife Society Bulletin* 33 (2): 677–687.

Dugat, S.L., Taylor, T.S., Matthews, N.S., and Gold, J.R. (2010). Values for triglycerides, insulin, cortisol, and ACTH in a herd of normal donkeys. *Journal of Equine Veterinary Science* 30: 141–144.

Ebedes, H. and Raath, J. (1999). Use of tranquilizers in wild herbivores. In: *Zoo & Wild Animal Medicine Current Therapy*, 4e (eds. M. Fowler and E. Miller), 575–584. Philadelphia, PA: Saunders Publishing.

Emami, M.R., Seifi, H., and Tavakoli, Z. (2006). Effects of totally intravenous thiopental anesthesia on cardiopulmonary and thermoregulatory system in donkeys. *Journal of Applied Animal Research* 29: 13–16.

Giorgi, M., Del Carlo, S., Sgorbini, M., and Saccomanni, G. (2009). Pharmacokinetics of tramadol and its metabolites M1, M2 and M5 in donkeys after intravenous and oral immediate release single-dose administration. *Journal of Equine Veterinary Science* 29: 569–574.

Grosenbaugh, D.A., Reinemeyer, C.R., and Figueiredo, M.D. (2011). Pharmacology and therapeutics in donkeys. *Equine Veterinary Education* 23 (10): 523–530.

Hampton, J.O., Robertson, H., Adams, P.J. et al. (2016). An animal welfare assessment framework for helicopter darting; a case study with a newly developed method for feral horses. *Wildlife Research* 43: 429–437.

Herman, C.L. (2009). The anatomical differences between the donkey and the horse. In: *Veterinary Care of Donkeys* (eds. N.S. Matthews and T.S. Taylor) www.ivis.org. https://www.ivis.org/library/veterinary-care-of-donkeys/anatomical-differences-between-donkey-and-horse.

Hoyer, M., de Jong, S., Verstappen, F., and Wolters, M. (2012). Standing sedation in captive zebra (*Equus grevyi* and *Equus burchellii*). *Journal of Zoo and Wildlife Medicine* 43 (1): 10–14.

Isaza, R. (2014). Remote drug delivery. In: *Zoo Animal and Wildlife Immobilization and Anesthesia*, 2e (eds. G. West, D. Heard and N. Caulkett), 155–169. Ames, IA: Wiley.

Kauffman, V., Soma, L., and Divers, T. (1989). Extrapyramidal side effects caused by fluphenazine decanoate in a horse. *Journal of the American Veterinary Medical Association* 195 (8): 1128–1130.

Klein, L. and Citino, S.S.B. (1995). Comparison of Detomidine/Carfentanil/Ketamine and Medetomidine/Ketamine Anesthesia in Grevy's Zebra. In: *Proceedings AAZV/WDA/AAWV Joint Conference*, 257–261.

Lamont, L.A. (2008). Multimodal pain management in veterinary medicine: the physiologic basis of pharmacologic therapies. *Veterinary Clinics of North America: Small Animal Practice* 38: 1173–1186.

Latzel, S.T. (2012). Subspecies studies: pharmacokinetics and pharmacodynamics of a single intravenous dose of xylazine in adult mules and adult Haflinger horses. *Journal of Equine Veterinary Science* 32 (12): 816–826.

Matthews, N.S. (2009). Anesthesia and analgesia for donkeys and mules. In: *Equine Anesthesia*, 2e (eds. W.W. Muir and J.A.E. Hubbell), 353–357. St. Louis, MO: Saunders Elsevier.

Matthews, N.S. and Myers, M.M. (1993). The use of tiletaine-zolazepam for darting feral horses. *Journal of Equine Veterinary Science* 13 (5): 264–267.

Matthews, N.S. and Thiemann, A.K. (2015). Appendix 2. Table of common drugs and approximate dosages for use in donkeys. In: *Robinson's Current Therapy in Equine Medicine*, 7e (eds. K.A. Sprayberry and N.E. Robinson), 949–953. St. Louis, MO: Elsevier Saunders.

Matthews, N.S., Taylor, T.S., and Hartsfield, S.M. (1997). Anaesthesia of donkeys and mules. *Equine Veterinary Education* **9**: 198–202.

Matthews, N.S., Peck, K.E., Taylor, T.S. et al. (2001). Pharmacokinetics of phenylbutazone and its major metabolite, oxyphenbutazone in miniature donkeys. *American Journal of Veterinary Research* 62: 673–675.

Matthews, N.S., Taylor, T.S., and Hartsfield, S.M. (2005). Anaesthesia of donkeys and mules. *Equine Veterinary Education* 7: 102–107.

Matthews, N.S., Petrini, K.R., and Wolff, P.L. (2010). Anesthesia of Przewalski's horses (*Equus przewalskii przewalskii*) with medetomidine/ketamine and antagonism with atipamezole. *Journal of Zoo and Wildlife Medicine* 26 (2): 231–236.

Mealy, K.L., Matthews, N.S., Peck, K.E. et al. (2004). Pharmacokinetics of R(−) and S(+) carprofen after administration of racemic carprofen in donkeys and horses. *American Journal of Veterinary Research* 65: 1479–1482.

Mostafa, M.B., Farag, K.A., Zomor, E., and Bashandy, M.M. (1995). The sedative and analgesic effects of detomidine (domosedan) in donkeys. *Journal of Veterinary Medicine A* 42: 351–356.

Paterson, J. (2014). Capture myopathy. In: *Zoo Animal and Wildlife Immobilization and Anesthesia*, 2e (eds. G. West, D. Heard and N. Caulkett), 171–179. Ames, IA: Wiley.

Plotka, E.D., Seal, U.S., Eagle, T.C. et al. (1987). Rapid reversible immobilization of feral stallions using etorphine hydrochloride, xylazine hydrochloride and atropine sulfate. *Journal of Wildlife Diseases* 23 (3): 471–478.

Read, M. (2002). Long acting neuroleptic drugs. International Veterinary Information Service. http://www.ivis.org/special_books/Heard/read/reference.asp. Retrieved September 2017

Regan, F.H., Hockenhull, J.C., Pritchard, J.C. et al. (2016). Identifying behavioral differences in working donkeys in response to analgesic administration. *Equine Veterinary Journal* 48: 33–38.

Shoukry, M., Seleh, M., and Fouad, K. (1975). Epidural anaesthesia in donkeys. *Veterinary Record* 97: 450–452.

Sinclair, M.D., Mealy, K.L., Matthews, N.S. et al. (2006). Comparative pharmacokinetics of meloxicam in clinically normal horses and donkeys. *American Journal of Veterinary Research* 67: 1082–1085.

Taylor, E.V., Baetge, C.L., Matthews, N.S. et al. (2008). Guaifenesin-ketamine-xylazine infusions to provide anesthesia in donkeys. *Journal of Equine Veterinary Science* 28: 295–300.

Van Dijk, P., Lankveld, D.P.K., Rijkenhuizen, A.B.M., and Jonker, F.H. (2003). Hormonal, metabolic and physiological effects of laparoscopic surgery using a detomidine-buprenorphine combination in standing horses. *Veterinary Anaesthesia and Analgesia* 30: 71–79.

Van Hoogmoed, L.M. and Galuppo, L.D. (2005). Laparoscopic ovariectomy using the endo-GI stapling device and endo-catch pouches and evaluation of analgesic efficacy of epidural morphine sulfate in 10 mares. *Veterinary Surgery* 34: 646–650.

Walzer, C. (2014). Non-domestic equids. In: *Zoo Animal and Wildlife Immobilization and Anesthesia*, 2e (eds. G. West, D. Heard and N. Caulkett), 523–531. Ames, IA: Wiley.

Woolnough, A.P., Hampton, J.O., Campbell, S. et al. (2012). Field immobilization of feral 'judas' donkeys (*Equus asinus*) by remote injection of medetomidine and ketamine and antagonism with atipamezole. *Journal of Wildlife Diseases* 48 (2): 435–443.

Zabek, M.A., Wright, J., Berman, D.M. et al. (2014). Assessing the efficacy of medetomidine and tiletamine-zolazepam for remote immobilization of feral horses (*Equus caballus*). *Wildlife Research* 41: 615–622.

15

Accident and Error Management
Daniel Pang

Department of Veterinary Clinical and Diagnostic Sciences, Faculty of Veterinary Medicine, University of Calgary, 3280 Hospital Drive NW, Calgary, Alberta, T2N 4Z6, Canada

Introduction

Errors, and their potential to lead to an adverse event, are common (see Table 15.1 for terminology). They have been described as part of the human condition, reflecting a normal aspect of cognitive function (Allnutt 2002; Reason 2008). If we accept that errors can occur in any system in which humans participate, we can consider how to create safer systems and organizations.

Awareness of error in human medicine received widespread attention with the publication of the Institute of Medicine's report "To Err is Human: Building a Safer Health System" (Kohn et al. 2000). This report marked a shift away from a culture of blame, moving from a focus on individual contributions to errors toward improving the systems in which humans work. To put it simply, systems should be designed "that make it hard for people to do the wrong thing and easy for people to do the right thing" (Kohn et al. 2000). Anesthesiologists were at the forefront of this shift in attitude in medicine, embracing a systems approach to preventing errors (Cooper et al. 1984, 2002). Such systems approaches were originally developed to minimize errors in complex organizations with the potential for catastrophic failures, such as the nuclear power and aviation industries. Similarities have been drawn between the roles of anesthetists and airline pilots: both groups are faced with an array of complex equipment, providing large quantities of information in real time, upon which decisions are made that are often time sensitive and under pressure (Allnutt 2002; Gaba et al. 2003; Ludders and McMillan 2017; Reason 2008). Some authors go further, proposing that managing anesthesia is more complex because of the additional dynamics of a patient (variable clinical presentations and inherent biological variability) and frequent requirement to perform simultaneous teaching and organizational tasks (Helmreich 2000; Reason 2008).

This chapter begins with an overview of error theory. It will compare traditional and current approaches to understanding the circumstances that lead to adverse events. This foundation forms the basis of a structured approach to adverse event analysis and prevention, with the goal of helping readers improve the systems in which they work. Finally, case examples from equine anesthesia are used to illustrate how accidents happen alongside strategies of how to deal with the consequences. While adverse events can have a considerable emotional and physical impact on patients and personnel, it is important to

Table 15.1 Definition of terms used in this chapter.

Term	Definition
Active failures	Unsafe acts: includes errors and violations (deliberate deviations from standard practice).
Adverse event (adverse incident, harmful incident, accident)	An action or event that caused harm to a patient (or personnel). Harm is variably defined but often recognized as changing the course of patient management, prolonged hospital stay, long-term disability, or death.
Error	Performance or activity that fails to achieve the intended outcome. Errors may be further classified as skill-based, decision-based, or perceptual-based.
Error wisdom	The ability of people on the frontline to recognize situations in which an error is likely.
High-reliability organization (HRO)	Organizations defined by the characteristics of successfully managing complex technologies under time pressure and to a high standard; achieved with a very low incidence of failure. Such organizations are alert to the possibility and prevention of failure. Prototypical examples are air traffic control, nuclear power plants, and aircraft carriers.
Human Factors Analysis and Classification System (HFACS)	An accident or adverse event investigation tool originally developed for the aviation industry. It is based on Reason's Swiss cheese accident model.
Patient safety incident	An event that could have resulted, or did result, in unnecessary harm.
Latent conditions	Factors within a system that may predispose an adverse event (e.g. work culture supporting dangerous practices, inadequate supervision of trainees, poorly functioning equipment).
Near miss incident	An incident (deviation from standard care) that did not result in harm to patient (or personnel) as a result of timely intervention or chance.

References: Ludders and McMillan (2017), Reason (2000, 2008), Runciman et al. (2009), and Wiegmann and Shappell (2005).

appreciate that the large majority of errors that result in an adverse event are preventable (Arbous et al. 2001; Cooper et al. 1984; Gibbs et al. 2017; Kohn et al. 2000; Macintosh 1949). This gives hope that the current situation can be improved through discussion, analysis, and learning from our errors.

Anesthetic Mortality and Error

A recent systematic review and meta-analysis showed significant and important decreases in peri-operative human anesthesia-related mortality internationally over the last five decades, despite an increase in baseline American Society of Anesthesiologists (ASA) status (Bainbridge et al. 2012). Mortality solely attributed to anesthesia has decreased 10-fold to around 3.4 per 100 000. Nevertheless, it has been estimated that over 70% of anesthesia-related deaths are preventable (Arbous et al. 2001; Cooper et al. 1984). In contrast to the relatively low incidence of anesthesia-related death, the incidence of adverse events in human medicine is as high as 4% in hospitalized patients, with the majority being associated with human error (Cooper et al. 1984; Gawande et al. 1999; Kohn et al. 2000). The veterinary literature regarding adverse events and near misses is extremely limited, with one study documenting a rate of 3.6% (n = 74/2028 anesthetized patients) in a university hospital anesthesia service (Hofmeister et al. 2014). Promisingly, this was reduced to 1.4% following changes in practice. A recent study of errors and adverse events (not limited to anesthesia) from two university hospitals (large and small animal) and a private referral and emergency hospital, found a 15% incidence of adverse events (n = 560 incident reports analyzed) (Wallis et al. 2019).

In addition to errors themselves, the complexity of anesthesia provision can magnify the consequences of errors. Administering anesthesia requires numerous interactions between anesthetist, patient, personnel, and equipment (Gaba et al. 1987; Reason 2005; Sutcliffe 2011). When these interactions are "loosely" coupled, change in one component has slow or minimal effects on its connecting component (e.g. a misunderstanding between services in case scheduling). Conversely, "tight" coupling allows little margin for error so that change in one component has a rapid or major impact on another (e.g. the rapid and potentially disastrous consequences of an unobserved breathing system disconnection) (Gaba et al. 1987). Furthermore, the complexity of interactions in complex systems can make it difficult to predict effects and outcome of changes between different components of a system. Extending the example of case scheduling, the time to clarify and reorganize case order for one service may lead to the late start of a higher risk case for another service so that case ends after hours, when key resources (experienced anesthesia and post-operative care personnel) may be limited.

Peri-operative Morbidity and Mortality in Horses

The occurrences of adverse events have been acknowledged in equine anesthesia and identified as an important area for development (Hartnack et al. 2013; Johnston et al. 2002). The Confidential Enquiry into Perioperative Equine Fatalities (CEPEF), a prospective observational epidemiological multi-center study, found a 7-day post-anesthesia mortality rate of 0.9% (out of 35 435 non-colic surgeries, 95% confidence interval 0.8–1.0%) (Johnston et al. 2002). Although the incidence of adverse events in equine anesthesia (other than

mortality) is unknown, Johnston et al. (2002) identified several factors in which error could play a role. These include time of day (odds ratio for midnight to 6 a.m. of 7.6; 95% confidence interval (CI) 2.2–26.7, odds ratio for 6 p.m. to midnight of 2.2; 95%CI 1.3–3.5) and day of the week (odds ratio of weekend of 1.5; 95%CI 1.0–2.3). The study suggested that fatigue and staffing levels could contribute to the risk associated with out-of-hours procedures (see the discussion on unsafe acts in the following text).

Error Theory

The likelihood of errors and possibility that they result in adverse events is predicated on two fundamental principles: (i) humans are error-prone, and (ii) conditions within the systems in which humans work often increase the risk of errors. These principles underlie current anesthesia (and aviation) safety literature. By understanding these two principles, we are better able to recognize how and why errors occur and develop strategies for their prevention (Allnutt 2002; Reason 2000, 2005, 2008).

Error Analysis

There are three broad approaches to understanding, analyzing, and preventing errors: (i) person-based approach, (ii) systems-based approach, or (iii) a combined approach (Reason 2000, 2008).

Person-Based Approach

This is the traditional and current model in the majority of veterinary clinics and hospitals, in which the search for the cause of an adverse event begins and ends with the person closest to the event. This is rational in the sense that within complex systems, such as anesthesia, human error accounts for the majority (>70%) of adverse events or near misses (Arbous et al. 2001; Cooper et al. 1984, 2002). The usual outcomes of this approach are to "blame and train" (to blame the individual and enforce additional training) or to "blame and shame" (Pang et al. 2018; Wiegmann and Shappell 2005). This approach conveniently ignores that errors are often made by highly trained, well-intentioned individuals, and fails to account for system and organizational influences that predispose the final act of human error (Allnutt 2002; Reason 2000, 2005, 2008; Wiegmann and Shappell 2005). As described by Ludders and Macmillan, the human is "the final common pathway for an error, thrust there by a flawed system" (Ludders and McMillan 2017).

Human error is unavoidable; it is therefore better to accept the fallibility of humans and act to minimize the factors that contribute to errors occurring, or the severity of their consequences (Allnutt 2002; Kohn et al. 2000; Reason 2000). Focusing on human error and blame has been likened to swatting mosquitoes: they can be swatted individually (and doing so may be satisfying) but is an ineffective long-term strategy. To eliminate mosquitoes, their source, the swamp, must be drained. In this analogy, the swamp represents the conditions within a system ("latent conditions," see below) that predispose it to error and draining it the act of identifying and removing these conditions (Reason 2005). Furthermore, allocating resources to control individuals (additional training, stricter rules and guidelines, etc.) is only successful when the individuals concerned are performing below the expected standard (those particularly error-prone, inexperienced, unmotivated, or badly trained) (Reason 2005). In recognizing this, it is logical to allocate resources to improving the system, an approach that yields long-term improvements.

Systems-Based Approach

Developed and successfully implemented by the nuclear power and aviation industries, systems-based approaches encompass humans (and their errors) alongside the systems in which they work (Allnutt 2002; Cooper et al. 1984, 2002; Kohn et al. 2000; Reason 2000). This holistic approach recognizes and accounts for human error but, more importantly, places these errors in the context of underlying systems factors, called latent conditions, that contribute to the frequency, likelihood, and consequences of error. Latent conditions comprise organizational influences, unsafe supervision, and preconditions for unsafe acts.

This is not to say that all responsibility for error lies with the "system," absolving humans of all responsibility (Reason 2008; Wiegmann and Shappell 2005). Reviewing the processes by which errors occur reveals that personal responsibility and error wisdom have a role to play. A more nuanced position is to recognize that while humans are central to the commission of errors, they are also critical in the prevention of errors or recovery from errors (Reason 2008).

The ability of humans to react and adapt is a valued characteristic and a defining feature of high-reliability organizations (HROs). This is exemplified by situations in which humans compensate successfully during complex technical procedures with a high risk of errors. Notably, study of such procedures, such as pediatric cardiac surgery, has also revealed that there is a limited ability to compensate for errors, even those that are minor i.e. resilience to error is limited (Carthey et al. 2003; De Leval et al. 2000; Reason 2000, 2008). Monitoring of human efforts is important, not only to identify unsafe acts and their underlying causes, but also to identify if humans are compensating unnecessarily for a flawed system.

Combining Person- and Systems-Based Approaches

Current frameworks for the study of errors and accidents strive for a balance between systems and person models. In anesthesia, these frameworks are based on the understanding that unsafe acts come from people in contact with a patient, but that local and organizational factors create the conditions for errors.

James Reason, a psychologist whose work is synonymous with the study of organizational safety, developed the Swiss cheese model of accidents (Reason 2008). Through its various iterations, it has become the most influential accident model in use (Figure 15.1) (Reason 2000, 2005, 2008). Reason's Swiss cheese model describes barriers, defenses, and safeguards through which an accident trajectory may penetrate to cause an adverse event. Each defensive layer represents a different factor within the system: organizational influences, unsafe supervision, preconditions for unsafe acts, and unsafe acts. Ideally, each layer would be solid, devoid of weaknesses; however, this does not reflect the reality of complex systems such as anesthesia. When enough weaknesses (holes) align, a series of events, which may be minor or innocuous when considered alone, culminate in an adverse event. These holes are usually dynamic; emerging, disappearing, and shifting as individual factors change, and are classified as latent conditions or active failures. Latent conditions are resident within a system, in place because of design or organizational decisions. They are usually in place for some time and can sometimes, but not always, be identified before they contribute to an adverse event. In contrast, active failures are unsafe acts, committed by a person and usually representing the tipping point that leads directly to an adverse event.

Most adverse events result from a combination of latent conditions and active failures.

Human Factors Analysis and Classification System

Building on Reason's Swiss cheese model, the Human Factors Analysis and Classification System (HFACS) was developed to define the holes within the model layers, with the goal of aiding accident investigation (Wiegmann and Shappell 2005). As such, the HFACS is a framework for analysis and investigation, comprising of four broad categories representing latent conditions and active failures (Figure 15.2) (Diller et al. 2014; Wiegmann and Shappell 2005). The HFACS should be viewed as an aid to facilitate a complete exploration of factors contributing to adverse events, rather than an exhaustive list. The HFACS is presented here in the order in which it would be applied during an adverse event investigation, i.e. beginning with the action most closely associated with the event, usually an unsafe act, and working through each level in turn, up to organizational influences.

Unsafe Acts

Unsafe acts have been variably categorized as slips, lapses, mistakes, errors (skill-based, decision and perceptual), and violations

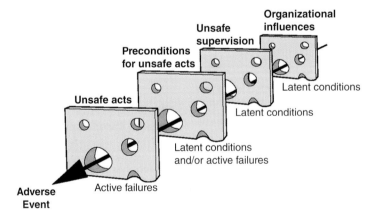

Figure 15.1 The Swiss cheese model describing barriers, defenses, and safeguards through which an accident trajectory must pass through to cause an adverse event. *Note:* not all layers (of cheese) need to be involved for an adverse event to occur.

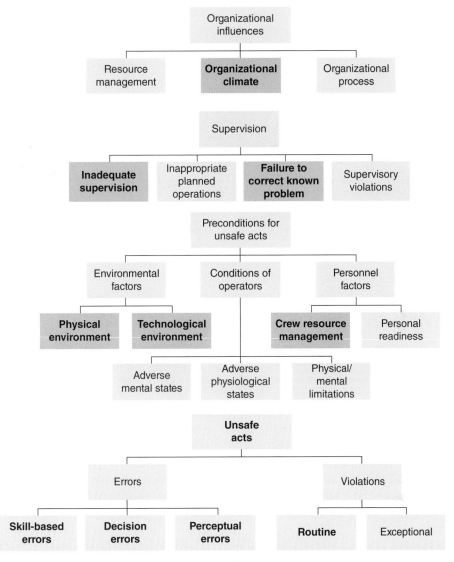

Figure 15.2 The Human Factors Analysis and Classification System (HFACS) for aiding accident investigation.

(Diller et al. 2014; Elbardissi et al. 2007; Reason 2005, 2008; Wiegmann and Shappell 2005). This confusing nomenclature represents different systems for classifying overlapping behaviors. Using the terminology of HFACS, there are three basic error types: skill-based, decision, and perceptual errors (Figure 15.2).

A skill-based error results from a failure of attention or memory when performing a routine, highly automated task, often in familiar circumstances. Examples of skill-based errors are common, e.g. not flushing an IV extension line before connection to an IV catheter, not giving antimicrobials (where indicated) before surgery begins, or placing oxygen tubing intranasally during recovery but failing to turn on the oxygen flowmeter. Skill-based errors were identified in over 50% of adverse events in a hospital setting (Diller et al. 2014). Medication errors can often be categorized as skill-based errors as they represent a routine task that is susceptible to attention or memory failure (Cooper et al. 1984; Mahajan 2010). They are often described as "wrong drug," "wrong dose," "wrong route," "wrong time" (Kohn et al. 2000). Medication errors were identified as the most common error type in a veterinary study, contributing to 54% of 560 reported incidents, and "wrong dose" was the most common example (58%) of medication error (Wallis et al. 2019).

A decision error is when an action goes as planned but the plan is inadequate. A normally good plan is misapplied because of time pressure (procedural error), a bad plan may be applied through an error of judgment or training (poor choice error), or a faulty plan is applied in the face of a novel (or poorly understood) situation (problem-solving error). Decision errors are extremely common, present in over 90% of adverse events (Diller et al. 2014). Not surprisingly, stage of training, experience, and supervision can play an important role in preventing or limiting these errors. Developing new plans in the face of novelty is prone to error because of limited mental resources, an incomplete or incorrect understanding of the situation and a tendency to fixate on a hypothesis while ignoring contradictory information. Unlike skill-based errors, decision errors are associated with tasks involving conscious effort and are susceptible to cognitive bias.

A perceptual error occurs when sensory input is limited (e.g. alarm silenced) or incorrect (e.g. visual illusion) and an incorrect response leads to an error. Trying to insert a hypodermic needle into an injection port by feel so as to avoid displacing surgical drapes and potentially disrupt a procedure, rather than using a light or lifting the drapes, may result in a stick injury. Perceptual errors appear to be less commonly encountered in medicine than aviation, identified in 15% of adverse events (Diller et al. 2014).

In contrast to errors, violations are deliberate deviations from safe or standard practice. Routine violations ("bending the rules") are habitual and often tolerated (e.g. driving a few miles or kilometers per hour in excess of the speed limit) (Wiegmann and Shappell 2005). They may be committed with the goal of improved efficiency, particularly where standard procedures are perceived to, or actually, inhibit efficient workflow (Diller et al. 2014). Examples could include using a smaller gauge needle to perform jugular IV injection and increasing the risk of intra-arterial injection or tolerating senior staff walking in and out of the OR in outdoor footwear while everyone else wears shoe covers. When routine violations are identified, this should trigger a search for a cause, which may include tolerance by a supervisor (supervisory violation), an absence of, or inadequate, policy (organizational process), and/ or a workplace culture of bending the rules (organizational climate). Routine violations occur frequently, recorded in 80% of adverse events (Diller et al. 2014). In contrast, exceptional violations, which are dramatic departures from standard practice, occur much less frequently. In anesthesia, they are typically associated with intentional violations of well-established standards of care (Diller et al. 2014). In general, the demographic of those most likely to violate are: young men, those with a high opinion of their skills (relative to others), those who are relatively experienced and not especially error-prone, those with a history of errors and adverse events, and those less affected by how they are viewed by others (Reason 2008).

Preconditions for Unsafe Acts

While unsafe acts are present at the majority of adverse events (80% in aviation and >90% in medicine), stopping the investigation at this level returns to a person-based system of blame (Diller et al. 2014; Wiegmann and Shappell 2005). Behind unsafe acts are predisposing preconditions as they apply to the operator (caregiver or anesthetist), personnel and environment (Figure 15.2).

Suboptimal operator performance can be created by an adverse mental or physiological state or physical/mental limitations. Mental fatigue (from sleep loss or other stressors) or distraction can easily predispose an individual to performing an unsafe act (Campbell et al. 2012). Distractions are commonplace, with one survey of 31 hours of anesthetic practice identifying a distracting event occurring on average of once every 4.5 minutes, and 22% of such events having a negative consequence for patient care (Campbell et al. 2012). Adverse physiological states represent illness, injury, or any other alteration (e.g. intoxication) that limits job performance. Adverse mental states are commonly reported (approximately 50% incidence) during adverse event investigations, whereas adverse physiological states are relatively rare (1%) (Diller et al. 2014). Physical/mental limitations refer to situations where the required task exceeds the ability of the individual. This may be as simple as having a hand that is too large to perform manual orotracheal intubation of a cow (leading to delayed intubation and potential aspiration of regurgitated fluid) or it may be a fundamental limitation. Occasionally, individuals that do not have an aptitude for anesthesia are encountered. While there may be organizational/institutional pressure to keep them in the service, this can put strain on other team members.

Personnel factors include team resource management and personal readiness (fitness for duty). Team resource management applies within and between teams. For example, a group of anesthesia providers may work well together, providing smooth, error-free anesthesia, but this is of limited value if there is poor coordination with other teams so that cases frequently run early or late, cases are presented for anesthesia unexpectedly or critical information (e.g. suspected drug reaction) is not shared. Good communication and coordination are key to good team resource management. Ineffective communication between team members constituted 70% of personnel factors (n = 448), followed by lack of teamwork (7%), and failure of leadership (4%) (Diller et al. 2014). In a review of 444 surgical

malpractice claims, of which 258 led to patient harm, 23% (n = 60) involved a breakdown of communication, almost all of which were verbal (Greenberg et al. 2007). Important contributing factors related to hierarchy (e.g. resident communication with more senior surgeon) and ambiguity regarding responsibility or leadership. In the majority of cases, information was either never transmitted (49%) or transmitted but inaccurately received (44%).

The frequency of communication failures in a study of six complex surgeries was high, with approximately one failure every eight minutes (13–48 failures per case) (Hu et al. 2012). Communication between disciplines failed twice as frequently as within a discipline and most failures were associated with absence of key individuals and failure to resolve an issue. Eighty-one percent of failures resulted in a loss of efficiency. Interestingly, this study was performed in a hospital where the Surgical Safety Checklist (SSC) was performed for all cases. As the SSC has been shown to reduce communication failures, delays, and morbidity/mortality, these findings suggest that failures may have been even more frequent without its use (Haynes et al. 2009; Lingard et al. 2008; Nundy et al. 2008). In veterinary medicine, communication breakdown was the second most common error type (approx. 30%), after medication error (approx. 60%), in contributing to reported incidents (Wallis et al. 2019).

Fitness for duty (which overlaps with adverse physiological states) is the expectation that individuals are able to perform at the expected level. Failures could result from fatigue or failure to adequately prepare for a scheduled case. Fitness for duty is a contributing factor to adverse events in medicine was uncommon (3%) (Diller et al. 2014). This contrasts with the high incidence of contributions from team resource management. Recognition of physical and mental health limitations must be coupled with the freedom to self-report without stigma or shame (Allnutt 2002).

Environmental factors comprise the physical and technological environment. In medicine and veterinary anesthesia, these apply to both personnel and patients. For example, noise during recovery from anesthesia could serve as a distraction to personnel and potentially affect the quality of recovery. Performing tasks in a darkened environment (e.g. during arthroscopy) can limit patient visibility, potentially leading to a perceptual error. Limited physical access to patients (e.g. surgery of the head/neck) can increase reliance on physiologic monitors and limit assessment of physical indicators of depth of anesthesia. Working in poorly designed environments (e.g. slippery flooring) or with poorly designed equipment (e.g. monitors that provide erroneous readings when heart rates are below 30 bpm) undoubtedly increase the risk of adverse events. Environmental factors were present in approximately 50% of human adverse events, with most instances related to a problem with equipment or environment design, though this may be higher in veterinary anesthesia (Diller et al. 2014).

Unsafe Supervision

Unsafe supervision has the potential to negatively influence quality of care and lead to an adverse event. When supervision is inadequate, there are deficiencies in guidance, training, leadership, and/or oversight. Unfortunately, most supervisors learn supervisory skills through experience alone without the benefit of formal instruction in teaching. As a result, it is common for supervisors, at least in the early stage of their careers, to supervise using the same style they experienced as trainees. This can lead to adverse events through inadequate oversight, excessive workload, and unrealistic expectations. Placing staff in situations without adequate oversight is more likely to lead to violations as they are forced to solve problems against a background of limited knowledge or training (Wiegmann and Shappell 2005). Planned inappropriate operations is the intentional request to increase work rate or type beyond the safe limits of an individual or team. This commonly occurs

when emergency procedures are added to a surgery list with the expectation that a full schedule of planned electives are also completed. Equally, staff shortages may lead to an excessive workload or to individuals performing cases for which they are not adequately trained or supervised. A failure to correct a known problem is when known deficiencies are ignored, often in the hope that they will disappear, or to avoid confrontation. This has widespread consequences, including supporting routine violations and continued use of unsafe equipment, which can lead to adverse events. Supervisory violations create an ideal situation for failure. Willfully disregarding established rules and procedures may directly lead to an adverse event or put others in the position of triggering an adverse event. For example, ignoring a clinic policy to have a minimum of three people present during the induction of general anesthesia will increase individual workload, risk, and likelihood of errors. Unsafe supervision contributed to approximately 50% of medical adverse events (Diller et al. 2014).

Organizational Influences

The final level of HFACS are the organizational influences. These undoubtedly contribute to accidents, though a clear chain of events may be difficult to establish and their contribution may be under-represented (Diller et al. 2014). Nonetheless, a large (n = 869 483 anesthetics), prospective, multi-center study of anesthetic mortality found that organizational factors contributed to mortality in 11–40% of cases (Arbous et al. 2001). Resource management relates to the use and allocation of human, financial, equipment, and facility resources. Decisions are often based on a conflict between safety and quality (individual care, equipment maintenance and replacement, staffing) versus quantity (caseload, workday length, and intensity). Proposed solutions, such as cross-training staff to perform multiple roles may not account for effects on team performance and minimal training requirements. The organizational climate is the workplace culture or atmosphere. Where this contradicts official policies or procedures, violations occur, indicating a problem with the policies or procedures themselves, or something affecting personnel behavior (culture, training, supervision, operator condition). Finally, the organizational process is the governance of daily activities, such as the establishment and application of policies, standard operating procedures, and checklists. Where deviation occurs, it indicates a problem in governance (e.g. incomplete checklist) or failure to adhere to standard practice.

Error Investigation

Investigations of adverse events have three goals: explanation, prediction, and remedies. Identifying and correcting problems at the preconditions and organizational levels provide the best value in terms of preventing future adverse events. However, it is important to keep in mind that the majority of organizations will have flaws, leading to the temptation to blame the system without establishing a plausible link to the adverse event. For example, sporadic clusters of cases of purulent nasal discharge following general anesthesia can easily trigger repeated sampling of anesthetic equipment for bacterial contamination, missing relationships between hospital occupancy rates, population demographics, and shared airspace. The HFACS system described above provides a comprehensive framework to understand and investigate how errors occur and identify targets for improvement. Simpler methods have also been described in veterinary medicine (Ludders and McMillan 2017; Pang et al. 2018). Adverse event investigations often take place in the form of morbidity and mortality conferences (M&MCs). When performed properly, these can be a valuable learning experience and drive improvement in care (Pang et al. 2018).

Error Prevention

Developing a Safety Climate

A safety climate may be defined as "the shared perceptions of practices, policies, procedures, and routines about safety in an organization" (Singer et al. 2010). In HROs, this climate permeates an organization at all levels, with a tangible effect on policy and practice. A general awareness of safety in human medicine was triggered by the 1999 Institute of Medicine report, "To Err Is Human." This was preceded by early recognition in anesthesia practice of the importance of individual components that fall under the umbrella of safety climate (Allnutt 2002; Cooper et al. 1984, 2002; Cooper 1984; Gaba et al. 1987; Kohn et al. 2000; Reason 2005). While considerable progress has been made, most notably with the widespread adoption and implementation of the World Health Organization's (WHO) SSC, the differences in safety climate between anesthesia and aviation (a prototypical example of a HRO) remain striking (Bergs et al. 2014; Haynes et al. 2009; Singer et al. 2010). A survey of naval aviators (all personnel, including commanding officers) and healthcare workers (senior managers, physicians, and other workers) in the United States (n = 34 206 respondents) found that the safety climate was perceived as significantly safer by the naval aviators (Singer et al. 2010). The authors suggested that these differences resulted from multiple factors, including the use of standard operating procedures, the existence of mechanisms for reporting safety hazards and adverse events, managerial and administrative support for safety, adherence to guidelines and standards of care for fitness for duty, and continuous training and assessment.

The recognition of safety climate within veterinary anesthesia is in its infancy, and there are few studies of the application or outcome of promoting safe practice (Armitage-Chan 2014; Hartnack et al. 2013; Hofmeister et al. 2014; McMillan 2014; Menoud et al. 2018). Hofmeister et al. (2014) reported promising results from a pre/ post-intervention observational study to identify adverse events and near misses over an 11.5-month period followed by the introduction of targeted interventions to reduce the recurrence of these incidents. Use of an anonymous reporting system identified 74 adverse events or near misses (3.6% of 2028 patients).

Checklists

The WHO SSC is the best known and most widely adopted peri-anesthetic checklist in use. In a landmark observational study involving eight hospitals in eight countries across the world, prospective data collected before and after implementation of the SSC showed a reduction in mortality and surgical infection from 1.5% to 0.8% and 6.2% to 3.4%, respectively (Haynes ct al. 2009). These findings have been repeated, with a recent meta-analysis supportive of the benefits of using the WHO SSC (Bergs et al. 2014). In addition to reductions in morbidity and mortality, the WHO SSC has resulted in cost savings, improved communication, and improved safety climate (Haynes et al. 2009, 2011; Kearns et al. 2011; Semel et al. 2010).

The WHO SSC comprises three sections, each corresponding to a different phase in the surgical pathway (before induction of anesthesia, before skin incision, before patient leaves operating room). Each section has items that are service specific (e.g. "Is the anesthetic machine and medication check complete?"; "Is the [surgical] site marked?") as well as those that ensure sharing of information and promote discussion (e.g. "What is the anticipated blood loss?"; "Are there any patient-specific concerns?"). Common to these sections, and key to the development of checklists in veterinary anesthesia, is specifying the personnel who should be present, the role of a single person responsible for managing the checklist, the requirement for verbal acknowledgment and confirmation of checklist items,

and the introduction of all personnel present (name and role, including trainees). These practices are believed to play a critical role in the successful or failed implementation of the WHO SSC in an individual institution and the overall impact on safety climate (Haynes et al. 2009).

There are several considerations key to successful implementation of a checklist system that is relevant to development and adoption for veterinary anesthesia and surgery (World Health Organization 2009; Alidina et al. 2018; Armitage-Chan 2014). (i) There must be public support from the administration and department/service chiefs for prioritizing safety and use of an SSC. (ii) Forming a team from a core, multidisciplinary group of interested personnel to establish and promote adoption of the checklist. (iii) The checklist should be modifiable. This promotes adaptation to local conditions and encourages team member involvement and support. When modifying the checklist, the principles of checklist development should be applied: the checklist should be concise, focused, brief (less than one minute per section), contain actionable items, be performed verbally, developed collaboratively, tested in a small/limited setting, and integrated into existing processes. (iv) Start small. Implement the checklist and track its use and performance on a limited scale (e.g. single operating room [OR] or with a single surgical team) before expanding its use after any necessary modifications are made. (v) Track process and outcome measures to monitor performance and identify problems early. The tools used in clinical audit would be ideal for this (Rose and Pang 2021). (vi) The checklist coordinator should be carefully selected. They must be able to work with key team members as they have the responsibility for ensuring completion and adherence to the checklist, including the power to stop progress to the next phase of the procedure.

As with veterinary anesthesia safety climate, there are few studies on the application or outcome of promoting safe practice, such as checklists (Hofmeister et al. 2014; McMillan 2014; Menoud et al. 2018). Menoud et al. (2018) used a consensus discussion (Delphi method) among veterinary anesthetists to develop a peri-anesthetic checklist based on the WHO SSC (Menoud et al. 2018). This work highlighted common obstacles encountered when attempting to introduce change associated with a checklist, including resistance to change, concerns regarding usefulness and relevance, and the time required to complete a checklist. Taken together, these underline the importance of garnering support, raising awareness and education of potential users. Such support is essential to achieving successful implementation of checklists and reaping the potential benefits in patient safety (Pickering et al. 2013).

Pre-anesthesia Checkout Procedure

The pre-anesthesia checkout (PAC) procedure comprises a protocol for checking components of anesthetic equipment paired with a checklist. In most instances, a physical checklist is used to prompt completion of all checks. Anesthetic equipment faults are relatively common, so a PAC is a simple, effective way to prevent a fault resulting in an adverse event (Barthram and Mcclymont 1992; Kendell and Barthram 1998). Anesthetic machine checks identify 30–60% of faults and approximately one-fifth of these may be serious, posing a direct risk to the patient (Barthram and Mcclymont 1992; Kendell and Barthram 1998). Additionally, completion of a PAC is associated with a decreased risk of anesthetic morbidity and mortality (odds ratio 0.64, 95%CI 0.43–0.95) (Arbous et al. 2005). Using the imagery of the Swiss cheese model, performing a PAC may be visualized as closing a hole in a defensive layer (Figure 15.1). As anesthesia equipment becomes increasingly complex and equipment varies considerably between clinics, it is impossible to provide a comprehensive, universal PAC guide (Association of Anaesthetists of Great Britain and Ireland

et al. 2012; Hartle 2013). Manufacturer guidelines should be followed for individual pieces of equipment. Table 15.2 presents an outline of key checks that should be completed, based on the most recent American Society of Anesthesiologists and Association of Anesthetists of Great Britain and Ireland guidelines (Anesthesiologists Society of Anesthesiologists 2008; Association of Anaesthetists of Great Britain and Ireland et al. 2012). A laminated copy of a PAC can be attached to each machine and completion of tasks confirmed by adding user initials and date as the checklist is completed. In addition to the pre-use PAC, it is important that anesthetic equipment is serviced regularly as per manufacturer requirements and a record of service kept.

Reporting

Adverse events and near misses are a well-recognized feature of equine anesthesia, but there are no widely accepted practices for reporting such incidents (Hartnack et al. 2013). All adverse events should be reported, allowing the opportunity for discussion, education, and action to prevent recurrence, often in the form of M&MCs (Pang et al. 2018). Reporting near misses is beneficial as it allows patterns to be identified early before an adverse event occurs. It is important that reports are collated and reviewed regularly, so that emerging patterns are identified, and the information shared. It may be helpful to classify reports according to type (e.g. medication error, hypoglycemia) to facilitate review (Hartnack et al. 2013; Pang et al. 2018). Reports should contain key information to identify what happened, when it took place, who (patient, personnel) was affected, and a description of the incident. Reports should be made as close to the incident as possible, helping ensure that information is accurate. Proper use of an anesthetic chart as a record of events will facilitate accurate reporting.

Table 15.2 Minimum recommended pre-anesthetic checkout procedure checklist for anesthetic and monitoring equipment prior to anesthesia of a patient.

Perform applicable manufacturer's recommendations on all equipment	
Power supply	Equipment plugged in a switched on
Gas supply	"Tug test"[a]
	Pipeline pressure adequate ($\geq$50 psig)
	Backup oxygen supply available
	Oxygen failure alarm working (if present)
	Flowmeter working
	Oxygen flush working
Breathing system[b]	"Leak test"[c]
	Breathing system patent[d]
	Connections correct and tight
	Vaporizer – fitted, filled, leak-free[e]
	Soda lime – check color, date of last change
	Backup breathing system available
Ventilator[b]	Alternative means of ventilation available[f]
	"Leak test"
	Appropriate setting for patient (or set to minimum value[g])
Scavenging system	Functional
Monitors	Switched on a functional
	Alarm limits and volumes set
Airway equipment[b,h]	Available and tested
Case-specific equipment?	e.g. Endoscope for assisted intubation
	Smaller ET tubes or nasotracheal intubation
Record completion of check	
TIME OUT immediately before anesthesia	Confirm: monitors on, ventilator or rebreathing bag connected, oxygen flow and ventilator setting appropriate, vaporizer filled

This applies to most common needs and configurations (use of central pipeline oxygen, active scavenging, and a ventilator).

[a] Pull on hosing connections and connection between hosing and gas supply terminal to ensure proper connection.

[b] Checked before each case. Any changes to equipment should trigger the full PAC to be completed.

[c] A pressure leak test assesses system integrity. A generic test is to occlude the breathing system y-piece, close the adjustable pressure limiting (APL, "pop off") valve, open the flowmeter until a pressure of 30 cmH$_2$O is achieved, close flowmeter, and confirm pressure is maintained. A leak <200 ml/min is acceptable (measured by slowly increasing oxygen flow until pressure is maintained). Open the APL valve at completion of the test unless the ventilator is immediately connected. Ventilator (ascending bellows): test system integrity by occluding y-piece and filling bellows via flowmeter. Once bellows is filled, close flowmeter and bellows should maintain filled/inflated position at the top of the bellows housing. Ventilator (descending bellows): occlude y-piece and lower bellows stop. Bellows should maintain position. A leak test for the anesthetic machine (bypassing the breathing system) is to attach a squeezed suction bulb to the common gas outlet. If the bulb remains collapsed for 10 seconds when it is released, this indicates no significant leak is present.

[d] System patency can be checked to a limited degree by visual inspection; ideally, a two-bag test is performed. Two-bag test: Attach a reservoir bag (test lung) to the y-piece, turn on fresh gas flow to 5 l/min and ventilate manually ensuring test lung inflates and deflates. Squeezing both reservoir bags checks APL valve function. Repeat test using ventilator (with fresh gas flow off or set to minimum).

[e] Set flowmeter to 5 l/min and occlude common gas outlet with vaporizer switched off. The flowmeter indicator should dip. Repeat test with vaporizer switched on.

[f] In equine anesthesia, this is usually a demand valve (for adults) or self-inflating bag (for foals).

[g] Setting a ventilator to minimum values prevents inadvertently delivering an excessive inspiratory volume or pressure to a patient at the start of a case.

[h] Varies between cases but typically includes mouth gag, ET tube, lubricant, cuff syringe, adhesive tape.

All members of staff should be able to submit an anonymous incident report. If there are concerns that anonymous reporting limits further analysis or investigation, confidentiality should be guaranteed. Creating a safety climate in which errors and accidents can be discussed in a non-punitive environment will encourage reporting (Hartnack et al. 2013; Hofmeister et al. 2014; Singer et al. 2010).

Audit

A clinical audit is a quality improvement tool used to evaluate and improve care (Langley et al. 2009; Mosedale 1998; Rose et al. 2016b; Rose and Pang 2021). It is an effective method for improving clinical care and has been widely adopted in human medicine, including for adverse events (Haynes et al. 2009; Pronovost et al. 2006; Shonfeld et al. 2011). Though often discussed in veterinary medicine, evidence of widespread use is low despite some successful applications (Hofmeister et al. 2014; Rose et al. 2016a, b; Viner 2010). The basic structure of a clinical audit is a four-step process: Plan, Do, Study, Act (Rose and Pang 2021). Plan is identifying a problem for study. This may be an outcome (e.g. movement during surgery) or a process (e.g. use of invasive blood pressure monitoring). Do is data collection. This could be, for example, the incidence of intra-operative movement or frequency that invasive blood pressure monitoring is performed. Study is data analysis. Clinical audits are observational intervention studies, so the analysis is based on a pre-/post-intervention comparison. Before an intervention is made, analysis can be as simple as visualizing collected data as a scatter plot or graph. For example, occurrences of intra-operative movement could be tracked over a six month period and plotted to show the overall incidence and any apparent clusters (these in turn may trigger further investigation or research). Act is to develop and enact recommendations based on the data collected and analyzed. A recommendation may be to continue current practice if no

problems are identified and performance satisfactory, or it may be to make a change in practice. For example, if intra-operative movement occurred more frequently in July, with new interns training in anesthesia, an intervention to improve training or supervision could be introduced. Any change should be followed by further data collection and analysis, to evaluate if the intervention has led to improvement and ensure it is maintained over time. Many studies to reduce adverse events follow this simple study design and have yielded impressive results (Haynes et al. 2009; Pronovost et al. 2006).

Recurrent Accident Patterns

Recurring patterns of similar accidents are prevalent in healthcare, and tend to have three features in common: (i) ever-present hazards (e.g. ability of horses to kick), (ii) local traps, characterized by factors leading people to commit an unsafe act (e.g. pressure from colleague(s) or immediate supervisor to begin procedure before adequate sedation is apparent), and (iii) the organizational climate that drives the creation of local traps (e.g. a desire to increase daily caseload). The goals of safety and productivity are commonly in conflict. In general, organizational drivers that set the scene for recurrent accidents are the opposite of those which characterize HROs.

Error Wisdom and Resilience

The ubiquity of human error is now widely accepted, leading to a shift in how adverse events and near misses are investigated and acted upon. However, it is increasingly recognized that humans frequently prevent adverse events, even in the face of considerable challenges (Carthey et al. 2003; De Leval et al. 2000; Reason 2008). They may be compensating for a flawed system or working in extremely demanding conditions (Carthey et al. 2003; De Leval et al. 2000). It has been proposed that individuals can be trained in "error wisdom," a way to recognize a situation in which an error is likely to occur (Reason 2004, 2008). This may be an effective means to quickly reduce error, particularly when fundamental organizational or workplace changes will take time to achieve. Reason has proposed a "three-bucket model" (Figure 15.3), representing the self (current state of the individual), context (nature of the context), and task (error potential of the task) (Reason 2004, 2008). The self is exemplified by the condition of the operator and personnel factors such as fatigue or illness. Context represents the environment in which the task is being performed, including distractions, patient transfer, time pressure, faulty, or limited equipment. Task refers to the likelihood of error varying at different steps of a task: things tend to be forgotten or overlooked toward the end of a task or when the preceding step does not cue the following step. Applying a tool such as the three-bucket model gives an individual the opportunity to step back and assess

a situation. As an anesthetist feels that the buckets are becoming full of bad (or brown) stuff, this should raise an internal alarm that an error, and potentially adverse event, is likely. For example, after a busy night on call (self), anesthetizing the first foal of the season when the foal anesthesia equipment has not been used recently (context) substantially increases the risk of error. Hopefully, the anesthetist elects to take steps to re-balance the situation (e.g. ask for help, discuss the planned course of action, prepare an alternative plan) rather than plowing ahead. Not all buckets need to be full for an error to occur and neither full nor empty buckets ensure error or safety, respectively.

Error wisdom can also be applied to cognitive bias (Table 15.3). In a series of simulated encounters in which 32 anesthesia residents participated, seven cognitive biases occurred with a greater than 50% incidence (Stiegler et al. 2012). Interestingly, faculty were able to predict the most common biases encountered, indicating that avoiding bias by metacognitive training ("thinking about thinking") may form a valuable part of residency training to limit cognitive bias (Croskerry 2002, 2003; Stiegler et al. 2012; Stiegler and Tung 2014).

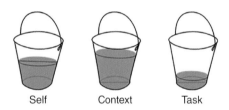

Self   Context   Task

Figure 15.3 The "three-bucket model" tool for identifying the potential for an error to occur and to enable the enhancement of safe practice.

Resilience

The ability of humans to prevent adverse events from occurring in demanding situations is finite.

Table 15.3 Cognitive biases frequently observed (>50%) during anesthesia simulator training for resident training.

Anchoring (tunnel vision/fixation)	Focusing on a single feature or event at the expense of other features or an evolving picture. May lead to premature closure.
Premature closure	Prematurely making a diagnosis or reaching a conclusion.
Confirmation bias	Only recognizing or seeking information that confirms the desired or expected diagnosis.
Commission bias	Performing an unnecessary action when inaction is indicated.
Overconfidence bias	Delay or failure in recognizing need for help or seeking help from inflated assessment of knowledge or ability.
Omission bias	Delay or failure to act when action is indicated.
Sunk costs	Commitment to a decision in the face of failure because of the time or effort invested.

Figure 15.4 Extension of the Swiss cheese model to demonstrate the ability of resilience to allowing an error to cause an adverse event. The mouse represents factors causing gradual erosion of the resilience.

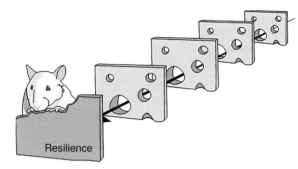

Resilience

Extending Reason's Swiss cheese model, resilience to allowing an error to cause an adverse event can be viewed as a solid slice of (cheddar) cheese that is gradually eroded by correcting, or compensating for, numerous errors (Figure 15.4). While it is clear that a major event (such as a horse moving intra-operatively) will lead to an adverse event if not corrected, a sufficient number of minor events (disrupting the flow of a procedure, which may have little impact on the patient) can eventually exhaust mental resources sufficiently to breach the human defense (Carthey et al. 2003; De Leval et al. 2000). Examples of such minor events could include: a difficult horse to sedate, working with new interns, miscommunication regarding induction time with the surgery team, scheduling multiple overlapping cases that require your attention, or replenishing drug infusion(s) during surgery.

Crisis Management

A crisis is a turning point, when a decisive change takes place leading to a positive or negative outcome (Runciman and Merry 2005). Crisis management focuses on the key features of detection, diagnosis, and action. The challenge for the anesthetist is to detect the impending or actual crisis, diagnose its cause, and act to support a positive outcome. The "COVER ABCD – A SWIFT CHECK" algorithm has been developed to stimulate structured, immediate action followed by specific written instructions (Table 15.4) (Runciman et al. 1993, 2005; Runciman and Merry 2005).

Research has shown that applying this algorithm would have led to an appropriate response in 60% of incidents within 40–60 seconds (Runciman et al. 1993), with a current recommendation to incorporate it into a regular, systematic scan during anesthesia. Should an abnormality be detected or a crisis present, this would then trigger the use of detailed, problem-specific sub-algorithms or checklists to achieve a diagnosis and institute treatment (Runciman et al. 2005). Currently, no sub-algorithm exists that is specific to equine anesthesia and thus would need to be developed. Importantly, if a problem is not rapidly solved

Table 15.4 The COVER ABCD – A SWIFT CHECK mnemonic for rapid response and regular scanning during anesthesia.

C	Circulation, Capnograph, and Color (saturation)
O	Oxygen supply and Oxygen analyzer
V	Ventilation (intubated patient) and Vaporizers
E	Endotracheal tube and Eliminate machine
R	Review monitors and Review equipment
A	Airway (with face or laryngeal mask)
B	Breathing (with spontaneous ventilation)
C	Circulation (in more detail)
D	Drugs (consider all administered or not administered)
A	be Aware[a] of Air[b] and Allergy

[a] Aware indicates patient awakening and a reminder to the anesthetist to be aware.
[b] Air indicates the presence of air as in embolism and pneumothorax. *A SWIFT CHECK*: regular scan of personnel, procedure, patient and physiologic monitors.

with use of the algorithm during anesthesia, then skilled and experienced help should be sought (Runciman et al. 2005).

A key consideration during crises is the role of clear, accurate, and concise communication. The importance of communication has been highlighted a determinant in successful checklist implementation and avoidance of adverse events (World Health Organization 2009; Carthey et al. 2003; De Meester et al. 2013; Diller et al. 2014; Greenberg et al. 2007; Haynes et al. 2009; Pronovost et al. 2006). Adopting the sterile cockpit concept (in which only essential communication takes place) to minimize distraction during critical phases (e.g. anesthetic induction and recovery) can improve communication (Broom et al. 2011; Wadhera et al. 2010). A simple method to enable effective communication is SBAR: Situation, Background, Assessment and Recommendation (Table 15.5). SBAR, designed by the military for efficient transfer of critical information between people who may sit on different levels of an organization's hierarchy, has been applied during patient transfer, to raise concerns over a patient's state and during peri-operative briefings (De Meester et al. 2013; Leonard et al. 2004).

In the context of equine anesthesia, an example use of SBAR might be:

S – I have a horse that has been recumbent in recovery for 75 minutes.
B – It is an 18 year old, gelding quarter horse that underwent colic surgery.

Table 15.5 Situation, Background, Assessment, and Recommendation (SBAR) method for improving communication.

Situation	What is going on with the patient?
Background	What is the clinical background or context?
Assessment	What do I think is the problem?
Recommendation	What would I do to correct it?

Source: Based on Leonard et al. (2004).

A – He has made three weak attempts, the last was around 20 minutes ago. He looks exhausted.
R – I am not sure what to do next.

While this may appear simplistic, the SBAR structure limits editorializing with unnecessary commentary or information ("I don't know why they waited so long to send him to surgery"; "You should have seen how long it took to close the skin").

High-Reliability Organizations

The practice of anesthesia shares characteristics common to HROs. These are a working environment that is complex, dynamic, nonroutine, intermittently intensely active, one with tightly coupled processes that are interactive with different levels of an organization and the necessity to perform exacting tasks under pressure (Gaba et al. 1987; Reason 2000; Sutcliffe 2011). In contrast to current anesthesia practice, HROs function with a near absence of catastrophic failure (Sutcliffe 2011). The three most widely recognized and studied HROs are aircraft carriers, nuclear power stations, and air traffic control centers. Much of the difference between anesthesia practice and HROs can be explained by how these organizations are structured and the actions and attitudes of people within them (Reason 2000; Sutcliffe 2011). Specifically, HROs build a culture of respectful interaction (trust, honesty, and respect), build a culture of heedful interrelation (awareness and understanding of how a person's actions and work affect those of others and how individual actions contribute toward an organization's goals), and establish processes and practices focused on minimizing errors. Processes necessary to establish an HRO include:

1) Preoccupation with failure – intelligent wariness is encouraged among members to recognize and recover errors. Potential

weaknesses are looked for proactively and information shared when errors occur

2) A reluctance to simplify interpretations – being open to alternative interpretations of information and situations in order to avoid complacency and a false sense of security.

3) Sensitivity to operations – described as situational awareness, seeing the big picture and how small changes can coalesce to affect it.

4) A commitment to resilience – resilience within an organization is cultivated as it is recognized that it is impossible to plan and prepare for every eventuality. Diversity within an organization in terms of individual training, experiences, and networks supports problem solving and recognition.

5) A deference to expertise – a feature of HROs is to give decision-making power to experts. This reflects a readiness to move away from a hierarchical structure where those at the top make the important decisions when faced with a problem, toward a focus on the person with the most relevant expertise. This is a powerful tool to address novel situations and recognizes the inevitable gaps in knowledge and experience.

Conclusion

Many of the ideas and suggestions presented in this chapter, in combination with institutional support, learning from mistakes, and understanding the conditions that predispose them, can encourage the development of anesthesia as an HRO.

Case Examples

Intra-arterial Injection

a) Event: An intern has asked if an adult horse scheduled for anesthesia can be sedated to facilitate jugular catheter placement as it will not stand still despite the help of experienced animal handlers. You agree and suggest a dose of xylazine. The intern leaves to prepare this as you continue to prepare for surgery. A few minutes later, a technician comes running to say the horse has collapsed. The horse is showing generalized seizure activity.

b) Immediate management

1) Ensure everyone present is out of harm's way. This may mean evacuating the immediate area and maintaining a barrier between the horse and people.

2) If it is safe to do so, padding can be placed under the horse's head to minimize trauma.

3) In most instances, convulsions will be self-limiting and short-lived (<5–10 minutes) but it is a sensible precaution to prepare an anti-convulsant (diazepam or midazolam, 0.05–0.1 mg/kg IV).

4) An alternative to benzodiazepine treatment is to induce general anesthesia. This controls the physical manifestations of convulsions and allows the animal to be transported to an area where it can be safely managed (supportive care: oxygen, vital signs monitoring) or potentially recover to standing (e.g. padded/bedded stall).

c) Considerations

1) Convulsions are caused by the direct effects of the injected drug on the brain (Christian et al. 1974). In some instances, damage may be severe and potentially irreversible with histopathological findings of hemorrhage, necrosis, and cerebral edema (Christian et al. 1974; Ludders and McMillan 2017).

2) Intra-arterial (IA) injections are usually associated with sedative agents such as alpha-2 adrenergic agonist agents or acepromazine as these are commonly injected without use of a catheter. (Note: catheters can be inadvertently placed in the carotid artery.)

3) A test injection comprising of a small volume (0.5 ml) of injectate can identify

inadvertent IA injection as reactions usually occur within 10 seconds of injection (Christian et al. 1974).

4) Reflection – Were standard procedures followed for injection (an assessment for procedure violation)? The carotid artery lies deep to the jugular vein so the angle of needle insertion should be shallow. The injection is usually performed around the junction of the upper and middle third of the neck, where there is slightly greater separation between the carotid artery and jugular vein. A larger gauge (e.g. 18G, 1 in.) needle is usually recommended in the hope that blood flow is more easily assessed. Was the needle detached from the syringe when inserted into the vessel? This can make it easier to assess if blood is dripping/flowing (venous) out or emerging as a jet (arterial). Additionally, some anesthetists prefer to direct the needle toward the heart as this may make it easier to visualize blood emerging under arterial pressure. With an 18G needle, blood flow may not be pulsatile (Gabel and Koestner 1963). Was lighting adequate to see blood flow from the needle hub? Assessing blood color is highly subjective and should not be used as the main determinant of venous versus arterial placement. Was the needle inserted up to the level of the hub? This is not always performed, but may limit needle migration as the syringe is attached and during injection. If standard procedure was not followed, why not – did an error or routine violation occur? Was the anesthetist adequately trained or supervised? Were there other preconditions present (e.g. distraction, time pressure) that may have led to the event?

Personnel Injury

Event: You are working a short period as a locum in a large, well-established equine hospital that has a steady surgical caseload. Things have been going very smoothly and the surgical and anesthesia teams are well organized and collegial. A young 450 kg stallion presenting for the next case, a head computed tomography (CT) for evaluation of nasal discharge, has been difficult to handle. He now appears well sedated with a lowered head and minimally responsive to noise, having received IV detomidine (15 mcg/kg), acepromazine (0.02 mg/kg), and butorphanol (0.02 mg/kg). The design of the induction area is such that each horse enters the padded area from one side, is induced behind a swing gate following closure of the sliding entry doors, and is transferred out of the opposite side of the induction area by hoist on to the operating/transport table. Standard practice at the clinic is to have two animal handlers present for induction, one at the head walking the horse into the induction area and the other to aid entry and manage the swing gate.

As the horse is walked on to the padded floor of the induction area, he becomes agitated and half turns as he attempts to reverse out. He is given time and space by the experienced handler at his head and appears to relax and his head returns to its lowered position. The second handler is standing by the entry doors, and you are waiting at the far side (head end) of the induction area with the anesthesia technician and an intern. As the horse has relaxed, you suggest trying again. The horse is hesitant but fully enters the induction area and allows himself to be positioned along the wall. The second handler, standing on the far side of the gate, pushes the swing gate toward the horse and half turns to slide close the entry doors. The movement/noise of the doors and/or sudden change in light levels as the doors are closed spooks the horse. He swings his rear away from the wall, contacts the swing gate, and reacts with a kick. This propels the gate toward the handler, hitting him in the chest and knocking him back against the half-closed entry door. The horse settles once he is no longer in contact with the gate and is calmed by the handler at his head.

a) Immediate management
1) Stop everything and assess the situation (any ongoing, immediate danger to personnel?).
2) Ask the second handler to leave the induction area through the entry doors so he is no longer placed between the horse and swing gate.
3) The horse still appears sedated. You assess his sensitivity to touch by running your hand over his back. As he shifts his hind feet in response, you decide to give more detomidine.
4) As the detomidine takes effect, the second handler, who is unharmed, is requested to wait outside the entry doors until you are satisfied with the level of sedation (you re-assess the horse's response to stimulation).
5) Once sedation appears acceptable, you request that the entry doors are closed from the outside by the second handler. You ask him to enter the induction area from the front (by the horse's head) and you confirm the level of sedation is acceptable with the handler at the horse's head before the second handler slowly closes and attaches the swing gate.
6) Induction then proceeds uneventfully.
b) Considerations
1) What went wrong? When working with horses, the possibility of unexpected reactions is always present, nevertheless the risk to personnel and horses can be minimized with clearly established procedures. For such procedures (often available as a standard operating procedure [SOP]) to be effective, they must be followed. The described scenario raises important questions about procedure, responsibility, training, and organizational climate.
2) In most clinics, the person responsible for the anesthetic induction process is the anesthetist. When the anesthetist is a new member of the team, this responsibility should be clearly established or devolved to another individual from the hospital with the appropriate experience. In this case, the anesthesia technician could have been given responsibility.
3) It is important to have a debrief following an accident or near miss event. This gives everyone the chance to review the event, discuss what happened, ensure there is a clear understanding of what went wrong, what was learned, and what can be done to prevent a recurrence. It is natural after such an event that everyone takes care to adhere to procedure. Over time, this level of heightened awareness will fade, and routine violations may occur unless a formal procedure is established and enacted for every case.
4) Ensure the event is reported as per clinic policy.
5) Reflection – It is important to establish if the decision to close the entry doors from inside the induction area with the handler placed between the swing gate and doors was an error or violation (routine or exceptional) of standard procedure. A documented procedure covering entry of horses did not exist for this hospital. Further investigation revealed numerous near misses had occurred over the years. Anecdotally, these were associated with the introduction of new personnel. Personnel learned the hospital's entry procedure through an informal process of experiential learning. The second animal handler was inexperienced and had not received formal instruction regarding the induction process. Following this incident, a standard operating procedure was established to cover the entry of horses to the induction area until the induction of general anesthesia. This SOP included overall responsibility, the steps at which critical decisions are made (entry to the

induction area, closing of entry doors and swing gate) and the physical positioning of personnel. Once the SOP was developed (with input from handlers, technicians, and anesthetists), all new/recent personnel received training. Did communication failures take place? When the horse was in the induction area, there was no clear communication about whether to proceed to the next step (closing the entry doors from the outside), wait, or assess the horse. The locum anesthetist is in a difficult position as he/she may not feel comfortable giving instruction to unfamiliar personnel; however, this is a critical moment in the process. Ideally, the roles of individuals should have been clearly established before the horse was brought for anesthesia. Should someone else have spoken up? Yes, though the existence of a hierarchical structure can suppress communication.

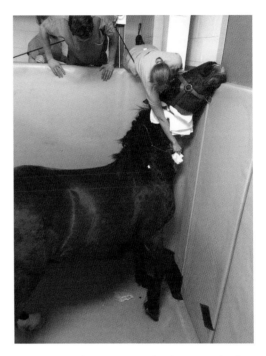

Figure 15.5 A horse recovering from anesthesia has disconnected the extension set from the intravenous jugular catheter. This puts the horse at risk for development of an air embolism.

Air Embolism

a) Event: Shortly after recovery to standing following anesthesia of a 650 kg horse, it is noticed that the IV jugular catheter has disconnected from the extension set and blood is dripping out intermittently (Figure 15.5).

b) Immediate management
   1) As the horse's head was in the box corner and the recovery box design allowed access, as well as a certain degree of head control using the attached rope, it was possible to reach in and remove the catheter.

c) Considerations
   1) Should the catheter be removed completely or reconnection to the IV line attempted? As it is early in the recovery period, the possibility that the horse stumbles and falls or injures itself remains. Therefore, maintaining easy IV access with a catheter is ideal. The decision to remove or reconnect the catheter should be based on accessibility and the risk to personnel. In this case, reaching in with both arms to reconnect the catheter may have increased the risk of falling or being pulled into the box. Compressing the vein during catheter removal will limit ongoing air entrainment, but is not always possible (Mirski et al. 2007).
   2) What are the risks of leaving the catheter disconnected? In this case, the catheter was placed with the tip toward the heart. This is standard practice at this institution to increase the probability of identifying inadvertent intra-arterial catheterization (pressurized arterial blood will be more easily identified than if the catheter is placed with the tip toward the head). The disadvantage of this placement technique is the possibility of air entrainment and creation of an air embolism should disconnection

occur. The rate of air entrainment depends on catheter gauge, vessel patency, and the pressure gradient between the catheter and right atrium. This is increased with the horse in a sternal or standing position, so that a large volume of air may enter rapidly. Experimentally, a flow rate of approximately 100 ml/s for a 14G needle with an inner diameter of 1.8 mm has been calculated (Flanagan et al. 1969). The risk of developing clinical signs is related to the rate of air entrainment, with slower rates allowing air to be transported to the pulmonary circulation and eliminated through respiration (Mirski et al. 2007). Volumes associated with clinical signs in horses are not well-defined, though tolerance of up to 0.25 ml/kg without clinical signs has been suggested (Muir and Hubbell 1991). Given the limited information regarding the volume of entrained air that might be tolerated without clinical signs (lethal volumes reported in other species are highly variable) and the role of speed of entrainment, it is not recommended to leave catheters disconnected unless the risk to personnel is unacceptably high.

3) How does venous air embolism manifest? Clinical signs vary in degree and severity depending on the volume of air in the circulation and organ systems affected. Due to the sporadic and anecdotal nature of case reports, determining risk or a relationship between air volume and symptom severity is difficult. Reported signs include central and peripheral nervous system deficits (vestibular disease, proprioceptive deficits, blindness, depressed mentation, excitement, convulsions), pruritis, kicking, flank biting, sweating, muscle fasciculations, collapse/recumbency, pulmonary edema, tachycardia, tachypnea, arrhythmias, cardiac arrest (Bradbury et al. 2005; Holbrook et al. 2007; Parkinson et al. 2018; Pelligrini-Masini et al. 2009; Sams and Hofmeister 2008). Life-threatening symptoms are caused by air emboli developing in the cerebrum, coronary circulation, or within the right side of the heart. The mechanism of cardiac arrest is usually attributed to air accumulation in the right heart (a mill-wheel murmur may be present), sufficient to create an airlock and prevent blood flow.

4) What is the treatment for venous air embolism? Treatment is primarily symptomatic depending on clinical signs. In theory, if air in the right ventricle is suspected or confirmed (echocardiography), it can be removed by aspiration using a catheter inserted into the cardiac chamber. Limited equipment availability and speed of onset of cardiac dysfunction and arrest tend to limit a successful intervention. In the presence of clinical signs, reported mortality is 19% (6/31 cases, retrospective study) from sudden death or euthanasia, with blindness, sweating, or recumbency associated with negative outcomes (Parkinson et al. 2018). The majority of cases will have a resolution of clinical signs approximately six hours after onset. In some cases, similar or new clinical signs may occur after initial resolution.

5) Reflection – Is this an isolated incident or is it a repeated occurrence – have incident reports been submitted? Luer lock fittings are standardized but this does not provide a guarantee that a lower quality batch of catheters or IV lines has been produced, or that products from different companies always provide a reliable connection. Equally, the catheter connection may have been loosened during transfer or never properly connected. Reported catheter disconnection rates vary from 0.7% to 2.7% (Parkinson et al. 2018).

Drug Administration Error – Wrong Drug

a) Event: You are about to induce the first case of the week, a bilateral hock arthroscopy in a 500 kg horse, and have reached the stage of induction of anesthesia. There is a busy day ahead, after a long weekend of on-call emergencies. You have just given 100 mcg/kg of romifidine IV and flushed the IV line with 10 ml of heparinized saline. As you place the syringes in your pocket, the yellow label of the flush syringe catches your eye. The label color at your clinic for heparinized saline is white. The yellow label reads "ketamine."

b) Immediate management
  1) Alert personnel that the horse is about to become anesthetized.
  2) Warn personnel that induction may be less smooth than usual, with increased limb rigidity and muscle tremors.
  3) As the horse is in the induction box, induction of anesthesia is continued, and diazepam given.

c) Considerations
  1) What is the likelihood of a "rough" induction? The onset of romifidine is several minutes, longer than that of ketamine or diazepam. Therefore, it is likely that the horse will exhibit some muscle rigidity and muscle tremors during induction, depending on the interval between the ketamine and diazepam (Muir et al. 1977). Muscle relaxation should occur as the romifidine and diazepam take effect.
  2) If the injection error occurred outside the induction box, is it safer to induce anesthesia or try and move the horse into the box? The onset time of ketamine is around 45 seconds and, during this time, the horse may not respond appropriately to commands or manipulations. Therefore, unless the induction box is adjacent it is probably safer to induce the horse and arrange transfer once the situation is controlled.

3) The use of color-coded labels is standard practice in many clinics. An international color scheme exists, with anesthetic induction agents assigned a yellow color. The use of a color, in addition to the printed drug name, helps minimize error resulting from misreading a plain or handwritten label. Despite the use of standardized label colors, wrong drug administrations ("syringe swap" or "substitution") continue to commonly occur (accounting for around 25% of medication errors), showing that labels are not read or misread, and the risk of a syringe swap increases with same size syringes (Cooper et al. 1984; Fasting and Gisvold 2000). In this case, the ketamine syringe was the same size as the saline flush syringe.

4) Should time have been taken to investigate the possibility of the correct agent (saline) being mislabeled? It may be tempting to do this, but the risk of injury (to the horse or personnel) outweighs the benefits of taking rapid control of the situation (proceeding with induction of anesthesia).

5) Should the prepared diazepam be given immediately upon recognizing the error? This depends on the likelihood that the syringe contents were correctly labeled as ketamine. If in doubt, it may be safer to avoid compounding the error by giving diazepam and creating a situation with a weak, ataxic, panicking horse. With an onset time of around 30–90 seconds for ketamine, the contents of the syringe will soon be known (Hall and Taylor 1981; Muir et al. 1977)!

6) Reflection – Was fatigue a precondition to this error? Working limits for medical staff exist in many countries to prevent fatigue created by work (of course, they do not control external factors, such as quality of rest at home). There are no similar standards in veterinary

medicine. The expectation that veterinary staff self-declare the presence of fatigue is limited as a result of organizational climate (common culture of working when tired), expectation to perform duties (resource management and organizational process) ability to recognize fatigue and knowledge of associated risks. Was pressure to work quickly a factor? Induction of general anesthesia is a time when numerous tasks must be performed correctly in the correct sequence. In aviation, a "sterile cockpit" is practiced, with only essential communications taking place to minimize the risk of distraction leading to an unsafe act (skill-based or decision error) (Broom et al. 2011; Campbell et al. 2012). Adding additional tasks (holding a conversation) or time pressure during this period is likely to cause a skill-based or decision error. Equally, responsibility of the anesthetic induction process rests with the anesthetist and it should be clear and accepted that performance of related tasks and speed is dictated by them. If a pre-induction/operative checklist is used, this is the time to raise and discuss concerns, not once the process has begun. Is it acceptable practice to carry both premedication and induction drugs at the same time? While this may be commonly done, keeping the syringes for premedication and induction in physically separate locations would have made this incident less likely; however, this does not address the issue of giving an injection without reading the syringe label.

Drug Administration Error – Wrong Dose

a) Event – You have anesthetized a 50 kg foal for an angular limb deformity surgical correction procedure. Surgery has begun well, and the surgeon has just reached the level of the periosteum when the foal suddenly flexes its neck and extends both forelimbs. You respond by injecting 1 ml (100 mg) of ketamine from the syringe connected to the IV line.

b) Immediate management

   1) Assess depth of anesthesia and turn down, or turn off, the vaporizer.

   2) As the foal is likely to be on a circle breathing system, turning up the oxygen flow rate will lead to a more rapid change in inspired volatile agent concentration.

   3) Calculate doses of atropine and epinephrine.

   4) Closely monitor depth of anesthesia and physiologic parameters to avoid a further lightening of anesthetic depth resulting from over-correction of the situation.

c) Considerations

   1) It is common practice for one to two doses of ketamine to be drawn up into a syringe, ready to be given quickly should a horse show an unacceptably light plane of anesthesia, such as nystagmus, an increase in muscle tone or movement. A typical bolus dose of ketamine for this application in an adult horse is 100–200 mg (approximately 0.2–0.5 mg/kg). In this case, the appropriate dose would be 10–25 mg.

   2) Of the different types of medication error that can occur, incorrect dosing is the most common (followed by "substitution"; administering the incorrect drug), accounting for approximately 30% of medication errors (Cooper et al. 2012; Cooper and Nossaman 2013).

   3) Ketamine has a relatively wide safety margin in part due to its sympathetic nervous system activity, so that this overdose is likely to be tolerated in a healthy animal. Nevertheless, the sudden increase in depth of anesthesia, combined with the cardiorespiratory depressant effects of a volatile anesthetic

agent, such as isoflurane, make accurate prediction of the response more difficult. Profound hypoventilation or apnea, muscular tremors, or nystagmus may occur. Large boluses of ketamine (6.6 mg/kg IV) shortly after xylazine (1.1 mg/kg IV) do not result in significant cardiovascular changes as compared to 2.2 mg/kg of ketamine (Muir et al. 1977).

4) As ketamine cannot be antagonized, the only option is to wait for the effects to wear off, monitoring depth of anesthesia closely to avoid a sudden lightening.

5) Reflection – Why was a large dose of rescue ketamine prepared? Preparing a standard drug dose/volume for a typical 400–600 kg adult horse may be a standard procedure for each case, so that once the planned action is begun there is a high likelihood it will be completed. When dealing with a less common size of patient could a list of pre-calculated drug doses have been helpful in avoiding this overdose? Some clinics calculate the dose and volume of drugs to be given in the event of an emergency (malignant arrhythmias, cardiac arrest). This can be helpful in a high-pressure, time-sensitive situation, perfect for predisposing an unsafe act, in this case a decision error. Additionally, in such high-pressure situations, there is a tendency to revert to learned behaviors such as giving the "standard" dose of ketamine suitable for a 500 kg adult horse. Limiting or preventing the possibility of doing this is more likely to be effective than relying on error-prone problem solving (decision error) under stress. Could a checklist have helped prevent this error? In addition to ensuring adequate preparation and readiness for planned procedures, the timeout when performing a checklist gives the chance for an automatic cycle of behavior to be broken, increasing the possibility of identifying a calculation error early.

Cardiovascular Compromise During Transfer/Sudden Position Change

a) Event: Following an uneventful anesthetic for multiple sarcoid removal for which an adult horse is positioned in lateral recumbency, the horse is hoisted into dorsal recumbency for transfer into the recovery box. Upon arrival in the recovery box (transfer time of 2–3 minutes) you immediately notice that mucous membranes are a very pale bluish-pink color. Palpating a peripheral pulse (facial artery) reveals bradycardia (now 24 beats/minute having been 32 beats/minute at the end of surgery), and the pulse is difficult to discern. The end-tidal isoflurane concentration at the end of surgery was 1.2% and end-tidal carbon dioxide concentration was 35 mmHg. The horse is apneic.

b) Immediate management

1) Begin intermittent positive pressure ventilation to remove isoflurane, promote recovery from anesthesia, and return of normal protective cardiac reflexes.

2) Monitor heart rate, oxygen saturation of hemoglobin, and arterial blood pressure (indirect technique).

3) Consider taking an arterial blood gas sample to evaluate $PaCO_2$ and PaO_2.

c) Considerations

1) What may have explained the sudden change in clinical picture? The combination of bradycardia and suspected hypotension in the absence of drug administration suggests possible activation of the Bezold-Jarisch reflex (Kinsella and Tuckey 2001; McMillan et al. 2012). This cardioinhibitory reflex is mediated by cardiac ventricular receptors sensitive to stretch (and chemicals). When activated, such as with a sudden reduction in venous return

associated with a postural change leading to reduced left ventricular filling, the afferent signal carried in the vagus nerve acts on the vasomotor center of the brain to inhibit sympathetic outflow. This promotes bradycardia, vasodilation, and hypotension (Campagna and Carter 2003; Kinsella and Tuckey 2001). It is unclear why the baroreceptor reflex does not provide a protective increase in sympathetic tone in response to a sudden reduction in venous return, though depression of baroreceptor reflex activity during volatile anesthesia may be a contributing factor in this case (Campagna and Carter 2003; Ebert et al. 1995). Additionally, vasodilation and pooling of blood in abdominal capacitance vessels may have promoted a reduction in venous return accompanying the postural change (Klein and Sherman 1977).

2) The Bezold-Jarisch reflex is usually short-lived but has been reported to last approximately one hour in an anesthetized dog (McMillan et al. 2012). In one report of a horse, it was believed to have resulted in cardiac arrest, triggered as a result of postural change during transfer to recovery at the end of anesthesia (Conde Ruiz and Junot 2018).

3) If reduced venous return is a contributing factor, the use of intermittent positive pressure ventilation (IPPV) may further reduce venous return if peak inspiratory pressure is high. However, the advantages conferred by ventilation and reducing isoflurane concentrations outweigh transitory reductions in venous return, particularly if care is taken when using a demand valve. Apnea at the end of equine anesthesia is not unusual. Horses are more sensitive to the respiratory depressant effects of isoflurane (reduced ventilatory response to carbon dioxide) than dogs and cats, so that the combination of isoflurane and end-tidal carbon dioxide concentrations in this case is likely to result in apnea until isoflurane levels decrease and carbon dioxide concentration increases. Administering fluids may help to offset the reduction in venous return.

4) Note: a similar clinical picture can occur if an alpha-2 adrenergic agonist is administered just before transfer. This creates a combination of vasoconstriction, reflex bradycardia, peripheral pulses that are difficult to palpate (reduced pulse pressure difference), and pale mucous membranes. In contrast to the presented scenario, hypertension would be present.

5) Reflection – Was the depth of anesthesia appropriate at the end of the procedure? As vasodilation and baroreflex depression are dose-dependent side effects of volatile anesthetics, it is possible that the risk of triggering a Bezold-Jarisch reflex is increased at deeper planes of anesthesia. The target depth of anesthesia at the point of transfer to recovery will depend on local factors, most notably the balance between safety of personnel if a horse moves and reducing volatile agent concentrations to a level that spontaneous breathing is present and protective physiologic reflexes return. What could be done to prevent this complication recurring? Available evidence on the incidence and contributing factors to triggering the Bezold-Jarisch reflex is sparse, making its occurrence difficult to predict. A cautious approach would be to avoid sudden changes in body position, particularly at deeper planes of anesthesia.

Tear in endotracheal (ET) Tube or Cuff

a) Event: Following an uneventful induction of general anesthesia in a 400 kg horse, followed by orotracheal intubation (26 mm internal diameter cuffed ET tube) by an anesthesia resident, you assist hoisting the horse on to the operating table in dorsal recumbency. As usual, the circle breathing system and ventilator is connected and switched following transfer. After delivery of the first breath, the ascending bellows fails to return to its resting position at the top of the bellows housing. This is not unusual, a common sign of a leak around the ET tube cuff. You inflate the cuff with 30 ml of air and watched the bellows as the next breath is delivered. The bellows is incompletely filled so only a partial inspired volume is delivered. Again, this is not unusual as the ventilator may take a few respiratory cycles to fill. You increase the oxygen flow rate to 10 l/min to hasten the process. The same pattern repeats itself over the subsequent eight breaths despite a further 60 ml of air being added to the cuff and no sensation of increasing resistance to injection as air is added (Figure 15.6).

b) Immediate management

1) The ventilator, anesthetic vaporizer, and oxygen flowmeter were switched off.
2) A nasogastric tube (approximately 1.5 cm outer diameter and 3 m long) was lightly lubricated and a replacement ET tube prepared (cuffed inflated to check for a leak and lubricated).
3) The breathing circuit was disconnected from the ET tube and capped, and the horse's head extended.
4) The nasogastric tube was inserted (rounded end first) through the endotracheal tube to the level of the middle of the neck and the ET tube removed while carefully holding the nasogastric tube in position.
5) The replacement ET tube was carefully threaded over the nasogastric tube and inserted into the trachea using the nasogastric tube as a guide. The nasogastric tube was then removed.
6) The anesthetic breathing system was reconnected, the cuff inflated, and the ventilator started.

c) Considerations

1) In a horse of this size, 30–60 ml of air is sufficient to create a sealed airway with a peak inspiratory pressure of approximately 25 cmH$_2$O.
2) What are common sources of airway leaks shortly after endotracheal intubation? Failure of an airtight seal is most

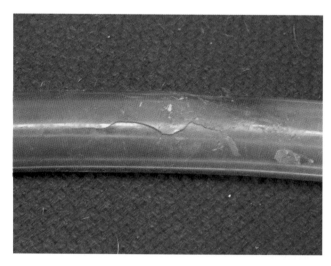

Figure 15.6 An approximately 7 cm tear in the wall of an endotracheal tube that resulted in an inability to mechanically ventilate a horse during anesthesia.

commonly caused by an under-inflated ET tube cuff or placement of a small tube (less likely in equine anesthesia). Other causes are a leak originating from the pilot tube or its cuff, an incompetent valve in the pilot tube cuff, or a defect in the ET tube wall.

3) Failure to create any degree of seal indicates a substantial leak. Incompetent valves usually provide a seal for a short time as air gradually leaks out. Large leaks are usually caused by a hole or tear in the cuff or damage to the ET tube wall.

4) As ET tubes age, the rubber can stiffen and deteriorate, making them more susceptible to damage. This process can be accelerated by autoclaving at high temperatures.

5) Although controlled ventilation was largely ineffective in this case, the provision of a high concentration of oxygen in the upper airway provides the opportunity for apneic oxygenation (Wong et al. 2017). During apnea, gas continues to be absorbed from the alveoli creating a pressure gradient that draws gas downward from the upper airway. If supplemental oxygen is provided, this can help to maintain oxygenation during a period of apnea, though the reliability of this mechanism in horses is unclear (Ambros et al. 2018; Blaze and Robinson 1987; Doodnaught and Pang 2017). Any spontaneous breaths would facilitate gas exchange but replacement of a high concentration of oxygen with room air and the tendency for horses to develop ventilation: perfusion mismatch under anesthesia could create hypoxemia.

6) Should the replacement ET tube be of the same diameter as the original? If the first ET tube was placed without difficulty, the same size of ET tube should pass. However, as it is not always possible to achieve good extension of the head and neck with the horse in dorsal recumbency or if there is any concern that sharp teeth may have damaged the tube, an ET tube one size smaller could be used.

7) Reflection – Was the ET tube examined before use? Checking the integrity and function of an ET tube cuff is a routine part of anesthetic practice – omitting this task is an unsafe act (error or violation). A visual inspection of ET tubes is quick and easy to perform, though this may not identify tubes that have reached the limit of their life and are susceptible to splitting during intubation. Was anything untoward noted during intubation? Intubation should always be performed gently, and the tube retracted slightly and re-ositioned should resistance be encountered. Was the person performing intubation appropriately trained/ supervised? Trainees often feel under pressure to perform intubations quickly as they are being watched and they are aware of the importance of rapidly securing an airway. It can be helpful to remind them that the horse is breathing and of the importance of being gentle to avoid tube or tissue damage (Heath et al. 1989; Touzot-Jourde et al. 2005). Was equipment to facilitate changing of the ET tube readily available? Though this is an uncommon complication, the equipment needed to exchange an ET tube is cheap, readily available, and makes the process relatively simple and rapid. Any reasonably stiff (ideally not rigid, to reduce the risk of inadvertent tracheal damage), pliable tube or rod can be used. A nasogastric tube works well, provided it is lightly lubricated to help it pass through the ET tube.

References

Alidina, S., Goldhaber-Fiebert, S.N., Hannenberg, A.A. et al. (2018). Factors associated with the use of cognitive aids in operating room crises: a cross-sectional study of US hospitals and ambulatory surgical centers. *Implementation Science* 13: 50.

Allnutt, M.F. (2002). Human factors in accidents. 1987. *Quality & Safety in Health Care* 11: 369–374.

Ambros, B., Carrozzo, M.V., and Jones, T. (2018). Desaturation times between dogs preoxygenated via face mask or flow-by technique before induction of anesthesia. *Veterinary Anaesthesia and Analgesia* 45: 452–458.

Anesthesiologists Society of Anesthesiologists (2008). 2008 ASA Recommendations for Pre Anesthesia Checkout. Internet: https://www.asahq.org/resources/clinical-information/2008-asa-recommendations-for-pre-anesthesia-checkout (accessed 21 August 2018).

Arbous, M.S., Grobbee, D.E., Van Kleef, J.W. et al. (2001). Mortality associated with anaesthesia: a qualitative analysis to identify risk factors. *Anaesthesia* 56: 1141–1153.

Arbous, M.S., Meursing, A.E., Van Kleef, J.W. et al. (2005). Impact of anesthesia management characteristics on severe morbidity and mortality. *Anesthesiology* 102: 257–268. quiz 491.

Armitage-Chan, E.A. (2014). Human factors, non-technical skills, professionalism and flight safety: their roles in improving patient outcome. *Veterinary Anaesthesia and Analgesia* 41: 221–223.

Association of Anaesthetists of Great Britain and Ireland (AAGBI), Hartle, A., Anderson, E. et al. (2012). Checking anaesthetic equipment 2012: association of anaesthetists of Great Britain and Ireland. *Anaesthesia* 67: 660–668.

Bainbridge, D., Martin, J., Arango, M. et al. (2012). Perioperative and anaesthetic-related mortality in developed and developing countries: a systematic review and meta-analysis. *Lancet* 380: 1075–1081.

Barthram, C. and Mcclymont, W. (1992). The use of a checklist for anaesthetic machines. *Anaesthesia* 47: 1066–1069.

Bergs, J., Hellings, J., Cleemput, I. et al. (2014). Systematic review and meta-analysis of the effect of the World Health Organization surgical safety checklist on postoperative complications. *The British Journal of Surgery* 101: 150–158.

Blaze, C.A. and Robinson, N.E. (1987). Apneic oxygenation in anesthetized ponies and horses. *Veterinary Research Communications* 11: 281–291.

Bradbury, L.A., Archer, D.C., Dugdale, A.H. et al. (2005). Suspected venous air embolism in a horse. *The Veterinary Record* 156: 109–111.

Broom, M.A., Capek, A.L., Carachi, P. et al. (2011). Critical phase distractions in anaesthesia and the sterile cockpit concept. *Anaesthesia* 66: 175–179.

Campagna, J.A. and Carter, C. (2003). Clinical relevance of the Bezold-Jarisch reflex. *Anesthesiology* 98: 1250–1260.

Campbell, G., Arfanis, K., and Smith, A.F. (2012). Distraction and interruption in anaesthetic practice. *British Journal of Anaesthesia* 109: 707–715.

Carthey, J., De Leval, M.R., Wright, D.J. et al. (2003). Behavioural markers of surgical excellence. *Safety Science* 41: 409–425.

Christian, R.G., Mills, J.H., and Kramer, L.L. (1974). Accidental intracarotid artery injection of promazine in the horse. *The Canadian Veterinary Journal* 15: 29–33.

Conde Ruiz, C. and Junot, S. (2018). Successful cardiopulmonary resuscitation in a sevoflurane anaesthetized horse that suffered cardiac arrest at recovery. *Frontiers in Veterinary Science* 5: 138.

Cooper, J.B. (1984). Toward prevention of anesthetic mishaps. *International Anesthesiology Clinics* 22: 167–183.

Cooper, L. and Nossaman, B. (2013). Medication errors in anesthesia: a review. *International Anesthesiology Clinics* 51: 1–12.

Cooper, J.B., Newbower, R.S., and Kitz, R.J. (1984). An analysis of major errors and equipment failures in anesthesia management: considerations for prevention and detection. *Anesthesiology* 60: 34–42.

Cooper, J.B., Newbower, R.S., Long, C.D., and Mcpeek, B. (2002). Preventable anesthesia mishaps: a study of human factors. 1978. *Quality & Safety in Health Care* 11: 277–282.

Cooper, L., Digiovanni, N., Schultz, L. et al. (2012). Influences observed on incidence and reporting of medication errors in anesthesia. *Canadian Journal of Anaesthesia* 59: 562–570.

Croskerry, P. (2002). Achieving quality in clinical decision making: cognitive strategies and detection of bias. *Academic Emergency Medicine* 9: 1184–1204.

Croskerry, P. (2003). Cognitive forcing strategies in clinical decision making. *Annals of Emergency Medicine* 41: 110–120.

De Leval, M.R., Carthey, J., Wright, D.J. et al. (2000). Human factors and cardiac surgery: a multicenter study. *The Journal of Thoracic and Cardiovascular Surgery* 119: 661–672.

De Meester, K., Verspuy, M., Monsieurs, K.G., and Van Bogaert, P. (2013). SBAR improves nurse-physician communication and reduces unexpected death: a pre and post intervention study. *Resuscitation* 84: 1192–1196.

Diller, T., Helmrich, G., Dunning, S. et al. (2014). The Human Factors Analysis Classification System (HFACS) applied to health care. *American Journal of Medical Quality* 29: 181–190.

Doodnaught, G.M. and Pang, D.S. (2017). Intubation following high-dose rocuronium in a cat with protracted laryngospasm. *JFMS Open Reports* 3 2055116917733642.

Ebert, T.J., Harkin, C.P., and Muzi, M. (1995). Cardiovascular responses to sevoflurane: a review. *Anesthesia and Analgesia* 81: S11–S22.

Elbardissi, A.W., Wiegmann, D.A., Dearani, J.A. et al. (2007). Application of the human factors analysis and classification system methodology to the cardiovascular surgery operating room. *The Annals of Thoracic Surgery* 83: 1412–1418. discussion 1418.

Fasting, S. and Gisvold, S.E. (2000). Adverse drug errors in anesthesia, and the impact of coloured syringe labels. *Canadian Journal of Anaesthesia* 47: 1060–1067.

Flanagan, J.P., Gradisar, I.A., Gross, R.J., and Kelly, T.R. (1969). Air embolus–a lethal complication of subclavian venipuncture. *The New England Journal of Medicine* 281: 488–489.

Gaba, D.M., Maxwell, M., and Deanda, A. (1987). Anesthetic mishaps: breaking the chain of accident evolution. *Anesthesiology* 66: 670–676.

Gaba, D.M., Singer, S.J., Sinaiko, A.D. et al. (2003). Differences in safety climate between hospital personnel and naval aviators. *Human Factors* 45: 173–185.

Gabel, A.A. and Koestner, A. (1963). The effects of intracarotid artery injection of drugs in domestic animals. *Journal of the American Veterinary Medical Association* 142: 1397–1403.

Gawande, A.A., Thomas, E.J., Zinner, M.J., and Brennan, T.A. (1999). The incidence and nature of surgical adverse events in Colorado and Utah in 1992. *Surgery* 126: 66–75.

Gibbs, N.M., Culwick, M., and Merry, A.F. (2017). A cross-sectional overview of the first 4,000 incidents reported to webAIRS, a de-identified web-based anaesthesia incident reporting system in Australia and New Zealand. *Anaesthesia and Intensive Care* 45: 28–35.

Greenberg, C.C., Regenbogen, S.E., Studdert, D.M. et al. (2007). Patterns of communication breakdowns resulting in injury to surgical patients. *Journal of the American College of Surgeons* 204: 533–540.

Hall, L.W. and Taylor, P.M. (1981). Clinical trial of xylazine with ketamine in equine anaesthesia. *The Veterinary Record* 108: 489–493.

Hartle, A.J. (2013). A reply. *Anaesthesia* 68: 877.

Hartnack, S., Bettschart-Wolfensberger, R., Driessen, B. et al. (2013). Critical incidence reporting systems – an option in equine anaesthesia? Results from a panel meeting. *Veterinary Anaesthesia and Analgesia* 40: e3–e8.

Haynes, A.B., Weiser, T.G., Berry, W.R. et al. (2009). A surgical safety checklist to reduce morbidity and mortality in a global population. *The New England Journal of Medicine* 360: 491–499.

Haynes, A.B., Weiser, T.G., Berry, W.R. et al. (2011). Changes in safety attitude and relationship to decreased postoperative morbidity and mortality following implementation of a checklist-based surgical safety intervention. *BMJ Quality and Safety* 20: 102–107.

Heath, R.B., Steffey, E.P., Thurmon, J.C. et al. (1989). Laryngotracheal lesions following routine orotracheal intubation in the horse. *Equine Veterinary Journal* 21: 434–437.

Helmreich, R.L. (2000). On error management: lessons from aviation. *BMJ* 320: 781–785.

Hofmeister, E.H., Quandt, J., Braun, C., and Shepard, M. (2014). Development, implementation and impact of simple patient safety interventions in a university teaching hospital. *Veterinary Anaesthesia and Analgesia* 41: 243–248.

Holbrook, T.C., Dechant, J.E., and Crowson, C.L. (2007). Suspected air embolism associated with post-anesthetic pulmonary edema and neurologic sequelae in a horse. *Veterinary Anaesthesia and Analgesia* 34: 217–222.

Hu, Y.Y., Arriaga, A.F., Peyre, S.E. et al. (2012). Deconstructing intraoperative communication failures. *The Journal of Surgical Research* 177: 37–42.

Johnston, G.M., Eastment, J.K., Wood, J., and Taylor, P.M. (2002). The confidential enquiry into perioperative equine fatalities (CEPEF): mortality results of phases 1 and 2. *Veterinary Anaesthesia and Analgesia* 29: 159–170.

Kearns, R.J., Uppal, V., Bonner, J. et al. (2011). The introduction of a surgical safety checklist in a tertiary referral obstetric centre. *BMJ Quality and Safety* 20: 818–822.

Kendell, J. and Barthram, C. (1998). Revised checklist for anaesthetic machines. *Anaesthesia* 53: 887–890.

Kinsella, S.M. and Tuckey, J.P. (2001). Perioperative bradycardia and asystole: relationship to vasovagal syncope and the Bezold-Jarisch reflex. *British Journal of Anaesthesia* 86: 859–868.

Klein, L. and Sherman, J. (1977). Effects of preanesthetic medication, anesthesia, and position of recumbency on central venous pressure in horses. *Journal of the American Veterinary Medical Association* 170: 216–219.

Kohn, L.T., Corrigan, J.M., Donaldson, M.S., and Committee on Quality of Healthcare in America (2000). *To Err Is Human*. Washington, DC: National Academy Press.

Langley, G., Moen, R., Nolan, K. et al. (2009). *The Improvement Guide: A Practical Approach to Enhancing Organizational Performance*, 2e. San Francisco, CA: Jossey-Bass.

Leonard, M., Graham, S., and Bonacum, D. (2004). The human factor: the critical importance of effective teamwork and communication in providing safe care. *Quality & Safety in Health Care* 13 (Suppl 1): i85–i90.

Lingard, L., Regehr, G., Orser, B. et al. (2008). Evaluation of a preoperative checklist and team briefing among surgeons, nurses, and anesthesiologists to reduce failures in communication. *Archives of Surgery* 143: 12–17.

Ludders, J.W. and McMillan, M. (2017). *Errors in Veterinary Anesthesia*, 1e. Ames, IA: Wiley.

Macintosh, R.R. (1949). Deaths under anaesthetics. *British Journal of Anaesthesia* 21: 107–136.

Mahajan, R.P. (2010). Critical incident reporting and learning. *British Journal of Anaesthesia* 105: 69–75.

McMillan, M. (2014). Checklists in veterinary anaesthesia: why bother. *The Veterinary Record* 175: 556–559.

McMillan, M.W., Aprea, F., and Leece, E.A. (2012). Potential Bezold-Jarisch reflex secondary to a 180° postural change in an anaesthetized dog. *Veterinary Anaesthesia and Analgesia* 39: 561–562.

Menoud, G., Axiak, F.S., Spadavecchia, C., and Raillard, M. (2018). Development and implementation of a perianesthetic safety checklist in a veterinary university small animal teaching hospital. *Frontiers in Veterinary Science* 5: 60.

Mirski, M.A., Lele, A.V., Fitzsimmons, L., and Toung, T.J. (2007). Diagnosis and treatment of vascular air embolism. *Anesthesiology* 106: 164–177.

Mosedale, P. (1998). Introducing clinical audit to veterinary practice. *In Practice* 20: 40–42.

Muir, W.W. and Hubbell, J.A.E. (1991). *Equine Anesthesia: Monitoring and Emergency Therapy*, 1e. St Louis, MO: Mosby.

Muir, W.W., Skarda, R.T., and Milne, D.W. (1977). Evaluation of xylazine and ketamine hydrochloride for anesthesia in horses. *American Journal of Veterinary Research* 38: 195–201.

Nundy, S., Mukherjee, A., Sexton, J.B. et al. (2008). Impact of preoperative briefings on operating room delays: a preliminary report. *Archives of Surgery* 143: 1068–1072.

Pang, D.S.J., Rousseau-Blass, F., and Pang, J.M. (2018). Morbidity and mortality conferences: a mini review and illustrated application in veterinary medicine. *Frontiers in Veterinary Science* 5: 43.

Parkinson, N.J., McKenzie, H.C., Barton, M.H. et al. (2018). Catheter-associated venous air embolism in hospitalized horses: 32 cases. *Journal of Veterinary Internal Medicine* 32: 805–814.

Pelligrini-Masini, A., Rodriguez, H.I., Stewart, A.J., and Divers, T.J. (2009). Suspected venous air embolism in three horses. *Equine Veterinary Education* 21: 79–84.

Pickering, S.P., Robertson, E.R., Griffin, D. et al. (2013). Compliance and use of the World Health Organization checklist in U.K. operating theatres. *The British Journal of Surgery* 100: 1664–1670.

Pronovost, P., Needham, D., Berenholtz, S. et al. (2006). An intervention to decrease catheter-related bloodstream infections in the ICU. *The New England Journal of Medicine* 355: 2725–2732.

Reason, J. (2000). Human error: models and management. *BMJ* 320: 768–770.

Reason, J. (2004). Beyond the organisational accident: the need for "error wisdom" on the frontline. *Quality & Safety in Health Care* 13 (Suppl 2): ii28–ii33.

Reason, J. (2005). Safety in the operating theatre – part 2: human error and organisational failure. *Quality & Safety in Health Care* 14: 56–60.

Reason, J. (2008). *The Human Contribution: Unsafe Acts, Accidents and Heroic Recoveries*, 1e. Burlington, VT: Ashgate Publishing.

Rose, N. and Pang, D. (2021). A practical guide to implementing clinical audit. *The Canadian Veterinary Journal* 62 (2): 145–152.

Rose, N., Kwong, G.P., and Pang, D.S. (2016a). A clinical audit cycle of post-operative hypothermia in dogs. *The Journal of Small Animal Practice* 57: 447–452.

Rose, N., Toews, L., and Pang, D.S. (2016b). A systematic review of clinical audit in companion animal veterinary medicine. *BMC Veterinary Research* 12: 40.

Runciman, W.B. and Merry, A.F. (2005). Crises in clinical care: an approach to management. *Quality & Safety in Health Care* 14: 156–163.

Runciman, W.B., Webb, R.K., Klepper, I.D. et al. (1993). The Australian Incident Monitoring Study. Crisis management–validation of an algorithm by analysis of 2000 incident reports. *Anaesthesia and Intensive Care* 21: 579–592.

Runciman, W.B., Kluger, M.T., Morris, R.W. et al. (2005). Crisis management during anaesthesia: the development of an anaesthetic crisis management manual. *Quality & Safety in Health Care* 14: e1.

Runciman, W., Hibbert, P., Thomson, R. et al. (2009). Towards an international classification for patient safety: key concepts and terms. *International Journal for Quality in Health Care* 21: 18–26.

Sams, L.M. and Hofmeister, E.H. (2008). Anesthesia case of the month. Treatment of colic of approximately 24 hours' duration. *Journal of the American Veterinary Medical Association* 232: 206–209.

Semel, M.E., Resch, S., Haynes, A.B. et al. (2010). Adopting a surgical safety checklist could save money and improve the quality of care in U.S. hospitals. *Health Affairs (Millwood)* 29: 1593–1599.

Shonfeld, A., Riyat, A., Kotecha, A., and Sacks, M. (2011). Critical care transfers: using audit to make a difference. *Anaesthesia* 66: 946–947.

Singer, S.J., Rosen, A., Zhao, S. et al. (2010). Comparing safety climate in naval aviation and hospitals: implications for improving patient safety. *Health Care Management Review* 35: 134–146.

Stiegler, M.P. and Tung, A. (2014). Cognitive processes in anesthesiology decision making. *Anesthesiology* 120: 204–217.

Stiegler, M.P., Neelankavil, J.P., Canales, C., and Dhillon, A. (2012). Cognitive errors detected in anaesthesiology: a literature review and pilot study. *British Journal of Anaesthesia* 108: 229–235.

Sutcliffe, K.M. (2011). High reliability organizations (HROs). *Best Practice & Research. Clinical Anaesthesiology* 25: 133–144.

Touzot-Jourde, G., Stedman, N.L., and Trim, C.M. (2005). The effects of two endotracheal tube cuff inflation pressures on liquid aspiration and tracheal wall damage in horses. *Veterinary Anaesthesia and Analgesia* 32: 23–29.

Viner, B. (2010). Clinical effectiveness. What does it mean for practitioners – and cats? *Journal of Feline Medicine and Surgery* 12: 561–568.

Wadhera, R.K., Parker, S.H., Burkhart, H.M. et al. (2010). Is the "sterile cockpit" concept applicable to cardiovascular surgery critical intervals or critical events? The impact of protocol-driven communication during cardiopulmonary bypass. *The Journal of Thoracic and Cardiovascular Surgery* 139: 312–319.

Wallis, J., Fletcher, D., Bentley, A., and Ludders, J. (2019). Medical errors cause harm in veterinary hospitals. *Frontiers in Veterinary Science* 6: 12.

Wiegmann, D.A. and Shappell, S.A. (2005). *A Human Factor Approach to Aviation Accident Analysis*, 1e. Burlington, VA: Ashgate Publishing Company.

Wong, D.T., Yee, A.J., Leong, S.M., and Chung, F. (2017). The effectiveness of apneic oxygenation during tracheal intubation in various clinical settings: a narrative review. *Canadian Journal of Anaesthesia* 64: 416–427.

World Health Organization (2009). *Implementation Manual WHO Surgical Safety Checklist 2009*. Geneva: World Health Organization.

Index

Page locators in **bold** indicate tables. Page locators in *italics* indicate figures.

Equine Anesthesia and Co-Existing Disease, First Edition. Stuart Clark-Price and Khursheed Mama.
© 2022 John Wiley & Sons, Inc. Published 2022 by John Wiley & Sons, Inc.